Therapeutics in Dermatology - Essentials for Clinical Practice

Aditya Kumar Bubna

Therapeutics in Dermatology - Essentials for Clinical Practice

Systemic Therapy: Volume 1

Springer

Aditya Kumar Bubna
Department of Dermatology
Katihar Medical College
Katihar, Bihar, India

ISBN 978-981-95-3790-7 ISBN 978-981-95-3791-4 (eBook)
https://doi.org/10.1007/978-981-95-3791-4

This Springer imprint is published by the registered company Springer Nature Singapore Pte Ltd.
The registered company address is: 152 Beach Road, #21-01/04 Gateway East, Singapore 189721, Singapore

I would like to dedicate this book to my mother, who has been an epitome of encouragement and love.

Proverbs 3:5, 6 *"Trust in the Lord with all your heart, Lean not on thy own understanding. Commit your ways to Him, and He will direct your paths."*

Preface to the First Edition

Dermatology as a branch has evolved swiftly in the last few decades, with an ever-expanding therapeutic arsenal, making it essential for all clinicians to be aware about various drugs and treatment modalities available for patient care.

Taking this into consideration, the concept of "Therapeutics in Dermatology: Essentials for Clinical Practice" emerged; a book that would comprehensively address all facets of different drugs, both topical and systemic, in dermatologic practice, and has taken almost 5 years for the author to complete writing this book.

As the amount of information is vast, it was considered to divide the book in to three volumes: Volumes 1 and 2 are dedicated to systemic therapy, and Volume 3 focuses on topical therapy.

Each drug in this book has been discussed under mechanism of action, pharmacokinetics, clinical uses, adverse effects and special considerations, with particular emphasis to practical prescribing information.

The chapter on biologic drugs is very meticulously discussed, such that the reader will not have to refer any other text, but get all information under one cover.

A separate chapter on steroid pulses in dermatology has been included, along with the chapter on systemic steroids for completion.

Also, drugs like anti-androgens and attenuated androgens that are often overlooked have been scrupulously discussed, allowing this feature of dermatologic pharmacology to get due importance.

Furthermore, miscellaneous drugs like rivaroxaban, sildenafil, anti-cholinergic agents and tranexemic acid, which have elaborated newer indications in dermatologic therapeutics, have been carefully evaluated, allowing the reader to obtain adequate information for the same.

Topical therapy too has been discussed in detail, with newer drugs like crisaborole, cysteamine, tirbanibulin and trifarotene being adequately described.

Though elaborate, a sincere effort has been taken to keep the language crisp and running, enabling the reader to maintain focus and interest.

Despite this, as an author, I do feel that room for improvement always exists, and it is my sincere appeal to readers to point the deficits, which certainly will be considered in the second edition of this book.

Katihar, Bihar, India

Aditya Kumar Bubna

Acknowledgements

- Dr. Vinayak Viplav, Senior Resident, AIIMS, Deoghar, for helping me with many of the illustrations in this book, as well as enabling me to procure various articles from different journals.
- My teachers, Dr. Sudha Rangarajan, Dr. Mahalakshmi Veeraraghavan, Dr. Shobana Subramanyam, Dr. Anandan Sankarasubramaniam, Dr. Murugan Sundaram, Dr. Adikrishnan Swaminathan and Dr. Krishnakanth Muralidharan, without whose mentorship and guidance, I do not think I would have been able to write this manuscript. I sincerely thank them from the bottom of my heart, and feel richly blessed to have such wonderful teachers.
- Dr. Nitin Patil, consultant dermatologist, NIT skin clinic, Pune, whose constant support, encouragement and advice in all steps of manuscript writing was very valuable.
- Dr. Anuradha Priyadarshini, Associate Professor (Department of Dermatology), Sri Ramachandra Medical College, Chennai, for her constant support.
- Dr. Leena Dennis Joseph, Professor (Department of Pathology), Sri Ramachandra Medical College, Chennai, for her constant support.

Competing Interests The author has no competing interests to declare that are relevant to the content of this manuscript.

Contents

Part I

Antimicrobial Drugs

Penicillins 1

Introduction

Penicillins belong to the class of β-lactam antibiotics. Originally penicillins were obtained from the fungus *Penicillium notatum*, but the present source is a high-yielding mutant *P. chrysogenum* [1].

Mechanism of Action

Penicillins are effective only against actively growing cell wall-synthesizing bacteria. Penicillins bind to penicillin-binding protein present in the bacterial cell wall and inhibit the synthesis of peptidoglycan (an important component of bacterial cell wall). This results in the release of autolysins and disruption of transpeptidation reaction in the bacterial cell wall, resulting in bacterial death [2].

The classification of penicillins is depicted in Table 1.1.

A. K. Bubna, *Therapeutics in Dermatology - Essentials for Clinical Practice*, https://doi.org/10.1007/978-981-95-3791-4_1

Table 1.1 Classification of penicillins

Natural penicillins	Penicillin G (benzyl penicillin)
	Penicillin V (acid-resistant alternative to penicillin G)
Semisynthetic penicillins	
Penicillinase-resistant penicillins	Methicillin Cloxacillin Dicloxacillin
Extended spectrum penicillins	
Aminopenicillins	Ampicillin Bacampicillin Amoxicillin
Carboxypenicillins	Carbenicillin Ticarcillin
Ureidopenicillins	Piperacillin Mezlocillin
β-Lactamase inhibitors	Clavulanic acid Sulbactam Tazobactam

Table 1.2 Pharmacokinetics of natural penicillins

Penicillin type	Pharmacokinetics
Penicillin G	It is generally administered intramuscularly However, sodium penicillin G (crystalline penicillin) can also be administered intravenously Penicillin G can also be given orally. However, owing to its acid-labile properties only one-third of the total dose is finally absorbed in the systemic circulation. Therefore, the oral route of administration is not employed After intramuscular injection, the peak plasma concentration is reached within 15–30 min The $t_{1/2}$ of penicillin G is 30 min Penicillin G is very slowly absorbed after intramuscular injection, and the average duration wherein its antimicrobial activity is seen in the plasma is 25 days Approximately 60% of penicillin G is bound to albumin Significant amounts of the drug appear in the liver, bile, kidneys, semen, joint fluid, lymph and intestine Excretion in mainly by glomerular filtration and tubular secretion
Penicillin V	Given orally It is acid stable It is well absorbed from the gut with a wide volume of distribution Renal excretion is the route for elimination

Natural Penicillins

The pharmacokinetics of natural penicillins is elaborated in Table 1.2.

Antimicrobial Spectrum

- *Streptococcus pyogenes/viridens/faecalis*
- *Pneumococci*
- *Meningococci*
- *Treponema pallidum*
- *Neisseria gonorrhoea*
- *Pasteurella multocida*

Indications and Dosing

The indications and dosing of penicillins are described in Table 1.3.

Table 1.3 Indications and dosing of penicillins

Indication	Dosing
Erysipelas	Mild cases: tab penicillin V 500 mg PO Q6H till lesions resolve Severe cases: inj crystalline penicillin 20,00,000 units IV Q6H till lesions resolve
Cellulitis	Inj crystalline penicillin 20,00,000 units IV Q6H till lesions resolve
Streptococcal perianal disease	Tab penicillin V 500 mg PO Q6H for 10 days
Anthrax	Inj crystalline penicillin 12–20 million units IV Q6H till appreciable reduction in lesions. May continue for a period of 6–8 weeks
Actinomycosis	Crystalline penicillin 10–20 million units IV Q6H for 6 weeks Some physicians prefer to continue tab pen V 500 mg (20–50 mg/kg in divided doses) Q6H for 2–3 months after the initial IV dosing of crystalline penicillin
Fusospirochaetal infections (trench mouth)	Tab penicillin V 500 mg Q6H for several days till the disease resolves
Lyme's disease (severe early disseminated disease or chronic disease)	Injection crystalline penicillin 18–24 million units IV Q4H per day for 14–28 days [3]
Primary, secondary and early latent syphilis [4]	Benzathine penicillinG 2.4 million units deep IM single dose (1.2 million units in each buttock) In children, benzathine penicillinG 50,000 IU/kg to the adult dose of 2.4 million units in a single dose Alternative regimen by WHO and NACO—procaine benzyl penicillin G 1.2 million units IM daily for 10 days (three vials each having a combination of 1 lakh units of benzyl penicillin G sodium and 3 lakh units of procaine penicillin G)

(continued)

Table 1.3 (continued)

Indication	Dosing
Late latent syphilis [4]	Three weekly injections of benzathine penicillinG 2.4 million units deep IM In children, three weekly injections of benzathine penicillinG at doses of 50,000 IU/kg to an adult dose of 2.4 million units IM Alternative regimen: procaine penicillin G 1.2 million units IM daily for 20 days
Neurosyphilis [4]	IV aqueous crystalline penicillin 18–24 million units daily for 14 days, OR Procaine penicillin G 2.4 million units IM daily for 14 days (only if the IV regimen cannot be administered)

IV intravenous, *IM* intramuscular, *PO* per oral

Contraindication

Hypersensitivity to penicillins.

Pregnancy prescribing status: category 'B'.

Drug Interactions

Probenecid blocks the secretion of penicillin in distal renal tubules, and therefore, concomitant administration of both drugs increases serum levels and duration of action of penicillins.

Adverse Effects

1. Penicillin allergy:

   - Penicillin reaction: Toxic or allergic.
   - Procaine reaction (Hoigne syndrome): This occurs secondary to inadvertent injection of crystals of procaine penicillin intravenously. It is characterized by an acute psychotic episode, severe anxiety, agitation, vertigo, seizures, visual and auditory hallucinations.
   - Jarisch–Herxheimer reaction: Flulike symptoms seen 2–12 h after injection benzathine penicillin in syphilis, but within 24 h. It is characterized by headache, fever, malaise, flushing and sweating. It lasts for 24 h. There can be a primary aggravation of existing syphilitic lesions. In late syphilis, the reactions are milder. Rarely serious adverse effects like glottic oedema, gummatous lesions and coronary artery occlusion may occur. Treatment is

supportive with IV fluids and non-steroidal anti-inflammatory drugs. It can be prevented by giving prednisolone at a dose of 30–40 mg, 2 days prior to the injection and continued 2–3 days after the administration of benzathine penicillin.
- Acute generalized exanthematous pustulosis.
- Stevens–Johnson syndrome/toxic epidermal necrolysis.
- Anaphylaxis.

2. Hematologic (on prolonged use).
   - Reversible neutropenia.
   - Anaemia.
   - Agranulocytosis.
   - Platelet dysfunction.
3. Gastrointestinal.
   - Diarrhoea.
   - Pseudomembranous colitis.

Penicillinase-Resistant Penicillins

Methicillin

Methicillin is a highly penicillinase-resistant penicillin. However, it is not acid resistant. It is given intravenously. Methicillin-resistant *Staphylococcus aureus* (MRSA) has become an emerging problem these days. The drugs used in treating MRSA include vancomycin and linezolid. Adverse effects with methicillin include haematuria, albuminuria and reversible interstitial nephritis. Methicillin has now been replaced by cloxacillin.

Cloxacillin and Dicloxacillin

Introduction

These congeneric semisynthetic penicillins are similar pharmacologically and thus conveniently considered together. Antimicrobial activity is mainly against *Staphylococcus aureus*. These agents are less effective against microorganisms sensitive to penicillin G and have no role against gram-negative organisms. Dicloxacillin is the most active, and many strains of *S. aureus* are inhibited by concentrations of 0.05–0.8 μg/ml. The comparable value for cloxacillin is 0.1–3 ng/ml.

Pharmacokinetics

Thirty to eighty per cent of both drugs are absorbed from the gastrointestinal tract. Greater than 90% of both drugs are bound to plasma albumin. They are preferentially given 1–2 h prior to meals so that better absorption is ensured. The $t_{1/2}$ of both drugs ranges between 30 and 60 min. The metabolism of both drugs occurs in the liver. Excretion is via the renal and biliary routes [1].

Indications [3]

- Impetigo.
- Folliculitis.
- Furunculosis.

Dosing

Both the drugs are dosed at 30–50 mg/kg body weight in four divided doses, for a period of 7–10 days.

Contraindication

- Hypersensitivity to the drug.

Pregnancy prescribing status: category 'B'.

Adverse Effects

Cutaneous

- Scarlatiniform, morbilliform rash.
- Urticarial rash.
- Vesicular and bullous eruptions.

Gastrointestinal

- Nausea.
- Vomiting.
- Diarrhoea.

Aminopenicillins.
Ampicillin.

Introduction

This is the prototype drug for aminopenicillins. It has an amino substitution in the side chain. Apart from being active against all organisms sensitive to penicillin G, it also has a wide antimicrobial spectrum against *H. influenza, E. coli, Proteus, Salmonella, Shigella* and *Helicobacter pylori.* Ampicillin gets destroyed by β-lactamase from both gram-positive and gram-negative organisms [1].

Mechanism of Action

Similar to other penicillins.

Antimicrobial Spectrum

- *Streptococcus viridens*
- Enterococci
- Pneumococci
- *Staphylococcus aureus*
- *Streptococcus pyogenes*
- *Salmonella*
- *Shigella*
- *Helicobacter pylori*

Table 1.4 Indications and dosing of ampicillin

Indications	Dosing
Gram-negative folliculitis [5]	Cap ampicillin 1gm/day for 7–14 days, in four divided doses, lowered then to a maintenance dose of 250 mg twice daily
Gonorrhoea: in cases of non-penicillinase-producing gonococcal infections	A single dose of 3.5gm of ampicillin along with 1gm of probenecid is adequate for urethritis
Impetigo	Cap ampicillin is given at a dose of 30–50 mg/kg body weight in four divided doses for 7–10 days
Folliculitis	Cap ampicillin is given at a dose of 30–50 mg/kg body weight in four divided doses for 7–10 days
Furuncle	Cap ampicillin is given at a dose of 30–50 mg/kg body weight in four divided doses for 7–10 days

Pharmacokinetics

Ampicillin is a stable acid with a good oral bioavailability. The $t_{1/2}$ of ampicillin is around 80 min. Oral absorption is adequate, though not complete. Excretion is primarily by the renal route, though a small amount of the drug is eliminated in the bile through enterohepatic circulation [1].

Indications and Dosing

The indications and dosing of ampicillin are described in Table 1.4.

Contraindication

- Hypersensitivity to the drug.

Pregnancy prescribing status: category 'B'.

Drug Interactions

- Hydrocortisone inactivates ampicillin if administered in the same solution.
- Probenecid retards renal excretion of ampicillin.
- Ampicillin may interfere with enterohepatic circulation of oral contraceptive pills.

Adverse Effects

Gastrointestinal

- Diarrhoea: alteration of gut flora due to incomplete absorption, leading to the unabsorbed portion of the drug irritating the lower intestine by causing marked alteration of gut flora.

Cutaneous

- Increased incidence of rash in AIDS patients, Epstein–Barr virus-infected patients and in patients with lymphocytic leukaemia.
- Concomitant administration of allopurinol also increases the incidence of rash.

Amoxicillin

Introduction

Amoxicillin is a penicillinase-susceptible semisynthetic penicillin which is a close chemical and pharmacologic relative of ampicillin. It is superior to ampicillin owing to its better oral absorption independent of food intake, along with higher and sustained concentrations being demonstrated in the blood. Furthermore, amoxicillin also has a better gastrointestinal tolerance compared to ampicillin [1].

Pharmacokinetics

Following oral dosing, peak plasma levels are obtained after 2 h. The $t_{1/2}$ of amoxicillin is 60–80 min. Twenty per cent of amoxicillin is bound to plasma proteins. Excretion of the drug is via the renal route [1].

Antimicrobial Spectrum

It is similar to ampicillin, except that it has less activity against *Shigella* and *H. influenzae*.

Indications and Dosing

The indications and dosing of amoxicillin are described in Table 1.5.

Table 1.5 Indications and dosing of amoxicillin

Indication	Dosing
Skin and skin structure infections	Cap amoxicillin given at a dose of 30–50 mg/kg body weight in three divided doses [6]. In severe cases, it can be combined with clavulanic acid [7]
Gonorrhoea: acute uncomplicated anogenital and urethral infections in males and females	Cap amoxicillin 3gms as a single oral dose In pre-pubertal children: Cap amoxicillin 50 mg/kg combined with probenecid 25 mg/kg and administered as a single oral dose. Since probenecid is contraindicated in children below 2 years; this regimen is to be avoided in this age group
H. pylori-associated duodenal ulcer	Triple antibiotic therapy: Cap amoxicillin 1gm, tab clarithromycin 500 mg, cap lansoprazole 30 mg Q12H for 14 days Dual therapy: Cap amoxicillin 1gm and cap lansoprazole 30 mg Q8H for 14 days

Contraindication

- Hypersensitivity to the drug.

Pregnancy prescribing status: category 'B'.

Drug Interactions [6]

- Clavulanic acid: increases the effects of amoxicillin and inhibits the development of resistance in β-lactamase-producing microbes.
- Probenecid: increases and prolongs blood amoxicillin concentrations.
- Methotrexate: amoxicillin decreases renal clearance of methotrexate and leads to renal impairment and toxicity.

Adverse Effects

Gastrointestinal

- Diarrhoea.
- Nausea.
- Vomiting.

Cutaneous

- Morbilliform exanthem.
- Urticaria and angioedema.
- Purpura.
- Erythema multiforme.
- Steven–Johnson syndrome.

Central Nervous System

- Dizziness.
- Headache.

Table 1.6 Details of carboxypenicillins

Name of the drug	Pharmacokinetics	Indications	Contraindication	Dosing	Adverse effects
Carbenicillin	Used IV or IM $t_{1/2} = 1$ h Excretion by renal route	Burn infections, Urinary tract infections, Septicaemia secondary to *Pseudomonas* and *Proteus* sp.	Hypersensitivity to the drug	1–2gm IM or 1–5gm IV Q6H in divided doses	Morbilliform rash, and if administered in high doses may interfere with platelet function, leading to bleeding
Ticarcillin 1) Semisynthetic penicillin 2) 2–4 times more active against *Pseudomonas* than carbenicillin 3) Marketed only in combination with clavulanic acid	Used IV or IM $t_{1/2} = 1$ h Excretion by renal route	Burn infections Urinary tract infections Septicaemia secondary to *Pseudomonas* and *Proteus* sp	Hypersensitivity to the drug	1–2gm IM or 1–5gm IV Q6H in divided doses	Morbilliform rash, and if administered in high doses may interfere with platelet function, leading to bleeding

Haematologic

- Reversible leucopoenia.
- Agranulocytosis.

Carboxypenicillins

The details of carboxypenicillins are described in Table 1.6.

Pregnancy prescribing status: category 'B'.

Ureidopenicillins

The details of ureidopenicillins are elaborated in Table 1.7.

Pregnancy prescribing status: category 'B'.

Clavulanic Acid

Introduction

Clavulanic acid (CA) is obtained from the fungus *Streptomyces clavuligerus*. It has a β-lactam ring but no antimicrobial activity of its own.

Mechanism of Action

CA is a progressive inhibitor of β-lactamase. It initially binds reversibly with the enzyme, following which, as time goes on, it begins to have a covalent association with β-lactamase and progressively inhibits it. It is therefore referred to as a suicide inhibitor. It also permeates the outer layers of the cell wall of gram-negative bacteria and inhibits β-lactamase located in the periplasm [8].

Pharmacokinetics

- CA is rapidly absorbed after oral administration.
- Its bioavailability is 60%.
- The $t_{1/2}$ is 1 h.
- It undergoes hydrolysis and decarboxylation before it undergoes renal elimination by glomerular filtration.

Table 1.7 Details of ureidopenicillins

Name of the drug	Pharmacokinetics	Indications	Contraindications	Dosing	Adverse effects
Piperacillin	Given IV usually Can also be given IM $t_{1/2} = 1$ h Excretion is via the renal route	Treating severe gram-negative infections in neutropenic, immunocompromised and burn patients Ecthyma gangrenosum	Hypersensitivity to the drug	100–150 mg/kg in three divided doses (maximum dose of 16gms per day)	Morbilliform drug rash Urticaria Headache Reversible leucopoenia
Mezlocillin	Given IV usually $t_{1/2} = 1$ h Excretion is via the renal route	Mainly for *Klebsiella* infections as it is better than carbenicillin for these microbes Also used for *E. faecalis* and is superior to ticarcillin	Hypersensitivity to the drug	Not available in India	Morbilliform drug rash Urticaria Headache Reversible leucopoenia

Indications

Combined with amoxicillin against

- β-lactamase-producing-resistant *Staphylococcus aureus* (but not MRSA that have altered penicillinase-binding proteins),
- *N. gonorrhoeae.*
- *H. influenzae.*
- *E. coli.*
- *Proteus* sp.
- *Klebsiella* sp.
- *Salmonella* and *Shigella.*

Addition of CA to ticarcillin extends its spectrum to *S. aureus*, gram-negative bacilli and *Bacteroides* sp., resembling imipenem in its activity.

Contraindication

Hypersensitivity to the drug.

Pregnancy prescribing status: category 'B'.

Dosing

- In uncomplicated urethritis of gonorrhoea (including penicillinase-producing *N. gonorrhoeae*): single dose of amoxicillin 3gm + CA 0.5gm + probenecid 1gm (this is highly curative).
- In other indications: tablet amoxicillin 250–500 mg + CA 125 mg PO Q8H for 7–10 days

  OR
  Injection amoxicillin 0.5–1 gm + CA 0.1–0.2 gm IV or deep IM Q8H for 7–10 days

Adverse Effects

- Poor gastrointestinal tolerance.
- Candidal stomatitis/vaginitis.
- Skin rash.

Sulbactam

Introduction

It is a semisynthetic β-lactamase inhibitor.

Mechanism of Action

The mechanism of action is similar to CA, only that it is 2–3 times less potent than CA.

Pharmacokinetics

Only used parenterally as oral absorption is erratic. Excretion is via the kidneys.

Antimicrobial Spectrum

- *S. aureus*.
- Anaerobes.

Availability and Dosing

It is available in combination with ampicillin for IV and IM use. Each vial contains ampicillin 1gm and sulbactam 0.5gm, administered Q8H or Q6H.

Adverse Effects

- Thrombophlebitis.
- Pain at the injection site.
- Rash.
- Diarrhoea.

Pregnancy prescribing status: category 'B'.

Tazobactam

- More effective against plasmid β-lactamases.
- Combined with piperacillin.

- Most effective against *Pseudomonas*.
- Dose is 0.5gm combined with piperacillin 4gm given IV over 30 min Q8H.

Pregnancy prescribing status: category 'B'.

Conclusion

Penicillins, though being a very old class of drugs, have an indispensable role in the management of a number of cutaneous infections. Therefore, all dermatologists need to be familiar with this class of drugs.

References

1. Petri WA Jr. Penicillins, cephalosporins and other β lactam antibiotics. In: Brunton LL, Chabner BA, Knollman BC, editors. Goodman and Gilman's the pharmacological basis of therapeutics. 12th ed. New York: McGraw Hill; 2012. p. 1477–503.
2. Deck DH, Winston LG. β lactam and other cell wall and membrane active antibiotics. In: Katzung BG, Tevor AJ. Basic and clinical pharmacology. 13th ed. New Delhi. McGraw Hill Education (India) Private Limited. 2015.p 769–787.
3. Lesher JL Jr, McConnel RC. Antimicrobial drugs. In: Bolognia JL, Jorizzo JL, Schaffer JV, editors. Dermatology. 3rd ed. London: Elsevier Saunders; 2012. p. 2105–29.
4. Sethuraman G, Sharma VK. Treatment of syphilis. In: Sharma VK, editor. Sexually transmitted diseases and HIV/AIDS. 2nd ed. New Delhi: Viva Books. p. 317–26.
5. Leyden JJ, Marples RR, Mills OH Jr, Kligman AM. Gram negative folliculitis—a compilation of antibiotic therapy in acne vulgaris. Br J Dermatol. 1973;88:533–8.
6. Kaur SP, Rao R, Nanda S. Amoxicillin: a broad spectrum antibiotic. Int J Pharm Pharm Sci. 2011;3:30–7.
7. Kar PK. A combination of amoxicillin and clavulanic acid in the treatment of pyoderma in children. Indian J Dermatol Venereol Leprol. 1996;62:91–4.
8. Tripathi KD. Beta lactam antibiotics. In: Tripathi KD, editor. Essentials of medical pharmacology. 7th ed. New Delhi: Jaypee brothers medical publishers private limited; 2013. p. 716–32.

Cephalosporins 2

Introduction

Cephalosporins, like penicillins, belong to the β-lactam group of antibiotics. They are derived from 'Cephalosporin c', a product obtained from the fungus *Cephalosporium acremonium* [1]. By isolating the active nucleus of Cephalosporin c, 7-aminocephalosporanic acid, and adding side chains to it, a number of semisynthetic compounds with antibacterial properties superior to the parent compound are obtained.

The classification of cephalosporins with the route of administration is outlined in Table 2.1.

A. K. Bubna, *Therapeutics in Dermatology - Essentials for Clinical Practice*, https://doi.org/10.1007/978-981-95-3791-4_2

Table 2.1 Classification of cephalosporins

Generation of cephalosporin	Drug name	Route of administration
First generation	Cefadroxil	PO (per oral)
	Cefazolin	IM/IV (intramuscular/intravenous)
	Cephalexin	PO
Second generation	Cefaclor	PO
	Cefprozil	PO
	Cefuroxime sodium	IM/IV
	Cefuroxime axetil	PO
Third generation	Cefdinir	PO
	Cefditoren	PO
	Cefixime	PO
	Cefpodoxime proxetil	PO
	Cefoperazone	IM/IV
	Cefotaxime	IM/IV
	Ceftazidime	IM/IV
	Ceftibuten	PO
	Ceftizoxime	IM/IV
	Ceftriaxone	IM/IV
Fourth generation	Cefipime	IM/IV
	Ceftaroline	IV
Cephamycins	Cefoxitin	IM/IV
	Cefotetan	IM/IV

Mechanism of Action

Similar to penicillins.

Pharmacokinetics

Orally administered cephalosporins are readily absorbed post intake. The $t_{1/2}$ of nearly all cephalosporins range from 1 to 2 h, except for ceftriaxone where the $t_{1/2}$ is 8 h, as a result of which, instead of a Q6H dose, a Q12H dose or a single dose is preferred. The metabolism occurs in the liver and elimination via the kidneys. Ceftriaxone also has good cerebrospinal fluid and aqueous humor penetration [1].

Indications

Various indications of cephalosporins are elucidated in Table 2.2.

Table 2.2 Indications and dosing of cephalosporins

Indication	Dosing schedule
Chancroid	Inj ceftriaxone 250 mg IM stat (WHO and NACO)
Uncomplicated gonococcal infection of the cervix, urethra and rectum	Tab cefixime 400 mg stat
Uncomplicated gonococcal infection of the pharynx	Inj ceftriaxone 125 mg IM stat
Disseminated gonococcal infection	Inj ceftriaxone 1gm IM/IV once daily for 7 days OR Inj cefotaxime 1gm IV Q8H for 7 days OR Inj ceftizoxime 1gm IV Q8H for 7 days
Gonococcal conjunctivitis	Inj ceftriaxone 1gm IM stat
Gonococcal meningitis	Inj ceftriaxone 1–2gm IV Q12H for 10–14 days
Gonococcal endocarditis	Inj ceftriaxone 1–2gm IV Q12H for 4 weeks
Ophthalmia neonatorum	Inj ceftriaxone 25–50 mg/kg IV or IM in a single dose. Dose should not exceed 125 mg
Pelvic inflammatory disease	Inj cefotetan 2gm IV Q12H for 7 days OR Inj cefoxitin 2gm IV Q6H for 7 days
Lyme's borreliosis [2] (a) Early localized disease (b) Early mild disseminated disease (c) Early severe disseminated disease	Inj cefuroxime axetil 500 mg (15 mg/kg) PO Q12H for 7–21 days (for early localised disease) Same as above except the duration needs to be extended up to 14–28 days (for early mild disseminated disease) Inj ceftriaxone 2gm (75–100 mg/kg) IV once daily for 14–28 days (for early severe disseminated disease) OR Inj cefotaxime 2gm (50–70 mg/kg) IV Q8H for 14–28 days
Impetigo, furunculosis, ecthyma	Cap cephalexin 30–50 mg/kg/day in four divided doses (Q6H) for 7–10 days OR Tab cefadroxil 30 mg/kg/day in two divided doses (Q12H) for 7–10 days OR Tab cefaclor 40 mg/kg/day in 2(Q12H) or 3(Q8H) divided doses for 7–10 days OR Tab cefuroxime axetil 20–30 mg/kg/day in 2(Q12H) divided doses for 7–10 days OR Tab cefixime 8 mg/kg/day in 2(Q12H) divided doses for 7–10 days OR Tab cefdinir 14 mg/kg/day in 2(Q12H) divided doses for 7–10 days

(continued)

Table 2.2 (continued)

Indication	Dosing schedule
Cellulitis, ecthyma pyogenicum	Cap cephalexin 30–50 mg/kg/day in four divided doses(Q6H) for 7–10 days OR Tab cefadroxil 30 mg/kg/day in two divided doses(Q12H) for 7–10 days OR Tab cefaclor 40 mg/kg/day in 2(Q12H) or 3(Q8H) divided doses for 7–10 days OR Tab cefuroxime axetil 20–30 mg/kg/day in 2(Q12H) divided doses for 7–10 days OR Tab cefixime 8 mg/kg/day in 2(Q12H) divided doses for 7–10 days OR Tab cefdinir 14 mg/kg/day in 2(Q12H) divided doses for 7–10 days OR Inj ceftriaxone 50 mg/kg/day given IM/IV as a once daily dose for 7–10 days

Contraindications

Absolute

Hypersensitivity to the drug.

Pregnancy prescribing status: category 'B'.

Drug Interactions

- Aminoglycosides: increase in the risk of nephrotoxicity with cephalosporins.
- Probenecid: reduction in renal clearance of cephalosporins.
- Proton pump inhibitors: reduces absorption of cephalosporins.
- Didanosine: reduction in absorption of cephalosporins.

Adverse Effects

Cutaneous

- Morbilliform eruptions.
- Urticaria.
- Anaphylaxis.
- Acute generalized exanthematous pustulosis.

Haematological

- Neutropenia.
- Thrombocytopenia.
- Haemolytic anaemia.
- Positive direct Coomb's test.

Gastrointestinal

- Diarrhoea.
- Vomiting.
- Nausea.
- Pseudomembranous colitis.

Conclusion

Cephalosporins are a group of drugs found to be immensely valuable in treating a number of cutaneous infections with a good toxicity profile.

References

1. Petri WA Jr. Penicillins, cephalosporins and other β lactam antibiotics. In: Brunton LL, Chabner BA, Knollman BC, editors. Goodman and Gilman's the pharmacological basis of therapeutics. 12th ed. New York: McGraw Hill; 2012. p. 1477–503.
2. Megraud F, Thijsen SFT. Curved and spiral bacilli: In: Cohen J, Powderly WG eds. Infectious diseases, 2nd ed. Philadelphia: Mosby, 2004.p. 2236–2239.

Quinolones

3

Introduction

These agents constitute an important group of drugs that demonstrate activity against a wide variety of infections [1].

Quinolones are classified in Table 3.1.

Table 3.1 Classification of quinolones

Generation	Drugs	Antimicrobial spectrum
First generation	Nalidixic acid	Gram-negative rods
Second generation	Ciprofloxacin, norfloxacin, ofloxacin, pefloxacin	Mainly against gram-negative rods, particularly anti-pseudomonal
Third generation	Levofloxacin, gatifloxacin, sparfloxacin	Gram-positive cocci, particularly pneumococci, and gram-negative rods
Fourth generation	Moxifloxacin, trovafloxacin	Gram-negative rods, gram-positive cocci, anaerobes and atypical mycobacteria

A. K. Bubna, *Therapeutics in Dermatology - Essentials for Clinical Practice*, https://doi.org/10.1007/978-981-95-3791-4_3

Mechanism of Action

These drugs inhibit bacterial DNA gyrase and topoisomerase IV. For gram-positive organisms, inhibition of topoisomerase is the major mechanism of action [2].

Pharmacokinetics

Quinolones are well absorbed after oral administration and distributed widely in body tissues. The bioavailability of quinolones ranges from 50 to 95%. The $t_{1/2}$ of most quinolones ranges from 3 to 5 h. The metabolism of these drugs occurs in the liver. Excretion is via the kidneys [2].

The indications and dosing are elaborated in Table 3.2.

Table 3.2 Indications and dosing of quinolones

Indication	Dosing
Chancroid	Tab ciprofloxacin 500mg PO Q12H for 3 days
Donovanosis	Tab ciprofloxacin 750mg Q12H for 3 weeks
Uncomplicated gonococcal infections of the cervix, urethra and rectum	Tab ciprofloxacin 500mg PO stat OR Tab ofloxacin 400mg PO stat OR Tab levofloxacin 250mg PO stat (along with tab azithromycin 1gm PO stat, if chlamydia infection is not ruled out)
Uncomplicated gonococcal infection of the pharynx	Tab ciprofloxacin 500mg PO stat (along with tab azithromycin 1gm PO stat, if chlamydia infection is not ruled out)
Disseminated gonococcal infection	Inj ciprofloxacin 400mg IV Q12H OR Inj ofloxacin 400mg IV Q12H The treatment needs to be continued for 24–48 h after improvement begins, following which the treatment is to be switched to the following to complete 1 week of antimicrobial therapy, that is, Tab ciprofloxacin 500mg PO Q12H OR Tab ofloxacin 400mg PO Q12H
Prostatitis	Tab ciprofloxacin 500mg PO Q12H for 4–12 weeks OR Tab norfloxacin 400mg PO Q12H for 4–12 weeks (in those patients not responding to co-trimoxazole)
Pseudomonal folliculitis Green nail syndrome Pseudomonal pyoderma Malignant otitis externa	Tab ciprofloxacin 500mg PO Q12H for 7 days OR Tab ofloxacin 400mg PO Q12H for 7 days
Ecthyma gangrenosum	Inj ciprofloxacin/ofloxacin 200mg IV Q12H, along with IV aminoglycosides, till visible improvement
Leprosy	Ofloxacin 400mg as an alternate drug has been utilized for leprosy resistant to dapsone and rifampicin wherein it is given for 24 months along with clofazimine 50mg, and either minocycline 100mg or clarithromycin 500mg for the first 6 months
Anthrax	Tab ciprofloxacin 500mg Q12H for 2 months
Schnitzler's syndrome	Tab pefloxacin 400mg Q12H[a] [3]

[a]Exact duration of treatment has not been defined.

Contraindications

Absolute

- Hypersensitivity to the drug
- Pregnancy and lactation
- Patients with QT prolongation on ECG

Relative

- Hypokalaemia

Pregnancy prescribing status: category ‘C’.

Drug Interactions

- Antacids containing magnesium, calcium, aluminium, iron and zinc salts prevent the absorption of quinolones.
- Quinolones increase the toxicity of theophylline and aminophylline owing to CYP1A2 inhibition.
- Quinolones increase the serum levels of warfarin.
- Quinolones, along with cyclosporine in renal transplant patients, can increase serum creatinine levels.
- Quinolones should be used with caution in patients taking erythromycin, antiarrhythmic agents and tricyclic antidepressants as they could cause QT prolongation.
- Gatifloxacin in combination with sulfonylureas can precipitate hypoglycaemia.

Adverse Effects

Cutaneous

- Phototoxicity.

Gastrointestinal System

- Changes in taste
- Abnormal liver function test

Renal

- Nephrotoxicity

Nervous System

- Headache
- Dizziness
- Light headedness
- Drowsiness
- Rarely seizures and raised intracranial tension
- Exacerbation of myasthenia gravis has been rarely described

Musculoskeletal System

- Rupture of tendo Achilles

Conclusion

Quinolones have demonstrated activity particularly against *Pseudomonas* and is therefore a valuable drug in this scenario. Given its acceptable safety profile, this class of drugs has proven its worth to the dermatologist.

References

1. Hooper DC. Quinolones. In: Mandell GL, Bennet JE, Dolin R, editors. Mandel, Douglas and Benett's, principles and practice of infectious diseases. 6th ed. New York: Churchill Livingstone; 2005. p. 451–67.
2. Petri WA Jr. Sulfonamides, trimethoprim-sulfamethoxazole, Quinolones and agents for urinary tract infections. In: Brunton LL, Chabner BA, Knollmann BC, editors. Goodman and Gilman's pharmacological basis of therapeutics. 12th ed. New York: McGraw Hill; 2012. p. 1463–76.
3. Asli B, Bienvenu B, Cordoliani F, et al. Chronic urticaria and monoclonal IgM gammopathy (Schnitzler syndrome): report of 11 cases treated with pefloxacin. Arch Dermatol. 2007;143:1046–50.

Macrolides

4

Introduction

These are a class of antimicrobial agents having a macrocyclic lactone ring with attached sugars. The members of this group include

- Erythromycin.
- Azithromycin.
- Roxithromycin.
- Clarithromycin.
- Telithromycin.

Mechanism of Action

Macrolides bind to the 50 s ribosomal subunit of bacterial cells and interfere with translocation. In this way, they inhibit bacterial protein synthesis. These agents are bacteriostatic in action [1]. These drugs have been used for a number of dermatologic indications and exhibit different actions for each, as stated below.

Acne

- Inhibition of IL-8 and neutrophilic chemotaxis [2, 3].

Bullous Pemphigoid

- Anti-inflammatory and immune-modulatory effects [4, 5].

A. K. Bubna, *Therapeutics in Dermatology - Essentials for Clinical Practice*, https://doi.org/10.1007/978-981-95-3791-4_4

Confluent and Reticulate Papillomatosis

- Inhibition of TNFα, IL-α and lymphocytic activity, thereby promoting immunomodulatory effects on keratinocytes [6].

Cyclosporine-Induced Gingival Hyperplasia

- Blockade of type 1 collagen synthesis and activation of matrix metalloproteinase (MMP)-2 levels [7].

Granulomatous Cheilitis

- Inhibition of inflammatory cytokines [8].

Immune Thrombocytopenic Purpura

- Immunomodulatory eradication of bacteria and elevation of platelet counts [9, 10].

Lupus Miliaris Disseminatus Faciei

- Anti-inflammatory properties and inhibition of vascular endothelial growth factor (VEGF) expression [11, 12].

Perioral Dermatitis, Pityriasis Rosea and Rosacea

- Inhibition of pro-inflammatory cytokines like IL-6, IL-8, IL-10 and TNFα [13–15].

Pityriasis Lichenoides

- Inhibition of lymphocytic activity [16, 17].

Psoriasis

- Inhibition of pro-inflammatory cytokines, reduction of neutrophilic activity and super antigen-producing ability of T lymphocytes [18–20].

SAPHO Syndrome

- Inhibition of pro-inflammatory cytokines [21].

Adult-Onset Still's Disease

- Anti-inflammatory and immunomodulatory properties [22].

The basic features and indications of macrolides are elaborated in Table 4.1.

Table 4.1 Pharmacokinetics, indications and dosing of macrolides

Drug	Pharmacokinetics	Indications	Dosage
Erythromycin	Erythromycin is incompletely but adequately absorbed from the gastrointestinal tract. As it is acid labile, it is administered as an enteric-coated tablet. It has a wide volume of distribution. The $t_{1/2}$ of erythromycin is 1.5 h. It is metabolized in the liver and majority of the drug is excreted in the bile; and a small amount undergoes renal excretion.	Chancroid	500 mg PO TID for 7 days [23]
		Donovanosis	500 mg PO QID for 2 weeks
		Non-gonococcal urethritis	500 mg PO QID for 7 days
		Acne vulgaris	500 mg PO thrice weekly on consecutive days for 6 months [2]
		Bullous pemphigoid	1000–3000 mg/day PO in 3–4 divided doses [4, 5]
		Confluent and reticulate papillomatosis	1000 mg/day PO in two divided doses for 6 weeks [6]
		Immune thrombocytopenic purpura (ITP)	600 mg /day PO [9]
		Perioral dermatitis	500 mg PO once daily for 7 days [13]

(continued)

Table 4.1 (continued)

Drug	Pharmacokinetics	Indications	Dosage
		Pityriasis rosea	250 mg/500 mg PO QID for 2 weeks [14]
		Pityriasis lichenoides	1000 mg/day PO in two divided doses for 4 weeks [17]
		Psoriasis	1000 mg PO in two divided doses for 4 weeks [19]
Azithromycin	It is rapidly absorbed on an empty stomach and is unique in being acid stable. It has a long terminal $t_{1/2}$ of >50 h. Excretion is mainly via the bile. Renal excretion of azithromycin accounts only for 10%.	Chancroid	1gm PO single dose [23]
		Donovanosis	1gm PO, once per week for 3 weeks
		Non-gonococcal urethritis	1gm PO single dose
		Acne vulgaris	500 mg PO thrice weekly on 3 consecutive days for 6 months [3]
		Confluent and reticulate papillomatosis	500 mg PO once daily for 6 weeks [6]
		Gingival hyperplasia secondary to cyclosporine	500 mg PO day 1, then 250 mg PO daily for another 4 days [7]
		Perioral dermatitis	500 mg PO once daily for 7 days[13]
		Pityriasis rosea	500 mg PO once daily for 7 days
		Pityriasis lichenoides	500 mg PO day 1, followed by 250 mg on days 2, 3, 4 and 5 for the first and third week of each month

(continued)

Table 4.1 (continued)

Drug	Pharmacokinetics	Indications	Dosage
		Psoriasis	500 mg PO once daily for 4 days, followed by a 10–day gap and then continue in the same fashion for 48 weeks [18]
		Rosacea	500 mg PO once daily for 3 consecutive days per week for 4 weeks [24]
		SAPHO syndrome	500 mg PO once daily for 6 successive days followed by 500 mg PO twice a week [21]
Roxithromycin	Better gastric tolerability. Good enteral absorption. $t_{1/2} = 12$ h. Elimination via the biliary route.	Confluent and reticulate papillomatosis	300 mg/day PO in two divided doses for 6 weeks
		Granulomatous cheilitis	150 mg/day PO once daily until clinical response is noted [25]
		Lupus miliaris disseminatus faciei (LMDF)	300 mg/day PO in two divided doses until clinical response is noted [26]
		Psoriasis	150 mg PO twice daily for 7 weeks

(continued)

Table 4.1 (continued)

Drug	Pharmacokinetics	Indications	Dosage
Clarithromycin	Rapidly absorbed from the gastrointestinal tract. Undergoes first-pass metabolism reducing its oral bioavailability to 50–55%. It may be given with food or without food, but the extended-release form is typically given once daily as a 1gm dose and administered after food to improve its bioavailability. $t_{1/2}$ is 6–9 h. Elimination is via the bile and urine.	Adult-onset still's disease	500 mg PO twice daily [22]
		Immune thrombocytopenic purpura	500 mg PO once daily [10]
		Perioral dermatitis	500 mg PO once daily for 7 days
		Confluent and reticulate papillomatosis	500 mg PO once daily for 6 weeks
		Acne vulgaris	250 mg PO twice daily for 7 days, followed by a 10- day gap, then to repeat the cycle again for a total of three such cycles [27]
		Infections caused by mycobacterium avium intracellulare in AIDS patients with CD4 counts <50 cells/mm3	500 mg PO twice daily, along with ethambutol 15 mg/kg/day once daily, with or without rifabutin; is an effective combination regimen [1]
Telithromycin	Oral 400 mg tablets available Bioavailability is 60% 60–70% of the drug is bound to plasma proteins $t_{1/2}$ is 9.8 h Cleared primarily by hepatic metabolism	-	-

Contraindications

Absolute

- Drug hypersensitivity.

Relative

- Hepatic impairment.

Pregnancy prescribing status: category 'B' (for erythromycin, azithromycin and roxithromycin) and Category 'C' (for clarithromycin and telithromycin).

Adverse Effects

Gastrointestinal

- Hepatotoxicity.
- Epigastric distress.
- Abdominal cramps.
- Nausea.
- Vomiting.

Cardiovascular

- Cardiac arrhythmias, especially with erythromycin and clarithromycin.

Others

- Fever.
- Eosinophilia.
- Drug rash.

Drug Interactions

- Carbamazepine
- Corticosteroids
- Cyclosporine
- Digoxin
- Ergot alkaloids
- Valproic acid
- Theophylline

→ The effects of these drugs are potentiated by erythromycin

- Cisapride
- Azoles
- Terfenadine
- Astemizole

→ Increased likelihood of torsades de pointes phenomenon

Monitoring Guidelines

Baseline

- Liver function tests.

Follow-Up

- In case of long-term treatment to repeat the same test once every 3 months.

Conclusion

Macrolides are a very important class of drugs in dermatology because of their potent anti-inflammatory effects.

References

1. MacDougall C, Chambers HF. Protein synthesis inhibitors and miscellaneous antibacterial agents. In: Bruton LL, Chabner BA, Knollmann BC. Goodman and Gilman's the pharmacological basis of therapeutics. 12th ed. New York. McGraw Hill. 2011. 1521–1547.
2. Labro MT. Antiinflammatory activity of macroides. A new therapeutic potential. J Antimicrob Chemother. 1998;41(Suppl B):37–41.
3. Kus S, Yucelten D, Hytug H. Comparison of the efficacy of azithromycin versus doxycycline in the treatment of acne vulgaris. Clin Exp Dermatol. 2005;30:215–20.
4. Fox BJ, Odom RB, Findlay RF. Erythromycin therapy in bullous pemphigoid: possible anti-inflammatory effects. J Am Acad Dermatol. 1982;7:504–10.
5. Altomare G, Capella GL, Fracchiola C, Frigerio E. Treatment of bullous pemphigoid with erythromycin. A reappraisal. Eur J Dermatol. 1999;9:583–5.

6. Tang HS, Oh CK, Cha JH, et al. Six cases of confluent and reticulate papillomatosis alleviated by various antibiotics. J Am Acad Dermatol. 2001;44:652–5.
7. Kim JY, Park SH, Cho KS, et al. Mechanism of azithromycin treatment on gingival overgrowth. J Dent Res. 2008;87:1075–9.
8. Ianaro A, Ialenti A, Maffia P, et al. Antiinflammatory activity of macrolide antibiotics. J Pharmacol Exp Ther. 2000;292:156–63.
9. Ohe M, Hashino S. Successful treatment with erythromycin for idiopathic thrombocytopenic purpura. Korean J Dermatol. 2011;46:139–42.
10. Ohe M, Kohno M. Three cases of idiopathic thrombocytopenic purpura showing a increase in platelet count following clarithromycin treatment. Rinsko Ketsueki. 2003;44:1044–6.
11. Koizumi N, Hatamochi A, Shinkai H. Treatment of lupus miliaris disseminates faciei with roxithromycin. Nishinihon J Dermatol. 2003;65:70–3.
12. Aoki D, Ueno S, Kubo F, et al. Roxithromycin inhibits angiogenesis of human hepatoma cells in vivo by suppressing VEGF production. Anticancer Res. 2005;25:133–8.
13. Goel NS, Burkhart CN, Morrell DS. Pediatric periorificial dermatitis: clinical course and outcomes in 222 patients. Pediatr Dermatol. 2015;32:333–6.
14. Bakar O, Demircay Z, Yuksel M, Haklar G, et al. The effect of azithromycin on reactive oxygen species in rosacea. Clin Exp Dermatol. 2007;32:197–200.
15. Sharma PK, Yadav TP, Gautam RK, et al. Erythromycin in pityriasis rosea: a double blind placebo controlled trial. J Am Acad Dermatol. 2000;42:241–4.
16. Truhan AP, Herbert AA, Esterly NB. Pityriasis lichenoides in children: therapeutic response to erythromycin. J Am Acad Dermatol. 1986;15:66–70.
17. Skinner RB, Levy AL. Rapid resolution of pityriasis lichenoides et varioliformis acuta with azithromycin. J Am Acad Dermatol. 2008;58:524–5.
18. Saxena VN, Dogra J. Long term oral azithromycin in chronic plaque psoriasis. A controlled trial. Eur J Dermatol. 2010;20:329–33.
19. Komine M, Tamaki K. An open trial of oral macrolide treatment for psoriasis vulgaris. J Dermatol. 2000;27:508–12.
20. Wakita H, Tikura Y, Furukawa F, et al. The macrolide antibiotic roxithromycin suppresses IFNγ mediated immunological functions of cultured normal human keratinocytes. Biol Pharm Bull. 1996;19:224–7.
21. Colina M, Lo Monaco A, Khodeir M, et al. Propionibacterium acnes and SAPHO syndrome. A case report and literature review. Clin Exp Rheumatol. 2007;25:457–60.
22. Saviola G, Benucci M, Abdi-Ali L, et al. Clarithromycin in adult onset stills disease. A study of six cases. Rheumatol Int. 2010;30:555–60.
23. Balachandran C, Pai SB. Chancroid. In: Sharma VK, editor. Sexually transmitted diseases and HIV/AIDS. 2nd ed. New Delhi: Viva Books; 2002. p. 337–46.
24. Fernandez-Obregon A. Oral use of azithromycin for the treatment of acne rosacea. Arch Dermatol. 2004;140:489–90.
25. Ishiguro E, Hatamochi A, Hamasaki Y, Ishikawa S, Yamazaki S. Successful treatment of granulomatous cheilitis with roxithromycin. J Dermatol. 2008;35:598–600.
26. Koizumi N. Treatment of lupus miliaris disseminatus faciei with roxithromycin. Nishinihon J Dermatol. 2003;65:70–3.
27. Rathi SK. Pulse clarithromycin therapy in severe acne vulgaris. Indian J Dermatol. 2002;47:234–5.

Tetracyclines

5

Introduction

These are a class of antibiotics having a nucleus with four cyclic rings that are obtained from soil actinomycetes. The drugs belonging to this group are tetracycline, doxycycline, demeclocycline, minocycline and lymecycline. A recent addition to the list is the drug sarecycline, that has a narrow spectrum of activity, as a result of which there are lesser chances of adverse effects.

Mechanism of Action

These drugs inhibit bacterial protein synthesis by binding to 30 s ribosomal subunit in the susceptible organism. It is usually bacteriostatic, but at higher concentrations may be bactericidal [1]. The mechanism of action for individual diseases is described below.

Acne [2–5]

- Blockage of bacterial products that stimulate inflammation.
- Inhibition of inflammatory mediators like interleukin (IL)-8 and MMP (matrix metalloproteinase).
- Scavenging action on reactive oxygen species.

Sarcoidosis

- Inhibition of T-cell proliferation and granuloma formation [6].

A. K. Bubna, *Therapeutics in Dermatology - Essentials for Clinical Practice*, https://doi.org/10.1007/978-981-95-3791-4_5

Immunobullous Dermatoses

- Inhibition of MMP and mast cell activation [7–9].

Kaposi Sarcoma

- Inhibition of MMP-2 and MMP-9 [10].

Lichen Planus

- Inhibition of T-lymphocyte responses [11, 12].

Lupus Miliaris Disseminatus Faciei

- Inhibition of T-cell proliferation and granuloma formation [4, 13].

Neutrophilic Dermatoses

- Inhibition of IL-8 and neutrophil activation [14, 15].

Pityriasis Lichenoides

- Inhibition of T-lymphocyte responses [16].

Prurigo Pigmentosa

- Inhibition of migration and/or function of neutrophils, as well as an active scavenging of reactive oxygen species [17, 18].

Red Scalp Disease

- Inhibition of MMP [19].

Red Scrotal Syndrome

- Inhibition of MMP [20].

Rosacea [21–23]

- Inhibition of neutrophilic migration.
- Direct scavenging effect on reactive oxygen species.
- Inhibitory effect on VEGF and nitric oxide, preventing excessive vascular dilatation and angiogenesis in rosacea.
- Improvement in epidermal hydration.
- Antagonistic effects on granuloma formation.

Pharmacokinetics

The pharmacokinetics of tetracyclines is elucidated in Table 5.1.

The indications and dosing are outlined in Table 5.2.

Table 5.1 Pharmacokinetics of various tetracyclines

Pharmacokinetic features	Tetracycline	Demeclocycline	Minocycline	Doxycycline
Oral absorption	Usually incomplete	Usually incomplete	Usually incomplete	Usually incomplete
Per cent of drug absorption on an empty stomach	60–80	60–80	100	95
Effect of milk and calcium-containing foods on absorption	Important factor; so, avoid these foods when administering tetracycline	Important factor; so, avoid these foods when administering demeclocycline	Unlikely to affect minocycline absorption	Unlikely to affect doxycycline absorption; yet avoid administration of antacids and calcium supplements
$t_{1/2}$	6–10 h	16 h	16–18 h	16–18 h
Plasma protein binding	Moderate	High	High	High
Metabolism	Hepatic	Hepatic	Hepatic	Hepatic
Major route for elimination	Renal	Renal	Renal	Renal
Other route for excretion	Biliary	Biliary	Biliary	Biliary

Table 5.2 Indications and dosing of tetracyclines

Indications	Dosing
Acne vulgaris	Doxycycline 50–100 mg PO (per oral) once or twice daily Minocycline 50–100 mg PO once or twice daily Lymecycline 408 mg PO once daily, Sarecycline (US FDA approved) 1.5mg/kg/day These drugs need to be continued for a period of at least 3 months to see effective results
Confluent and reticulate papillomatosis	Minocycline 200 mg PO once daily for 6 weeks
Sarcoidosis	Minocycline 200 mg PO once daily The exact duration of treatment in sarcoidosis cannot be determined
Immunobullous disorders that include bullous pemphigoid, linear IgA bullous dermatosis, pemphigus vulgaris, pemphigus foliaceus, Hailey Hailey disease and cicatricial pemphigoid.	Tetracycline 1500 mg PO per day in two or three divided doses Minocycline 100 mg PO once daily Doxycycline 100 mg PO twice daily Along with tab niacinamide 500 mg Q8H The duration of treatment is prolonged and could even extend for 6–12 months
Lichen planus	Tetracycline 500 mg PO twice daily Doxycycline 100 mg PO twice daily These drugs need to be continued for a minimum of at least 3 months for effective results
Lupus miliaris disseminatus faciei	Minocycline 100 mg PO once daily The drug needs to be continued for a minimum of at least 3 months for effective results
Sweet's syndrome and pyoderma gangrenosum	Doxycycline 100 mg PO twice daily Minocycline 200–300 mg PO per day either as a single dose or two divided doses. Treatment is often prolonged
Pityriasis lichenoides	Tetracycline 500 mg PO twice daily for 6 weeks
Prurigo pigmentosa	Doxycycline 200 mg PO in two divided doses for 6 weeks Minocycline 200 mg PO in two divided doses for 6 weeks
Red scalp disease	Lymecycline 300 mg/day PO once daily till resolution of lesions
Red scrotal syndrome	Doxycycline 100 mg/day PO once daily for 3–6 weeks
Rosacea	Doxycycline 100 mg PO once daily for 3 months Minocycline 100 mg PO once daily for 3 months
Primary, secondary and early latent syphilis (in penicillin allergic patients)	Doxycycline 100 mg PO twice daily for 2 weeks Tetracycline 500 mg PO four times daily for 2 weeks
Endemic treponematosis (in penicillin allergic patients)	Tetracycline 500 mg PO four times daily for 5 days
Donovanosis	Tetracycline 500 mg PO four times daily for 2–3 weeks Doxycycline 100 mg PO twice daily for 3 weeks and until all lesions have completely cleared

(continued)

Table 5.2 (continued)

Indications	Dosing
Uncomplicated gonococcal infection of the pharynx	Doxycycline 100 mg PO twice daily for 7 days
Non-gonococcal urethritis	Doxycycline 100 mg PO twice daily for 7 days
Lymphogranuloma venerum [24, 25]	Doxycycline 100 mg PO twice daily for 3 weeks Tetracycline 500 mg PO four times daily for 3 weeks Minocycline 300 mg PO initially as a single dose, followed by 200 mg PO twice daily for 10 days
Pelvic inflammatory disease	Doxycycline 100 mg PO twice daily for 2 weeks, usually in combination with metronidazole and ceftriaxone

Contraindications

Absolute

- Hypersensitivity to the drug.
- Pregnancy and lactation.

Relative

- Children.
- Renal/hepatic insufficiency.

Pregnancy prescribing status: category 'D'.

Drug Interactions

- Simultaneous use of tetracyclines along with diuretics is to be avoided as there can be an elevation of blood urea levels.
- Injectable tetracyclines and penicillin should not be mixed as inactivation occurs.
- Proton pump inhibitors increase gastric pH and reduce tetracycline absorption.
- Tetracyclines increase serum levels of digoxin, lithium and warfarin.

Adverse Effects

Gastrointestinal

- Fatty liver.
- Jaundice.
- Fatal fulminant hepatitis.

Renal

- Renal toxicity occurs usually in patients with pre-existing renal disease.
- All tetracyclines, except doxycycline, accumulate in renal tubules and enhance renal failure.

Cutaneous

- Phototoxicity (particularly with demeclocycline).
- Fixed drug eruption (particularly with tetracycline).
- Diffuse muddy brown pigmentation (with minocycline).
- Minocycline hypersensitivity syndrome, including lupus like syndrome.
- Very rarely rashes and angioedema.

Teeth

- Ill-formed teeth more susceptible to caries if taken from mid pregnancy to 5 months of intrauterine life.
- If given to children between 3 months and 6 years of age, the crown of permanent anterior dentition could be severely affected. Repeated courses are more damaging.

Bones

- If given during pregnancy or early childhood, there is temporary suppression of bone growth.

Nervous System

- Diabetes insipidus.
- Vertigo (minocycline).
- Nystagmus.
- Increased intracranial tension.

Antianabolic Effect

- Reduces protein synthesis with an overall catabolic effect.

Conclusion

Tetracyclines comprise a versatile group of drugs in treating a number of dermatologic disorders.

References

1. MacDougall C, Chambers HF. Protein synthesis inhibitors and miscellaneous antibacterial agents. In: Bruton LL, Chabner BA, Knollmann BC. Goodman and Gilman's the pharmacological basis of therapeutics. 12th ed. New York. McGraw Hill. 2011. 1521–1547.
2. Monk E, Shalita A, Siegel DM. Clinical applications of non-antimicrobial tetracyclines in dermatology. Pharm Res. 2011;63:130–45.
3. Sarici G, Cinar S, Armutcu F, et al. Oxidative stress in acne vulgaris. J Eur Acad Dermatol Venereol. 2010;24:763–7.
4. Skidmore R, Kovach R, Walker C, et al. Effects of subantimicrobial dose doxycycline in the treatment of moderate acne. Arch Dermatol. 2003;139:459–64.
5. Bahrami F, Morris DL, Pourgholami MH. Tetracyclines: drugs with huge therapeutic potential. Mini Rev Med Chem. 2012;12:44–52.
6. Bachales H, Senet P, Cadranel J, et al. The use of tetracyclines for the treatment of sarcoidosis. Arch Dermatol. 2001;137:69–73.
7. McCarty M, Fivenson D. Two decades using the combination of tetracycline derivatives and niacinamide as steroid sparing agents in the management of pemphigus: defining a niche for low toxicity agents. J Am Acad Dermatol. 2014;71:475–9.
8. Le Sache-de PL, Raynaud E, Bouchardeau A, et al. Familial benign chronic pemphigus and doxycycline: a review of 6 cases. J Eur Acad Dermatol Venereol. 2014;28:370–3.
9. Shan XF, Zhang FR, Tian HQ, et al. A case of linear IgA dermatosis successfully treated with tetracycline and niacinamide. Int J Dermatol. 2016;55:e216–7.
10. Richards C, Pantanowitz L, Dezube BJ. Antimicrobial and non-antimicrobial tetracyclines in human cancer trials. Pharmacol Res. 2011;63:151–6.
11. Hantash BM, Kanzler MH. The efficacy of tetracycline antibiotics for the treatment of lichen planus: an open label clinical trial. Br J Dermatol. 2007;156:758–60.
12. Kloppenburg M, Verweij CL, Mittenburg AM, et al. The influence of tetracyclines on T cell activation. Clin Exp Immunol. 1995;102:635–41.
13. Estero T, Faria A, Alves R, et al. Lupus miliaris disseminatus faciei. A case report. Dermatol Online J. 2010;16:10.
14. Joshi RK, Atukorala DN, Abarmi A, et al. Successful treatment of sweet's syndrome with doxycycline. Br J Dermatol. 1993;128:584–6.
15. Berth-Jones J, Tan SV, Graham Brown RA, et al. The successful use of minocycline in pyoderma gangrnosum—a report of 7 cases and review of the literature. J Dermatolog Treat. 1989;128:584–6.
16. Piamphongsant T. Tetracycline for the treatment of pityriasis lichenoides. Br J Dermatol. 1974;91:319–22.
17. Kim TI, Choi JW, Jeong KH, et al. Pustular prurigo pigmentosa treated with doxycycline. J Dermatol. 2016;43:965–6.
18. Matsumoto C, Kinoshita M, Baba S et al. Vesicular prurigo pigmentosa cured by minocycline. J Eur Acad Dermatol Venereol Leprol 2001; 15: 354–356.
19. Oberholzer PA, Nobbe S, Kolm I, et al. Red scalp disease—a rosacea like dermatoses of the scalp? Successful therapy with oral tetracycline. Dermatology. 2009;219:178–81.
20. Wollina U. Red scrotal syndrome. J Dermatol Case Rep. 2011;5:38–41.

21. Baldwin HE. Diagnosis and treatment of rosacea. State of the art. J Drugs Dermatol. 2012;11:725–30.
22. Perret LJ, Tait CP. Non antibiotic properties of tetracyclines and their clinical application in dermatology. Australas J Dermatol. 2014;55:111–8.
23. Ni Raghallaigh S, Powell FC. Epidermal hydration levels in patients with rosacea improves after minocycline therapy. Br J Dermatol. 2014;171:259–66.
24. Sexually transmitted diseases. Treatment guigelines. 2006. www.cdc-gov
25. Sowmini CN, et al. Minocycline in the treatment of lymphogranuloma venerum. J Am Vener Dis Assoc. 1976;2:19–22.

Clindamycin

6

Introduction

Clindamycin (CLIND) is a synthetic derivative of lincomycin. It has been isolated from *Streptomyces* species [1].

Mechanism of Action

Infections

CLIND binds with the 50 s ribosomal subunit of bacteria and inhibits bacterial protein synthesis [1]. Antibacterial spectrum includes *Staphylococcus aureus, Streptococcus pneumoniae, Streptococcus pyogenes, Streptococcus viridens,* anaerobic *streptococci, Peptostreptococci, Peptococci, Bacteriodes* spp. and *Fusobacteria* [1].

CLIND delineates anti-inflammatory properties, because of which it is utilized for various dermatologic disorders as stated below.

Acne and Rosacea [2–4]

- Modulates cytokine production in lipopolysaccharide-stimulated macrophages.
- Reduces TNFα and IL-1β concentrations.
- Increases IL-6 concentrations.

A. K. Bubna, *Therapeutics in Dermatology - Essentials for Clinical Practice*, https://doi.org/10.1007/978-981-95-3791-4_6

Folliculitis Decalvans

- Suppresses chemotaxis of neutrophils secondary to complement activation, thereby reducing potential inflammation [5].

Fox–Fordyce Disease

- The mechanism here is similar to that seen in folliculitis decalvans [6, 7].

Hidradenitis Suppurativa

CLIND enhances the uptake of microbes by host phagocytes and suppresses chemotaxis of neutrophils secondary to complement activation, thereby reducing inflammation in hidradenitis suppurativa [8, 9].

Pharmacokinetics

CLIND has good oral bioavailability. It penetrates soft tissues very well. The $t_{1/2}$ is 3 h. It is metabolized in the liver and excreted via the bile and urine [1].

Clinical Uses

Cellulitis

CLIND is given to patients who exhibit penicillin sensitivity in the following manner:

(a) Where outpatient antibiotic treatment can be given: 600 mg intravenous (IV) Q8H till lesions subside.
(b) Where hospital admission is a must: 900 mg IV Q8H till lesions subside.

Bacterial Vaginosis

- Clindamycin 300 mg PO Q12H for 7 days.
- OR
- Clindamycin ovules 100 mg intravaginally once at bed time for 3 days.
- OR
- Clindamycin 2% vaginal cream 5gm intravaginally at bed time for 7 days.

Acne

- Topical clindamycin 1% gel twice daily for 3 months or till lesions resolve.

Rosacea

- Topical clindamycin 1% gel twice daily for 3 months or till lesions resolve.

Folliculitis Decalvans and Hidradenitis Suppurativa

- Clindamycin 300 mg PO Q12H, along with rifampicin 300 mg PO Q12H for 10–12 weeks.

Fox–Fordyce Disease

- Topical clindamycin 1% gel twice daily till lesions resolve.

Impetigo, Ecthyma, Folliculitis and Furunculosis

- Clindamycin 300 mg PO Q12H for 7 days.

Contraindications

Absolute

- Hypersensitivity to the drug.

Relative

- Colitis.

Pregnancy prescribing status: category 'B'.

Drug Interactions

- Erythromycin and chloramphenicol: should not be used along with CLIND as their therapeutic efficacy is diminished.

- CLIND can potentiate neuromuscular effects of botulinum toxin or other neuromuscular blockers.

Adverse Effects

- Pseudomembranous colitis.
- Elevated liver enzymes.
- Hypersensitivity reactions: eosinophilia, thrombocytopenia and Stevens–Johnson syndrome.

Conclusion

CLIND is an important drug in the dermatologic therapeutic armamentarium.

References

1. MacDougall C, Chambers HF. Protein synthesis inhibitors and miscellaneous antibacterial agents. In: Bruton LL, Chabner BA, Knollmann BC. Goodman and Gilman's the pharmacological basis of therapeutics. 12th ed. New York. McGraw Hill. 2011. 1521–1547.
2. Del Rosso JQ, Schmidt NF. A review of the anti-inflammatory properties of clindamycin in the treatment of acne vulgaris. Cutis. 2010;85:15–24.
3. Weinkle AP, Doktor V, Emer J. Update on the management of rosacea. Clin Cosmet Investig Dermatol. 2015;8:159–77.
4. Breneman D, Savin R, VandePol C, et al. Double blind randomized vehicle controlled trial of once daily benzoyl peroxide/clindamycin topical gel in the treatment of patients with moderate to severe rosacea. Int J Dermatol. 2004;43:381–7.
5. Powell JJ, Dawber RP, Gatter K. Folliculitis decalvans including tufted folliculitis: clinical, histological and therapeutic findings. Br J Dermatol. 1999;140:328–33.
6. Yost J, Robinson M, Meehan SA. Fox Fordyce disease. Dermatol Online J. 2012;18:28.
7. George A, Bhatia A, Thomas E. Fox Fordyce disease: a report of 2 cases responding to topical clindamycin. Indian J Dermatol Venereol Leprol. 2015;81:87–8.
8. Van der Zee HH, Boer J, Prens EP, et al. The effect of combined treatment with oral clindmycin and oral rifampicin in patients with hidradenitis suppurativa. Dermatology. 2009;219:143–7.
9. Pasquale JR, Tan JS. Non antimicrobial effects of antibacterial agents. Clin Infect Dis. 2005;40:127–35.

Metronidazole

7

Introduction

Metronidazole is a nitroimidazole drug that was first introduced in the market as an antiprotozoal agent. With progression of time, there have been a number of applications of metronidazole discovered in the field of dermatology and venereology.

Mechanism of Action

As an Antiprotozoal and Antibacterial Agent for Bacteria like Bacteroides and Clostridium Species

Once taken up by the bacteria and sensitive protozoa, metronidazole gets nonenzymatically reduced to ferredoxin. This reduced metabolite obtained is up taken by DNA molecules of the concerned pathogen, and unstable molecules that form finally have toxic implications on microbes [1].

Rosacea

Apart from its antibiotic properties, metronidazole impedes leukocyte chemotaxis and there is selective suppression of cell-mediated immunity [2]. Furthermore, it inhibits release of free radicals, along with an inhibitory influence on the mite, *Demodex brevis* [3, 4].

A. K. Bubna, *Therapeutics in Dermatology - Essentials for Clinical Practice*,
https://doi.org/10.1007/978-981-95-3791-4_7

Lichen Planus

- Immunomodulatory effects [5].

Acne

- Immunomodulatory/anti-inflammatory/antipruritic properties, and the ability to inhibit generation of free radicals [6–8].

Cutaneous Metastatic Crohn Disease

- Antibacterial and anti-inflammatory effects [9].

Periorificial Dermatitis

- Anti-inflammatory and immunomodulatory effects, along with its antagonistic action on neutrophils regarding the generation of free radicals [10, 11].

Seborrheic Dermatitis

- Anti-inflammatory properties and the ability to inhibit generation of free radicals [12–15].

Pharmacokinetics

Metronidazole, after oral intake, is promptly absorbed and widely distributed in the tissues. With the exception of placenta, metronidazole penetrates well into all body fluids, including vaginal secretions, seminal fluid, saliva, breast milk and cerebrospinal fluid. The $t_{1/2}$ of metronidazole is around 8 hours. Less than 20% of the drug is bound to plasma proteins. The metabolism of metronidazole occurs in the liver, where two metabolites are released, namely an acidic derivative and a hydroxy compound. Glucuronide formation has also been encountered as a part of metronidazole metabolism. Excretion of the drug is mainly through the kidneys [16].

The indications and dosing of metronidazole are described in Table 7.1.

Table 7.1 Indications and dosing of metronidazole

Indication	Dosing details
Amoebiasis	Tab metronidazole 750 mg PO Q8H for 10 days OR Tab metronidazole 500 mg IV Q6H for 10 days [17]
Giardiasis	Tab metronidazole 400 mg PO Q8H for 5–7 days OR Tab metronidazole 2gm PO once daily for 3 days
Trichomoniasis (FDA approved)	Tab metronidazole 500 mg PO Q12H for 7 days OR Tab metronidazole 2gm PO stat dose
Bacterial vaginosis	Tab metronidazole 400 mg or 500 mg PO Q12H for 7 days OR Tab Metronidazole 2gm PO stat dose
Anaerobic bacterial infections like *Peptococcus, Peptostreptococcus, Bacteroides* and *Fusobacterium species*	Tab metronidazole 500 mg PO Q6H or Q8H for 7–14 days OR Tab metronidazole 500 mg IV Q8H for 7–14 days
Fournier's gangrene	Dose similar to the one described for anaerobic bacterial infections; however, metronidazole is administered with β-lactamase inhibitor penicillins for this indication
Perioral dermatitis	Tab metronidazole 250 mg PO Q12H for 4–6 weeks Topical metronidazole gel 0.75% and 1% is also helpful
Acne, seborrheic dermatitis, rosacea	As a topical 0.75%, 1% and 2% gel
Lichen planus	Tab metronidazole 400–500 mg PO Q12H that can be continued for a period of 2–3 months
Cutaneous metastatic Crohn disease	Metronidazole 20 mg/kg IV per day in divided doses

Contraindications

Absolute

- Hypersensitivity to the drug.
- First trimester of pregnancy.

Relative

- Impaired liver function.

Pregnancy prescribing status: category 'B' (but better avoided in the first trimester).

Drug Interactions

- Metronidazole increases circulating levels of cyclosporine, tacrolimus and phenytoin.
- Metronidazole potentiates the anticoagulant effect of warfarin.
- In combination with protease inhibitors or if consumed with alcohol, metronidazole may produce a disulfiram-like reaction.
- If used with reverse transcriptase inhibitors, metronidazole increases the risk of developing peripheral neuropathy.

Adverse Effects

Cutaneous

- Morbilliform eruptions.
- Pruritus.

Gastrointestinal System

- Metallic taste in the mouth.
- Nausea.
- Vomiting.

Renal

- Dark urine.
- Dysuria.

Nervous System

- Sensory neuropathy.
- Confusion.
- Seizures.
- Headache.
- Syncope.

Hematological

- Transient leucopoenia.

Conclusion

In dermatology, metronidazole has proven to be a valuable drug with multiple uses. Besides, it is economical for patients. Further, it has an acceptable safety profile.

References

1. Deck DH, Winston LG. Miscellaneous antimicrobial agents: disinfectants, antiseptics and sterilants. In: Katzung BG, Trevor AJ, editors. Basic and clinical pharmacology. 13th ed. New Delhi: McGraw Hill Education(India) Private Limited; 2012. p. 865–72.
2. Burkhart CN, Katz KA. Other topical medications. In: Goldsmith LA, Katz SI, Gilchrest BA, Paller AS, Leffel DJ, Wolff K, editors. Fitzpatrick's dermatology in general medicine. 8th ed. New York: McGraw Hill; 2012. p. 2697–707.
3. Del Rosso JQ. A status report of the medical management of rosacea: focus on topical therapeutics. Cutis. 2002;70:271–5.
4. Schmadel LK, McEvoy GK. Topical metronidazole: a new therapy for rosacea. Clin Pharm. 1990;9:94–101.
5. Buyuk AY, Kavala M. Oral metronidazole treatment for lichen planus. J Am Acad Dermatol. 2000;43:260–2.
6. Kirchoff T, Merkesdal S, Rosenthal S, Prokop M, Chavan A, Wagner A, et al. Diagnostic management of patients with SAPHO syndrome. Use of MR imaging to guide bone biopsy at CT for microbiological and histological work up. Eur Radiol. 2003;13:2304–8.
7. Nishimuta K, Ito Y. Effects of metronidazole and tinidazole ointments on models for inflammatory dermatosis in mice. Arch Dermatol Res. 2003;294:544–51.
8. Khodaeiani E, Fouladi RF, Yousefi N, Amirnia M, Babaeinijad S, Shokri J. Efficacy of 2% metronidazole gel in moderate acne vulgaris. Indian J Dermatol. 2012;57:279–81.
9. Khan KJ, Ullman TA, Ford AC, Abreu MT, Abadir A, Marshall JK, et al. antibiotic therapy in inflammatory bowel disease: a systematic review and metaanalysis. Am J Gastroenterol. 2011;106:661–73.
10. Boeck K, Abeck D, Werfel S, Ring J. Perioral dermatitis in children—clinical presentation, pathogenesis—related factors and response to topical metronidazole. Dermatology. 1997;195:235–8.
11. Rodriguez-Caruncho C, Bielsa I, Fernandez-Figueras MT, Ferrandiz C. Childhood granulomatous perioral dermatitis with good response to oral metronidazole. Pediatr Dermatol. 2013;30:e98–9.
12. Zip CM. Innovative use of topical metronidazole. Dermatol Clin. 2010;28:525–34.
13. Bikowski J. Facial seborrheic dermatitis: a report on current status and therapeutic horizons. J Drugs Dermatol. 2009;8:125–33.
14. McFalda WL, Roebuck HL. Rational management of papulopustular rosacea with concomitant facial seborrheic dermatitis. A case report. J Clin Aesthet Dermatol. 2011;4:40–2.
15. Seckin D, Gurbuz O, Akin O. Metronidazole 0.75% gel vs ketoconazole 2% cream in the treatment of facial seborrheic dermatitis: a randomized double blind study. J Eur Acad Dermatol Venereol. 2007;21:345–50.
16. Lamp KL, Freeman CD, Klutman NE, Lacy MK. Pharmacokinetics and pharmacodyanamics of nitroimidazole antimicrobials. Clin Pharmacokinet. 1999;36:353–73.
17. Rosenthal PJ. Antiprotozoal drugs. In: Katzung BG, Trevor AJ, editors. Basic and Clinical Pharmacology. 13th ed. New Delhi: McGraw Hill Education(India) Private Limited; 2012. p. 886–907.

Rifampicin

8

Introduction

Rifampicin (RFP) is a semisynthetic derivative of rifamycin B, an antimicrobial agent produced by *Streptomyces mediterranei*. It is a broad-spectrum antimicrobial agent and inhibits growth of most gram-positive bacteria, as well as many gram-negative organisms. However, it has other valuable properties, apart from its antimicrobial effects.

Mechanism of Action

RFP is used in various dermatological conditions with a different mode of action for each, as described below.

Leprosy and Cutaneous Tuberculosis

RFP binds to the β subunit of DNA-dependent RNA polymerase and suppresses RNA synthesis, thereby exhibiting bactericidal properties toward *Mycobacterium leprae, M. tuberculosis, M. intracellulare* and *M. avium* [1].

Psoriasis

- Immunosuppressive and anti-inflammatory effects [2, 3].

A. K. Bubna, *Therapeutics in Dermatology - Essentials for Clinical Practice*, https://doi.org/10.1007/978-981-95-3791-4_8

Hidradenitis Suppurativa

- Alteration in the capacity of human monocytes to secrete inflammatory cytokines [4].
- Reduction of NF-κβ activity and Th-17 differentiation, thus modulating T-cell responses [5].

Pruritus Secondary to Cholestasis

- RFP enhances the metabolism of bilirubin and its breakdown products. Further, it induces phase I, II and III biotransformation enzymes and transporters, such as CYP3A4, UGT1A1, SULTA1 and MRP2 [6–8].

Tufted Folliculitis and Folliculitis Decalvans

- Anti-inflammatory, immunomodulatory and antibacterial effects [9].

Dermatitis Cruris Pustulosa et Atrophicans

- Antimicrobial and anti-inflammatory effects [10].

Pharmacokinetics

RFP is well absorbed orally on an empty stomach with a bioavailability of 70%. Food reduces RFP absorption, and therefore, it needs to be always given on an empty stomach. The $t_{1/2}$ of RFP is 2–5 hours. The metabolism of RFP takes place in the liver. Excretion is mainly via the bile, and a small amount of RFP is eliminated via the renal route [1].

Clinical Uses

Leprosy

- RFP is a part of both paucibacillary (PB) and multibacillary (MB) multidrug therapy (MDT) regimens.
- The dose of RFP is 600 mg that is administered on the first day of each pulse. For PB-MDT, there are 6 pulses; and for MB-MDT, 12 pulses are given.
- Further RFP in leprosy has also demonstrated positive effects in the healing of trophic ulcers as an adjunct drug.
- The schedule of PB-MDT and MB-MDT is outlined in Table 8.1.

Table 8.1 World Health Organization (WHO) drug schedule for leprosy

Type of leprosy	WHO drug regimen
Paucibacillary	Oral rifampicin 600 mg once every month for 6 months Oral dapsone 100 mg every day for 6 months Schedule needs to be completed over a period of 6–9 months
Multibacillary	Oral rifampicin once every month for 12 months Oral dapsone 100 mg every day for 12 months Oral clofazimine 300 mg once every month for 12 months, along with 50 mg each day for 12 months Schedule needs to be completed over a period of 12–18 months

Hidradenitis Suppurativa

- In hidradenitis suppurativa, RFP is administered in combination with clindamycin.
- RFP 600 mg PO once daily along with clindamycin 300 mg PO twice daily is given for a period of 10–12 weeks [5].

Psoriasis

- RFP is dosed at 300 mg PO twice daily; the exact duration of treatment cannot be specified owing to variability in responses seen in different patients [11].

Pruritus Secondary to Cholestasis

- RFP is given at a dose of 300 mg/day for this indication [12].

Tufted Folliculitis and Folliculitis Decalvans

- RFP (300 mg PO Q12H) is given along with clindamycin (3000 mg PO Q12H). Other agents that can be combined with RFP include co-trimoxazole, doxycycline, tetracycline, clarithromycin, minocycline and isotretinoin [13].

Cutaneous Tuberculosis

RFP is administered at a dose of 8–12 mg/kg/day, with a maximum dose not exceeding 600 mg/day. For newly diagnosed patients, RFP is administered for 6 months along with other antitubercular drugs. In case the patient has been previously treated, RFP needs to be given in the same dose for a period of 8 months along with other antitubercular drugs like isoniazid, pyrazinamide, ethambutol and streptomycin.

Adverse Effects

- Hepatitis: a major adverse effect, which is generally seen in patients with pre-existing liver disease. It is dose related and infrequent with doses ≤600 mg/day.
- Cutaneous syndromes characterized by flushing, pruritus and rash have been reported.
- Flu-like syndrome.
- Gastrointestinal effects like nausea, vomiting and abdominal cramps with or without diarrhoea.
- Rarely shock and renal failure.

Pregnancy prescribing status: category 'C'.

Drug Interactions

As RFP is a microsomal enzyme inducer, it enhances the metabolism of a number of drugs and therefore dose adjustments are needed.

Some of those drugs include

- Warfarin.
- Oral contraceptive pills.
- Sulfonylureas.
- Corticosteroids.
- HIV protease inhibitors.
- Fluconazole.
- Ketoconazole.
- Clarithromycin.
- Metoprolol.

Conclusion

RFP overall is a valuable drug not just for infections, but also diseases associated with chronic inflammation.

References

1. Gumbo T. Chemotherapy of tuberculosis, mycobacterium avium complex disease and leprosy. In: Brunton LL, Chabner BA, Knollman BC, editors. Goodman and Gilman's the pharmacological basis of therapeutics. 12th ed. New York: McGraw Hill; 2011. p. 1549–70.
2. Nilson BS. Rifampicin: An immunosuppressant? Lancet. 1971;2:374.
3. Dajani BM, Canady MS, Thompson JS, et al. Rifampicin; An immunosuppressant? Lancet. 1972;2:1094.

4. Mendonca CO, Griffiths CE. Clindamycin and rifampicin combination therapy for hidradenitis suppurativa. Br J Dermatol. 2006;154:977–8.
5. Gener G, Canoui-Poitrine F, Revuz JE, Faye O, Poli F, Gabison G, Pouget F, Viallette C, Wolkenstein P, Bastuji-Garin S. Combination therapy with clindamycin and rifampicin for hidradenitis suppurativa: a series of 116 consecutive patients. Dermatology. 2009;219:148–54.
6. Le Cluyse EL. Pregnane X receptor: molecular basis for species differences in CYP3A induction by xenobiotics. Chem Biol Interact. 2001;134:283–9.
7. Marschall HU, Wagner M, Zollner G, et al. Complementary stimulation of hepatobiliary transport and detoxification systems by rifampicin and ursodeoxycholic acid in humans. Gastroenterology. 2005;129:476–85.
8. Khurana S, Singh P. Rifampicin is a safe treatment for pruritus due to chronic cholestasis: a meta-analysis of prospective randomized controlled trials. Liver Int. 2006;26:943–8.
9. Powell JJ, Dawber RP, Gatter K. Folliculitis decalvans including tufted folliculitis: clinical, histological and therapeutic findings. Br J Dermatol. 1999;140:328–33.
10. Kaimal S, D'Souza M, Kumari R. Dermatitis cruris pustulosa et atrophicans. Indian J Dermatol Venereol Leprol. 2009;75:348–55.
11. Kazandjieva J, Kamarashev J, Hinkov G, et al. Rifampicin and psoriasis. Akt Dermatol. 1997;23:78–81.
12. Mela M, Mancuso A, Burroughs AK. Review article: pruritus in cholestatic and other liver diseases. Aliment Pharmacol Ther. 2003;17:857–70.
13. Rambhia PH, Conic RRZ, Murad A, Atanaskova-Mesinkovska N, Piliang M, Bergfeld W. Updates in therapeutics for folliculitis decalvans: a systematic review with evidence-based analysis. J Am Acad Dermatol. 2019;80:794–801.e1.

Vancomycin

9

Introduction

Vancomycin (VAN) is a tricyclic glycopeptide antibiotic produced by *Streptococcus orientalis* and *Amycolatopsis orientalis*. It is active only against gram-positive bacteria. VAN has a molecular weight of 1450Daltons. It is water soluble and quite stable.

Mechanism of Action

VAN inhibits bacterial cell wall synthesis by firmly binding to the D-Ala-D-Ala terminus of nascent peptidoglycan pentapeptide. Once this occurs, inhibition of trans glycosylation takes place, which prevents further elongation and crosslinking of peptidoglycan chains, thus weakening bacterial cell wall and making it susceptible to lysis. [1]

Pharmacokinetics

VAN is poorly absorbed from the intestinal tract and therefore for cutaneous infections needs to be administered by the intravenous route. An hourly intravenous infusion of 1gm of VAN produces blood levels of 15–30mcg/ml for 1–2 hours. The $t_{1/2}$ of VAN is 6 h. Elimination of VAN is via the kidneys [1]. Therefore, caution needs to be exercised while administering VAN in patients with poor renal function.

A. K. Bubna, *Therapeutics in Dermatology - Essentials for Clinical Practice*,
https://doi.org/10.1007/978-981-95-3791-4_9

Indications

VAN is indicated for complicated and severe skin and soft tissue infections where gram-positive organisms, including hospital-acquired methicillin-resistant *Staphylococcus aureus* (MRSA), are the leading pathogens [2].

Dosing

VAN hydrochloride is marketed as a sterile powder that needs to be reconstituted for intravenous use. The time for each infusion is 1 h to avoid any adverse reaction as a result of the infusion.

The recommended adult dose of VAN is 30–45 mg/kg/day in 2–3 divided doses.

For paediatric patients, the dose of VAN is elucidated in Table 9.1 [3, 4].

For patients with impaired renal function, dose adjustments are mandated and intermittent dosing may be considered [2].

Vancomycin Resistance

VAN-resistant *Staphylococcus aureus* and coagulase-negative S*taphylococci* have been identified. Resistance is attributed to multiple mutations that encode enzymes in the biosynthetic pathway of bacterial cell walls [5]. Other predisposing factors for VAN resistance include prior treatment courses with low plasma VAN levels that precipitate treatment failure with VAN intermediate strains.

Adverse Effects

Cutaneous

- Macular skin lesions.
- Red man syndrome that is characterized by extreme flushing and is not an allergic reaction but a direct toxic effect of VAN on mast cells, causing them to release histamine.
- Urticarial reactions as a result of rapid intravenous infusion of VAN.

Table 9.1 Paediatric dosing of vancomycin

Paediatric population	Vancomycin dosage
Newborns	15 mg/kg initially Followed by 10 mg/kg every 12 hourly
Infants (8–30 days old)	15 mg/kg initially Followed by 10 mg/kg every 8 hourly
Infants (> 30 days old)	10–15 mg/kg every 6 hourly

General

- Fever.
- Chills.
- Tachycardia.
- Hypotension.

Auditory

- Ototoxicity resulting in permanent hearing impairment has been encountered with VAN. This occurs when drug concentrations in plasma exceed 60–100mcg/ml of VAN.

Renal

- Nephrotoxic effects.

Pregnancy prescribing status: category 'C'.

Drug Interactions

Nephrotoxic drugs like aminoglycosides are contraindicated with VAN as they can increase the risk of kidney damage.

Conclusion

VAN has been a very useful drug employed for managing MRSA-associated cutaneous infections. However, with the emergence of resistant strains of VAN, newer antimicrobials would need to be considered in their management.

References

1. Deck DH, Winston LG. Beta lactam and other cell wall and membrane active antibiotics. In: Katzung BG, Trevor AJ, editors. Basic and clinical pharmacology. 13th ed. New Delhi: McGraw Hill Education (India) Private Limited; 2015. p. 769–87.
2. Gasbarre CC, Schmitt SK, Tomecki KJ. Antibiotics. In: Goldsmith LA, Katz SI, Gilchrist BA, Paller AS, Leffell D, Wolff K, editors. Fitzpatrick's dermatology in general medicine. 8th ed. New York: McGraw Hill; 2012. p. 2776–87.
3. MacDougall C, Chambers HF. Protein synthesis inhibitors and miscellaneous antibacterial agents. In: Brunton LL, Chabner BA, Knollmann BC, editors. Goodman and Gilmans. The pharmacological basis of therapeutics. 12th ed. New York: McGraw Hill; 2011. p. 1521–47.

4. Frymoyer A, Hersh AL, Benet LZ, et al. Currant recommended dosing of vancomycin for children with invasive methicillin resistant staphylococcus aureus infections is inadequate. Pediatr Infect Dis. 2009;28:398–402.
5. Weigel LM, Clewell DB, Gill SR, et al. Genetic analysis of a high level vancomycin resistant isolate of *Staphylococcus aureus*. Science. 2003;302:1569–71.

Newer Antimicrobials

10

Introduction

These days an alarming rate of antimicrobial resistance is being encountered in our day-to-day clinical practice, thereby posing a serious threat to treatment. In particular, emerging resistance to vancomycin and teicoplanin; drugs considered apt for the management of gram-positive infections unresponsive to other antibiotics have now become more common. Strains of vancomycin-resistant *enterococci* (VRE) and vancomycin intermediate-resistant *Staphylococcus aureus* (VISA) have also been separately identified [1–3]. *Staphylococcus aureus* and *Streptococcus pyogenes* specifically are responsible for the majority of uncomplicated and complicated cutaneous infections. Uncomplicated infections include simple abscesses, impetiginized dermatoses, cellulitis and furuncles. Complicated infections include surgical wound infections, infected burns and ulcers, erysipelas, necrotizing fasciitis and severe carbunculosis. These complicated infections can be an important factor increasing patient morbidity and mortality. Owing to these implications, an ongoing search continues for an appropriate antimicrobial agent that will help obtain a solution to this predicament [4]. Some of the newer drugs utilized and under investigation include linezolid, daptomycin, quinupristin/dalfopristine, tigecycline, oritavancin and dalbavancin.

Linezolid

Introduction

Linezolid belongs to the oxazolidinone group of antimicrobial agents. Oxazolidinones were first recognized by DuPont Pharmaceuticals in 1987. However, it was only in the 1990s that linezolid was identified [5]. Finally in April 2000, linezolid was approved by the US FDA [6].

A. K. Bubna, *Therapeutics in Dermatology - Essentials for Clinical Practice*,
https://doi.org/10.1007/978-981-95-3791-4_10

Mechanism of Action

Linezolid binds to the 23 s region of 50 s ribosomal subunit in bacteria and restricts the initiation phase of translation. This prevents the formation of initiation complexes, thereby frustrating protein synthesis. Because of this unique mechanism of action, linezolid further prevents synthesis of staphylococcal and streptococcal virulence factors like haemolysins, coagulases and protein A. Besides, rRNA methylases in bacteria that serve in producing bacterial resistance do not affect linezolid, and in this way potentiate the drug's antimicrobial effects [7, 8].

Pharmacokinetics

In a normal host, bioavailability of linezolid is complete. Though consumption after food may slightly reduce its absorption, the amount of drug reaching the systemic circulation is unaltered. Linezolid therefore can either be taken on an empty stomach or after meals. The $t_{1/2}$ of linezolid is 5–7 hours, and it is 31% bound to plasma proteins. The metabolism is by oxidation, following which two inactive metabolites are generated. Cytochrome P_{450} enzyme system does not interfere with the metabolism of linezolid. The major route of linezolid elimination is via the kidneys [9, 10].

Indications

The US FDA has approved linezolid for the following conditions:

- Various gram-positive infections.
- Hospital and community-acquired pneumonias.
- Complicated/uncomplicated skin infections.
- VRE infections.

Dosage Regimens

- For uncomplicated skin infections, 400 mg of linezolid is administered every 12 hours for 10–14 days.
- In complicated infections, 600 mg of linezolid is given either intravenously or orally once every 12 hours. On occasions, the duration of treatment could exceed 14 days wherein the treating clinician best decides on the time span for the same.

  While switching from intravenous to oral route, no drug adjustments are required because of the near-complete bioavailability of linezolid [7].

In Vitro Activity

Following in vitro studies, linezolid demonstrated efficacy against many gram-positive bacteria that were resistant to other antibiotics, including methicillin-resistant *Staphylococcus aureus* (MRSA), VRE and *Streptococcus pneumonia* resistant to penicillins. Though linezolid is mainly bacteriostatic, it demonstrates bactericidal properties against *Clostridium perfringens, Bacteroides fragilis* and some strains of *Streptococcus pneumonia* [11–13]. Apart from its activity against many antibiotic-resistant gram-positive organisms, it also exhibits broad-spectrum activity against some *mycobacteria*, gram-negative anaerobes and gram-positive cocci [14].

Moderate inhibition in the growth of *Haemophilus influenzae* and *Moraxella catarrhalis* has also been delineated by linezolid. However, linezolid is ineffective against *Pseudomonas aeruginosa* and *Enterobacteriaceae* [15].

Adverse Effects

- Common side effects include diarrhoea, headache and nausea [16].
- Reversible thrombocytopenia and anaemia are other extremely rare complications. The risk of linezolid-induced thrombocytopenia is usually increased in patients with renal failure. The mechanism underlying this has not been elucidated though [17, 18]. Anaemia, on the other hand, occurs secondary to the blockade of mitochondrial respiration in cells [19].
- Pseudomembranous colitis is another adverse effect reported with linezolid.
- In patients with uncontrolled hypertension, caution needs to be exercised while administering linezolid [20].
- Accordingly, if linezolid has been administered for >28 days, signs for peripheral and optic neuropathy need to be monitored [21].

Pregnancy prescribing status: category 'C'.

Drug Interactions

In patients receiving serotonergic and/or adrenergic agents, there is a likelihood of interaction with linezolid as it is a non-selective reversible blocker of monoamine oxidase. Therefore, caution is mandated in this circumstance [21].

Newer Oxazolidinone

Tedizolid is the second oxazolidinone approved by the US FDA and can be of much value against gram-positive microbes, both in hospital and outpatient setups [22]. In vitro activity of tedizolid is superior to linezolid against *staphylococci* and *enterococci* [23].

Conclusion

Linezolid has indeed proven its importance in managing a number of bacterial infections resistant to basic antibiotics. The advantages of linezolid include its excellent clinical efficacy (only 0.05% resistance), good cutaneous penetration, 100% bioavailability and an acceptable safety profile. However, resistance to this drug is slowly emerging. Therefore, post-marketing surveillance to detect emerging linezolid resistance should be regarded as a prudent public health practice.

Daptomycin

Introduction

Daptomycin is a parenterally administered cyclic lipopeptide antibiotic, obtained after fermentation of a strain of *Streptomyces roseosporus,* and has demonstrated potent antibacterial activity against a number of gram-positive bacteria, especially MRSA and VRE [24].

Mechanism of Action

Daptomycin has a very specific mechanism of action, acting on all phases of bacterial growth. Based on a calcium-dependent mechanism, it attaches itself to the bacterial cytoplasmic membrane, eventuating in rapid bacterial cell membrane disruption, without the drug having to penetrate into the cytoplasm [25–27]. Apart from this, daptomycin impedes bacterial protein synthesis, as well as synthesis of DNA, RNA and lipoteichoic acid. This attribute of daptomycin makes it notably proficient in treating deep-seated infections, and bacteria existing within biofilms, that are recalcitrant to conventional antibiotics [27].

Pharmacokinetics

Daptomycin demonstrates linear pharmacokinetics, given its once-daily schedule, with minimal accumulation [28]. Following repeated once-daily administration, a steady state of the drug is attained by the third dose. Daptomycin has a $t_{1/2}$ of

8–9 hours [29]. Excretion of daptomycin is via the kidneys [30]. In patients with creatine clearance of <30 ml/min and in those undergoing peritoneal and haemodialysis, adjusting the dose of daptomycin is suggested [31, 32]. Daptomycin does not cross cell membranes and is primarily distributed in the extracellular fluid. Ninety-two per cent of the drug reversibly binds to plasma proteins [33]. As hepatic metabolism of daptomycin is limited, other drugs that undergo hepatic metabolism interact minimally with it.

In Vitro Activity

Daptomycin has proven to have bactericidal properties against both *Staphylococcus aureus* and *Enterococcus faecalis*. It is observed that the bactericidal activity of daptomycin is accentuated when concentrations are ≥4 times the minimum inhibitory concentration [34]. Moreover, as long as the therapeutic levels of daptomycin are maintained, acquisition of spontaneous resistance will be rare.

Clinical Indications

Recently, daptomycin has been approved for the treatment of complicated skin and soft tissue infections, caused by MRSA and methicillin-susceptible *Staphylococcus aureus* (MSSA).

Dosage Regimen

The dose recommended here is 4 mg/kg intravenously once daily for 7–14 days [35]. However, in difficult-to-treat infections, a higher dose of daptomycin >6 mg/kg/day may be advocated to obtain better bacterial clearance and reduce the risk of an upcoming bacterial infection [36, 37]. The Infectious Disease Society of America (IDSA) guidelines recommend daptomycin in a dosage of 10 mg/kg/day in patients who have persistent bacteraemia secondary to MRSA with associated vancomycin unresponsiveness [38].

Daptomycin in Combination with Other Antimicrobial Agents

Despite antimicrobial therapy being appropriately advocated, bacteraemia secondary to MRSA needs confrontation [39]. In order to increase the efficacy of daptomycin and prevent occurrence of resistance, administering high-dose daptomycin, along with other antibacterial agents, has been recommended according to the IDSA guidelines [38]. Combination of daptomycin with beta-lactams has offered many advantages. Beta-lactams amplify the negative charge on bacterial cell walls, following which they inactivate penicillin-binding protein 1, and facilitate better binding of daptomycin with bacteria, and in this way improves drug efficacy [40–42]. Other successful combinations employed with daptomycin for targeting MRSA infections include rifampicin, co-trimoxazole, fosfomycin, tigecycline and linezolid. [43–46]

Daptomycin Resistance

Resistance to daptomycin by *S. aureus* and *Enterococci* has been documented [47–49]. The most common factors involved in bacterial resistance to daptomycin include

- Changes in fluidity of bacterial cell membrane owing to dysregulation of dlt A transcription. Because of this alteration, attachment of daptomycin to the target site is diminished [50, 51].
- Occurrence of mutations in genes involved in the synthesis of bacterial cell membrane phospholipid. This is particularly observed in *S. aureus* and *E. faecalis* [52].

Adverse Effects

Daptomycin has been shown to have a good safety profile in various studies [53, 54]. The commonly observed side effects include nausea, headache and constipation [55]. Elevated levels of creatinine phosphokinase after administering multiple daily injections of daptomycin have been reported, with a risk of skeletal muscle toxicity. However, usage of once-daily dosing of daptomycin reduces this risk [56, 57].

Pregnancy prescribing status: category ‘B’.

Conclusion

Daptomycin appears to be a promising and safe antimicrobial drug. One particular advantage seen is its use in the outpatient department, wherein it can be administered with ease as a two-minute intravenous bolus. Moreover, though there has been documentation about daptomycin resistance, it is not so common. As it can be combined with other antibiotics, the chances of resistance can be further minimized.

Quinupristin/Dalfopristin

Introduction

Quinupristin/dalfopristin is a parenterally administered streptogramin antibacterial agent consisting of two semisynthetic pristinamycin derivatives. Although both quinupristin and dalfopristin have individual antimicrobial properties, when used together they exhibit synergy.

Mechanism of Action

Though bacteriostatic individually, quinupristin and dalfopristin when combined become bactericidal [58]. After entering bacterial cells, both bind to different sites of the 50 s ribosomal subunit, and irreversibly antagonize protein synthesis [59, 60]. Dalfopristin inhibits substrate attachment to the P and A sites of 50S ribosomal subunits by blocking peptidyl transferase (an early step of bacterial protein synthesis), and quinupristin acts on the late step of bacterial protein synthesis by inhibiting elongation of protein chains. Quinupristin/dalfopristin accumulate in significant amounts in phagocytic cells, with marked levels of efficacy being obtained [61].

Pharmacokinetics

Quinupristin/dalfopristin after intravenous administration gets widely distributed. The $t_{1/2}$ of quinupristin and dalfopristin is 60 minutes and 30 minutes, respectively. Besides, regardless of penicillin susceptibility, the post-antibiotic effect of quinupristin/dalfopristin is prolonged >7.4 hours against streptococci. Elimination of quinupristin/dalfopristin is via the faecal route through bile. In patients with chronic renal failure, clearance of quinupristin/dalfopristin maybe slightly reduced [62].

In Vitro Activity

Quinupristin/dalfopristin exhibits bactericidal activity against MRSA, vancomycin-resistant *Enterococcus faecalis* (VREF) and *Streptococcus pnuemoniae* in vitro, along with bacteriostatic properties against *E. faecium* [63]. Quinupristin/dalfopristin also demonstrates synergistic activity with other antibiotics, namely rifampicin and doxycycline in vitro against MRSA and VREF, respectively.

Clinical Indications

In 1995, quinupristin was approved for emergency use. It is particularly observed to be beneficial for infections secondary to VREF.

FDA Indications

- Serious infections associated with VREF bacteraemia.
- Complicated cutaneous infections caused by methicillin-susceptible *Staphylococcus aureus* (MSSA) and/or *Streptococcus pyogenes* [64, 65].

Dosage Regimen

A dose of 7.5 mg/kg intravenously (IV) twice daily for 7 days is administered for complicated skin and soft structure infections, and can be escalated up to thrice daily for bacteraemic patients. In hepatic insufficiency, 5 mg/kg IV twice daily is recommended. For elderly and renal impaired patients, no adjustment in dosing is mandated [10].

Adverse Effects

Injection site pain, along with inflammation during drug administration, is witnessed in around 55% of patients. Other reported toxicities encountered include atrophy, oedema, haemorrhage, hypersensitivity and thrombophlebitis [66, 67]. Gastrointestinal (GI) toxicity like vomiting and diarrhoea is also reported, along with mild arthralgias, myalgias and cutaneous rash [68, 69].

Contraindication and Drug Interactions

- Known hypersensitivity to the drug.
- As quinupristin/dalfopristin has been shown to block biotransformation rates of cytochrome P_{450} substrates, drugs like vinca alkaloids, benzodiazepines, calcium channel blockers and corticosteroids should be used with caution.
- Drugs prolonging the QT interval like terfenadine, cisapride, astemizole and diisopyramide are to be carefully administered in this setting [69].

Resistance

VREF resistance has been encountered here, though not very common [70, 71].

Pregnancy prescribing status: category 'B'.

Conclusion

Quinupristin/dalfopristin forms a unique alternative for managing many resistant microbial infections. Owing to demonstrable post-antibiotic effect and infrequent resistance, it has proven outstanding for treating these infections. However, prior to advocating its use, the clinical efficacy needs to be weighed against the likelihood of potential adverse effects. In patients where other potential treatment options are unviable, quinupristin/dalfopristin can be considered the treatment of choice.

Tigecycline

Introduction

Tigecycline is a glycylglycine antibiotic. In June 2005, it was approved by the US FDA to treat complicated skin and skin structure infections in adults caused by MRSA, MSSA, *S. pyogenes*, *Bacteroides fragilis* and *E. faecalis*. Glycylglycines are semisynthetic derivatives of antibiotics belonging to the tetracycline group. Here, a glycyclamide moiety is positioned at the D-ring, ninth position of the base molecule. This adaptation helps in maintaining steadfastness of tigecycline against resistance mechanisms developed for tetracyclines [72, 73].

Mechanism of Action

Tigecycline is bacteriostatic in nature. It binds to the 30 s ribosomal subunit and obstructs entry of aminoacyl t-RNA molecules to the A site of ribosomes [74].

Pharmacokinetics

After intravenous administration, tigecycline expresses a linear pharmacokinetics. Approximately 71–89% of tigecycline is plasma protein bound. Following an intravenous dose, the serum levels of tigecycline initially decline swiftly as it gets dispersed in body tissues. The mean $t_{1/2}$ of tigecycline is around 43 hours. The major route of elimination is by biliary and faecal excretion, with small amounts being eliminated by the kidneys [74].

In Vitro Activity

A broad spectrum of activity in vitro against MRSA, VRE and methicillin-resistant *Staphylococcus epidermidis* has been demonstrated by tigecycline. Tigecycline is not effective against *Pseudomonas* strains [74].

Clinical Indications

Tigecycline is indicated for complicated skin and soft tissue infections. Its efficacy has been synonymous with vancomycin and aztreonam combination therapy as demonstrated in two double-blind phase III comparison studies [75].

Dosage Regimen

Regimen begins as an initial dose of 100 mg that is succeeded by 50 mg once every 12 hourly. Intravenous infusions are dispersed over 30–60 minutes every 12 hourly. The recommended duration is 5–14 days. In patients with severe hepatic derangement, dosage of tigecycline is adjusted, wherein it is initially administered as a 100 mg intravenous infusion, followed by 25 mg every 12 hourly instead of 50 mg. No dose adjustment is required in patients with renal disease [10].

Adverse Effects

- Nausea.
- Vomiting.
- Altered laboratory parameters like prolonged prothrombin time and partial thromboplastin time without remarkable bleeding episodes.
- Hyperbilirubinemia.
- Photosensitivity.
- Pancreatitis.
- Teratogenic.
- Pseudotumor cerebri.

As it is similar to tetracycline structurally, a few of the adverse effects of tetracycline are simulated by tigecycline. Therefore, in patients with tetracycline hypersensitivity, patients need to be carefully monitored when administering tigecycline [76].

Drug Interactions

Tigecycline should not be administered concomitantly with amphotericin B, diltiazem and warfarin [10].

Pregnancy prescribing status: category ‘D’.

Conclusion

Tigecycline has shown promise especially as an initial empiric treatment for serious dermatologic infections unresponsive to conventional antibiotics [76].

Oritavancin

Introduction

Oritavancin is an analogue of vancomycin previously referred to as LY3333328. It is a synthetic derivative of chloroeremomycin, a naturally occurring glycopeptide [77]. It is composed of both hydrophobic and lipophilic groups and belongs to the lipoglycopeptide group of antibacterial drugs. Other drugs belonging to this category include dalbavancin and telavanin [78, 79]. On the disaccharide sugar of oritavancin, a 4′ chlorobiphenylmethyl substitute is attached, making it structurally unique to chloroeremomycin [77]. This change in its structure imparts improved activity against VRE and MRSA [80].

Mechanism of Action

Oritavancin has the ability to dimerize, which potentiates its ability to bind to the peptidoglycan bacterial cell wall. The sequence of events that follow binding of oritavancin to the bacterial cell wall is represented in Fig. 10.1 [81–85]. Owing to sundry mechanisms displayed by oritavancin in bacterial killing, it demonstrates both swift concentration-dependent bacterial destruction and at the same time is effective against biofilm-producing gram-positive bacteria [86].

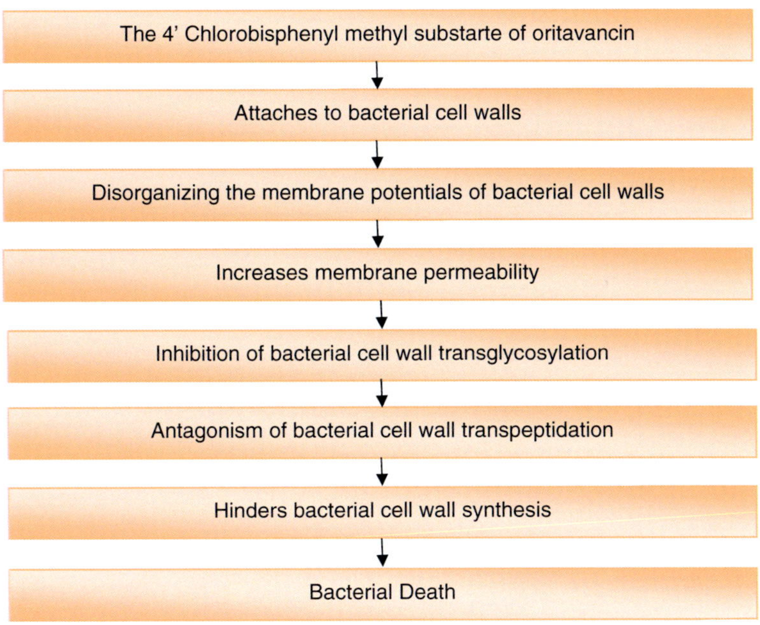

Fig. 10.1 Mechanism of action of oritavancin

Pharmacokinetics

Oritavancin is only administered intravenously, owing to poor absorption from the gastrointestinal tract. It exhibits linear pharmacokinetics and has a $t_{1/2}$ of 393 hours. Eighty-five per cent of oritavancin is bound to plasma proteins. Oritavancin maybe a weak inducer or antagonist of cytochrome P_{450} enzyme. Renal route is the major gateway for oritavancin elimination [87, 88].

In Vitro Activity

Oritavancin has demonstrated antimicrobial activity against VRE, *Micrococcus* species, *Listeria monocytogenes*, *Corynebacterium* species, *Peptostreptococcus*, *Streptococcus pyogenes,* as well as *Streptococcus intermedius* [89]. It has also shown synergism when combined with gentamycin, linezolid, moxifloxacin and rifampicin against *Staphylococci* [90].

Clinical Indications

It is approved by the US FDA for the treatment of acute bacterial skin and skin structure infections, particularly those caused by MRSA, VISA, VRE and vancomycin-resistant *Staphylococcus aureus*.

Dosage Regimen

A single intravenous dose of 1200 mg over 3 h in adult patients is the employed protocol.

Adverse Effects [91, 92]

- Nausea: most common.
- Rise in the levels of alanine aminotransferase.
- Delayed hypersensitivity reactions can be encountered.

Drug Interactions

As oritavancin is a weak inducer or inhibitor of cytochrome P_{450} enzyme, its inhibitory effect on warfarin mandates monitoring of international normalized ratio.

Pregnancy prescribing status: category ‘C’.

Conclusion

As it is administered as a single dose, it facilitates patient compliance and can be a valuable consideration for outpatient parenteral antimicrobial therapy (OPAT). Further, with its better side effect profile and antimicrobial activity against many vancomycin-resistant organisms, it serves as a significant replacement in managing these infections.

Dalbavancin

Introduction

Dalbavancin in a semisynthetic lipoglycopeptide antibiotic. It has been derived from an antibiotic A-40926, which is a natural antibiotic resembling teicoplanin produced by *Nonumuria* sp. [93, 94] Structurally, dalbavancin possesses an extended lipophilic side chain not observed in A-40926, which enhances its effectiveness in attaching to the cell membranes of bacteria, increasing its potency, extending its half-life and permitting extended dosing intervals [95].

Mechanism of Action

Owing to amidation of the carboxyl side group of dalbavancin, it demonstrates better anti-staphylococcal action. The mechanism of action for dalbavancin is similar to that of oritavancin [96, 97].

Pharmacokinetics

Dalbavancin is only administered parenterally. Like oritavancin, dalbavancin demonstrates a dose-related linear pharmacokinetics. It has a $t_{1/2}$ of 346 hours, thereby the interval between doses can be extended. Ninety-five per cent of the drug is bound to albumin. Excretion is mainly via the faecal route, although 33% of the drug is excreted unchanged in the urine [98–100].

In Vitro Activity

Dalbavancin has demonstrated in vitro activity to a wide range of gram-positive organisms like *Staphylococcus aureus, Streptococcus pyogenes, Enterococcus faecium, Enterococcus faecalis* and *Streptococcus agalactiae.* However, clinical activity against *Enterococcus* has not been seen with dalbavancin. An 8–16-fold greater activity against *Staphylococci* and *Streptococci* is observed in vitro by dalbavancin compared to vancomycin [101–103].

Clinical Indications

It has been recently approved by the US FDA for acute bacterial skin and skin structure infections (ABSSSIs). Activity of dalbavancin is seen against gram-positive pathogens mentioned earlier, including MRSA.

Dosing Regimen

It is administered as an initial intravenous dose of 1000 mg followed by 500 mg 1 week later to complete the entire treatment course for ABSSSIs. However, in patients with a creatine clearance of <30 ml/min, dosing of dalbavancin is adjusted to 750 mg initially, followed by 375 mg after 1 week. In hepatic insufficiency, dalbavancin clearance is unaffected, not requiring any dose adjustment [104].

Adverse Effects

Common side effects include [105]

- Nausea.
- Headache.
- Vomiting.
- Rash.
- Pruritus.

Dalbavancin has not been associated with nephrotoxicity till date. As dalbavancin has a prolonged $t_{1/2}$, there has been speculation about its long-term safety profile. Till date, after 28 days of administration of dalbavancin, no adverse effects have been documented. However, long-term data are limited for the same [106].

Pregnancy prescribing status: category 'C'.

Conclusion

In conclusion, dalbavancin has proven to be a promising drug in treating resistant gram-positive bacterial infections. With a better therapeutic and safety profile compared to vancomycin, it presents an extremely valuable therapeutic alternative. Though resistance to dalbavancin has been reported, it is extremely rare and has been observed in less than 1% of isolates [101, 102].

References

1. Lohray BB, Baskaran S, Rao BS, et al. A short synthesis of oxazolidinone derivatives linezolid and eperezolid: a new class of antibacterials. Tetrahedron Lett. 1999;40:4855–6.
2. Mutnick AH, Biedenbach DJ, Turnidge JD, et al. Spectrum and potency of evaluation of a new oxazolidinone, linezolid: report from the SENTRY antimicrobial surveillance program, 1998–2000. Diagn Microbiol Infect Dis. 2002;43:65–73.
3. Centers for Disease Control and Prevention(CDC). Reduced susceptibility of staphylococcus aureus to vancomycin-Japan, 1996. MMWR Morb Mortal Wkly Rep. 1997;46:624–6. Vancomycin.
4. Chein JW, Kucia ML, Salata RA. Use of linezolid, an oxazolidinone, in the treatment of multidrug resistant gram positive bacterial infections. Clin Infect Dis. 2000;30:146–51.
5. Livermore DM. Linezolid in vitro: mechanism and antibacterial spectrum. J Antimicrob Chemother. 2003;51(Suppl 2):9–16.
6. Brickner SJ, Barbachyn MR, Hutchinson DK, et al. Linezolid(Zyvox) the first member of a completely new class of antimicrobial agents for treatment of serious gram positive infections. J Med Chem. 2008;51:1981–90.
7. Swaney SM, Aoki H, Ganoza MC, Shinabarger DL. The oxazolidinone linezolid inhibits initiation of protein synthesis in bacteria. Antimicrob Agents Chemother. 1998;42:3251–5.
8. Gemmell CG, Ford CW. Virulence factor expression by gram positive cocci exposed to subinhibitory concentrations of linezolid. J Antimicrob Chemother. 2002;50:665–72.
9. Slatter JG, Stalker DJ, Feenstra KL, Welshman IR, Bruss JB, Sams JP, et al. Pharmacokinetics, metabolism and excretion of linezolid following an oral dose of [(14)C] linezolid to healthy human subjects. Drug Metab Dispos. 2001;29:1136–45.
10. Mikhail M, Weinberg JM. New antimicrobials. In: Wolf R, Davidovici BB, Parish JL, Parish LC, editors. Emergency dermatology. 1st ed. Cambridge: Cambridge University Press; 2011. p. 18–33.
11. Eliopoulos GM, Wennersten CB, Gold HS, Mollering RC Jr. In vitro activities in new oxazolidinone antimicrobial agents against enterococci. Antimicrob Agents Chemother. 1996;40:1745–7.
12. Ford CW, Hamel JC, Wilson DM, et al. In vivo activities of U-100592 and U-100766, novel oxazolidinone antimicrobial agents, against experimental bacterial infections. Antimicrob Agents Chemother. 1996;40:1508–13.
13. Jorgenson JH, McElmeel ML, Tippy CW. In vitro activities of the oxazolidinone antibiotics U-100592 and U-100766 against staphylococcus aureus and coagulase negative staphylococcus species. Antimicrob Agents Chemother. 1997;41:465–7.
14. Mercier RC, Penzak SR, Rybak MJ. In vitro activities of an investigational quinolone, glycycline, glycopeptides, streptogramin and oxazolidinone tested alone and in combinations against vancomycin resistant enterococcus faecium. Antimicrob Agents Chemother. 1997;41:2573–5.
15. Noskin GA, Siddiqui F, Strosor V, et al. In vitro activities of linezolid against important gram positive bacterial pathogens including vancomycin resistant enterococci. Antimicrob Agents Chemother. 1999;43:2059–62.
16. Clement D, Markham A. Linezolid. Drugs. 2000;59:815–27.
17. Lin YH, Wu VC, Tsai IJ, et al. High frequency linezolid associated thrombocytopenia among patients with renal insufficiency. Int J Antimicrob Agents. 2006;28:345–51.
18. Attasi K, Hershberger E, Alam R, et al. Thrombocytopenia associated with linezolid therapy. Clin Infect Dis. 2002;34:695–8.
19. Bernstein WB, Trotta RF, Rector JT, et al. Mechanisms for linezolid induced anemia and thrombocytopenia. Ann Pharmacother. 2003;37:517–20.

20. French G. Safety and tolerability of linezolid. J Antimicrob Chemother. 2003;51 Suppl 2:ii45-53.
21. Narita M, Tsuji BT, Yu VL. Linezolid associated peripheral and optic neuropathy, lactic acidosis and serotonin syndrome. Pharmacotherapy. 2007;27:1189–97.
22. Moran GJ, Fang E, Corey GR, et al. Tedizolid for 6 days versus linezolid for 10 days for acute bacterial skin and skin structure infections (ESTABLISH-2): a randomized double blind phase 3, non-inferiority trial. Lancet Infect Dis. 2014;14:696–705.
23. Livermore DM, Mushtaq S, Warner M, et al. Activity of oxazolidinone TR-700 against linezolid susceptible and resistant staphylococci and enterococci. J Antimicrob Chemother. 2009;63:713–5.
24. Van Hal SJ, Paterson DL. New gram-positive antibiotics better than vancomycin? Curr Opin Infect Dis. 2011;24:515–20.
25. Nakhate PH, Yadav VK, Pathak AN. A review on daptomycin; the first US FDA approved lipopeptide antibiotics. J Sci Innov Res. 2013;2:970–80.
26. LaPlante KL, Rybak MJ. Daptomycin-a novel antibiotic against gram positive pathogens. Expert Opin Pharmacother. 2004;5:2321–31.
27. Hancock RE. Mechanisms of action of newer antibiotics for gram positive pathogens. Expert Opin Pharmacother. 2005;5:209–18.
28. Benvenuto M, Benziger DP, Yankelev S, Vigliani G. Pharmacokinetics and tolerability of daptomycin at doses up to 12 milligrams per kilogram of body weight once daily in healthy volunteers. Antimicrob Agents Chemother. 2006;50:3245–9.
29. Baietto L, Corcione S, Pacine G, Di Perri GD' Avolio A, De Rosa FG. A 30 years review on pharmacokinetics of antibiotics: is the right time for pharmacogenetics? Curr Drud Metab 2014; 15: 581–598.
30. Gostelow M, Gonsalez D, Smith PB, Cohen-Wolkowicz M. Pharmacokinetics and safety of recently approved drugs used to treat methicillin resistant staphylococcus aureus infections in infants, children and adults. Expert Rev Clin Pharmacol. 2014;7:327–40.
31. Dvorchik B. Moderate liver impairment has no influence on daptomycin pharmacokinetics. J Clin Pharmacol. 2004;44:715–22.
32. Schriever CA, Fernandez C, Rodvold KA, Danziger LH. Daptomycin: a novel cyclic lipopeptide antimicrobial. Am J Health Syst Pharm. 2005;62:1145–58.
33. Estes KS, Derendorf H. Comparison of the pharmacokinetic properties of vancomycin, linezolid, tigecyclin and daptomycin. Eur J Med Res. 2010;15:533–43.
34. Rybak MJ, Hershberger E, Moldovan T, Gruez RG. In vitro activities of daptomycin, vancomycin, linezolid and quinipristin-dalfopristin against staphylococci and enterococci, including vancomycin intermediate and resistant strains. Antimicrob Agents Chemother. 2000;44:1062–6.
35. Strahilevitz J, Rubinstein E. Novel agents for resistant gram-positive infections-a review. Int J Infect Dis. 2002;6(Suppl 1):s38–46.
36. Wu G, Abraham T, Rapp J, Vastey F, Saad N, Balmir E. Daptomycin: evaluation of a high dose strategy. Int J Antimicrob Agents. 2011;38:192–6.
37. Bassetti M, Nicco E, Ginocchio F, Ansaldi F, deFlorentiis D, Viscoli C. High dose daptomycin in documented staphylococcus infections. Int J Antimicob Agents. 2010;36:459–61.
38. Liu C, Bayer A, Cosgrove SE, et al. Clinical practice guidelines by the infectious disease society of America for the treatment of methicillin resistant staphylococcus aureus infection in adults and children: executive summary. Clin Infect Dis. 2011;52:285–92.
39. Sakoulas G, Moise PA, Casapao AM, et al. Antimicrobial salvage therapy for persistent staphylococcal bacteremia using daptomycin plus ceftaroline. Clin Ther. 2014;36:1317–33.
40. Ortwine JK, werth BJ, Sakoulas G, Rybak MJ. Reduced glycopeptides and lipopeptide susceptibility in staphylococcus aureus and the seasaw effect: taking advantage of the back door left open? Drug Resist Updat. 2013;16:73–9.
41. Berti AD, Sakoulas G, Nizet V, Tewhey R, Rose WE. Beta lactam antibiotics targeting PBP1 selectively enhance daptomycin activity against methicillin resistant staphylococcus aureus. Antimicrob Agents Chemother. 2013;57:5005–12.

42. Berti AD, Theisen E, Sauer JD, et al. Penicillin binding protein 1 is important in the compensatory response of staphylococcus aureus to daptomycin induced membrane damage and is a potential target for beta lactam daptomycin synergy. Antimicrob Agents Chemother. 2015;60:451–8.
43. Claeys KC, Smith JR, Casapao AM, et al. Impact of the combination of daptomycin and trimethoprim-sulfamethoxazole on clinical outcomes in methicillin resistant staphylococcus aureus infections. Antimicrob Agents Chemother. 2015;59:1969–76.
44. Dhand A, Sakoulas G. Daptomycin in combination with other antibiotics for the treatment of complicated methicillin resistant staphylococcus aureus bacteremia. Clin Ther. 2014;36:1303–16.
45. Kelesidis T, Humphries R, Ward K, Lewinski MA, Yang OO. Combination therapy with daptomycin, linezolid and rifampicin as treatment option for MRSA meningitis and bacteremia. Diagn Microbiol Infect Dis. 2011;71:286–90.
46. Ahmad NM, Rojtman AD. Successful treatment of daptomycin non susceptible methicillin resistant staphylococcus aureus bacteremia with addition of rifampicin to daptomycin. Ann Pharmacother. 2010;44:918–21.
47. Diederen BM, Van Duijn I, Willemse P, Kluytmansin JA. In vitro activity of daptomycin against methicillin resistant staphylococcus aureus, including heterogeneously glycopeptide resistant strains. Antimicrob Agents Chemother. 2006;50:3189–91.
48. Lewis JS 2nd, Owens A, Cadena J, Sabol K, Patterson JE, Jorgensen JH. Emergence of daptomycin resistance in enterococcus faecium during daptomycin therapy. Antimicrob Agents Chemother. 2005;49:1664–5.
49. Munoz-Price LS, Lolans K, Quinn JP. Emergence of resistance to daptomycin during treatment of vancomycin resistant enterococcus faecalis infection. Clin Infect Dis. 2005;41:565–6.
50. Mishra NN, Bayer AS, Weidenmaier C, et al. Phenotypic and genotypic characterization of daptomycin resistant methicillin staphylococcus aureus strains: relative roles of mprF and dlt operons. PLoS One. 2004;9:e107426.
51. Tran TT, Munita JM, Arias CA. Mechanism of drug resistance: daptomycin resistance. Ann N Y Acad Sci. 2015;1354:32–53.
52. Humphries RM, Pollett S, Sakoulas G. A current perspective on daptomycin for the clinical microbiologist. Clin Microbiol Rev. 2013;26:759–80.
53. Aikawa N, Kusachi S, Mikamo H, et al. Efficacy and safety of intravenous daptomycin Japanese patients with skin and soft tissue infections. J Infect Chemother. 2013;19:447–55.
54. Pertel PE, Eisenstein BI, Link AS, et al. The efficacy and safety of daptomycin vs vancomycin for treatment cellulitis and erysipelas. Int Clin Pract. 2009;63:368–75.
55. Fowler VG Jr, Boucher HW, Corey GR, et al. Daptomycin versus standard therapy for bacteremia and endocarditis caused by staphylococcus aureus. N Engl J Med. 2006;355:653–65.
56. Hanberger H, Nillson LE, Maller R, Isaksson B. Pharmacodyanamics of daptomycin and vancomycin on enterococcus faecalis and staphylococcus aureus demonstrated by studies of initial killing and post antibiotic effect and influence of Ca^{2+} and albumin on these drugs. Antimicrob Agents Chemother. 1991;35:1710–6.
57. Dvorchik BH, Brazier D, DeBruin MF, Arbeit RD. Daptomycin pharmacokinetics and safety following administration of escalating doses once daily to healthy subjects. Antimicrob Agents Chemother. 2003;47:1318–23.
58. Bouanchaud DH. In vitro and in vivo synergic activity and fractional inhibitory concentration(FIC) of the components of a semisynthetic streptogramin, RP59500. J Antimicrob Chemother. 1992;30(Suppl A):95–9.
59. Bryson HM, Spencer CM. Quinupristin-dalfopristin Drugs. 1996;52:406–15.
60. Cocito C, Di-Giambattista M, Nyssen E, Vannuffel P. Inhibition of protein synthesis by streptogramins and related antibiotics. J Antimicrob Chemother. 1997;39 Suppl A:7–13.
61. Desnottes JF, Diallo N. Cellular uptake and intracellular bactericidal activity of RP 59500 in murine macrophages. J Antimicrob Chemother. 1992;30(Suppl A):107–15.
62. Lambs HM, Figgit DP, Faulds D. Quinupristin/dalfopristin: A review of its use in the management of serious gram positive infections. Drugs. 1999;58:1061–97.

63. Baudoux P, Lemaire S, Denis O, Tulkens PM, VanBambeke F, Glupczynski Y. Activity of Quinupristin/dalfopristin against extracellular and intracellular staphylococcus aureus with various resistance phenotypes. J Antimicrob Chemother. 2010:1228–36.
64. Landman D, Quale JM. Management of infections due to resistant enterococci: A review of therapeutic options. J Antimicrob Chemother. 1997;40:161–70.
65. Linden PK, Pasculle AW, McDevitt D, Kramer DJ. Effect of Quinupristin/dalfopristin on the outcome of vancomycin resistant enterococcus faecium bacteremia: comparison with a control cohort. J Antimicrob Chemother. 1997;39(Suppl A):145–51.
66. Nichols RL, Graham DR, Barriere SL, et al. Treatment of hospitalized with complicated gram positive skin and skin structure infections: two randomized, multicentre studies of quinupristin/dalfopristin versus cefazolin, oxacillin or vancomycin. Synercid skin and skin structure infection group. J Antimicrob Chemother. 1999;44:263–73.
67. Moellering RC, Linden PK, Reinhardt J, et al. The efficacy and safety of quinupristin/dalfopristin for the treatment of infections caused by vancomycin resistant enterococcus faecium. Synercid emergency use study group. J Antimicrob Chemother. 1999;44:251–61.
68. Oslen KM, Rebuck JA, Rupp ME. Arthralgias and myalgias related to quinupristin-dalfopristin administration. Clin Infect Dis. 2001;32:e83–6.
69. Rubinstein E, Prokocimer P, Talbot GH. Safety and tolerability of quinupristin/dalfopristin: administration guidelines. J Antimicrob Chemother. 1994;44(Suppl A):37–46.
70. Eliopoulos GM. Quinupristin-dalfopristin and linezolid: evidence and opinion. Clin Infec Dis. 2003;36:473–81.
71. Abbanat D, Macielag M, Bush K. Novel antibacterial agents for the treatment of serious gram positive infections. Expert Opin Investig Drugs. 2003;12:379–99.
72. Garrison MW, Neumiller JJ, Setter SM. Tigecycline: an investigational glycylglycine antimicrobial with activity against resistant gram positive organisms. Clin Ther. 2005;27:12–22.
73. Bergeron J, Ammirati M, Danley D, et al. Glycylglycines bind to the high affinity tetracycline ribosomal binding site and evade $Tet_{(M)}$ and $Tet_{(O)}$ mediated ribosomal protection. Antimicrob Agents Chemother. 1996;40:2226–8.
74. MacDougall C, Chambers HF. Protein synthesis inhibitors and miscellaneous antibacterial agents. In: Brunton LL, Chabner BA, Knollmann BC, editors. Goodman and Gilman's the pharmacological basis of therapeutics. 12th ed. New York: McGraw Hill; 2011. p. 1521–47.
75. Ellis-Grosse EJ, Babinchak T, Dartois N, et al. The efficacy and safety of tigecycline in treatment of skin and skin structure infections: results of a 2 double blind phase 3 comparison studies with vancomycin-aztreonam. Clin Infect Dis. 2005;41(Suppl 5):s341–53.
76. Fraise AP. Tigecycline: the answer to beta lactam and fluoroquinolone resistance? J Infect. 2006;53:293–300.
77. Allen NE. From vancomycin to oritavancin: the discovery and development of a novel lipoglycopeptide antibiotic. Antinfect AgentsMed Chem. 2010;9:23–47.
78. Hanel GG, Schweizer F, Karlousky JA. Oritavancin: mechanism of action. Clin Infect Dis. 2012;54(Suppl 3):S214–9.
79. Guskey MT, Tsuji BT. Comparative review of the lipoglycopeptides oritavancin, dalbavancin and telavanin. Pharmacotherapy. 2010;30:80–94.
80. Belley A, Harris R, Beveridge T, et al. Ultrastructural effects of oritavancin on methicillin resisatant staphylococcus aureus and vancomycin resistant enterococcus. Antimicrob Agents Chemother. 2009;53:800–4.
81. Belley A, McKay GA, Arhin FF, et al. Oritavancin disrupts membrane integrity of staphylococcus aureus and vancomycin resistant enterococci to effect rapid bacterial killing. Antimicrob Agents Chemother. 2010;54:5369–71.
82. Patti GJ, Kim SJ, Yu TY, et al. Vancomycin and oritavancin have different modes of action in enterococcus faecium. J Med Biol. 2009;392:1178–91.
83. Allen NE, Nicas TI. Mechanism of action of oritavancin and related glycopeptides antibiotics. FEMS Microbiol Rev. 2003;26:511–32.

84. Belley A, Neesham-Grenon E, McKay G, et al. Oritavancin kills stationary phase in biofilm staphylococcus aureus cells in vitro. Antimicrob Agents Chemother. 2009;53:918–25.
85. Kim SJ, Singh M, Schafer J. Oritavancin binds to isolated protoplast membranes but not intact protoplasts of Staphylococcus aureus. J Mol Biol. 2009;391:414–25.
86. Zhanel GG, Schweizer F, Karlowsky JA. Oritavancin: mechanism of action. Clin Infect Dis. 2012;54:s214–9.
87. Rubino CM, Van Wart SA, Bhavnani SM, et al. Oritavancin population pharmacokinetics in healthy subjects and patients with complicated skin and skin structure infections or bacteremia. Antimicrob Agents Chemother. 2009;53:4422–8.
88. Bhavnani SM, Owen JS, Loutit JS, et al. Pharmacokinetics, safety and tolerability of ascending single intravenous doses of oritavancin administered to healthy human subjects. Diagn Microbiol Infect Dis. 2004;50:95–102.
89. Mendes RE, Farrell DJ, Sader HS, Jones RN. Oritavancin microbiologic features and activity results from the surveillance program in the United States. Clin Infect Dis. 2012;54(suppl 3):S203–13.
90. Belley A, Neesham-Grenon E, Arhin FF, McKay GA, Parr TR Jr, Moeck G. Assessment by time kill methodology of the synergistic effects oritavancin in combination with other antimicrobial agents against staphylococcus aureus. Antimicrobial Agents Chemother. 2008;52:3820–2.
91. Corey GR, Kabler H, Mehra P, et al. SOLO II investigators single dose oritavancin versus 7-10 days of vancomycin in the treatment of acute bacterial skin infections. N Engl J Med. 2014;370:2180–90.
92. Corey GR, Good S, Jlang H, et al. SOLO II investigators single dose of oritavancin versus 7-10 days of vancomycin in the treatment of gram positive acute bacterial skin and skin structure infections: the SOLO II non-inferiority study. Clin Infect Dis. 2015;60:254–62.
93. Kim A, Kuti JL, Nicolau DP. Review of dalbavancin, a novel semisynthetic lipoglycopeptide. Expert Opin Investig Drugs. 2007;16:717–33.
94. Malabarba A, Goldstein BP. Origin, structure and activity in vitro and in vivo of dalbavancin. J Antimicrob Chemother. 2005;55(Suppl 2):ii15–20.
95. Zhanel GG, Calic D, Schweizer F, et al. New lipoglycopeptide: a comparative review of dalbavancin, oritavancin and telavancin. Drugs. 2010;70:859–86.
96. Nagarajan R. Structure-activity relationships of vancomycin type glycopeptides antibiotics. J Antibiot. 1993;46:1181–95.
97. Trevino J, Bayon C, Arda a, et al. New insights into glycopeptides antibiotic binding to cell wall precursors using SPR and NMR spectroscopy. Chemistry. 2014;20:7363–72.
98. Leighton A, Gottleib AB, Dorr MB, et al. Tolerability, pharmacokinetics and serum bacterial activity of intravenous dalbavancin in healthy volunteers. Antimicrob Agents Chemother. 2004;48:940–5.
99. Dorr MB, Jabes D, Cavaleri M, et al. Human pharmacokinetics and rationale for once weekly dosing of dalbavancin, a semisynthetic glycopeptides. J Antimicrob Chemother. 2005;55(Suppl 2):ii25–30.
100. Dowell JA, Goldstein BP, Buckwalter M, Stogniew M, Damle B. Pharmacokinetic-pharmacodyanamic modeling of dalbavancin, a novel glycopeptides antibiotic. J Clin Pharmacol. 2008;48:1063–8.
101. Jones RN, Flamm RK, Sader HS. Surveillance of dalbavancin potency and spectrum in the United States (2012). Diagn Microbiol Infect Dis. 2013;76:122–3.
102. Jones RN, Sader HS, Flamm RK. Update of dalbavancin spectrum and potency in the USA: report from the SENTRY antimicrobial surveillance program(2011). Diagn Microbiol Infect Dis. 2013;75:304–7.
103. Chong YP, Park SJ, Kim HS, et al. In vitro activities of ceftobiprole, dalbavancin, daptomycin, linezololid, tigecycline against methicillin resistant staphylococcus aureus blood isolates: stratified analysis by vancomycin MIC. Diagn Microbiol Infect Dis. 2012;73:264–6.

104. Marbury T, Dowell JA, Seltzer E, Buckwalter M. Pharmacokinetics of dalbavancin in patients with renal or hepatic impairment. J Clin Pharmacol. 2009;49:465–76.
105. Raad I, Darouiche R, Vazquez J, et al. Efficacy and safety of weekly dalbavancin therapy for catheter related blood stream infection caused by gram positive pathogens. Clin Infect Dis. 2005;40:374–80.
106. Boucher HW, Wilcox M, Talbot GH, Puttagunta S, Das AF, Dunne MW. Once weekly dalbavancin versus daily conventional treatment for skin infection. N Engl J Med. 2014;370:2169–70.

Part II

Antiviral Drugs

Acyclovir and Valacyclovir

11

Acyclovir: Introduction

Acyclovir is an acyclic guanosine derivative with clinical activity against herpes simplex virus (HSV) 1, HSV 2 and varicella zoster virus (VZV) with 10 times higher potency against HSV 1 and 2 [1]. It also demonstrates weak in vitro activity against Epstein–Barr virus (EBV), cytomegalovirus (CMV) and human herpes virus (HHV) 6 [1].

Mechanism of Action

Acyclovir interacts with viral thymidine kinase and gets converted to acyclovir monophosphate. Host cell enzymes further add two more phosphates to acyclovir converting it to acyclovir triphosphate, which is taken up by viral particles. Acyclovir triphosphate further interacts with viral DNA polymerase, preventing uptake of host 2′ deoxyguanosine monophosphate by replicating viruses, thereby halting viral replication [1].

Pharmacokinetics

Oral bioavailability of acyclovir is around 10–30% [2]. Acyclovir can also be administered intravenously. It is widely distributed in the body, attaining CSF concentrations corresponding to 50% of the plasma concentration. Besides, acyclovir also penetrates the cornea. It has a $t_{1/2}$ of 2–3 hours. Excretion is via glomerular filtration and tubular secretion. Dose reduction is therefore advisable in renal dysfunction [1].

A. K. Bubna, *Therapeutics in Dermatology - Essentials for Clinical Practice*,
https://doi.org/10.1007/978-981-95-3791-4_11

Indications

FDA Approved

- Primary and secondary genital herpes simplex infection.
- Suppressive therapy for herpes simplex.
- Varicella.
- Herpes zoster.
- Intravenous acyclovir in immunocompromised patients with disseminated HSV or VZV (in patients with severe herpes zoster) [3].

Off-Label

- Prevention of recurrent herpes associated with erythema multiforme.
- Eczema herpeticum.
- Primary herpes gingivostomatitis.
- Herpetic whitlow.
- Neonatal herpes.
- EBV-related oral hairy leukoplakia.

Contraindications

Absolute

- Hypersensitivity to the drug.

Relative

- Impaired renal function.

Pregnancy prescribing status: category 'B'.

Dosing

The dosing schedule of acyclovir is highlighted in Table 11.1.

In patients with renal disease, dose adjustment with acyclovir is required, which is mentioned in Table 11.2.

Table 11.1 Dosing schedule of acyclovir

Indication	Details with all regimens currently employed
Primary genital herpes [4]	Tab acyclovir 200 mg PO five times daily for 10 days OR Tab acyclovir 400 mg PO three times daily for 10 days
Recurrent genital herpes [4]	Tab acyclovir 400 mg PO three times daily for 5 days OR Tab acyclovir 800 mg PO two times daily for 5 days OR Tab acyclovir 800 mg PO three times daily for 2 days
Chronic suppression of herpes [4]	Tab acyclovir 400 mg PO two times daily
Herpes zoster	Tab acyclovir 800 mg PO five times daily for 7–10 days
Varicella	In patients >40 kg: tab acyclovir 800 mg PO four times daily for 5 days In patients <40 kg: tab acyclovir 20 mg/kg (800 mg maximum) PO three times daily for 5 days
Mucocutaneous herpes simplex in immunocompromised patients, including HIV infected	Acyclovir 5 mg/kg (if age > 10 years) or 10 mg/kg (if age < 10 years) IV Q8H for 7 days Tab acyclovir 400 mg PO 3–5 times a day for 14–21 days
Disseminated herpes zoster	Acyclovir 5–10 mg/kg IV Q8H for 7–10 days In paediatric patients <12 years: 20 mg/kg IV Q8H for 7–10 days
HSV encephalitis	Acyclovir 10 mg/kg IV Q8H for 10 days.

Table 11.2 Dosing adjustments of acyclovir in patients having renal impairment

Indication	Creatinine clearance (ml/min)	Adjusted dose
Primary genital herpes	< 10	Tab acyclovir 200 mg PO twice daily
Recurrent genital herpes	<10	Tab acyclovir 200 mg PO twice daily
Chronic suppression of herpes	<10	Tab acyclovir 200 mg PO twice daily
Herpes zoster	10–20	Tab acyclovir 800 mg PO thrice daily
	<10	Tab acyclovir 800 mg PO twice daily
Immunocompromised patients with mucocutaneous herpes and disseminated zoster	25–50	Injection acyclovir 5–10 mg/kg IV Q12H
	10–24	Injection acyclovir 5–10 mg/kg IV Q24H
	<10	Injection acyclovir 2.5–5 mg/kg IV Q24H

Drug Interactions

- Amphotericin B: increases serum levels of acyclovir.
- Cisplatin: increases the risk of acyclovir nephrotoxicity.
- Probenecid: increases serum levels of acyclovir.
- Zidovudine: increases serum levels of acyclovir.
- Theophylline: increases serum levels of acyclovir.
- Interferons: may worsen potential neurologic side effects of acyclovir.

Adverse Effects

Gastrointestinal

- Nausea.
- Abdominal pain.
- Diarrhoea.

Dermatologic

- Morbilliform eruptions.
- Urticaria and angioedema.
- Steven–Johnson syndrome.

Haematologic

- Leucopoenia.
- Thrombocytopenia.
- Aplastic anaemia.

Nervous System

- Headache.
- Vertigo.
- Lethargy.
- Confusion.

Cardiovascular

- Hypertension.
- Tachycardia.

Renal

- Reversible crystalluria-induced nephropathy typically in patients with pre-existing renal dysfunction and dehydration.

Acyclovir Resistance

The main mechanism responsible for acyclovir resistance is deficient or absent viral thymidine kinase secondary to an underlying mutation. Rarely, mutations may be seen in viral DNA polymerase. In such cases, foscarnet and cidofovir become the alternatives that need utilization.

Conclusion

Acyclovir is a safe and effective antiviral drug.

Valacyclovir: Introduction

Valacyclovir is an ester prodrug of acyclovir. The main advantage over acyclovir is its improved bioavailability (55–70%). This is facilitated by peptide transporters that actively transport valacyclovir in the intestine [1]. The anti-herpes virus profile of valacyclovir is similar to acyclovir.

Mechanism of Action

In the intestine, valacyclovir is acted upon by esterases and is completely converted to acyclovir. Therefore, its antagonistic mechanics against herpes virus is similar to acyclovir [1].

Indications and Contraindications

Similar to acyclovir. **Pregnancy prescribing status**: category 'B'.

Dosing Schedule

The dosing schedule of valacyclovir is elucidated in Table 11.3.

In patients with renal disease, dose adjustments in valacyclovir are needed and are tabulated in Table 11.4.

Table 11.3 Dosing schedule of valacyclovir

Indication	Details with all regimens currently employed
Primary genital herpes [4]	Tab valacyclovir 1gm PO two times daily for 10 days
Recurrent genital herpes [4]	Tab valacyclovir 500 mg PO two times daily for 3 days OR Tab valacyclovir 1gm PO once daily for 5 days
Chronic suppression of herpes [4]	Tab valacyclovir 500 mg (if <10 outbreaks per year) or 1 gm (if >10 outbreaks per year) PO once daily
Herpes zoster	Tab valacyclovir 1gm PO three times daily for 7 days
Varicella	Tab valacyclovir 20 mg/kg (max: 1gm) PO three times daily for 5 days
Mucocutaneous herpes simplex in immunocompromised patients, including HIV infected	Tab valacyclovir 1 gm PO 2–3 times daily for 7 days and continue till lesions heal
Recurrent orolabial herpes	Tab valacyclovir 2gm PO two times daily for 1 day

Table 11.4 Dosing adjustments of valacyclovir in patients having renal impairment

Indication	Creatinine clearance (ml/min)	Adjusted dose
Primary genital herpes	10–29	Tab valacyclovir 1gm PO once daily
	< 10	Tab valacyclovir 500 mg PO once daily
Recurrent genital herpes	< 30	Tab valacyclovir 500 mg PO once daily
Chronic suppression of herpes	< 30	Tab valacyclovir 500 mg PO once daily or once in 2 days
Herpes zoster	30–49	Tab valacyclovir 1gm PO two times daily
	10–29	Tab valacyclovir 1gm once daily
	< 10	Tab valacyclovir 500 mg once daily
Recurrent orolabial herpes	30–49	Tab valacyclovir 1gm two times daily
	10–29	Tab valacyclovir 500 mg two times daily
	< 10	Tab valacyclovir 500 mg one stat dose

Drug Interactions

- Metformin and glyburide: in patients with impaired renal function, valacyclovir may cause lactic acidosis.
- Probenecid: reduces the rate of conversion of valacyclovir to acyclovir.
- Theophylline: increases serum levels of valacyclovir.
- Zidovudine: increases serum levels of valacyclovir.

Adverse Effects

Same as acyclovir.

Valacyclovir Resistance

Same as acyclovir.

Conclusion

Valacyclovir is superior to acyclovir, with a better dosing profile as well as patient compliance.

References

1. Acosta AP, Flexner C. Antiviral drugs(non retroviral). In: Brunton LL, Chabner BA, Kollmann BC, editors. Goodman and Gilman's the pharmacologic basis of therapeutics. 12th ed. New York: McGraw Hill; 2012. p. 1593–622.
2. Wagstaff AJ, Faulds D, Goa KL. Acyclovir: a reappraisal of its anti viral activity, pharmacokinetic properties and therapeutic efficacy. Drugs. 1994;47:153–205.
3. Evans TY, Tyring SK. Advances in antiviral therapy in dermatology. Dermatol Clin. 1998;16:409–20.
4. Nath AK, Thappa DM. Newer trends in management of genital herpes. Indian J Dermatol Venereol Leprol. 2009;75:566–74.

Famciclovir

12

Introduction

Famciclovir is the diacetyl ester prodrug of 6-deoxy penciclovir lacking antiviral properties intrinsically. It needs to be converted to penciclovir to exhibit antiviral effects [1].

Mechanism of Action

After oral administration, famciclovir gets rapidly deacetylated and oxidized by first-pass metabolism to form penciclovir. Penciclovir is the active metabolite obtained from famciclovir, which exhibits antiviral properties against HSV 1, HSV 2, VZV and EBV. Like acyclovir, penciclovir gets phosphorylated after interacting with viral thymidine kinase and then completely inhibits viral DNA polymerase, thereby antagonizing the synthesis of viral DNA [2].

Pharmacokinetics

The advantage of administering famciclovir over penciclovir orally is its good bioavailability of 75%. In the intestine, famciclovir gets deacetylated and is rapidly converted to penciclovir [3]. Food slows down penciclovir absorption. However, it does not reduce the overall bioavailability. Penciclovir has a $t_{1/2}$ of 2 h. More than 90% of the drug is excreted unchanged in the urine, with a meagre amount being eliminated in the faeces.

A. K. Bubna, *Therapeutics in Dermatology - Essentials for Clinical Practice*,
https://doi.org/10.1007/978-981-95-3791-4_12

Indications [4, 5]

FDA Approved

- Primary genital herpes.
- Recurrent genital herpes.
- Chronic suppression of herpes.
- Herpes zoster.
- Mucocutaneous herpes simplex in immunocompromised patients (including HIV infected patients).
- Recurrent orolabial herpes.

Off-Label

- Herpes-associated erythema multiforme.
- Eczema herpeticum.
- Primary herpetic gingivostomatitis.
- Herpetic whitlow.
- EBV-related oral hairy leukoplakia.

Contraindications

Absolute

Drug hypersensitivity.

Relative

Patients with renal disease.**Pregnancy prescribing status**: category 'B'.

Dosing

The dosing schedule of famciclovir is elaborated in Table 12.1.

The dose adjustments of famciclovir in patients with renal disease are mentioned in Table 12.2.

Table 12.1 Dosing schedule of famciclovir

Indication	Details of dosing schedule
Primary genital herpes	Tab famciclovir 250 mg PO three times daily for 10 days
Recurrent genital herpes	Tab famciclovir 125 mg PO two times daily for 5 days OR Tab famciclovir 1gm PO two times daily for 1 day OR Tab famciclovir 500 mg PO, one dose followed by 250 mg twice daily for 2 days
Chronic suppression of herpes	Tab famciclovir 250 mg PO two times daily
Herpes zoster	Tab famciclovir 500 mg PO three times daily for 7 days
Mucocutaneous herpes simplex in immunocompromised patients, including HIV infected	Tab famciclovir 500 mg PO two times daily for 5–10 days
Recurrent orolabial herpes	Tab famciclovir 1500 mg stat dose

Table 12.2 Dose adjustment of famciclovir in patients with renal impairment

Indication	Creatinine clearance (ml/min)	Adjusted dose
Primary genital herpes	20–39	Tab famciclovir 125 mg two times daily
	< 20	Tab famciclovir 125 mg once daily
Recurrent genital herpes	40–59	Tab famciclovir 500 mg two times daily for 1 day
	20–39	Tab famciclovir 500 mg one stat dose
	< 20	Tab famciclovir 250 mg one stat dose
Chronic suppression of herpes	20–39	Tab famciclovir 125 mg two times daily
	< 20	Tab famciclovir 125 mg once daily
Herpes zoster	40–59	Tab famciclovir 500 mg two times daily
	20–39	Tab famciclovir 500 mg once daily
	< 20	Tab famciclovir 250 mg once daily
Recurrent orolabial herpes	40–59	Tab famciclovir 750 mg one stat dose
	20–39	Tab famciclovir 500 mg one stat dose
	< 20	Tab famciclovir 250 mg one stat dose
Immunocompromised patients with mucocutaneous herpes	20–39	Tab famciclovir 500 mg once daily
	< 20	Tab famciclovir 250 mg once daily

Drug Interactions

In vitro studies with raloxifene, a potent aldehyde oxidase inhibitor, have demonstrated a reduction in the conversion of famciclovir to penciclovir. However, the magnitude of this interaction has not been calculated.

Adverse Effects

Cutaneous

- Pruritus.

Nervous System

- Paraesthesia.
- Headache.
- Fatigue.

Gastrointestinal System

- Nausea.
- Vomiting.
- Diarrhoea.
- Flatulence.

Resistance

Resistant variants reflecting mutations in DNA polymerase and thymidine kinase have been studied in vitro, but the incidence is relatively low. It is seen that thymidine kinase-deficient acyclovir-resistant herpes virus are cross-resistant to penciclovir [6].

Conclusion

Famciclovir is a safe and effective antiviral drug.

References

1. Acosta AP, Flexner C. Antiviral drugs (non-retroviral). In: Brunton LL, Chabner BA, Kollmann BC, editors. Goodman and Gilman's the pharmacologic basis of therapeutics. 12th ed. New York: McGraw Hill; 2012. p. 1593–622.
2. Safrin S. Antiviral agents. In: Katzung BG, Trevor A, editors. Basic and clinical pharmacology. 13th ed. New Delhi: Mc Graw Hill education (India) private limited; 2012. p. 835–64.
3. Gill KS, Wood MJ. The clinical pharmacokinetics of famciclovir. Clin Pharmacokinet. 1996;31:1–8.
4. Sacks SL, Wilson B. Famciclovir/penciclovir. Adv Exp Med Biol. 1999;458:135–47.
5. Tyring SK, Beutner K, Tucker BA, et al. Antiviral therapy for herpes zoster. Arch Fam Med. 2000;9:863–9.
6. Bacon TH, Levin MJ, Leary JJ, et al. Herpes simplex virus resistance to acyclovir and penciclovir after two decades of antiviral therapy. Clin Microbiol Rev. 2003;16:114–28.

13 Cidofovir

Introduction

Cidofovir is a cytidine nucleotide analogue antiviral drug with antagonizing properties against human herpes virus (HHV), human papilloma virus (HPV), pox virus and adenovirus [1].

Mechanism of Action

As cidofovir gets phosphorylated by host enzymes, it is active against those mutant viruses deficient in thymidine kinase. The diphosphate salt of cidofovir exhibits dual activity against the viral agent. First, it acts as a potent inhibitor of viral DNA polymerase; and secondly, it acts as an alternative substrate for viral DNA polymerase, thereby getting incorporated into viral DNA chains and competitively antagonizing viral DNA synthesis [2].

Pharmacokinetics

Cidofovir has a low oral bioavailability, owing to its di-anionic nature at physiological pH [3]. Following intravenous administration, dosing declines in a biphasic manner. The terminal $t_{1/2}$ of cidofovir is 2.6 h. Two active metabolites of cidofovir have been demonstrated. The active metabolite, cidofovir diphosphate, has a prolonged intracellular half-life of 17–65 h, whereas cidofovir phosphocholine, the second metabolite, has a half-life of 87 h, thereby serving as an intracellular reservoir of the active drug. Clearance of cidofovir is by glomerular filtration and tubular secretion. Ninety per cent of the drug is recovered unchanged in the urine, without significant metabolism [4].

A. K. Bubna, *Therapeutics in Dermatology - Essentials for Clinical Practice*,
https://doi.org/10.1007/978-981-95-3791-4_13

Indications

FDA-Approved

- Cytomegalovirus (CMV) retinitis.

Off-Label

- Resistant HSV and CMV infections.
- Severe warts (in a dose of 3–5 mg/kg as a single IV dose given every 1–2 weeks) [5].

Contraindications

Absolute

- Hypersensitivity to the drug.
- Pregnancy.

Relative

- Renal tubular dysfunction.

Pregnancy prescribing status: category 'C'.

Availability

- Injectable solution of 75 mg/ml supplied as a non-preserved hypertonic solution in a single-use clear glass vial.

Dosing

CMV Retinitis

- *Induction phase*: 5 mg/kg IV over 1 h once per week for 2 weeks.
- *Maintenance treatment*: 5 mg/kg IV every 2 weeks until CD4 counts become greater than 100 (usually after 6 months of HAART).
- If serum creatinine increases more than 0.3–0.4 mg/dl above baseline, then the dose needs to be reduced to 3 mg/kg IV; if serum creatinine levels >0.4 mg/dl above baseline, then treatment needs to be discontinued.

- Serum creatinine, urinary protein and WBC total and differential count need to be monitored prior to each dose. Visual acuity and intraocular tension require close evaluation similarly.
- *Concomitant therapy*: Probenecid 2gms to be given 3 h prior to each cidofovir dose, and 1gm at least 2 h and 8 h after completion of 1 h of the cidofovir infusion. Ingestion of food prior to each dose of probenecid may reduce dose-related nausea and vomiting.
- Hydration: Patients must receive at least 1 litre of 0.9% NS solution IV prior to each infusion of cidofovir. It should be administered over 1–2 h. A second litre can be infused immediately following cidofovir infusion if well tolerated.

Drug Interactions

Administration of cidofovir with other potentially nephrotoxic agents is to be avoided, namely amphotericin B, aminoglycosides, pentamidine, foscarnet and NSAIDs. Cidofovir and ganciclovir are poorly tolerated in combination at full doses [4]. Valproic acid has been reported to impair the antiviral activity of cidofovir.

Adverse Effects

Gastrointestinal

- Nausea.

Cutaneous

- Rash.
- Alopecia.
- Fever.

General

- Fever.
- Myalgia.

Renal

- Renal tubular damage.
- Proteinuria.

- Azotaemia.
- Metabolic acidosis.
- Fanconi's syndrome.

Ocular

- Uveitis.
- Ocular hypotony.

Genetic

- Mutagenic.
- Gonadotoxic.
- Embryotoxic.

Cidofovir Resistance

In CMV, resistance to cidofovir occurs due to mutations in the viral DNA polymerase. Low-level resistance to cidofovir develops in up to 30% of CMV retinitis patients by the end of 3 months of therapy.

Conclusion

Cidofovir is an effective drug in those cases of herpes virus infection, resistant to acyclovir and its analogues.

References

1. Hitchcock M, Jaffe H, Martin J, Stagg R. Cidofovir, a new agent with potent anti herpes virus activity. Antivir Chem Chemother. 1996;7:115–27.
2. Safrin S. Antiviral agents. In: Katzung BG, Trevor A, editors. Basic and clinical pharmacology. 13th ed. New Delhi: Mc Graw Hill education (India) private limited; 2012. p. 835–64.
3. Cundy K. Clinical pharmacokinetics of the antiviral nucleotide analogues cidofovir and adefovir. Clin Pharm. 1999;36:127–43.
4. Acosta AP, Flexner C. Antiviral drugs (nonretroviral). In: Brunton LL, Chabner BA, Kollmann BC, editors. Goodman and Gilman's the pharmacologic basis of therapeutics. 12th ed. New York: McGraw Hill; 2012. p. 1593–622.
5. Mackintosh L, Parker A, Leman J. Intravenous cidofovir for the treatment of florid cutaneous warts in association with graft versus host disease. Br J Dermatol. 2012;167:116.

Foscarnet

14

Introduction

Foscarnet (phosphonoformic acid) is an inorganic pyrophosphate analogue that is antagonistic for all herpes virus and HIV [1].

Mechanism of Action

Foscarnet directly interacts with herpes virus DNA polymerase, RNA polymerase and HIV reverse transcriptase, thereby blocking pyrophosphate-binding sites of these enzymes apart from hindering cleavage of pyrophosphate from deoxynucleotide phosphates. Besides, in vitro activity against HSV, VZV, EBV, CMV, HHV 6, HHV 8 and HIV 1 and 2 is demonstrated with foscarnet [2].

Pharmacokinetics

As oral bioavailability of foscarnet is poor, only intravenous preparations are available for the same. Following an intravenous infusion of foscarnet (60 mg/kg every 8 h), peak and trough plasma concentrations are 450–575 µm and 80–150 µm, respectively. It is generally administered by an infusion pump in a dilute solution over 1–2 h. The $t_{1/2}$ of foscarnet includes an initial phase of 4–8 hours and a terminal phase of 88 hours. Twenty per cent of the dose gets deposited in the bone and 80% is excreted by the kidneys, mandating dose adjustments in patients with renal dysfunction [1].

A. K. Bubna, *Therapeutics in Dermatology - Essentials for Clinical Practice*, https://doi.org/10.1007/978-981-95-3791-4_14

Indications

- CMV retinitis in AIDS patients.
- CMV colitis.
- CMV polyradiculopathy in combination with ganciclovir.
- Acyclovir-resistant HSV infections.
- Ganciclovir-resistant CMV infections.

Contraindications

Absolute

- Drug hypersensitivity.
- Pregnancy.

Relative

- Renal dysfunction.

Pregnancy prescribing status: Category 'C'. It is suggested that female patients of childbearing potential should use effective contraception during therapy, and male patients should not father a child during therapy and for up to 6 months after the last dose.

Dosing

The dosing schedule is mentioned in Table 14.1.

Table 14.1 Dosing schedule for foscarnet

Indication	Dosage	Route	Duration
CMV retinitis [3]	Induction phase: 90 mg/kg Q12H	IV	14–21 days
	Maintenance phase: 90 mg/kg Q24H	IV	Until CD4 counts >100 on 6 months of HAART
Acyclovir-resistant HSV infection [3]	40 mg/kg Q8H	IV	2–3 weeks or till full clinical resolution
	60 mg/kg Q12H	IV	2–3 weeks or till full clinical resolution

Monitoring of Therapy

Renal toxicity is the major concern for foscarnet. Therefore, patient's renal profile needs vigilant monitoring. Saline hydration prior to administering foscarnet and a slow infusion of the drug can reduce nephrotoxicity [3].

Adverse Effects

Renal

- Renal impairment.

Metabolic

- Hyper/hypocalcaemia.
- Hypomagnesemia.
- Hypokalaemia.
- Hypo/hyperphosphatemia.

Gastrointestinal

- Nausea.
- Vomiting.
- Elevation of liver enzymes.

Haematological

- Anaemia.

Nervous System

- Headache.
- Hallucinations.
- Seizures.
- Nephrogenic diabetes insipidus.

Genitourinary

- Genital ulceration.

Resistance

This has been described secondary to point mutations in the viral DNA polymerase gene and HIV 1 reverse transcriptase enzyme.

Conclusion

Foscarnet is of value especially in conditions resistant to acyclovir, valacyclovir and famciclovir.

References

1. Acosta AP, Flexner C. Antiviral drugs(non retroviral). In: Brunton LL, Chabner BA, Kollmann BC, editors. Goodman and Gilman's the pharmacologic basis of therapeutics. 12th ed. New York: McGraw Hill; 2012. p. 1593–622.
2. Safrin S. Antiviral agents. In: Katzung BG, Trevor A, editors. Basic and clinical pharmacology. 13th ed. New Delhi: Mc Graw Hill Education (India) Private Limited; 2012. p. 835–64.
3. Elston DM. Antiviral drugs. In: Goldsmith LA, Katz SI, Gilchrist BA, Pallar AS, Leffell DJ, Wolff K, editors. Fitzpatricks's dermatology in general medicine. 8th ed. New York: McGraw Hill; 2012. p. 2787–96.

Part III

Antifungal Drugs

15 Azole Antifungals

Itraconazole: Introduction

Itraconazole (ITRA) is a triazole antifungal agent that was synthesized in 1980. It has broad-spectrum activity against a number of mycoses, which include dermatophytosis, superficial candidiasis, sporotrichosis, histoplasmosis, penicillinosis, coccidioidomycosis, blastomycosis and allergic and invasive aspergillosis [1].

Mechanism of Action

ITRA inhibits the cytochrome P450 enzyme 14α demethylase, thereby preventing ergosterol biosynthesis from lanosterol. This leads to reduction in the ergosterol content and accumulation of methylated precursors that cause profound disruption in the normal balance of sterols in fungal cell membranes, leading to fungal cell death [2].

Furthermore, owing to the comparatively large side chain in ITRA, closer and tighter binding between the drug and the active site of 14α demethylase occurs, facilitating better fungal destruction [3].

Pharmacokinetics

ITRA requires an acidic environment for proper absorption, which forms the basis for its administration with food or acidic soft drinks [4]. It is seen that oral bioavailability of ITRA doubles following food consumption [5].

The metabolism of ITRA takes place in the liver via the CYP isoenzyme CYP3A4, with production of an active metabolite hydroxyl-itraconazole which also

A. K. Bubna, *Therapeutics in Dermatology - Essentials for Clinical Practice*,
https://doi.org/10.1007/978-981-95-3791-4_15

possesses antifungal properties, comparable to the parent compound. The concentrations of hydroxyl-itraconazole are approximately twice as that of the parent compound [6].

Excretion of ITRA occurs majorly in the bile [7], with lesser portions eliminated via the urine and faeces [8].

In the skin, major routes of ITRA delivery are by passive diffusion from blood in keratinocytes and excretion by sebaceous glands. It is seen that ITRA levels in sebum become measurable after 4 days of drug intake and are 5–10 times higher than the corresponding peak plasma levels [9].

ITRA in nails reaches the nail matrix via the bloodstream and then diffuses from the nail bed to the nail plate. Further, drug levels of ITRA accumulate and remain in the nail for 6–9 months after drug cessation (reservoir effect), posing an added advantage for the same [10].

The indications and dosing regimens are elaborated in Table 15.1.

Table 15.1 Indications and dosing regimens for itraconazole

Clinical condition	Dosing regimen
Tinea corporis	200 mg PO Q12H for 7 days
Tinea cruris	200 mg PO Q12H for 7 days
Pityriasis versicolor	200 mg PO Q12H for 7 days
Tinea pedis/manuum	100 mg PO once daily for 30 days OR 200 mg PO Q12H for 7 days
Onychomycosis	200 mg PO once daily for 3 months OR Pulse therapy: 200 mg PO Q12H for 7 days at monthly intervals; two such pulses for finger nails and three such pulses for toe nail involvement
Oropharyngeal candidiasis	200 mg PO once daily and continued for 7–14 days after clinical resolution
Vulvovaginal candidiasis	200 mg PO Q12H for 1 day
Coccidioidomycosis	200 mg PO Q12H or Q8H continued until clinical resolution (may take months to years)
Histoplasmosis	In mild-to-moderate acute pulmonary histoplasmosis and step-down therapy for severe disease: 200 mg PO Q8H for 3 days, followed by 200 mg PO Q12H for 6–12 weeks In chronic cavitary pulmonary histoplasmosis: 200 mg PO Q12H for 3 days, followed by 200 mg PO once daily or twice daily for at least 1 year
Sporotrichosis	Lymphocutaneous disease: 200 mg PO once daily for 2–4 weeks after clinical resolution (usually 3–6 months) Osteoarticular/non-life-threatening pulmonary disease: 200 mg Q12H for at least 12 months
Blastomycosis	200 mg PO Q8H for 3 days, and then once daily or Q12H for 6–12 months

(continued)

Table 15.1 (continued)

Clinical condition	Dosing regimen
Chronic pulmonary aspergillosis	200 mg PO once daily or Q12H; usually lifelong treatment is mandated
Allergic bronchopulmonary aspergillosis	200 mg PO Q12h for 4–6 months, followed by 4–6 months tapered dose, with a longer course for relapses
Prophylaxis in HIV and neutropenia due to haematological malignancy or bone marrow transplantation	200 mg PO once daily, and to twice daily if proven low circulating neutrophil levels OR Oral solution 5 mg/kg in two divided doses continued until neutrophil count or CD4+ count recovers
Penicillium marneffei	Consolidation therapy in severe disease: 200 mg PO Q12H for 10 weeks Mild to moderate disease: 200 mg PO Q12H as monotherapy for 8 weeks and then 200 mg PO once daily until CD4 counts are >100/μl for over 6 months
Palmoplantar pustulosis	100 mg PO once daily for 4 weeks, followed by 100 mg PO on alternate days for the next 4 weeks

Use of Itraconazole in Special Populations

Renal Insufficiency

Limited data are available on the use of oral ITRA in patients with renal impairment. A study utilizing a single 200 mg dose of intravenous ITRA in 19 patients with renal impairment concluded that there was no significant effect of haemodialysis or peritoneal dialysis on ITRA pharmacokinetics [11].

Hepatic Insufficiency

As ITRA predominantly gets metabolized in the liver, patients with hepatic impairment receiving ITRA require assiduous monitoring. In a pharmacokinetic study utilizing a single 100 mg PO dose of ITRA in cirrhotic subjects, it was concluded that there was an increase in the elimination half-life in these patients when compared to healthy volunteers (37 ± 17 versus 16 ± 5 h, respectively). Therefore, while prescribing ITRA in this setting, careful consideration should be given in the dosing pattern [12].

Neonates and Children

There is relative paucity of data elucidating the utility of ITRA in infants and older children. A single intravenous or oral dose of ITRA solution of 2.5 mg/kg/day in children aged 7 months to 17 years is well tolerated, but results in considerable variability in drug exposure [13].

Oral ITRA solution given 2.5 mg/kg twice daily has been found to be effective in treating oropharyngeal candidiasis in HIV-positive children [14] and for the prevention of invasive fungal infection in children with neutropenia [15].

In Recalcitrant and Widespread Fungal Skin Infections

Dermatophytosis

For recalcitrant tinea infections, extending the course of ITRA for another 2–3 months until complete healing may be considered a good alternative [16]. Supportive treatment with topical antifungal agents needs to be concurrently administered.

Malassezia

A maintenance regimen with oral ITRA (200 mg PO on the first 2 days of each month for 4–6 months after the initial treatment with 200 mg PO Q12H for 7 days) is an effective prophylaxis in seborrheic dermatitis and patients with Malassezia-positive atopic dermatitis of the face and neck [17].

Contraindications

Absolute

- Hypersensitivity to the drug.
- Left-sided heart disease.

Relative

- Hepatic dysfunction.
- Lactation.

Pregnancy prescribing status: category ‘C’.

Adverse Effects

Cutaneous

- Morbilliform eruptions.
- Pruritus.
- Urticaria.

- Alopecia.
- Steven–Johnson syndrome.
- Infusion site reactions (parenteral administration).

Gastrointestinal

- Anorexia.
- Nausea.
- Vomiting.
- Abdominal pain.
- Hepatic dysfunction.

Cardiac

- Congestive cardiac failure (rarely).
- Pulmonary oedema (rarely).

Nervous System

- Peripheral neuropathy.

General

- Fatigue.
- Headache.
- Dizziness.
- Fever.
- Oedema.

Drug Interactions

- Astemizole, terfenadine, cisapride: can result in *torsades de pointes*.
- Warfarin: elevation of warfarin levels.
- Cyclosporine: increase in levels of cyclosporine, thereby increasing the chance for nephrotoxicity, neurotoxicity and hypertension.
- Rifampicin: reduction in plasma levels of ITRA.
- Phenytoin: reduction in plasma levels of ITRA.
- Sildenafil: increase in plasma levels of sildenafil when used concomitantly with ITRA.

- Atorvastatin, simvastatin: can result in rhabdomyolysis and myopathy when administered with ITRA.
- Phenobarbitone, carbamazepine, isoniazid, nevirapine: reduction in levels of ITRA.

Monitoring Guidelines

Baseline

- Liver function tests.

Follow-Up

- Liver function tests to be done every month till progression of treatment.

Conclusion

The broad-spectrum antifungal activity of ITRA makes it a valuable antifungal drug. However, emergence of resistance has become a major concern with ITRA. Therefore, ITRA needs to be appropriately and judiciously used in patients with dermatophytosis in dosing schedules recommended by experts, along with employing other supportive measures that augment superior therapeutic outcomes.

Fluconazole: Introduction

Fluconazole (FLU) is a first-generation triazole antifungal drug. It is given either orally or intravenously and has a wide spectrum of activity against most *Candida* spp., *Cryptococcus neoformans*, some dimorphic fungi and dermatophytes, among others.

Mechanism of Action

FLU inhibits fungal cytochrome P450 enzyme 14α demethylase. This blockade prevents conversion of lanosterol to ergosterol (an essential component of fungal cytoplasmic membranes), with subsequent accumulation of 14α methyl sterols within fungal cells and eventual destruction of the fungal pathogen. FLU is primarily fungistatic but exhibits fungicidal properties against *Cryptococcus neoformans* in a dose-dependent manner [18, 19].

Pharmacokinetics

Following oral administration, FLU is rapidly absorbed, with achievement of steady-state levels (in the absence of loading dose) after 4–5 days of oral or intravenous administration, and a plasma protein-binding capacity of 11%. FLU has good penetration into body fluids and tissues, including cerebrospinal fluid (CSF), skin, nails and peritoneal fluid [20, 21]. The $t_{1/2}$ of FLU is around 30 hours. Elimination of FLU is via the kidneys, with 80% of the drug being recovered in the kidneys unchanged [22, 23].

The indications and dosing of FLU are elaborated in Table 15.2 [24].

Table 15.2 Indications and dosing of fluconazole

Indication	Adult dosing of fluconazole	Paediatric dosing of fluconazole
Oropharyngeal candidiasis	200 mg PO on day 1, followed by 100 mg once daily for ≥2 weeks	6 mg/kg on day 1, followed by 3 mg/kg every 24–72 hours for 2 weeks (if the patient is less than 2 weeks old, the dosing is every 24–72 hours; if the patient is more than 2 weeks old, then the dosing is every 24 h)
Oesophageal candidiasis	200 mg PO on day 1, followed by 100 mg once daily for at least 3 weeks; to treat for another 2 weeks after symptoms resolve	6 mg/kg on day 1, followed by 3–12 mg/kg every 24–72 hours for 3 weeks (if the patient is less than 2 weeks old, the dosing is every 24–72 hours; if the patient is more than 2 weeks old, then the dosing is every 24 hours)
Systemic candidiasis	400 mg on day 1, followed by 200 mg/day for ≥4 weeks or at least 2 weeks after resolution	6–12 mg/kg every 24–72 hours for 28 days (if the patient is less than 2 weeks old, the dosing is every 24–72 hours; if the patient is more than 2 weeks old, then the dosing is every 24 hours)
Cryptococcal meningitis (acute therapy)	400 mg on day 1, followed by 200–400 mg once daily IV Treatment is to be continued for 10–12 weeks after CSF culture is negative	12 mg/kg IV on day 1, followed by 6–12 mg/kg every 24–72 hours as per the age of the child Treatment to be continued for 10–12 weeks after CSF culture is negative
Cryptococcal meningitis (suppressive therapy)	200 mg/day	–

(continued)

Table 15.2 (continued)

Indication	Adult dosing of fluconazole	Paediatric dosing of fluconazole
Prophylaxis of candidiasis in bone marrow transplantation	400 mg/day	10–12 mg/kg/day as a single dose Maximum dose per day not to exceed 600 mg
Vaginal candidiasis	150 mg PO stat dose	–
Pityriasis versicolor	400 mg PO stat dose OR 300 mg PO stat dose, with a possible second dose within a week depending on the clinical response	–
Tinea corporis/cruris	150 mg PO once weekly for 2–4 weeks	–
Tinea pedis	Pulse dose of 150 mg PO once a week for 2–6 weeks	
Tinea capitis	–	6 mg/kg/day for 2–3 weeks
Onychomycosis	Pulse dose: Finger nail: 150 mg/week for 9 months Toe nail: 150 mg/week for 12 months	–

Contraindications

Absolute

- Hypersensitivity to the drug.

Relative

- Hepatic impairment.
- Renal impairment.

Pregnancy prescribing status: category 'D'.

Adverse Effects

Gastrointestinal

- Nausea.
- Vomiting.
- Abdominal pain.
- Diarrhoea.

Hepatic

- Elevated hepatic transaminases.
- In some cases, fatal hepatotoxic side effects seen.

Cutaneous

- Exfoliative dermatitis.
- Angioedema.
- Drug rash.
- Steven–Johnson syndrome.

Drug Interactions

- Astemizole, cisapride, terfenadine and erythromycin: Increased risk of cardiac arrhythmias and therefore should be avoided [25].
- Rifampicin: Reduces FLU levels significantly and also has hepatotoxic side effects and so needs to be used with appropriate monitoring.
- Cyclosporine: FLU has been infrequently associated with increase in cyclosporine concentrations in renal transplant recipients [26, 27]. However, increased cyclosporine levels following FLU administration have not been associated with cyclosporine toxicity. Careful monitoring of cyclosporine in patients receiving both agents is therefore recommended [28].
- Phenytoin: Phenytoin metabolism is inhibited when FLU is simultaneously administered, and therefore appropriate monitoring is required.

Conclusion

FLU is an effective antifungal agent for a number of important mycoses. FLU can be considered to be the therapy of choice in oropharyngeal and oesophageal candidiasis in immunocompromised patients. Further, the useful role of FLU in patients with cryptococcal meningitis cannot be undermined. Moreover, with a safer toxicity profile compared with amphotericin-B, FLU has an added advantage.

Ketoconazole: Introduction

Ketoconazole is an imidazole derivative that was approved by the FDA in 1981 as an antifungal drug. However, in 2013, the drug was taken off the European and Australian market due to the risk of severe hepatic side effects, with strict restrictions for its use in the USA and Canada. In India, though, ketoconazole is still available.

Mechanism of Action

The antifungal mechanism of ketoconazole is outlined in Fig. 15.1 [29]. Further, ketoconazole exhibits anti-androgenic effects by inhibiting the synthesis of adrenal steroids like aldosterone, cortisol and testosterone following antagonism of cytochrome P-450 enzymes.

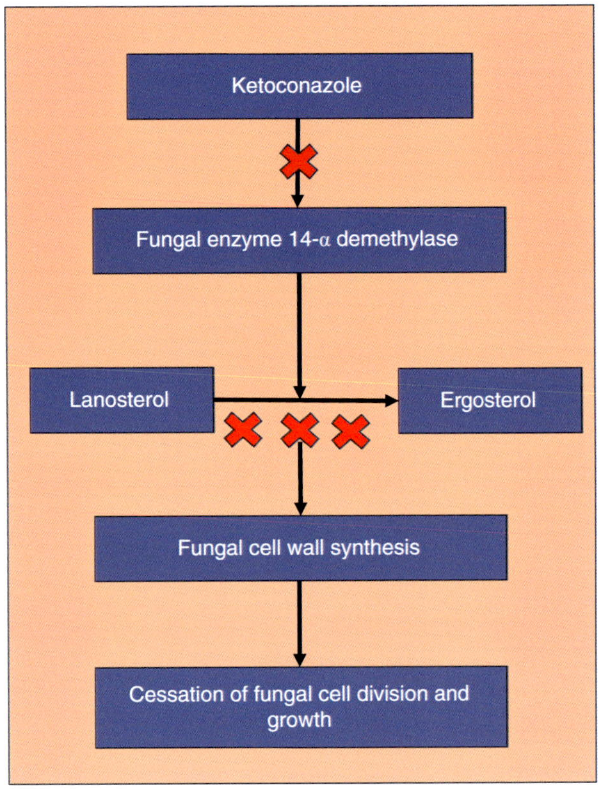

Fig. 15.1 Antifungal mechanism of action of ketoconazole

Pharmacokinetics

Following oral intake, ketoconazole is rapidly absorbed in the gastrointestinal tract and reaches the stratum corneum via the eccrine sweat apparatus and/or passive diffusion, where it binds to keratinocytes and surface lipids. Besides, ketoconazole persists in the skin at therapeutic concentrations for up to 10 days after a dose of 200 mg/day for 10 days. The $t_{1/2}$ of ketoconazole is 2 hours during the first 10 hours and slows thereafter, as plasma elimination of the drug is biphasic. The metabolism of ketoconazole is through the hepatic route, and excretion is majorly via the bile into the intestinal tract, with subsequent elimination occurring through the faeces. Around 13% of the drug undergoes renal elimination [30].

Clinical Uses

Dermatophytosis

Ketoconazole is used in treating dermatophytosis at dosages ranging from 200 to 400 mg/day. The 400 mg/day dose is given only in recalcitrant cases of dermatophytosis. Responses to ketoconazole occur within 2 weeks, and this duration can be used as a cutoff to predict the success of ketoconazole treatment [31]. Besides, ketoconazole (200 mg/day) demonstrates greater efficacy than griseofulvin (250 mg/day, ultra-micronized preparation) in the treatment of dermatophytosis, with fewer relapses [32].

If by 2 weeks clinical responses are not observed with the 200 mg/day dose of ketoconazole, the dose can be escalated to 400 mg/day with proper monitoring of the hepatic profile. If still responses fail to occur by 2 weeks, it is labelled as therapeutic failure. Complete clinical responses, though, are observed by 8 weeks for most patients.

Also, skin of palms and soles responds less readily than skin in other parts of the body to ketoconazole [33].

Pityriasis Versicolor

Ketoconazole is generally employed only for recalcitrant or severe disfiguring/disabling pityriasis versicolor (PV). Doses of 400 mg/week for 2 weeks or 200 mg/day for 2–5 weeks have produced good rates of mycological cure [34].Further, ketoconazole 400 mg/day or 200 mg/day for 3 days, once monthly for 6 months, is effective as a prophylactic treatment for patients who typically suffer recurrent outbreaks of PV [34].

Deep Fungal Infections

Ketoconazole has been used for the treatment of blastomycosis, mycetoma coccidioidomycosis, histoplasmosis, chromoblastomycosis and paracoccidiodomycosis, with doses ranging from 400 to 800 mg/day. However, careful monitoring is warranted while using the 800 mg daily dose. Ketoconazole, however, is an alternative second-line treatment for these infections. The exact duration of ketoconazole therapy is not clearly defined, depending majorly on the clinical response, even extending up to 1–3 years in certain circumstances [35].

Seborrheic Dermatitis

For seborrheic dermatitis (SD), ketoconazole is given at 200 mg/day for 4 weeks [36]. Besides, topical use of ketoconazole as a 2% cream is also of value in SD.

Leishmaniasis

Reports have outlined ketoconazole to be effective in the treatment of cutaneous leishmaniasis (CL). In the report by Kumaresan and Kumar [37], ketoconazole administered at a dose of 100 mg/day (in one patient) and 200 mg Q12H (in 2 patients) was successful in achieving clinical cure in all three patients with localized CL as a first-line therapeutic agent, following 3 months of treatment.

In another report, ketoconazole (600 mg/day for 28 days) was comparable to sodium stibogluconate (20 mg antimony/kg, with maximum of 850 mg antimony/day for 20 days) in treating CL, secondary to *L. brasiliensis*, making the authors suggest its utility as an initial line of management for the same [38]. Besides, the use of ketoconazole in Post Kala Azar Dermal Leishmaniasis has also been elaborated. It is suggested that ketoconazole acts by interfering with the synthesis of ergosterol that is present in large concentrations in the cell wall of *Leishmania* spp. [37]

Subcorneal Pustular Dermatoses (SCPD)

In an anecdotal report, ketoconazole (200 mg/day) was effective in treating SCPD in a 30-year-old woman who was unresponsive to dapsone and betamethasone (3 mg on alternate days). Improvement was noticed as early as 3 days, with complete remission at 2 weeks. Though unclear, it is suggested that ketoconazole may outline immunomodulatory effects that can help in SCPD [39].

Acne

As ketoconazole has antiandrogenic properties, it is but logical for its use in treating hormonal acne. However, in order to exhibit antiandrogenic effects, higher doses ranging from 400 to 500 mg/day are essential.

Ghetti et al. [40] reported ketoconazole (300mgQ12H) for 3 months in bringing about satisfactory results in three patients with hormonal acne. Besides, ketoconazole has been used as an off-label drug in the treatment of hirsutism as well [41].

Adverse Effects

Gastrointestinal

- Nausea and vomiting
- Epigastric pain

Hepatic

- Elevated hepatic transaminases (in 5–10% cases)
- Toxic hepatitis (in 1/10,000 patients)

Cutaneous

- Rash
- Pruritus

Rare

- Gynaecomastia
- Headache
- Somnolence
- Thrombocytopenia
- Leucopoenia
- Haemolytic anaemia

Use in Special Populations

Pregnancy

At high doses, ketoconazole (80 mg/kg/day) has demonstrated teratogenic and embryotoxic properties in animal studies, despite it crossing the placental barrier poorly, posing a risk to the developing foetus, and its use should be avoided.

Lactation

Owing to published data, not much is available regarding the use of ketoconazole in lactation. However, if required by the mother, it may not be a reason to discontinue breastfeeding.

Paediatrics

In children, ketoconazole can be given based on body weight if needed and careful monitoring of the hepatic profile.

Geriatric

Ketoconazole can be given with proper hepatic monitoring if at all needed. If hepatic enzymes are >2 of the upper limit, ketoconazole needs to be withheld.

Drug Interactions

As ketoconazole is a potent inhibitor of CYP3A4, plasma concentrations of drugs metabolized by CYP3A4 may increase and should not be concomitantly used. Those include terfenadine, cisapride, macrolides, alprazolam, midazolam, triazolam, quinidine, ergot alkaloids and statins. Besides, when used with these drugs, there is a likelihood of precipitation of torsades de pointes.

Levels of ketoconazole can be drastically reduced when used with rifampicin, isoniazid, gastric acid suppressants and nevirapine; dose adjustment may be needed.

Monitoring Guidelines

Baseline

Liver function tests (LFT).
Electrocardiogram (ECG).

Follow-Up

LFT: weekly for 1 month and then monthly for 6 months.

ECG: within 1 week after starting treatment and later if indicated clinically.

Conclusion

Ketoconazole, though an old drug, is valuable in the management of fungal infections resistant to other azole drugs. The only drawback is its hepatotoxic potential because of which its usage needs caution.

Voriconazole: Introduction

Voriconazole (VORI) is a new second-generation triazole antifungal drug that can be administered both orally and intravenously. It is effective for treating candidiasis, invasive aspergillosis and also non-dermatophyte moulds like *Fusarium* and *Scedosporium* spp. Besides, it is well tolerated.

Mechanism of Action

VORI selectively inhibits the fungal cytochrome P450-dependent enzyme 14α sterol demethylase, thereby interrupting an essential step in ergosterol biosynthesis. VORI is 250-fold active against the fungal demethylase enzyme than against mammalian P450-dependent steroid hormone biosynthesis [42].

Pharmacokinetics

As mentioned earlier, VORI is available in both intravenous and oral formulations.

The intravenous formulation is solubilized in sulfobutylether β-cyclodextrin sodium (SBECD) and is infused over 1–2 hours. In adults, steady plasma levels after intravenous infusion of 3–6 mg/kg twice daily range from 3 to 6 mcg/ml [43]. Only after 5 days of receiving VORI at the above dose do patients achieve a steady-state concentration. However, if a loading dose of 6 mg/kg is given every Q12H for a total of two doses, then steady-state concentrations are achieved within 1 day [44]. Following the loading dose, a maintenance dose of 4 mg/kg every 12 hourly is continued.

Oral bioavailability of VORI is estimated to be 96%, which may therefore permit switching between intravenous and oral formulations, when appropriate clinically. As the presence of high-fat food affects absorption of VORI by approximately 50%, it is best to administer the drug either 1 hour before or after meals [44].

The pharmacokinetics of VORI in adults is non-linear, with 58% of VORI being bound to plasma proteins, as well as having a large volume of distribution. The metabolism of VORI takes place in the liver by hepatic cytochrome P450 isoenzymes, CYP2C19, CYP2C9 and CYP3A4. CYP2C19 is the major metabolic pathway for VORI and depends on genetic characteristics. It is seen that as many as 20% of non-Indian Asians have low CYP2C19 activity and can achieve VORI levels as much as four times higher than noted in homozygous subjects who metabolize the drug more extensively. However, dose adjustments regarding this feature have not been propounded. Excretion of 80% of VORI is via the urine and the remaining undergoes faecal elimination [44].

Clinical Uses

Aspergillosis

VORI is approved for the treatment of invasive aspergillosis. Dening et al. [45], in their study, demonstrated a favourable response to VORI in 60% of their patients with acute invasive aspergillosis. The dose administered was intravenous VORI 6 mg/kg Q12H on day 1, followed by 3 mg/kg twice daily for 6–27 days and subsequent administration of oral VORI 200 mg Q12H for 24 weeks.

A subsequent randomized trial compared VORI with standard amphotericin B (AMB) for primary treatment of invasive aspergillosis [46]. Out of the 277 patients who had confirmed invasive aspergillosis, 144 were randomized to receive VORI and 133 were randomized to receive AMB. More than 80% of patients in both treatment groups had haematological malignancies or had received stem cell transplants. Complete or partial responses at week 12 were noted in 53% patients of the VORI group and in 32% of the AMB group. The survival rate was 71% in the VORI group and 58% in the AMB group. VORI was thus found to be superior to AMB in treating patients with invasive aspergillosis.

Pseudallescheria and Scedosporium Infections

VORI is licensed for treating *Pseudallescheria boydii* and *Scedosporium apiospermum* infections in patients refractory or intolerant to other therapies. These pathogens particularly infect immunosuppressed patients who have had an allogenic stem cell transplant [47, 48] and are resistant to AMB. Though VORI has demonstrated successful outcomes for *Pseudallescheria boydii* and *Scedosporium apiospermum* in pulmonary, disseminated and central nervous system (CNS) infections, activity against *Scedosporium proliferans* (an organism found mostly in Spain and Australia) is modest [49–53].

Fusarium Infections

VORI is approved for treating *Fusarium* infections refractory to other drugs, though reports are limited [54]. A case of keratitis secondary to *Fusarium solani* was cured with surgery, topical VORI therapy and 8 weeks of high-dose orally administered VORI [55].

Candida Infections

VORI is used as an off-label drug for oesophageal candidiasis in immunocompromised patients. The dose of VORI is 200 mg PO Q12H for 2–6 weeks, which is extended for another 7 days after clinical resolution [56]. In cases refractory to fluconazole, VORI has proved to be a valuable alternative [57].

Cryptococcosis

VORI has shown excellent in vitro activity against *C. neoformans,* with good levels being attained in the cerebrospinal fluid [58, 59].

However, in a case report of relapsing cryptococcal meningitis due to fluconazole-resistant fungi in an advanced case of HIV infection, maintenance therapy with VORI was unsuccessful in preventing recurrences [60]. Currently, therefore, VORI is not recommended for treating patients with cryptococcosis.

Endemic Mycosis

VORI has demonstrated activity against *B. dermatitidis*, *C. immitis* and *H. capsulatum* and was also effective in an animal model of pulmonary blastomycosis [61–63]. However, reports regarding the effectiveness of VORI for the above indications are based solely on individual reports and therefore cannot be fully recommended in treating endemic mycoses.

Dosing

An intravenous loading dose of 6 mg/kg at 12 hourly intervals should be administered on day 1, followed by a maintenance dose of 4 mg/kg 12 hourly. VORI should be administered at a maximum rate of 3 mg/kg/hour over 1–2 hours. Maintenance therapy can be switched to oral VORI at a dose of 200 mg/day 12 hourly (for patients ≥40 kg) or 100 mg 12 hourly (for patients ≤40 kg).

If therapy is initiated with oral VORI, a loading dose of VORI 400 mg 12 hourly (for patients ≥40 kg) and 200 mg 12hourly (for patients ≤40 kg) should be administered on day 1. Administration of a loading dose on day 1 results in peak plasma concentrations close to steady states within 24 hours. Treatment duration depends on clinical and mycologic response. Oral VORI should be taken at least an hour before or after a meal.

Contraindications

Absolute

- Hypersensitivity to the drug.

Relative

- Hepatic impairment.
- Renal impairment.

Pregnancy prescribing status: category 'D'.

Adverse Effects

Ocular

- Abnormal vision.
- Photophobia.
- Chromatopsia.

Visual disturbances usually occur around half an hour after administration of VORI and resolve spontaneously within 1 hour and are the most common during the first week of treatment. These reactions are usually transient and reversible, seldom necessitating treatment cessation.

Cutaneous

- Pruritus.
- Maculopapular rash.
- Photosensitivity reactions in long-term treatment.
- Rarely TEN and SJS.

Hepatic

- Abnormal liver function tests.
- Rarely serious hepatitis and hepatic failure leading to death.

Cardiovascular System

- Tachycardia.
- Hypo/hypertension.

Gastrointestinal

- Nausea.
- Vomiting.
- Diarrhoea.
- Cholestatic jaundice.

Metabolic

- Hypokalaemia.
- Peripheral oedema.

Infusion Reactions

- Anaphylactic reactions like flushing, fever, sweating and tachycardia have occurred rarely, immediately upon instituting VORI infusion.

Drug Interactions

- Rifampicin: reduces bioavailability of VORI, so their co-administration is contraindicated.
- Carbamazepine and phenobarbital: they significantly reduce bioavailability of VORI.
- Ergot alkaloids: VORI increase their concentrations precipitating ergotism, and therefore, their co-administration is contraindicated.
- Terfenadine, cisapride, astemizole, pimozide and quinidine: they are contraindicated with VORI because of precipitation of QTc prolongation and rarely *torsades de pointes*.

- Statins: VORI can increase plasma levels of statins, and therefore, careful monitoring is required while administering both drugs together.
- Sulfonylureas: VORI may increase plasma levels of glipizide, tolbutamide and glyburide precipitating hypoglycaemia, and therefore, careful monitoring of plasma glucose is mandated when administering both drugs together.
- Sirolimus: VORI increases blood levels of sirolimus extensively, and therefore, their co-administration is contraindicated.

Administration Guidelines

No dose adjustment is necessary based on gender or age ≥ 12 years. However, a maintenance dose of 4 mg/kg intravenously (or the closest equivalent in oral form) every 12 hours is recommended for children aged between 2 and 12 years of age.

Patients with mild-to-moderate hepatic cirrhosis (Child–Pugh Class A or B) should receive standard dosing of VORI but maintenance dose should be halved [64].

Patients with moderate-to-severe renal dysfunction (creatinine clearance <50 ml/min) may experience accumulation of the vehicle SBECD when VORI is administered via the intravenous route. In such patients, oral VORI can be given until the benefit of intravenous VORI outweighs the risk. Serum creatinine levels should be closely monitored in these patients and a shift to oral therapy can be considered.

Conclusion

VORI is a valuable and important addition to the limited armamentarium of antifungal drugs in systemic mycoses. As it is available in both oral and intravenous preparations, this serves as an added advantage.

Posaconazole: Introduction

Posaconazole (POSA) is a triazole antifungal agent with a wide spectrum of activity that includes *Candida* and *Cryptococcus* species, many moulds and some endemic fungi. POSA differs in structure from the compact triazoles, fluconazole and voriconazole in part by virtue of its extended side chain, a feature shared with itraconazole. On the other hand, POSA differs from itraconazole by the presence of a furan ring and substitution of chlorine with fluorine. This extended side chain of POSA provides additional points of contact with the azole target, CYP51 [65].

Mechanism of Action

POSA acts on the enzyme 14α demethylase and inhibits it, resulting in decreased ergosterol content in fungal cell membranes, accumulation of toxic methylated intermediates within fungal cells with resultant disruption of fungal cell membrane function, growth inhibition and, in some cases, even cell death.

An additional advantage with POSA is the presence of multiple hydrophobic contacts resulting from the interaction of the extended side chain within a channel of CYP51, which potentiates enhanced binding affinities and may account for the preservation of activity of POSA against fungi resistant to fluconazole and voriconazole (form mutations at the active site in close proximity to the heme moiety of demethylase) [66, 67].

Pharmacokinetics

POSA is available as a cherry-flavoured suspension (40 mg/ml), tablets and as an intravenous (IV) infusion.

Consuming POSA after a non-fat or a high-fat meal improves its bioavailability 2.6-fold to 4.0-fold, respectively. Absorption of POSA is unaffected by changes in gastric pH [68]. Greater POSA exposure is seen when the drug is administered in divided doses rather than a single dose [65]. POSA is highly lipophilic with a large volume of distribution. Around 98% of the drug is bound to plasma proteins. Steady-state concentrations of POSA are achieved after 7–10 days [69]. The $t_{1/2}$ of POSA is 35 hours. Metabolism occurs in the liver by glucuronidation. Renal clearance plays a minor role in the removal of POSA, with the faecal route being primarily responsible for drug elimination.

Indications

FDA-Approved

- Oropharyngeal candidiasis.
- Prophylaxis for invasive aspergillosis and *Candida* infections in patients ≥13 years of age who are at high risk of developing these infections; in adult and adolescent haematopoietic stem cell transplant recipients with graft versus host disease (GVHD), and in persons with haematologic malignancies and prolonged neutropenia due to chemotherapy.

Off-Label

- Zygomycete infections.
- Salvage therapy for patients with invasive aspergillosis and coccidioidomycosis.
  1. In an elderly lung transplant patient with pneumonia secondary to *Fusarium* proliferation, the efficacy of POSA was reported [70].
  2. In a case of ocular fusariosis, good response to POSA was outlined [71].
  3. Similarly, a case of disseminated phaehyphomycosis responding completely to POSA [72] and six patients with histoplasmosis responding successfully to POSA with failed previous therapies was reported [73].
  4. Coccidioidomycosis has also shown favourable responses with POSA [74].

Dosing

The dosing schedule for POSA is elaborated in Table 15.3.

Table 15.3 Dosing schedule for posaconazole

Clinical condition	Dosing
Prophylaxis for invasive aspergillosis and candida infections	Oral suspension: 200 mg (5 ml) PO Q8H Tablet: 300 mg PO Q12H (day 1), then 300 mg PO once daily from day 2 Injection: loading dose 300 mg IV Q12H on day 1, followed by maintenance dose of 300 mg IV once daily from day 2 (duration of therapy is based on recovery from neutropenia or immunosuppression)
Oropharyngeal candidiasis	Oral suspension: loading dose of 100 mg (2.5 ml) Q12H on day 1, followed by maintenance dose of 100 mg once daily for 13 days
Oropharyngeal candidiasis refractory to fluconazole and itraconazole	Oral suspension: 400 mg (10 ml) Q12H (duration is based on the severity of patients' underlying disease and clinical response)

Contraindications

Absolute

- Hypersensitivity to the drug.

Relative

- Hepatic impairment.
- Renal impairment.

Pregnancy prescribing status: category 'C'.

Adverse Effects

Gastrointestinal

- Nausea.
- Vomiting.
- Abdominal pain.
- Diarrhoea.

Cutaneous

- Rashes.

Central Nervous System

- Headache.
- Blurred vision.
- Tremors.

Cardiovascular

- Hypertension.

Renal

- Increased creatinine levels.

Hepatic

- Elevated hepatic transaminases.

General

- Anorexia.
- Dizziness.
- Fatigue.

Drug Interactions

- Cyclosporine: as POSA inhibits cytochrome P4503A4 enzyme, cyclosporine dose should be reduced to approximately 3/fourth of the original dose.
- Terfenadine, astemizole, cisapride, pimozide, quinidine, halofantrine: contraindicated with POSA as it can lead to *torsades de pointes*.
- Phenytoin: reduction of phenytoin dose is required on concomitant POSA administration.
- Rifabutin: avoid concomitant administration with POSA as it inhibits CYP3A4 enzyme.

Conclusion

POSA is a valuable alternative for oropharyngeal candidiasis that is refractory to fluconazole and itraconazole. Further, in immunocompromised individuals with systemic mycoses, POSA has demonstrated good efficacy.

References

1. Lestner J, Hope WW. Itraconazole: an update on pharmacology and clinical use for treatment of invasive and allergic fungal infections. Expert Opin Drug Metab Toxicol. 2013;9:911–26.
2. Lamb DC, Kelly DE, Venkateswarlu K, et al. Generation of complete, soluble and catalytically active sterol 14 alpha demethylase reductase complex. Biochemistry. 1999;38:8733–8.
3. Ji H, Zhang W, Zhou Y, et al. A three dimensional model of lanosterol 14 alpha demethylase of candida albicans and its interaction with azole antifungals. J Med Chem. 2000;43:2493–505.
4. Jaruratanasirikul S, Kleepkaew A. Influence of an acidic beverage (coca-cola) on absorption of itraconazole. Eur J Clin Pharmacol. 1997;52:235–7.

5. Zimmerman T, Yeates RA, Laufen H, et al. Influence of concomitant food intake on the oral absorption of two triazole antifungal agents, itraconazole and fluconazole. Eur J Clin Pharmacol. 1994;46:147–50.
6. Barine JA, Koh JG, Bierman RH, et al. Food interaction and steady state pharmacokinetics of itraconazole in healthy male volunteers. Antimicrob Agents Chemother. 1993;37:778–84.
7. Hardin TC, Graybill JR, Fetchick R, et al. Pharmacokinetics of itraconazole following oral administration to normal volunteers. Antimicrob Agents Chemother. 1988;32:1310–3.
8. Poirier J, Mcheymol G. Optimization of itraconazole therapy using target drug concentrations. Clin Pharmacokinet. 1998;35:461–73.
9. Cauwenbergh G, Degreef H, Heykants J, et al. Pharmacokinetic profile of orally administered itraconazole in human skin. J Am Acad Dermatol. 1988;18(2 Pt 1):263–8.
10. Matthieu L, De Doncker P, Cauwenbergh G, et al. Itraconazole penetrates the nail via the nail matrix and the nail bed – An investigation in onychomycosis. Clin Exp Dermatol. 1991;16:374–6.
11. Boelaert J, Schurgers M, Matthys E, et al. Itraconazole pharmacokinetics in patients with renal dysfunction. Antimicrob Agents Chemother. 1988;32:1595–7.
12. Heykants J, Van Peer A, Van De Velde V, et al. The clinical pharmacokinetics of itraconazole: An overview. Mycoses. 1989;32(Suppl 1):67–87.
13. Abdel-Rahman SM, Jacobs RF, Massarella J, et al. Single dose pharmacokinetics of intravenous itraconazole and hydroxypropyl-beta-cyclodextrin in infants, children and adolescents. Antimicrob Agents Chemother. 2007;51:2668–73.
14. Groll AH, Wood L, Roden M, et al. Safety pharmacokinetics and pharmacodynamics of cyclodextrin itraconazole in pediatric patients with oropharyngeal candidiasis. Antimicrob Agents Chemother. 2002;46:2554–63.
15. Foot AB, Veys PA, Gibson BE. Itraconazole oral solution as antifungal prophylaxis in children undergoing stem cell transplantation for hematologic disorders. Bone Marrow Transplant. 1999;24:1089–93.
16. De Doncker P, Pande S, Richarz U, et al. Itraconazole: What clinicians should know? Indian J Drugs Dermatol. 2017;3:4–10.
17. Caputo R. Itraconazole (sporonox) in superficial and systemic fungal infections. Expert Rev Anti Infect Ther. 2003;1:531–42.
18. Pfizer Australia Pvt Ltd. Diflucan (Australian approved product information). West Ryde (NSW): Pfizer Australia; 2004.
19. Nicky L, Conrad M, Kabanda T, et al. Dose response effect of high dose fluconazole for HIV associated cryptococcal meningitis in south western Uganda. Clin Infect Dis. 2008;47:1556–61.
20. Foulds G, Brennan DR, Wajszczuk C, et al. Fluconazole penetration into cerebrospinal fluid in humans. J Clin Pharmacol. 1988;28:363–6.
21. Tucker RM, Williams PL, Arathoon EG, et al. Pharmacokinetics of fluconazole in cerebrospinal fluid and serum in human coccidioidal meningitis. Antimicrob Agents Chemother. 1988;32:369–73.
22. Brammer KW, Farrow PR, Faulkner JK. Pharmacokinetics and tissue penetration of fluconazole in humans. Rev Infect Dis. 1990;12(Suppl 3):S318–26.
23. Dudley MN. Clinical pharmacology of fluconazole. Pharmacotherapy. 1990;10(Suppl 6):S141–5.
24. Zervos M, Silverman J, Meunier F. Fluconazole in fungal infection. A review. Infect Dis Clin Pract. 1994;3:94–101.
25. "US Pharmacist". Retrieved on 2015-01-28.
26. Kruger HU, Schuler ZR, et al. Absence of significant interaction of fluconazole with cyclosporine. J Antimicrob Chemother. 1989;24:781–6.
27. Canafox DM, Graves NM, Dm H, et al. Increased cyclosporine levels as a result of simultaneous fluconazole and cyclosporine therapy in renal transplant recipients: a double blind randomized pharmacokinetic and safety study. Transplant Proc. 1991;23:1041–2.
28. Sugar AM, Saunders C, Idelson-Beldon A, et al. Interaction of fluconazole and cyclosporine. Ann Intern Med. 1989;110:844.

29. Van Tyle JH. Ketoconazole. Mechanism of action, spectrum of activity, pharmacokinetics, drug interactions, adverse reactions and therapeutic use. Pharmacotherapy. 1984;4:343–73.
30. Daneshmend TK, Warnock DW. Clinical pharmacokinetics of ketoconazole. Clin Pharmacokinet. 1988;14:13–34.
31. Arora P, Sardana K, Kulhari A, Kaur R, Rawat D, Panesar S. Real world analysis of response rate and efficacy of Oral Ketoconazole in patients with recalcitrant tinea Corporis and Cruris. Am J Trop Med Hyg. 2021;106:38–44.
32. Legendre R, Steltz M. A multi-center, double-blind comparison of ketoconazole and griseofulvin in the treatment of infections due to dermatophytes. Rev Infect Dis. 1980;2:586–91.
33. Heel RC, Brogden RN, Carmine A, Morley PA, Speight TM, Avery GS. Ketoconazole: a review of its therapeutic efficacy in superficial and systemic fungal infections. Drugs. 1982;23:1–36.
34. Gupta AK, Batra R, Bluhm R, Faergemann J. Pityriasis versicolor. Dermatol Clin. 2003;21:413–29.
35. Azoles-Ketoconazole. In: AHFS drug information 2005. Bethesda, MD; American Society of Health-System Pharmacists 2005. P510–P516.
36. Gupta AK, Ryder JE, Nicol K, Cooper EA. Superficial fungal infections: an update on pityriasis versicolor, seborrheic dermatitis, tinea capitis, and onychomycosis. Clin Dermatol. 2003;21:417–25.
37. Kumaresan M, Kumar P. Localized cutaneous leishmaniasis in South India: successful treatment with ketoconazole. Indian J Dermatol Venereol Leprol. 2007;73:361–2.
38. Saenz RE, Paz H, Berman JD. Efficacy of ketoconazole against Leishmania braziliensis panamensis cutaneous leishmaniasis. Am J Med. 1990;89:147–55.
39. Verma KK, Pasricha JS. Ketoconazole as a therapeutic modality in subcorneal pustular dermatosis. Acta Derm Venereol. 1997;77:407–8.
40. Ghetti P, Patrone P, Tosti A. Ketoconazole in the treatment of acne in women. Arch Dermatol. 1986;122:629.
41. Işik AZ, Gökmen O, Zeyneloğlu HB, Senoz S, Zorlu CG. Low dose ketoconazole is an effective and a relatively safe alternative in the treatment of hirsutism. Aust N Z J Obstet Gynaecol. 1996;36:487–9.
42. Ghannoum MA, Kahn DM. Voriconazole—better chances for patients with invasive mycoses. Eur J Med Res. 2002;7:242–56.
43. Hoffman HL, Rathburn RC. Review of the safety and efficacy of voriconazole. Exoert Opin Investig Drugs. 2002;11:409–29.
44. Purkins L, Wood N, Ghahramani R, et al. Pharmacokinetics and safety of voriconazole following intravenous to oral dose escalation regimens. Antimicrob Agents Chemother. 2002;46:2456–3.
45. Denning DW, Ribaud P, Milpied N, et al. Efficacy and safety of voriconazole in the treatment of acute invasive aspergillosis. Clin Infect Dis. 2002;34:563–71.
46. Herbrecht R, Denning DW, Patterson TF, et al. Voriconazole versus amphotericin B for primary therapy of invasive aspergillosis. N Engl J Med. 2002;347:408–15.
47. Revankar SG, Patterson JE, Sutton DA, et al. Disseminated phaeohyphomycosis: review of an emerging mycosis. Clin Infect Dis. 2002;34:467–76.
48. Marr KA, Carter RA, Cripper F, et al. Epidemiology and outcome of mold infections in hematopoietic stem cell transplant patients. Clin Infect Dis. 2002;34:909–17.
49. Nesky MA, McDougal EC, Peacock JE Jr. Pseudallescheria boydii brain abscess successfully treated with voriconazole and surgical drainage: case report and literature review of central nervous system pseudallescheriasis. Clin Infect Dis. 2000;31:673–7.
50. Munoz P, Marin M, Tornero P, et al. Successful outcome of Scedosporium apiospermum disseminated infection treated with voriconazole in a patient receiving corticosteroid therapy. Clin Infect Dis. 2000;31:1499–501.
51. Poza G, Montoya J, Redondo C, et al. Meningitis caused by Pseudallescheria boydii treated with voriconazole. Clin Infect Dis. 2000;30:981–2.

52. Jabado N, Cassaniva JL, Haddad E, et al. Invasive pulmonary infection due to Scedosporium apiospermum in two children with chronic granulomatous disease. Clin Infect Dis. 1998;27:1437–41.
53. Carrillo AJ, Guarro J. In vitro activities of four triazoles against Scedosporium spp. Antimicrob Agents Chemother. 2001;45:2151–3.
54. Perfect JR, Lustar I, Gonzalex-Ruiz A. Voriconazole for the treatment of resistant and rare fungal pathogens [abstract 303]. In: Program and abstracts of the 38th annual meeting of the infectious disease Society of America. New Orleans; 2000.
55. Reis A, Sundmachar R, Tintelnot K, et al. Successful treatment of ocular invasive mold infection (fusariosis) with the new antifungal agent voriconazole. Br J Ophthalmol. 2000;84:932–3.
56. Ally R, Schurmann D, Kreisel W, et al. A randomized double blind double dummy, multicentric trial of voriconazole and fluconazole in the treatment of esophageal candidiasis in immunocompromised patients. Clin Infect Dis. 2001;33:1447–54.
57. Hegener P, Troke P, Fatkenheuer G, et al. Treatment of fluconazole resistant candidiasis with voriconazole in patients with AIDS. AIDS. 1998;12:2227–8.
58. Hoban DJ, Zhanel GC, Karlousky JA. In vitro susceptibilities of candida and Cryptococcus neoformans isolated from blood cultures of neutropenic patients. Antimicrob Agents Chenother. 1999;43:1463–4.
59. Pfaller MA, Zhang J, Messer SA, et al. In vitro activities of voriconazole, fluconazole and itraconazole against 566 clinical isolated of Cryptococcus neoformans from United States and Africa. Antimicrob Agents Chemother. 1999;43:169–71.
60. Friese G, Discher T, Fussle R, et al. Development of azole resistance during fluconazole maintenance therapy for AIDS associated cryptococcal disease. AIDS. 2001;15:2344–5.
61. Espinel-Ingroff A. In vitro activity of the new triazole voriconazole (UK-109,496) against opportunistic filamentous and dimorphic fungi and common emerging yeast pathogens. J Clin Microbiol. 1998;36:198–202.
62. Li RK, Ciblak MA, Nordoff N, et al. In vitro activities of voriconazole, itraconazole and amphotericin B against Blastomyces dermatitidis, Coccidioides immitis and Histoplasma capsulatum. Antimicrob Agents Chemother. 2000;44:1734–6.
63. Sugar AM, Liu X. Efficacy of voriconazole in treatment of murine pulmonary blastomycosis. Antimicrob Agents Chemother. 2001;45:601–4.
64. Tan KKC, Wood N, Weil A. Multiple dose pharmacokinetics of voriconazole in chronic hepatic impairment [abstract A-16]. In: IN: program and abstracts of the 6th Interscience conference on antimicrobial agents and chemotherapy. Toronto, Ont: American Society of Microbiology; 2000. p. 23.
65. Xiao L, Madison V, Chau AS, et al. Three dimensional models of wild type and mutated forms of cytochrome P-450 14α sterol demethylase from aspergillus fumigates and Candida albicans provide insights into posaconazole binding. Antimicrob Agents Chemother. 2004;48:568–74.
66. Munayyer HK, Mann PA, Chau S, et al. Posaconazole is a potent inhibitor of sterol 14α demethylation in yeasts and molds. Antimicrob Agents Chemother. 2004;48:3690–6.
67. Heimark L, Shipkova P, Grace J, et al. Mechanism of azole antifungal activity as determined by liquid chromatographic/mass spectrometric monitoring ergosterol biosynthesis. J Mass Spectrom. 2002;37:265–9.
68. Courtney R, Radwanski E, Lim J, et al. Pharmacokinetics of posaconazole co-administered with antacid in fasting and non-fasting healthy men. Antimicrob Agents Chemother. 2004;48:804–8.
69. Ezzet F, Wexler D, Radwanski E, et al. Oral bioavailability of posaconazole in fasted healthy subjects: comparison between three regimens and basis for clinical dosage recommendations. Clin Pharmacokinet. 2005;44:211–20.
70. Herbrecht R, Kressler R, Kravanja C, et al. Successful treatment of Fusarium proliferation pneumonia with posaconazole in a lung transplant recipient. J Heart Lung Transplant. 2004;23:1451–4.

71. Tu EY, DL MC, Bealty RF, et al. Successful treatment of resistant ocular fusariosis with posaconazole (SCH-56952). Am J Ophthalmol. 2007;143:222–7.
72. Negroni R, Helou SH, Petri N, et al. Case study: posaconazole treatment of disseminated phaeohyphomycosis due to Exophiala spinifera. Clin Infect Dis. 2004;38:e15–20.
73. Restreppo A, Toban A, Clark B, et al. Salvage treatment of histoplasmosis with posaconazole. J Infect. 2007;54:319–27.
74. Anstead JM, Corcoran G, Lewis J, et al. Refractory coccidioidomycosis treated with posaconazole. Clin Infect Dis. 2005;40:1770–6.

Terbinafine

16

Introduction

Terbinafine (TBF) belongs to the allylamine class of antifungal drugs. Oral TBF was first introduced in the United Kingdom in February 1991 and approved by the US FDA for treating onychomycosis in May 1996. TBF is available both as oral and topical preparations.

Mechanism of Action

TBF inhibits the fungal enzyme squalene epoxidase (a complex membrane-bound enzyme system that is not a part of cytochrome P-450 superfamily) [1]. This results in the deficiency of ergosterol within fungal cells and accumulation of squalene, a toxic compound, which eventuates in fungal death.

Pharmacokinetics

Greater than 70% of TBF is absorbed orally. Absorption of TBF is unaffected by food. Owing to its highly lipophilic and keratophilic nature, TBF gets extensively distributed within the adipose tissue, dermis, epidermis and nails. The metabolism of TBF occurs in the liver by N-demethylation and oxidation of the tertiary butyl group. Around 15 metabolites of TBF have been identified, with none of them possessing any antifungal activity [2–4]. The plasma concentration–time profile of TBF is triphasic [5]. After 4 weeks of TBF 250 mg/day, the mean terminal half-life is 22 days in the plasma. In the dermis–epidermis, hair and nails, the mean elimination half-life of TBF ranges from 24 to 28 days [4].

A high concentration of TBF well above the minimum inhibitory concentration (MIC) for most dermatophytes is reached in the skin within hours of therapy

A. K. Bubna, *Therapeutics in Dermatology - Essentials for Clinical Practice*, https://doi.org/10.1007/978-981-95-3791-4_16

initiation [6, 7]. TBF is primarily delivered to the stratum corneum via sebum and to a lesser extent it gets incorporated into basal keratinocytes and in this way reaches the stratum corneum [8]. In contrast, TBF remains undetectable in eccrine sweat.

Even after discontinuation of TBF therapy, it still remains in the skin above the MIC concentrations for most dermatophytes for 2–3 weeks.

In the distal nail plate, TBF can be detected within 1 week of initiating therapy, and following 6 and 12 weeks of oral therapy with TBF, it remains in the nail plate of finger and toe nails for 30 and 36 weeks, respectively, at concentrations above the MIC for most cutaneous fungal infections [9, 10].

As TBF undergoes extensive hepatic metabolism, in patients with hepatic dysfunction dose adjustment may be required [5]. Excretion of TBF is via the kidneys; therefore, if serum creatinine levels exceed 300 μmol/L or when creatinine clearance is ≤50 mL/min, then the oral dose of TBF should be approximately halved [11].

Clinical Uses

Onychomycosis

Oral TBF has been approved by the US FDA as a continuous therapy for 12 and 6 weeks for dermatophyte onychomycosis of toe nails and finger nails, respectively [12]. In some patients with poor nail outgrowth during the first few weeks of treatment, a longer course of TBF may be required. In such instances, some clinicians prefer to treat toe nail onychomycosis for 16 weeks instead of 12 weeks.

Gupta et al. [13] employed another dosing schedule with TBF for onychomycosis. They administered two 4-week courses utilizing 250 mg of TBF with a 1-month interval between the two courses. They found this regimen to be equally effective as the continuous TBF schedule and more efficacious than pulse itraconazole for treating toe nail onychomycosis.

A regimen of three weekly pulses of TBF (250 mg twice daily for 1 week every month) alone or in combination with topical TBF is also effective in dermatophyte onychomycosis [14, 15].

Alternative protocols for treating onychomycosis with TBF are also reported. Shuster and Munro [16] administered 1000 mg of TBF in various schedules for onychomycosis, details of which are elaborated in Table 16.1.

It is seen in vitro that TBF is fungicidal against dermatophytes, *Aspergillus fumigatus*, *Scopulariopsis brevicaulis* and *Candida parapsilosis* and fungistatic against *C. albicans*. Further, TBF is found to be more effective than griseofulvin and itraconazole in the treatment of finger nail and toe nail onychomycosis [17–19].

For candidal onychomycosis, TBF may need to be dosed at 250 mg/day for 4 months rather than the conventional 3 months, which is usually sufficient for dermatophyte toe nail infections [20].

For treating onychomycosis secondary to non-dermatophyte moulds, more experience is needed to delineate the exact dosing protocol [21].

Table 16.1 Dosing schedule of terbinafine in the study by Shuster and Munro

Author	Number of patients	Dosing schedule with terbinafine	Results
Shuster and Munro [16]	5 patients	1000 mg stat dose	No improvement
	2 patients	1000 mg, 2 doses given at 2 weekly intervals	One patient showed a clear response One patient showed no improvement
	4 patients	1000 mg, 3 doses given at 2 weekly intervals	In all patients, lesions cleared completely

In the paediatric population, TBF is administered at a dose of 3–6 mg/kg/day for 6 and 12 weeks for finger and toe nail onychomycosis, respectively.

Tinea Capitis

TBF is approved by the FDA for treating tinea capitis in children older than 4 years.

The dosing of TBF for tinea capitis in children is as follows:

- <25 kg: 125 mg/day for 6 weeks.
- 25–35 kg: 187.5 mg/day for 6 weeks.
- Over 35 kg: 250 mg/day for 6 weeks.

Tinea Corporis and Cruris

In adults, the dosing of TBF for tinea corporis and tinea cruris is 250 mg/day ranging from 2 to 4 weeks [22, 23]. In children, the dose ranges from 3 to 6 mg/kg/day for 2–4 weeks.

Tinea Pedis

TBF is particularly effective in treating moccasin foot variant of tinea pedis. The dose is similar to that of tinea corporis/cruris except that the duration may extend from 2 to 6 weeks [24, 25].

Other Dermatomycoses

Other dermatomycosis where TBF is effective include tinea imbricata [26], Majocchi's granuloma [27], cutaneous sporotrichosis [28] and black piedra [29].

A suggested dosing schedule is as follows:

- Weight > 40 kg: 250 mg/day.
- Weight 20–40 kg: 125 mg/day.
- Weight < 20 kg: 62.5 mg/day.

Contraindications

Absolute

- Drug hypersensitivity

Relative

- Pregnancy (category 'B') and lactation
- Chronic or active hepatic impairment (if clinical or laboratory evidence of liver injury exists, TBF should be discontinued)
- Renal impairment (creatinine clearance <50 mL/min)
- Immunodeficiency or immunosuppression (in these patients, complete blood count at baseline and every 6 weeks while under treatment is recommended. TBF should be discontinued if neutrophil count is less than $1000/mm^3$).

Adverse Effects

Gastrointestinal

- Diarrhoea
- Nausea/vomiting
- Flatulence
- Abdominal pain
- Taste disturbances

Cutaneous

- Erythema or rash
- Pruritus
- Urticaria
- Rarely TEN and SJS, fixed drug eruption, exacerbation of psoriasis and erythema annulare centrifugum

Central Nervous System

- Headache

Hepatobiliary

- Asymptomatic reversible elevation of hepatic enzymes
- Rarely symptomatic liver injury with TBF that may be idiosyncratic or cholestatic, manifested as jaundice and pruritus [30, 31]

Others

- Tiredness
- Fatigue
- Pain (back, knees, legs)

Drug Interactions

- Rifampicin: increases clearance of TBF by 100%.
- Cyclosporine: TBF increases clearance of cyclosporine by 15%.
- Terfenadine: reduces TBF clearance by 16%.

Monitoring

If patients are taking TBF for more than 6 weeks, then LFT and complete blood counts need to be monitored. However, no firm monitoring guidelines regarding this aspect have been suggested.

Conclusion

TBF is a valuable drug for treating numerous fungal infections.

References

1. Ryder NS. Terbinafine: mode of action and properties of squalene epoxidase inhibition. Br J Dermatol. 1992;126(Suppl 39):2–7.
2. Stephen A, Czok R, Male O. Terbinafine: initial clinical results. In: Fromtling RA, editor. Recent trends in the discovery, development and evaluation of antifungal agents. Barcelona: JR Prous Science Publishers SA; 1987. p. 511–20.

3. Kovarik JM, Kirkesseli S, Humbert H, et al. Dose proportional pharmacokinetics of terbinafine and its N-demethylated metabolite in healthy volunteers. Br J Dermatol. 1992;126(Suppl 39):8–13.
4. Zehende H, Denouel J, Faergemann J, et al. Elimination kinetics of terbinafine from human plasma and tissues following multiple dose administration and comparison with 3 main metabolites. Drug Invest. 1994;8:203–10.
5. Jensen JC. Pharmacokinetics of Lamisil in humans. J Dermatol Treat. 1990;1(Suppl 2):15–8.
6. Lever LR, Dykes PJ, Thomas R, et al. How orally administered terbinafine reaches the stratum corneum. J Dermatol Treat. 1990;1:23–5.
7. Faergemann J, Zehender H, Jones T, et al. Terbinafine levels in serum, stratum corneum, dermis-epidermis (without stratum corneum), hair, sebum and eccrine sweat. Acta Derm Venereol (Stockh). 1990;71:322–6.
8. Faergemann J, Zehender H, Denouel J, et al. Levels of terbinafine in plasma, stratum corneum, dermis-epidermis (without stratum corneum), sebum, hair and nails during and after 250 mg terbenafine orally once per day for four weeks. Acta Derm Venereol (Stockh). 1993;73:305–9.
9. Faergemann J, Zehender H, Millerioux L, et al. Levels of terbinafine in plasma, stratum corneum, dermis-epidermis (without stratum corneum), sebum, hair and nails during and after 250 mg terbinafine orally once daily for 7 and 14 days. Clin Exp Dermatol. 1994;19:121–6.
10. Schatz F, Brautigam M, Dobrowolski E, et al. Nail incorporation kinetics of terbinafine in onychomycosis patients. Clin Exp Dermatol. 1995;20:377–83.
11. Terbenafine product monograph. East Hanover: Sandoz Pharmaceuticals; 1996 April.
12. Terbenafine product monograph. Dorval: Sandoz Canada Inc; 1995 November. p. 1–33.
13. Gupta AK, Lynch LE, Kogan N, et al. The use of an intermittent terbinafine regimen for the treatment of dermatophyte toe nail onychomycosis. J Eur Acad Dermatol Venereol. 2009;23:256–62.
14. Takahota Y, Hiruma M, Shiraki Y, et al. Treatment of dermatophyte onychomycosis with three pulses of terbinafine (500 mg/day for a week). Mycoses. 2009;52:72–6.
15. Nakano N, Hiruma M, Shiraki Y, et al. Combination of pulse therapy with terbinafine tablets and topical terbinafine cream for the treatment of dermatophyte onychomycosis. A pilot study. J Dermatol. 2006;33:753–8.
16. Shuster S, Munro C. Single dose treatment of fungal nail disease. Lancet. 1992;133:329–47.
17. Haneke E, Tausch I, Brautigam M, Weidinger G, Welzel D, LAGOS III Study Group. Short duration treatment of finger nail dermatophytosis: a randomized, double-blind study with terbinafine and griseofulvin. J Am Acad Dermatol. 1995;32:72–7.
18. Faergemann J, Anderson C, Hersle K, et al. Double-blind parallel group comparison of terbinafine and griseofulvin in the treatment of toe nail onychomycosis. J Am Acad Dermatol. 1995;32:750–3.
19. Brautigam M, Notting S, Schopf RE, et al. Randomized double-blind comparison of terbinafine and itraconazole for treatment of toe nail tinea infection. BMJ. 1995;311:919–22.
20. Segal R, Kritzman A, Cividalli L, et al. Treatment of candida nail infection with terbinafine. J Am Acad Dermatol. 1996;35:958–61.
21. Notting S, Brautigam M, Weidinger G. Terbinafine in onychomycosis with involvement by non-dermatophyte fungi. Br J Dermatol. 1994;130(Suppl 43):16–21.
22. Cole GW, Sticklin G. A comparison of a new oral antifungal terbinafine with griseofulvin therapy for tinea corporis. Arch Dermatol. 1989;125:1537–9.
23. Del Palacio Hernanz A, Gomez SL, Lastra FG. A comparative double-blind study of terbinafine (Lamisil) and griseofulvin in tinea corporis and tinea cruris. Clin Exp Dermatol. 1990;15:210–6.
24. Savin RC. Oral terbinafine versus griseofulvin in the treatment of moccasin type tenia pedis. J Am Acad Dermatol. 1990;23(Suppl):807–9.
25. Savin RC. Successful treatment of chronic tinea pedis (moccasin type) with terbinafine (Lamisil). Clin Exp Dermatol. 1989;14:116–9.

26. Budimulja U, Kuswadji K, Bramono S, et al. A double blind randomized, stratified controlled study of the treatment of tinea imbricate with oral terbinafine or itraconazole. Br J Dermatol. 1994;130:29–31.
27. Gupta AK, Prussick R, Sibbald RG, et al. Terbinafine in the treatment of Majocchi's granuloma. Int J Dermatol. 1995;34:489.
28. Hull PR, Vismer HF. Treatment of cutaneous sporotrichosis with terbinafine. Br J Dermatol. 1992;126:51–5.
29. Gip L. Black Piedra: the first case treated with terbinafine (Lamisil). Br J Dermatol. 1994;130:26–8.
30. Lowe G, Green C, Jennings P. Hepatitis associated with terbinafine treatment [Letter]. Br Med J. 1993;306:248.
31. Hepatobiliary reactions with terbinafine hydrochloride. Can Med Assoc J. 1996;154:62–3.

Griseofulvin

17

Introduction

Griseofulvin is a heterocyclic benzofuran systemic antifungal agent with a wide variety of applications in dermatology, apart from the management of cutaneous dermatophytosis.

Mechanism of Action

Orally administered, griseofulvin enters the dermatophyte nuclei and inhibits microtubule function in fungal cells by binding to specific sites on the microtubular protein, thereby disrupting mitotic tubule assembly. In addition to binding with tubulin, the drug also interacts with microtubule-associated protein [1]. It is to be noted that griseofulvin is a fungistatic drug and is effective only against growing cells [2].

Antifungal Spectrum

Griseofulvin is effective only against dermatophytes, that is, *Epidermophyton*, *Microsporum* and *Trichophyton* species. It is ineffective against *Candida* and *Malassezia* species [2].

Pharmacokinetics

Griseofulvin is only given orally. Post-intake, peak plasma concentrations are achieved within 4 h. As griseofulvin has a very low water solubility, its rate of absorption is slightly irregular. This disadvantage can be tackled by consuming

A. K. Bubna, *Therapeutics in Dermatology - Essentials for Clinical Practice*, https://doi.org/10.1007/978-981-95-3791-4_17

griseofulvin with a fatty meal or micro fining the drug particles [1]. Within 4–8 h of griseofulvin administration, it is detected in the horny layer of the skin. Further, sweat and trans epidermal water loss facilitate griseofulvin transfer to the stratum corneum. One significant feature observed is that griseofulvin tends to get retained in dermatophyte-infected cells. Griseofulvin undergoes hepatic metabolism by methylation and is excreted in the urine [1, 2].

Indications

Griseofulvin has a wide variety of applications in dermatology and is discussed in Table 17.1 [3–10].

Table 17.1 Applications of griseofulvin in dermatology

Clinical indication	Details
Cutaneous dermatophytosis	Used for dermatophytosis of the skin, hair and nails It is the drug of choice for tinea capitis in children *Trichophyton rubrum* and *T. mentagrophytes* may require higher than conventional doses of griseofulvin to demonstrate clinical efficacy Dosing is 10–20 mg/kg body weight per day in 2–3 divided doses Duration of treatment for cutaneous and hair dermatophytosis is 4–6 weeks Duration of treatment from finger nail onychomycosis is 6–9 months Duration of treatment for toe nail onychomycosis is 12 months
Molluscum contagiosum	It is effective in molluscum contagiosum because of its immunomodulatory property It is given at a dose of 500–750 mg daily in patients over 14 years of age, and 250 mg daily in younger patients for 4–6 weeks [3, 4]
Lichen planus	It is effective in lichen planus because of its immunomodulatory property Griseofulvin given at a dose of 500 mg/day demonstrated good results in one study [5]. However, in another study, results were not satisfactory [6]
Raynaud's phenomenon	Griseofulvin given at a dose of 1 g twice daily in patients with Raynaud's phenomenon demonstrates clinical improvement after 4 weeks of drug intake. This can be attributed to the vasodilatory property of griseofulvin [7]
Wells syndrome	Griseofulvin is employed as a treatment option in eosinophilic cellulitis [8] A case report for the same, wherein 500 mg of griseofulvin was administered in two divided doses, demonstrated complete lesional resolution after 1 month of therapy. This can be attributed to the leucopenic effects of griseofulvin [9]
Pigmented purpuric dermatosis	Successful treatment of pigmented purpuric dermatosis with griseofulvin has been reported by Tamaki et al. [10]

Contraindications

Absolute

- Drug hypersensitivity

Relative

- Hepatic disease
- Gastrointestinal disturbances
- Patients who consume alcohol as griseofulvin causes alcohol intolerance

  Pregnancy prescribing status: category 'C'

Drug Interactions

- Griseofulvin facilitates warfarin metabolism by inducing hepatic CYPs. An adjustment in the dose of griseofulvin is therefore mandated.
- Griseofulvin also reduces efficacy of oestrogen-containing oral contraceptive pills by a similar mechanism.
- Patients on phenytoin and phenobarbitone may require increasing the dose of griseofulvin as they reduce oral absorption of griseofulvin.

Adverse Effects

Nervous System

- Headache
- Peripheral neuropathy
- Lethargy
- Mental confusion
- Syncope
- Vertigo
- Blurring of vision

Gastrointestinal System

- Hepatotoxicity
- Nausea
- Vomiting
- Heartburn

- Flatulence

Haematological

- Leucopoenia
- Neutropenia
- Punctate basophilia
- Monocytosis

Cutaneous

- Urticaria and angioedema
- Photosensitivity
- Erythema multiforme-like rash
- Vesicular/morbilliform eruptions
- Serum sickness-like picture

Renal

- Albuminuria
- Cylindruria without evidence of renal insufficiency

Conclusion

Griseofulvin is an extremely beneficial drug in the dermatologic armamentarium. However, with the advent of newer antifungal agents, the availability of this drug in the market has reduced.

References

1. Benner JE. Antifungal agents. In: Brunton LL, Chabner BA, Knollmann BC, editors. Goodman and Gilman's the pharmacological basis of therapeutics. 12th ed. New York: McGraw Hill; 2011. p. 1571–91.
2. Robertson DB, Maibach HI. Dermatologic pharmacology. In: Katzung BG, Trevor AJ, editors. Basic and clinical pharmacology. 13th ed. New Delhi: McGraw Hill Education (India) private limited; 2015. p. 1033–51.
3. Singh OP, Kanwar A. Griseofulvin therapy in molluscum contagiosum. Arch Dermatol. 1977;113:1615.
4. Kapur TR. Griseofulvin therapy in molluscum contagiosum. A case report. Indian J Dermatol Venereol Leprol. 1976;42:90.

5. Sehgal VN, Bickchandani R, Koranne RV, Nayar M, Saxena HM. Histopathological evaluation of griseofulvin therapy in lichen planus. A double-blind controlled study. Dermatologica. 1980;161:22–7.
6. Massa MC, Rogers RS III. Griseofulvin therapy of lichen planus. Acta Derm Venereol. 1981;61:547–50.
7. Sabri S, Roberts VC, Higgins RF, Cotton LT, Williams DI, Wilson LC. A double-blind clinical trial of griseofulvin in patients with Raynaud's phenomenon. Postgrad Med J. 1973;49:641–3.
8. Räßler F, Lukács J, Elsner P. Treatment of eosinophilic cellulitis (Wells syndrome) – a systematic review. J Eur Acad Dermatol Venereol. 2016;30:1465–79.
9. Sharma PK, Gautam RK, Sharma AK. Eosinophilic cellulitis—a case study and management with griseofulvin. Indian J Dermatol Venereol Leprol. 1995;61:163–4.
10. Tamaki K, Yasaka N, Osada A, Shibagaki N, Furue M. Successful treatment of pigmented purpuric dermatosis with griseofulvin. Br J Dermatol. 1995;132:159–60.

Amphotericin B

18

Introduction

Amphotericin B (AmB) is a natural polyene macrolide, extracted via fermentation from the soil actinomycete *Streptomyces nodosus*. Though developed primarily for the treatment of life-threatening systemic fungal infections, presently the utility of AmB has extended to the management of complicated cutaneous and visceral leishmaniasis. Besides, there are reports describing the use of AmB in subcutaneous mycoses, onychomycosis and superficial fungal infections with promising outcomes [1].

Mechanism of Action

The mechanism of action of AmB is represented in Fig. 18.1 [2]. Additionally, in leishmaniasis, other mechanisms postulated for AmB include (a) cholesterol sequestration in the host membrane, thereby blocking interaction of the parasite with host macrophages (mandatory for initiation and perpetuation of infection); [3, 4] (b) lipid peroxidation, with subsequent protozoal destruction; (c) antagonism of endosome–lysosome fusion; [5, 6] (d) apoptosis [7] and (e) promotion of IFNγ production, which helps in macrophage activation [6].

A. K. Bubna, *Therapeutics in Dermatology - Essentials for Clinical Practice*, https://doi.org/10.1007/978-981-95-3791-4_18

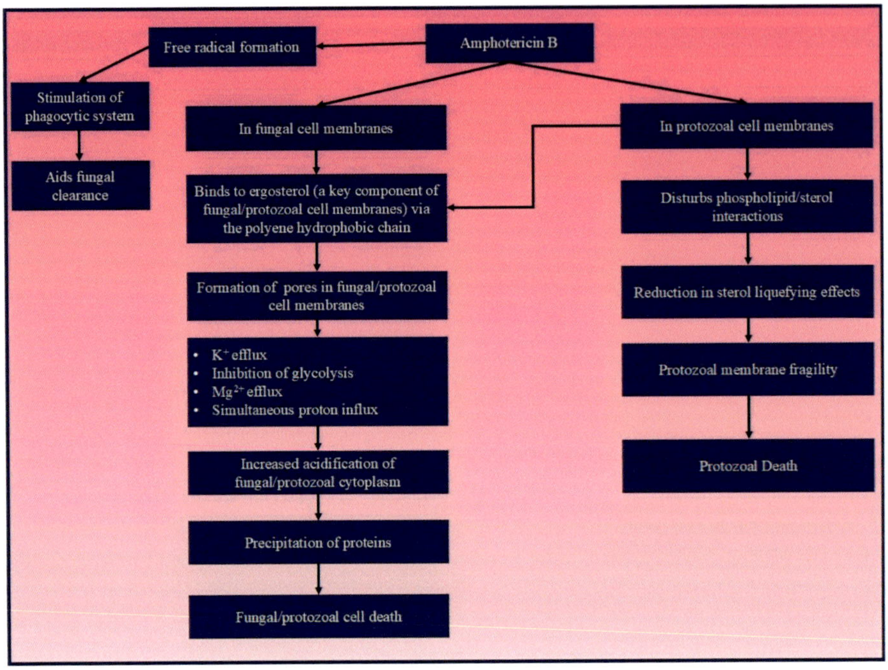

Fig. 18.1 Mechanism of action of amphotericin B

Clinical Uses

Invasive Fungal Infections

The incidence of invasive fungal infections (IFIs) has increased remarkably in recent years. Furthermore, existing comorbidities like neutropenia, human immunodeficiency virus (HIV)/acquired immunodeficiency syndrome (AIDS) and cancer are often encountered in patients presenting with IFIs, with an increased predisposition for resistance to antifungal agents [8–10].

AmB continues to be the reference drug in treating IFIs even today, essentially due to its broader gamut of action. Because of the association of several adverse effects with the conventional formulation of AmB (d-AmB), various newer AmB preparations have now been developed with an effort to reduce the toxic effects encountered following usage of d-AmB. All newer formulations are lipid-based; advanced by the favourable lipid solubility of AmB [11].

These formulations include (a) liposomal AmB (L-AmB), (b) AmB colloid dispersion (ABCD) and (c) AmB lipid complex (ABLC).

Table 18.1 depicts the salient points related to them [8, 12–18].

Various IFIs where AmB is utilized are elaborated in Table 18.2 [19–22].

Table 18.1 Salient points related to the lipid formulations of amphotericin B

	Liposomal AmB	AmB colloid dispersion	AmB lipid complex
Components	Unilamellar lipid structure consisting of AmB complexed with three major components, soy phosphatidylcholine, distearoylphosphatidylglycerol and cholesterol, in a ratio of 2:1:1:0.8	Disc-like lipid structure consisting of AmB and cholesteryl sulfate at a 1:1 molar ratio	Ribbon-like lipid structure consisting of AmB complexed with L-α-dimyristoyl-phosphatidyl glycerol at a 1:7:3 molar ratio
Year of approval by the US FDA	1977	1996	1995
Standard dose	3 mg/kg/day	3–4 mg/kg/day	5 mg/kg/day
Pharmacokinetics	Achieves extraordinarily high serum concentrations relative to those achieved by other formulations and has a $t_{1/2}$ of 152 h Less than 10% of the drug is excreted unchanged in the urine and faeces Because of the small size of the particles in this preparation, substantial escapc from the mononuclear phagocytic system results in a higher C_{max} and higher area under curve (AUC)	Serum levels of AmB colloid dispersion are lower than liposomal AmB owing to its larger size and poor dissociation Besides, its property of getting rapidly engulfed by the macrophage phagocytic system results in a lower C_{max} and AUC	Serum levels of AmB lipid complex are quite low, yet distribution to certain organs such as the lungs are reported to exceed those of other formulations Because it is a larger molecule and engulfed rapidly by macrophages, it delineates a lower C_{max}, low AUC and high volume of distribution

Cutaneous Mucormycosis

Cutaneous mucormycosis (CM) is an emerging mycotic infection commonly encountered in immunosuppressed individuals and patients with uncontrolled diabetes. It often occurs following direct inoculation through trauma with a non-specific presentation, closely mimicking other dermatologic disorders [23]. Although d-AmB is the therapy of choice, lipid formulations are often utilized owing to their favourable toxicity profile [24]. In fact, studies reveal AmB to be the most active drug against mucorales, with minimum inhibitory concentrations (MICs) of ≤1 mg/mL in the majority of tested strains [25]. Apart from AmB therapy, surgical debridement and control of underlying immunosuppression become equally important in the management of CM. Besides, within 5 days of diagnosis, therapy needs to be initiated.

Table 18.2 Utility of amphotericin B for invasive fungal infections

Infection	Treatment regimen(s)
Cryptococcal meningitis	According to the current WHO guidelines, d-AmB (1 mg/kg/day) plus flucytosine (100 mg/kg/day) for 7 days, followed by fluconazole (1200 mg/day) for 7 days [1] However, in a phase 3 RCT, a single dose of L-AmB (10 mg/kg/day), along with 2 weeks treatment with flucytosine (100 mg/kg/day) and fluconazole (1200 mg/day), was non-inferior to the WHO-recommended treatment for HIV-associated cryptococcal meningitis (with fewer adverse effects) [19]
Candidemia and invasive candidiasis in non-neutropenic patients	Lipid formulation AmB (3–5 mg/kg daily) is a reasonable alternative if there is intolerance, limited availability or resistance to other antifungal agents (strong recommendation; high-quality evidence) and transition from AmB to fluconazole is recommended after 5–7 days among patients who have isolates that are susceptible to fluconazole, who are clinically stable and in whom repeat cultures on antifungal therapy are negative (strong recommendation; high-quality evidence) [20]
Neutropenic candidemia	Lipid formulation AmB (3–5 mg/kg daily) is an effective but less attractive alternative because of the potential for toxicity (strong recommendation; moderate-quality evidence) [20]
Chronic disseminated candidiasis (hepatosplenic)	Initial therapy with lipid formulation AmB (3–5 mg/kg/day) (strong recommendation; low-quality evidence) [20]
Empiric treatment for suspected invasive candidiasis in non-neutropenic patients in the intensive care unit	Lipid formulation AmB (3–5 mg/kg/day) is an alternative, if there is intolerance to other antifungal agents (strong recommendation; low-quality evidence) [20]
Neonatal candidiasis, including central nervous system infection	AmB deoxycholate (1 mg/kg/day) (strong recommendation; moderate-quality evidence) Lipid formulation AmB (3–5 mg/kg/day) is an alternative but should be used with caution, particularly in the presence of urinary tract involvement (weak evidence; low-quality evidence) [20]
Invasive aspergillosis	According to the infectious disease Society of America (IDSA) guidelines, AmB deoxycholate as well as lipid formulations are recommended in invasive aspergillosis when voriconazole is not feasible. AmB deoxycholate is suitable for resource-limited settings, while lipid formulations are preferred in cases of azole intolerance or contraindication [21] Liposomal AmB (3 mg/kg/day) offers a rate of response similar to voriconazole in the first-line treatment of invasive aspergillosis [22]

The recommended dosing of d-AmB in immunosuppressed patients with CM is 1–1.5 mg/kg/day, and for immunocompetent patients it is 0.5–1 mg/kg/day. L-AmB is dosed at 5–10 mg/kg/day, and ABLC is administered at 5–7.5 mg/kg/day in both immunosuppressed and immunocompetent individuals [26]. The duration of treatment is still not determined, with some authors suggesting to continue therapy till clinical/radiological resolution, and others recommending a treatment period of 6–8 weeks [26, 27].

Interestingly, successful use of L-AmB has been documented in an extremely preterm infant (<28 weeks) who developed primary CM, along with polymicrobial sepsis, within the first 10 days of life. L-AmB was given for a period of 4 weeks with resultant spontaneous sloughing of the fungal eschar and no long-term sequelae as a consequence to CM [28].

Furthermore, use of topical AmB, both as combination and monotherapy for CM, has been described [29, 30].

In a 6-month-old infant with leukaemia, severe necrotizing skin and soft tissue mucormycosis of the chest wall outlined successful response with systemic L-AmB, local wound control, surgical resection and topical AmB. Topical AmB was added because the response to systemic L-AmB alone was inadequate, and addition of the topical formulation was found critical in facilitating wound healing [29].

Also, AmB 3% cream as an individual therapy was found to be highly effective in treating vaginal mucormycosis in a 56-year-old woman. She was started on a once-daily application schedule for 3 weeks with satisfactory clinical responses. However, symptoms relapsed after therapy cessation, for which 3% AmB cream was restarted for another month and gradually tapered as an alternate-day schedule for 2 months with complete clinical and mycological cure, even at 12 months of follow-up [30].

Chromoblastomycosis

Chromoblastomycosis represents a cutaneous/subcutaneous mycotic infection caused by a group of dematiaceous (black) fungi and occurs following traumatic skin inoculation, with the majority of lesions involving the lower extremities of outdoor workers [31].

Currently, existing trials regarding its treatment are limited, with oral itraconazole and terbinafine constituting the primary therapeutic pillars for chromoblastomycosis. Unfortunately, cure rates are low with the above drugs, and high rates of relapse make management very challenging [32]. The utility of AmB in chromoblastomycosis has been described in two reports [33, 34].

In the first report, intravenous L-AmB for 1 month was helpful in attaining mycological cure in a 37-year-old woman with chromoblastomycosis of the right breast. Following this, the patient was maintained on itraconazole (200 mg/day) and 5-flucytosine (4 g/day) for 12 months with no relapse [33].

In the second report, intralesional AmB (obtained by dissolving 25 mg of AmB in 20 mL of sterilized water and 5 mL of 2% lidocaine solution to make 1 mg/mL of AmB) given once weekly for 19 weeks, along with 500 mg/day of oral terbinafine, was successful in attaining clinical cure of chromoblastomycosis in a 75-year-old farmer who had the disease for 12 years and was unresponsive to oral itraconazole, cryotherapy and complete surgical excision [34].

Despite these promising reports, more robust clinical trials are mandated in relation to the precise dosing schedule of AmB and its combination with other antifungals for treating chromoblastomycosis.

Blastomycosis

Blastomycosis is a chronic granulomatous and suppurative systemic mycosis primarily affecting the lungs, with involvement of the skin, bones and central nervous system in disseminated forms [35]. Although itraconazole is employed as the first-line drug for most cases, AmB proves to be valuable in widespread and disseminated forms of the disease. Furthermore, in cases unresponsive to itraconazole, substitution of AmB in the therapeutic regimen has demonstrated efficacy [36].

Histoplasmosis

Histoplasmosis is a highly infectious mycosis caused by *Histoplasma capsulatum* that primarily affects the lungs. Although most pulmonary lesions heal spontaneously in immunocompetent hosts, in immunosuppressed individuals this progresses to disseminated histoplasmosis, with mucocutaneous involvement serving as an important diagnostic clue [37]. The regimen of AmB in the management of histoplasmosis is represented in Table 18.3 [38, 39].

Recently, in a randomized controlled trial (RCT), a single high dose of L-AmB (10 mg/kg) in HIV/AIDS-related disseminated histoplasmosis was documented to be non-inferior to the standard therapy with AmB. Besides, a single induction dose

Table 18.3 Regimens of AmB in the treatment of various forms of histoplasmosis

Serial no.	Histoplasmosis variant	Amphotericin B recommendation
1	Diffuse pulmonary histoplasmosis in an immunocompetent host	AmB 0.7 mg/kg/day (or one of the lipid preparations at a dose of 3 mg/kg/day) should be used initially in those patients with more severe manifestations who require ventilatory supportive therapy If AmB is being exclusively used because the patient cannot tolerate treatment with oral medications, a total course of ≤35 mg/kg is recommended, but this situation is expected to be rare
2	Chronic pulmonary histoplasmosis	AmB (0.7 mg/kg/day) is recommended in those patients with ventilatory insufficiency, general debilitation, inability to take itraconazole, inability to achieve detectable concentrations of itraconazole in blood or failure to improve clinically after at least 12 weeks of itraconazole therapy In patients unable to tolerate the dose of AmB, the dose can be reduced to 0.5–0.6 mg/kg/day or one of the lipid formulations may be substituted. If AmB is administered for the full course of therapy, at least 35 mg/kg needs to be given at doses of 0.7 mg/kg three times a week, if tolerated. In case of intolerability, treatment can be switched to itraconazole (200 mg once or twice daily)

(continued)

Table 18.3 (continued)

Serial no.	Histoplasmosis variant	Amphotericin B recommendation
3	Disseminated histoplasmosis in immunocompetent hosts and immunocompromised hosts without AIDS	AmB (0.7 mg/kg/day) is recommended for patients who are sufficiently ill to require hospitalization Most patients respond quickly with AmB and then can be treated with itraconazole. The transition from AmB to itraconazole can occur after the patient becomes afebrile and does not require ventilatory support, intravenous fluids/nutrition and is able to consume oral drugs If AmB is required for the full course, total dosage should be 35 mg/kg given over 2–4 months
4	Patients with AIDS as the cause of immunosuppression	AmB (0.7–1 mg/kg/day) is given for an initial period of 12 weeks (an intensive phase) to induce remission of clinical illness Following the intensive phase, AmB is replaced with itraconazole (200 mg once or twice daily) for the chronic maintenance phase for life, or AmB (0.7 mg/kg IV) once weekly can be used as an alternative, and should only be reserved for those patients who cannot take itraconazole
5	CNS histoplasmosis	AmB (0.7–1 mg/kg/day) to complete a 35 mg/kg total dose over 3–4 months is considered the treatment of choice, followed by fluconazole 800 mg/day for 9–12 months to reduce the risk of relapse Liposomal AmB (3–5 mg/kg/day or every other day) administered over 3–4 months may be given to patients who have failed therapy with AmB, followed by fluconazole Liposomal AmB has been associated with higher concentrations in the blood and brain than d-AmB or other lipid formulations
6	Granulomatous mediastinitis	AmB (0.7–1 mg/kg/day) as an initial therapy followed by itraconazole (200 mg once or twice daily) after sufficient improvement for outpatient treatment

would considerably reduce drug acquisition costs (almost fourfold) and help in simplifying treatment [39]. However, more robust clinical trials are needed to confirm these findings.

Cutaneous Fusariosis

Fusariosis is a complex infection caused by the pathogenic fungus *Fusarium* spp., which is commonly found in soil and water, and transmitted to humans following traumatic inoculation. Based on the host's immune status, the clinical presentation in fusariosis differs. In immunocompetent individuals, localized and superficial symptoms confined to the skin are observed, whereas invasive and disseminated presentations are encountered in immunosuppressed patients. Prolonged periods of neutropenia predispose the development of disseminated fusariosis, which is associated with high mortality [40]. d-AmB (1–1.5 mg/kg/day) in combination with terbinafine (250 mg TID) and subsequent intravenous L-AmB (5 mg/kg/day) has demonstrated efficacy in treating a case of disseminated infection with *Fusarium oxysporum* following chemotherapy for acute myelogenous leukaemia [41]. Further, in a granulocytopaenic patient with myelodysplastic syndrome post peripheral blood stem cell transplant, combination of L-AmB (3 mg/kg/day) and terbinafine (250 mg TID) outlined efficacy in treating fusariosis, following failure with voriconazole [42].

Interestingly, successful combination of voriconazole and AmB in treating a case of disseminated fusariosis in a patient with neutropenic fever has been reported [43].

Although voriconazole still remains the first-line choice of fusariosis at present, some fusarium species like *F. proliferatum* have elucidated low susceptibility to it, which may explain the reason for therapeutic failure with voriconazole [42]. In such scenarios, AmB proves to be a valuable alternative, and if combined with other antifungals, superior outcomes can be expected.

Protothecosis

Human protothecosis is an algal infection due to the environmentally ubiquitous achlorophyllic algae; *Prototheca* spp. Clinically, it presents in three forms: (a) cutaneous lesions, (b) olecranon bursitis and (c) disseminated/systemic infections [44]. Therapy for protothecosis remains debatable, with various treatment regimens being tried. Besides, data for most treatments in protothecosis are drawn from isolated case reports, limited case series and in vitro studies. To add to the conundrum, there are no prospective studies comparing specific treatments for the same.

Among the available treatments, AmB displays the best activity against *Prototheca* spp. For cutaneous lesions, systemic as well as topical use of AmB has been attempted [45]. For olecranon bursitis, intrabursal administration of AmB is suggested in patients ineligible for bursectomy [46]. In systemic disease, intravenous AmB (including liposomal preparations) is considered the drug of choice. The dosing is similar to that used for invasive mycotic infections. Responses to AmB, though, may be variable. Combination therapy with doxycycline, fluconazole, voriconazole and itraconazole may be beneficial in recalcitrant cases [47–51].

Congenital and Neonatal Candidiasis

Congenital candidiasis (CC) is a rare entity, manifesting within the first 6 days of life. It usually occurs following intrauterine candidal infection and maybe localized, involving the skin alone, or have a generalized presentation resulting in respiratory distress and meningitis, with ultimate sepsis and death [52].

Systemic treatment with AmB (0.5–1 mg/kg/day) is the preferred line of management in neonates with disseminated systemic candidiasis, respiratory distress and/or sepsis. Lipid-associated preparations of AmB (3.5 mg/kg/day) are reserved for those cases with invasive candidiasis and severe pre-existing renal insufficiency.

Further, for infections involving the CNS, 5-flucytosine (50–10 0 mg/kg/day) is used in combination with AmB. Currently, no controlled trials exist delineating the exact duration of therapy. However, it is suggested that treatment needs continuation for a minimum of 21–28 days [53, 54].

Genital Candidiasis

Vulvovaginal candidiasis (VVC) is one of the most common infections of the female genital tract [55]. Topical AmB has demonstrated efficacy in the treatment of refractory VVC due to *C. glabrata* and *C. krusei*. In the two reports on *C. glabrata* VVC, AmB 100 mg plus flucytosine 1 g in Aquagel (in a total 8 g dose) was given by a vaginal applicator for 14 nights. Following completion of treatment, all patients outlined significant symptomatic improvement as well as negative cultures for the yeast pathogen [56, 57].

In the publication on *C. krusei* VVC, 3% amphotericin gel (containing d-AmB with Aquagel lubricant gel and propylene glycol) was developed and administered intravaginally for 14 days. Although patient's symptoms resolved after 1 month of therapy, vaginal cultures remained positive [58].

Oral Candidiasis

The use of d-AmB oral suspension has been recommended by the IDSA to treat oral candidiasis refractory to fluconazole [20].

Pityriasis Versicolor

Pityriasis versicolor (PV) is a mild yet chronic superficial cutaneous mycosis caused by *Malassezia* yeasts. Currently, several topical azole compounds constitute the cornerstone of PV therapy [59]. Though never utilized for this indication, lipophilic properties of AmB may contribute towards its favourable effects for the same.

In a comparative study by Ghahartars and colleagues, topical AmB 0.4% was found to be equally effective as clotrimazole 1% in obtaining clinical and mycologic cure for PV [60]. However, based on this anecdotal report, drawing significant conclusions would be unpractical. Therefore, it becomes imperative for robust clinical trials to determine the potential consequences and safety profile for the utility of liposomal topical preparations of AmB in PV.

Onychomycosis

Onychomycosis is an umbrella term encompassing all fungal nail infections. Currently, oral itraconazole and terbinafine are the recommended first-line drugs for onychomycosis [61]. However, owing to adverse effects and concomitant drug interactions, their utility in many individuals may not be suitable, making it mandatory to consider alternative approaches to tackle these issues. In such scenarios, the use of topical antifungal agents proves valuable. Despite their lower potencies and limited on-site penetration, topical therapy for onychomycosis may offer some advantages like (a) better site selectivity, (b) avoidance of systemic adverse effects and (c) easy application at the site of fungal infection. Presently, topical therapy of onychomycosis consists of amorolfine, ciclopirox olamine and azoles, with conflicting outcomes [62].

The role of topical AmB in onychomycosis has recently been exemplified in two reports [63, 64].

In the first report, a topical formulation consisting of 0.3% AmB in 30%. Dimethyl sulfoxide (DMSO) cream (group A, n = 10) was compared with 30% DMSO cream (group B, n = 9) for the treatment of non-dermatophyte onychomycosis. Following 36 weeks of daily treatment, clinical cure was seen in 70% of patients in group A and 22% patients in group B. Besides, mycological cure rates were observed in 80% and 44.4% of patients in groups A and B, respectively [63].

In the second report, topical nanoliposomal AmB 0.4% gel was utilized for treating onychomycosis in 12 patients for a period of 12–36 weeks, wherein the drug was applied twice daily over the entire surface of the affected nails, including a 6 mm margin around the cuticle. At 12 weeks, 50% showed complete clinical cure (CCC), 16.66% outlined an effective clinical response (ECR) and 16.66% denoted a partial clinical response (PCR). Mycological cure (MC) was observed in 50% of patients at week 12. At week 24, CCC and MC were elucidated in 91.66% patients, with 8.33% delineating no response. Besides, apart from temporary nail detachment in one patient, no other adverse events were reported. Notably, in one patient nanoliposomal AmB was effective in attaining CCC of fluconazole-resistant onychomycosis at week 12 [64]. Furthermore, it is documented that the MICs of non-liposomal AmB is lower for *C. albicans*, *C. glabrata*, *T. rubrum* and *F. solani,* making it a potential quasi-efficient alternative for onychomycosis, demanding lower doses and having the advantage of topical use without any off-target systemic side effects [64]. Nevertheless, more studies are essential to strengthen these observations.

Dermatophytosis

Currently, no clinical studies exist on the use of AmB in vivo for dermatophyte infections, although in vitro studies have demonstrated susceptibility testing of dermatophytes to AmB. Interestingly, variable results from these studies have been documented.

Yenişehirli et al. demonstrated terbinafine to be the most effective drug against *T. rubrum* and *T. verrucosum,* followed by AmB. However, for *T. mentagrophytes* and *E. floccosum*, AmB was better than miconazole, ketoconazole and griseofulvin, but inferior to terbinafine and itraconazole [65].

In another evaluation, AmB was inferior to caspofungin and itraconazole but superior to ketoconazole and fluconazole against all dermatophytes tested [66]. Interestingly, Coelho et al. [67] elucidated AmB to be the most superior drug against microconidia of *T. rubrum* and *T. tonsurans* in comparison to fluconazole, terbinafine, itraconazole and griseofulvin. Despite these positive findings, clinical application of this data warrants caution because in vitro susceptibility may not always translate to in vivo efficacy.

Nevertheless, topical AmB may at least in part provide a solution to the annoying issue of recalcitrant dermatophytes. However, it cannot be overlooked that AmB remains the primary drug for invasive life-threatening fungal infections, and it would be prudent to restrict its use only to very specific cases, where it is justified.

Cutaneous Leishmaniasis

Leishmaniasis is a protozoal disease transmitted by sandfly vectors and is endemic in 88 countries, commonly in tropical and subtropical regions. Clinical manifestations of leishmaniasis range from aggressive cutaneous ulcers to systemic multi-organ disease (that constitute visceral leishmaniasis) [68].

Currently, systemic therapy for cutaneous leishmaniasis (CL) is only recommended in old-world CL with mucosal involvement or in patients with complicated cutaneous lesions defined as (i) ≥ 3 lesions, (ii) lesions with diameters>30 mm, (iii) lesions in anatomic locations unsuitable for local treatment and (iv) lesions refractory to local therapy [69, 70].

The common drugs currently employed for systemic therapy in leishmaniasis include pentavalent antimony, AmB, fluconazole and miltefosine. To date, no prospective clinical trials comparing the efficacy of any of these drugs for complicated CL have been conducted, with the choice of therapy relying solely on retrospective case descriptions and case series. d-AmB and lipid-bound AmB products are well-established treatments for visceral leishmaniasis (VL) [71]. However, in complicated CL, there is no clear consensus regarding its systemic use, as well as the optimal dosing schedule. Besides, in this scenario, L-AmB is preferable, owing to reduced nephrotoxicity, and its ability to specifically target macrophages in which leishmania parasites develop [72]. Presently, the dosing schedule stated by the American Society of Tropical Medicine for VL is employed for this indication and consists of intravenous L-AmB (3–4 mg/kg/day) on days 1–5, 10 and 17 and then weekly until healing or a cumulative dose of 40 mg/kg is achieved [73].

Besides, in uncomplicated CL, use of intralesional and topical AmB has demonstrated propitious outcomes (Table 18.4) [74–77]. Moreover, as it is administered locally, the chances of systemic side effects with AmB are minimal. Although spontaneous healing of lesions may occur in uncomplicated CL, treatment is recommended to accelerate cure and reduce scar formation, especially at cosmetically important sites [78].

Table 18.4 Studies outlining the utility of topical and intralesional amphotericin B for uncomplicated cutaneous leishmaniasis

S no.	Authors	Study type	Details	Remarks
1	Goyonlo et al. [74]	Prospective study	93 patients were included in the study Of them, 79 were unresponsive to intralesional meglumine antimoniate AmB deoxycholate diluted with 10 mL distilled water and 0.1–0.3 mL from this solution was again diluted with 2–3 parts of distilled water and injected intralesionally once a week until lesions resolved The average number of injections ranged from 10.31 ± 5.41	Complete remission was seen in 63.5% of patients with urban leishmaniasis, 66.7% with rural leishmaniasis and 54.6% with lupoid leishmaniasis at the end of 12 weeks Partial remission was seen in 20.6% of patients with urban leishmaniasis, 33.3% with rural leishmaniasis and 22.7% with lupoid leishmaniasis at 12 weeks No response was observed in 15.9% patients with urban leishmaniasis and 22.7% patients with lupoid leishmaniasis No recurrence was observed in patients with rural leishmaniasis At <6 months, recurrence was seen in four patients with urban leishmaniasis and two patients with lupoid leishmaniasis At 6–12 months, recurrence was seen in two patients with lupoid leishmaniasis At >12 months, recurrence was observed in two patients with lupoid leishmaniasis Side effects were negligible and did not lead to premature treatment discontinuation in any of the patients
2	Goswami et al. [75]	Prospective study comparing the efficacy of two dosages of intralesional amphotericin B (2.5 mg/mL and 5 mg/mL)	Group A (n = 25) received 2.5 mg/mL of intralesional AmB per week for 8 weeks Group B (n = 25) received 5 mg/mL of intralesional AmB per week for 8 weeks	At the end of 8 weeks, complete response, partial response and no response were seen in 72%, 20% and 8% of patients, respectively, in group A In group B, complete response, partial response and no response at 8 weeks were seen in 56%, 28% and 16% of patients, respectively At the end of 12 weeks, group A patients outlined complete, partial and no response in 88%, 8% and 4% of patients, respectively At the end of 12 weeks, group B patients portrayed complete, partial and no response in 64%, 24% and 12% of patients, respectively Side effect reported was only pain at injection site that did not last for >30 min and did not warrant treatment discontinuation

3	Layegh et al. [76]	Comparative clinical trial evaluating the efficacy of topical liposomal amphotericin B versus intralesional meglumine antimonate for treating cutaneous leishmaniasis	50 patients were given topical liposomal AmB (3–7 drops twice daily for 8 weeks) of which 11 did not adhere ($n = 39$) 60 patients were given intralesional meglumine antimoniate (once weekly, maximum 2 mL for 8 weeks) of which 23 did not adhere ($n = 37$)	At 8 weeks, in the AmB group 56.4% patients achieved clinical cure, whereas 67.6% patients in the meglumine antimoniate group obtained clinical cure Besides, at 6 months of follow-up no recurrence of lesions was reported Side effects were limited to pruritus in the AmB group and erythema and oedema in the meglumine antimoniate group, which were transient and did not demand therapy discontinuation
4	Lopez et al. [77]	An open-label, randomized non-comparative phase Ib/II clinical trial evaluating the efficacy of topical 3% AmB cream for uncomplicated cutaneous leishmaniasis	80 patients were included in the study and allocated 1:1 in two groups ($n = 40$ in each) to receive 3% Amb cream thrice daily for 4 weeks in group A and 3% AmB cream twice daily for 4 weeks	Definite cure at 90 days was seen in 39.4% of patients in group A and 35.3% of patients in group B No adverse events were reported

Post Kala-Azar Dermal Leishmaniasis

Post Kala-azar Dermal Leishmaniasis (PKDL) is a complication of VL characterized by macular, maculopapular and nodular rash in a patient apparently cured, inadequately treated or untreated for VL [79]. L-AmB is the second-line treatment for PKDL in patients where miltefosine is contraindicated [80].

Miltefosine (given at 2.5 mg/kg/day in children and 100 mg/day in adults) further is advantageous over AmB because of its oral route of administration. However, the major disadvantage with miltefosine is its high cost. Besides, d-AmB (dosed at 1 mg/kg for 60–80 infusions) is often associated with nausea, vomiting, fever, rigour and other toxicities accounting for patient non-compliance [81]. To tackle this issue, low-dose d-AmB (0.5 mg/kg/day) for 20 infusions, for three courses, at an interval of 15 days between each course has been attempted with promising results, as well as shortening the duration of hospitalization and minimising drawbacks related to its tolerability [82]. Furthermore, these days, L-AmB is being used for treating PKDL with lesser toxicity compared to d-AmB.

In a randomized open-label study comparing L-AmB versus miltefosine for PKDL, the final cure rate as per protocol analysis was 74.5% and 86.9% for L-AmB and miltefosine, respectively. Further, relapse of PKDL was observed in 25.5% patients in the L-AmB group and 13% patients belonging to the miltefosine group. Besides, none of the patients in both groups developed any serious untoward effects [83].

Interestingly, combination therapy with L-AmB and miltefosine has been assessed for PKDL by Ramesh et al. [80] In their exposition, the above concoction (consisting of three injections of L-AmB 5 mg/kg on days 1, 8 and 15, and capsule miltefosine 100 mg/day for 45 days) was compared with miltefosine monotherapy (for 90 days) and demonstrated rapid decline in parasite load along with 100% clinical cure and no reports of relapse. However, in the miltefosine monotherapy group, although gradual reduction in parasite load and ultimate clinical cure was attained, 25% of patients relapsed at 18 months of follow-up [80]. Given the promising report of this collaboration, more clinical trials are warranted to substantiate the above finding. Moreover, the briefer duration of therapy, along with minimal side effects, encourages further application of this therapy for the treatment of PKDL.

Adverse Effects

In ~80% of patients, infusion-related adverse effects and nephrotoxicity are documented. As AmB interacts with cholesterol in human cell membranes, toxicity is precipitated. Common adverse effects include

- Hypokalaemia, hypomagnesemia and anaphylaxis [84].
- Nephrotoxicity, which correlates with conventional AmB use. However, renal damage is reversible post cessation of AmB. Besides, avoiding concomitant

nephrotoxic drugs and appropriate hydration can reduce the incidence of nephrotoxicity with AmB. Also, liposomal formulations of AmB considerably lower chances of renal toxicity compared to d-AmB. Vasoconstriction of afferent renal arterioles results in decreased renal blood flow and GFR accounting for nephrotoxicity [85].
- Long-term AmB administration is associated with normochromic, normocytic anaemia secondary to low erythropoietin concentrations [86].
- Initial doses of AmB often precipitate, fever, headache cheilitis, hypotension, tachypnoea and vomiting within 2–6 h of transfusion. Transient substernal chest pain and flank pain have also been described, which resolves on discontinuation and administration of intravenous diphenhydramine. This is observed predominantly with d-AmB and ABCD, and rarely with L-AmB and AMLC, and occurs following release of pro-inflammatory cytokines like IL-1β, TNFα, IL-6 and IL-8, after recognition via toll-like receptors and transmembrane signalling protein CD14 [8].
- Cutaneous reactions mainly comprise urticarial reactions and thrombophlebitis at the injection site. Drug rash with eosinophilia and systemic symptoms and cutaneous vasculitis have also been described with L-AmB [8, 87, 88]. The suggested aetiology of urticarial eruptions is liposomal activation of the complement cascade and subsequent release of C3a and C5a [89].
- Rare side effects include new-onset dilated cardiomyopathy with associated heart failure, which subsides within 6 months of treatment discontinuation. Other unusual toxicities include hyperbilirubinemia, elevated hepatic transaminases, pancreatitis and pseudo-hypophosphatemia (observed even with L-AmB) [89].

Use in Special Population

Pregnancy

During pregnancy, AmB should be used only when indicated. According to IDSA guidelines, for invasive candidiasis in pregnancy, AmB is the drug of choice. Further, potential adverse effects on the foetus can be reduced by using the ideal body weight of the mother rather than the total body weight. Also, it would be preferrable to use the liposomal formulation owing to minimal risk of teratogenicity [90].

Lactation

AmB can be used during lactation. Because AmB is (a) highly protein bound, (b) possesses a large molecular weight and (c) is poorly absorbed, the probability of its secretion in breast milk is minimal [91].

Paediatric Patients

All preparations of AmB have been used in children with documented safety and efficacy. However, its usage in neonates still needs elucidation [92].

Geriatric Patients

ABLC given to elderly patients at a dose of 5 mg/kg/day is not associated with significant adverse events [21].

Patients with Renal and Hepatic Impairment

No dose adjustment is needed in patients with renal impairment based on creatinine clearance estimate. L-AmB has been successfully dispensed in patients with pre-existing renal impairment. The effect of L-AmB in patients with hepatic impairment is not known [21].

Storage and Administration

This is elaborated in Table 18.5.

Table 18.5 Storage and administration guidelines for amphotericin B

	AmB deoxycholate	Liposomal AmB
Storage requirements	Stored in dry form at 2–8 °C away from light	Stored in dry form at 2–8 °C away from light
Reconstitution	50 mg vial + 10 mL sterile water, to obtain a solution containing 5 mg/mL	50 mg vial + 12 mL sterile water, to obtain a solution containing 4 mg/mL
Further dilution	With 500 mL of 5% dextrose to obtain 0.1 mg/mL	With 5% dextrose to provide a solution containing: 1–2 mg/mL (adults) 0.2–0.5 mg/mL (infants and children)
Test dose	0.1 mg/kg (not exceeding 1 mg) given by infusion over 20–60 min	0.1 mg/kg (not exceeding 1 mg) given by infusion over 20–60 min
Administration	Infuse over 2–6 h via a distal vein Administer immediately after preparation	Infuse over 2–6 h via a distal vein Administer immediately after preparation
Premedication	For infusion-related reactions: Paracetamol Diphenhydramine Corticosteroids (30 min before infusion)	For infusion-related reactions: Paracetamol Diphenhydramine Corticosteroids (30 min before infusion)

(continued)

Table 18.5 (continued)

	AmB deoxycholate	Liposomal AmB
Monitoring requirements	Daily serum creatinine (as nephrotoxicity is commonly observed) Regular electrolyte monitoring (K^+, Mg^{2+}, Ca^{2+}, PO_4^-) Maintenance of proper hydration For infusion-related reactions (15 min-3 h) Signs of hypokalaemia	Regular electrolyte monitoring (K^+, Mg^{2+}, Ca^{2+}, PO_4^-) Maintenance of proper hydration For infusion-related reactions (15 min-3 h) Signs of hypokalaemia
Dose adjustment	If serum creatinine >2.5 mg/dL: Reduce dose by 50% OR Switch to L-AmB	Based on clinical response
Special consideration	Higher risk of nephrotoxicity Requires careful monitoring of renal function	Better renal tolerance Preferred in patients with/at risk of renal dysfunction
Emergency monitoring	For suspected hypokalaemia (muscle cramps, drowsiness): Immediate ECG Serum K^+ measurement Prompt correction of electrolytes Adequate hydration	For suspected hypokalaemia (muscle cramps, drowsiness): Immediate ECG Serum K^+ measurement Prompt correction of electrolytes Adequate hydration

Drug Interactions

As AmB is not metabolized by the cytochrome P_{450} pathway, documented drug–drug interactions are few. Cyclosporine and tacrolimus used in kidney transplant can increase the toxicity of AmB, with an increased risk of hypokalaemia occurring with concomitant use of digoxin and corticosteroids [93].

Amphotericin B Resistance

Fortunately, AmB resistance is rare compared to other antifungal agents. However, resistance has been encountered. The following mechanisms have been outlined to delineate the same: (a) reduction in polyene-induced oxidative stress, which allows better AmB tolerability and is commonly encountered with *Aspergillus terreus* [94]; (b) an increase in 1,3α-glucan and 1,3β-glucan fraction that leads to an alteration of the fungal cell wall with subsequent AmB resistance and is exhibited in infections with *Aspergillus flavus* and *Candida tropicalis* [95, 96]; and (c) mutation in the ERG genes in various *Candida* spp. that alter the sterol composition of the fungal cell membrane, thereby preventing AmB in producing its antifungal effects [97].

Novel Oral AmB Formulations

To date, oral AmB formulations are at various stages of preclinical development, with some making it to human clinical investigations. The oral AmB lipid-based formulation has been specifically designed to reduce limitations existing with intravenous formulations as per the treatment of systemic mycoses and VL [98].

This formulation consists of a self-emulsifying mixture of monoglycerol oleate, lauroyl polyoxyl-32 glyceride and D-α-tocopherol polyethylene glycol succinate (that serves as a penetration enhancer). Besides, this formulation further stabilizes the less-toxic monomeric form of AmB [98].

Recently, two human phase I clinical studies have been completed. In the phase Ia human clinical study, the primary end point of safety and tolerability of the oral AmB formulation (in capsule form) following administration of all single ascending doses were met, including no signs of kidney, liver and gastrointestinal adversities [99].

In the phase Ib human clinical study, all repeated doses of the oral AmB formulation were well tolerated with no serious adverse events, including no signs of gastrointestinal, renal and hepatic toxicities [99].

Besides, the self-nanoemulsifying drug delivery system was utilized for AmB encapsulation in order to enhance its oral bioavailability [100]. With the above promising findings, oral AmB could revolutionize the management of many of the tropical dermatoses owing to (a) easier administration, (b) reduced toxicity, (c) cost efficacy and (d) the ability to be stored at room temperature.

Conclusion

AmB is a valuable drug for the treatment of many tropical dermatoses. With research going on regarding oral preparations of the drug, its utility could become more widespread owing to the ease of administration.

References

1. Agarwal A, Kar BR. Amphotericin-B in dermatology. Indian Dermatol Online J. 2022;13:152–8.
2. Yang TS, Ou KL, Peng PW, Liou BC, Wang WT, Huang YC, et al. Quantifying membrane permeability of amphotericin B ion channels in single living cells. Biochim Biophys Acta. 2013;1828:1794–801.
3. Pucadyil TJ, Chattopadhyay A. Cholesterol: a potential therapeutic target in Leishmania infection? Trends Parasitol. 2007;23:49–53.
4. Chattopadhyay A, Jafurulla M. A novel mechanism for an old drug: amphotericin B in the treatment of visceral leishmaniasis. Biochem Biophys Res Commun. 2011;416:7–12.
5. Inselmann G, Kutzschbach A, Heidemann HT. Amphotericin B and sodium deoxycholate induced impairment of renal p-aminohippurate accumulation (PAH) and effect on lipid peroxidation in the rat kidney. Ren Fail. 1992;14:17–21.

6. Vertut-Doï A, Ohnishi SI, Bolard J. The endocytic process in CHO cells, a toxic pathway of the polyene antibiotic amphotericin B. Antimicrob Agents Chemother. 1994;38:2373–9.
7. Lee N, Bertholet S, Debrabant A, Muller J, Duncan R, Nakhasi HL. Programmed cell death in the unicellular protozoan parasite Leishmania. Cell Death Differ. 2002;9:53–64.
8. Hamill RJ. Amphotericin B formulations: a comparative review of efficacy and toxicity. Drugs. 2013;73:919–34.
9. De Pauw BE. Increasing fungal infections in the intensive care unit. Surg Infect. 2006;7:S93–6.
10. Miceli MH, Díaz JA, Lee SA. Emerging opportunistic yeast infections. Lancet Infect Dis. 2011;11:142–51.
11. Cifani C, Costantino S, Massi M, Berrino L. Commercially available lipid formulations of amphotericin B: are they bioequivalent and therapeutically equivalent. Acta Biomed. 2012;83:154–63.
12. Stone NR, Bicanic T, Salim R, Hope W. Liposomal amphotericin B (AmBisome®): a review of the pharmacokinetics, pharmacodynamics, clinical experience and future directions. Drugs. 2016;76:485–500.
13. Bekersky I, Fielding RM, Dressler DE, Lee JW, Buell DN, Walsh TJ. Pharmacokinetics, excretion, and mass balance of liposomal amphotericin B (AmBisome) and amphotericin B deoxycholate in humans. Antimicrob Agents Chemother. 2002;46:828–33.
14. Dora CL, Souza LC. New commercial formulations of amphotericin B. Rev Cienc Med Campinas. 2005;14:187–97.
15. Larabi M, Gulik A, Dedieu JP, Legrand P, Barratt G, Cheron M. New lipid formulation of amphotericin B: spectral and microscopic analysis. Biochim Biophys Acta. 2004;1664:172–81.
16. Moen MD, Lyseng-Williamson KA, Scott LJ. Liposomal amphotericin B: a review of its use as empirical therapy in febrile neutropenia and in the treatment of invasive fungal infections. Drugs. 2009;69:361–92.
17. Tiphine M, Letscher-Bru V, Herbrecht R. Amphotericin B and its new formulations: pharmacologic characteristics, clinical efficacy, and tolerability. Transpl Infect Dis. 1999;1:273–83.
18. Andes D, Safdar N, Marchillo K, Conklin R. Pharmacokinetic-pharmacodynamic comparison of amphotericin B (AMB) and two lipid-associated AMB preparations, liposomal AMB and AMB lipid complex, in murine candidiasis models. Antimicrob Agents Chemother. 2006;50:674–84.
19. Jarvis JN, Lawrence DS, Meya DB, Kagimu E, Kasibante J, Mpoza E, et al. Single-dose liposomal amphotericin B treatment for cryptococcal meningitis. N Engl J Med. 2022;386:1109–20.
20. Pappas PG, Kauffman CA, Andes DR, Clancy CJ, Marr KA, Ostrosky-Zeichner L, et al. Clinical practice guideline for the management of candidiasis: 2016 update by the Infectious Diseases Society of America. Clin Infect Dis. 2016;62:e1–50.
21. Noor A, Preuss CV. Amphotericin B. 2024 Feb 28. In: StatPearls [internet]. Treasure Island: StatPearls Publishing; 2024 Jan. Available from: https://www.ncbi.nlm.nih.gov/books/NBK482327/
22. Karthaus M. Leitliniengerechte Therapie der invasiven Aspergillose [Guideline based treatment of invasive aspergillosis]. Mycoses. 2010;53:36–43. German.
23. Bonifaz A, Vázquez-González D, Tirado-Sánchez A, Ponce-Olivera RM. Cutaneous zygomycosis. Clin Dermatol. 2012;30:413–9.
24. Shoham S, Magill SS, Merz WG, Gonzalez C, Seibel N, Buchanan WL, et al. Primary treatment of zygomycosis with liposomal amphotericin B: analysis of 28 cases. Med Mycol. 2010;48:511–7.
25. Chowdhary A, Kathuria S, Singh PK, Sharma B, Dolatabadi S, Hagen F, et al. Molecular characterization and in vitro antifungal susceptibility of 80 clinical isolates of mucormycetes in Delhi, India. Mycoses. 2014;57:97–107.
26. Blyth CC, Gilroy NM, Guy SD, Chambers ST, Cheong EY, Gottlieb T, et al. Consensus guidelines for the treatment of invasive mould infections in haematological malignancy and haemopoietic stem cell transplantation, 2014. Intern Med J. 2014;44:1333–49.

27. Skiada A, Lanternier F, Groll AH, Pagano L, Zimmerli S, Herbrecht R, et al. Diagnosis and treatment of mucormycosis in patients with hematological malignancies: guidelines from the 3rd European Conference on Infections in Leukemia (ECIL 3). Haematologica. 2013;98:492–504.
28. Lowe CD, Sainato RJ, Stagliano DR, Morgan MM, Green BP. Primary cutaneous mucormycosis in an extremely preterm infant successfully treated with liposomal amphotericin B. Pediatr Dermatol. 2017;34:e116–9.
29. Di Pentima MC, Chan S, Powell J, Napoli JA, Walter AW, Walsh TJ. Topical amphotericin B in combination with standard therapy for severe necrotizing skin and soft-tissue mucormycosis in an infant with bilineal leukemia: case report and review. J Pediatric Hematol Oncol. 2014;36:e468–70.
30. Sobel JD. Vaginal mucormycosis: a case report. Infect Dis Obstet Gynecol. 2001;9:117–8.
31. Elgart GW. Chromoblastomycosis. Dermatol Clin. 1996;14:77–83.
32. Tuffanelli L, Milburn PB. Treatment of chromoblastomycosis. J Am Acad Dermatol. 1990;23:728–32.
33. Park SG, Oh SH, Suh SB, Lee KH, Chung KY. A case of chromoblastomycosis with an unusual clinical manifestation caused by Phialophora verrucosa on an unexposed area: treatment with a combination of amphotericin B and 5-flucytosine. Br J Dermatol. 2005;152:560–4.
34. Ranawaka RR. Treatment of chromoblastomycosis with a combination of debulking surgery, intralesional amphotericin B, and oral terbinafine. Int J Dermatol. 2021;60:1040–1.
35. Saccente M, Woods GL. Clinical and laboratory update on blastomycosis. Clin Microbiol Rev. 2010;23:367–81.
36. Ortega-Loayza AG, Nguyen T. Cutaneous blastomycosis: a clue to a systemic disease. An Bras Dermatol. 2013;88:287–9.
37. Chang P, Rodas C. Skin lesions in histoplasmosis. Clin Dermatol. 2012;30:592–8.
38. Wheat J, Sarosi G, McKinsey D, Hamill R, Bradsher R, Johnson P, et al. Practice guidelines for the management of patients with histoplasmosis. Infectious Diseases Society of America. Clin Infect Dis. 2000;30:688–95.
39. Pasqualotto AC, Lana DD, Godoy CSM, Leitão TDMJS, Bay MB, Damasceno LS, et al. Single high dose of liposomal amphotericin B in human immunodeficiency virus/AIDS-related disseminated histoplasmosis: a randomized trial. Clin Infect Dis. 2023;77:1126–32.
40. Marr KA, Carter RA, Crippa F, Wald A, Corey L. Epidemiology and outcome of mould infections in hematopoietic stem cell transplant recipients. Clin Infect Dis. 2002;34:909–17.
41. Rothe A, Seibold M, Hoppe T, Seifert H, Engert A, Caspar C, et al. Combination therapy of disseminated Fusarium oxysporum infection with terbinafine and amphotericin B. Ann Hematol. 2004;83:394–7.
42. Neuburger S, Massenkeil G, Seibold M, Lutz C, Tamm I, le Coutre P, et al. Successful salvage treatment of disseminated cutaneous fusariosis with liposomal amphotericin B and terbinafine after allogeneic stem cell transplantation. Transpl Infect Dis. 2008;10:290–3.
43. Ho DY, Lee JD, Rosso F, Montoya JG. Treating disseminated fusariosis: amphotericin B, voriconazole or both? Mycoses. 2007;50:227–31.
44. Huerre M, Ravisse P, Solomon H, Ave P, Briquelet N, Maurin S, et al. Human protothecosis and environment. Bull Soc Pathol Exot. 1993;86:484–8.
45. Leimann BC, Monteiro PC, Lazéra M, Candanoza ER, Wanke B. Protothecosis. Med Mycol. 2004;42:95–106.
46. Boyd AS, Langley M, King LE Jr. Cutaneous manifestations of Prototheca infections. J Am Acad Dermatol. 1995;32:758–64.
47. Mayhall CG, Miller CW, Eisen AZ, Kobayashi GS, Medoff G. Cutaneous protothecosis. Successful treatment with amphotericin B. Arch Dermatol. 1976;112:1749–52.
48. Torres HA, Bodey GP, Tarrand JJ, Kontoyiannis DP. Protothecosis in patients with cancer: case series and literature review. Clin Microbiol Infect. 2003;9:786–92.
49. Sands M, Poppel D, Brown R. Peritonitis due to Prototheca wickerhamii in a patient undergoing chronic ambulatory peritoneal dialysis. Rev Infect Dis. 1991;13:376–8.

50. Polk P, Sanders DY. Cutaneous protothecosis in association with the acquired immunodeficiency syndrome. South Med J. 1997;90:831–2.
51. Lass-Flörl C, Mayr A. Human protothecosis. Clin Microbiol Rev. 2007;20:230–42.
52. Khambadkone SM, Dixit KM, Divekar A, Joshi SM, Irani SF, Desai M. Congenital candidiasis. Indian Pediatr. 1996;33:512–6.
53. Jagtap SA, Saple PP, Dhaliat SB. Congenital cutaneous candidiasis: a rare and unpredictable disease. Indian J Dermatol. 2011;56:92–3.
54. Aruna C, Seetharam K. Congenital candidiasis. Indian Dermatol Online J. 2014;5(Suppl 1):S44–7.
55. Agatensi L, Franchi F, Mondello F, Bevilacqua RL, Ceddia T, De Bernardis F, et al. Vaginopathic and proteolytic Candida species in outpatients attending a gynaecology clinic. J Clin Pathol. 1991;44:826–30.
56. Shann S, Wilson J. Treatment of Candida glabrata using topical amphotericin B and flucytosine. Sex Transm Infect. 2003;79:265–6.
57. White DJ, Habib AR, Vanthuyne A, Langford S, Symonds M. Combined topical flucytosine and amphotericin B for refractory vaginal Candida glabrata infections. Sex Transm Infect. 2001;77:212–3.
58. Chamorro-de-Vega E, Gil-Navarro MV, Perez-Blanco JL. Treatment of refractory Candida krusei vaginitis with topical amphotericin B. Med Clin (Barc). 2016;147:565–6.
59. Gupta AK, Foley KA. Antifungal treatment for pityriasis versicolor. J Fungi (Basel). 2015;1:13–29.
60. Ghahartars M, Hosseini H, Khedri M, Sadati MS. Comparison of the efficacies of topical liposomal amphotericin B and topical clotrimazole in the treatment of pityriasis versicolor. Dermatol Pract Concept. 2024;14:e2024083.
61. Lipner SR, Scher RK. Onychomycosis: clinical overview and diagnosis. J Am Acad Dermatol. 2019;80:835–51.
62. Gupta AK, Paquet M, Simpson FC. Therapies for the treatment of onychomycosis. Clin Dermatol. 2013;31:544–54.
63. Leeyaphan C, Suiwongsa B, Komesmuneeborirak P, Kiratiwongwan R, Wongdama S, Prasong W, et al. Effectiveness and safety of topical amphotericin B in 30% dimethyl sulfoxide cream versus 30% dimethyl sulfoxide cream for nondermatophyte onychomycosis treatment: a pilot study. Indian J Dermatol Venereol Leprol. 2022;88:494–9.
64. Firooz A, Zamani S, Ghadrei A, Ayatollahi A, Tamimi P, Khamesipour A, et al. Evaluation of efficacy and safety of topical nanoliposomal amphotericin B 0.4% gel as a potential treatment for onychomycosis: an interventional pilot clinical study. Dermatol Ther. 2023;2023:9955124.
65. Yenişehirli G, Tunçoğlu E, Yenişehirli A, Bulut Y. In vitro activities of antifungal drugs against dermatophytes isolated in Tokat, Turkey. Int J Dermatol. 2013;52:1557–60.
66. Aktas AE, Yigit N, Aktas A, Gozubuyuk SG. Investigation of in vitro activity of five antifungal drugs against dermatophytes species isolated from clinical samples using the E-test method. Eurasian J Med. 2014;46:26–31.
67. Coelho LM, Aquino-Ferreira R, Maffei CM, Martinez-Rossi NM. In vitro antifungal drug susceptibilities of dermatophytes microconidia and arthroconidia. J Antimicrob Chemother. 2008;62:758–61.
68. Herwaldt BL. Leishmaniasis. Lancet. 1999;354:1191–9.
69. Blum J, Lockwood DN, Visser L, Harms G, Bailey MS, Caumes E, et al. Local or systemic treatment for New World cutaneous leishmaniasis? Re-evaluating the evidence for the risk of mucosal leishmaniasis. Int Health. 2012;4:153–63.
70. Blum J, Buffet P, Visser L, Harms G, Bailey MS, Caumes E, et al. LeishMan recommendations for treatment of cutaneous and mucosal leishmaniasis in travelers, 2014. J Travel Med. 2014;21:116–29.
71. Minodier P, Retornaz K, Horelt A, Garnier JM. Liposomal amphotericin B in the treatment of visceral leishmaniasis in immunocompetent patients. Fundam Clin Pharmacol. 2003;17:183–8.

72. Musa AM, Khalil EA, Mahgoub FA, Hamad S, Elkadaru AM, El Hassan AM. Efficacy of liposomal amphotericin B (AmBisome) in the treatment of persistent post-kala-azar dermal leishmaniasis (PKDL). Ann Trop Med Parasitol. 2005;99:563–9.
73. Aronson N, Herwaldt BL, Libman M, Pearson R, Lopez-Velez R, Weina P, et al. Diagnosis and treatment of leishmaniasis: clinical practice guidelines by the Infectious Diseases Society of America (IDSA) and the American Society of Tropical Medicine and Hygiene (ASTMH). Clin Infect Dis. 2016;63:e202–64.
74. Goyonlo VM, Vosoughi E, Kiafar B, Nahidi Y, Momenzadeh A, Taheri AR. Efficacy of intralesional amphotericin B for the treatment of cutaneous leishmaniasis. Indian J Dermatol. 2014;59:631.
75. Goswami P, Ghiya BC, Kumar V, Rekha S, Mehta RD. Comparison of efficacy of two different concentrations of intralesional amphotericin B in the treatment of cutaneous leishmaniasis; a randomized controlled trial. Indian Dermatol Online J. 2019;10:627–31.
76. Layegh P, Rajabi O, Jafari MR, Emamgholi Tabar Malekshah P, Moghiman T, Ashraf H, et al. Efficacy of topical liposomal amphotericin B versus intralesional meglumine antimoniate (glucantime) in the treatment of cutaneous Leishmaniasis. J Parasitol Res. 2011;2011:656523.
77. López L, Vélez I, Asela C, Cruz C, Alves F, Robledo S, et al. A phase II study to evaluate the safety and efficacy of topical 3% amphotericin B cream (Anfoleish) for the treatment of uncomplicated cutaneous leishmaniasis in Colombia. PLoS Negl Trop Dis. 2018;12:e0006653.
78. Murray HW, Berman JD, Davies CR, Saravia NG. Advances in leishmaniasis. Lancet. 2005;366:1561–77.
79. Zijlstra EE, Musa AM, Khalil EA, el-Hassan IM, el-Hassan AM. Post-kala-azar dermal leishmaniasis. Lancet Infect Dis. 2003;3:87–98.
80. Ramesh V, Dixit KK, Sharma N, Singh R, Salotra P. Assessing the efficacy and safety of liposomal amphotericin B and miltefosine in combination for treatment of post kala-azar dermal leishmaniasis. J Infect Dis. 2020;221:608–17.
81. Thakur CP, Narain S, Kumar N, Hassan SM, Jha DK, Kumar A. Amphotericin B is superior to sodium antimony gluconate in the treatment of Indian post-kala-azar dermal leishmaniasis. Ann Trop Med Parasitol. 1997;91:611–6.
82. Rabi Das VN, Siddiqui NA, Pal B, Lal CS, Verma N, Kumar A, et al. To evaluate efficacy and safety of amphotericin B in two different doses in the treatment of post kala-azar dermal leishmaniasis (PKDL). PLoS One. 2017;12:e0174497.
83. Pandey K, Pal B, Siddiqui NA, Lal CS, Ali V, Bimal S, et al. A randomized, open-label study to evaluate the efficacy and safety of liposomal amphotericin B (AmBisome) versus miltefosine in patients with post-kala-azar dermal leishmaniasis. Indian J Dermatol Venereol Leprol. 2021;87:34–41.
84. Usami E, Kimura M, Kanematsu T, Yoshida S, Mori T, Nakashima K, et al. Evaluation of hypokalemia and potassium supplementation during administration of liposomal-amphotericin B. Exp Ther Med. 2014;7:941–6.
85. Sawaya BP, Briggs JP, Schnermann J. Amphotericin B nephrotoxicity: the adverse consequences of altered membrane properties. J Am Soc Nephrol. 1995;6:154–64.
86. Vaish E, Gupta KK, Ansari SA, Singh KK. Amphotericin B induced pancytopenia. J Family Med Prim Care. 2022;11:5692–5.
87. Cagatay AA, Taranoglu O, Alpay N, Tufan F, Karadeniz A, Kapmaz M, et al. Amphotericin B-induced cutaneous leucocytoclastic vasculitis: case report. Mycoses. 2008;51:81–2.
88. Hagihara M, Yamagishi Y, Hirai J, Koizumi Y, Kato H, Hamada Y, et al. Drug-induced hypersensitivity syndrome by liposomal amphotericin-B: a case report. BMC Res Notes. 2015;8:510.
89. Groll AH, Rijnders BJA, Walsh TJ, Adler-Moore J, Lewis RE, Brüggemann RJM. Clinical pharmacokinetics, pharmacodynamics, safety and efficacy of liposomal amphotericin B. Clin Infect Dis. 2019;68:S260–74.
90. O'Grady N, McManus D, Briggs N, Azar MM, Topal J, Davis MW. Dosing implications for liposomal amphotericin B in pregnancy. Pharmacotherapy. 2023;43:452–62.

91. Drugs and Lactation Database (LactMed®) [Internet]. Bethesda: National Institute of Child Health and Human Development; 2006. Amphotericin B 2021 Mar 17.
92. Pandey K, Pal B, Siddiqui NA, Rabi Das VN, Murti K, Lal CS, et al. Efficacy and safety of liposomal amphotericin B for visceral leishmaniasis in children and adolescents at a tertiary care center in Bihar, India. Am J Trop Med Hyg. 2017;97:1498–502.
93. Nett JE, Andes DR. Antifungal agents: spectrum of activity, pharmacology, and clinical indications. Infect Dis Clin N Am. 2016;30:51–83.
94. Posch W, Blatzer M, Wilflingseder D, Lass-Flörl C. Aspergillus terreus: novel lessons learned on amphotericin B resistance. Med Mycol. 2018;56:73–82.
95. Seo K, Akiyoshi H, Ohnishi Y. Alteration of cell wall composition leads to amphotericin B resistance in Aspergillus flavus. Microbiol Immunol. 1999;43:1017–25.
96. Mesa-Arango AC, Rueda C, Román E, Quintin J, Terrón MC, Luque D, et al. Cell wall changes in amphotericin B-resistant strains from Candida tropicalis and relationship with the immune responses elicited by the host. Antimicrob Agents Chemother. 2016;60:2326–35.
97. Carolus H, Pierson S, Lagrou K, Van Dijck P. Amphotericin B and other polyenes-discovery, clinical use, mode of action and drug resistance. J Fungi (Basel). 2020;6:321.
98. Wasan E, Mandava T, Crespo-Moran P, Nagy A, Wasan KM. Review of novel oral amphotericin B formulations for the treatment of parasitic infections. Pharmaceutics. 2022;14:2316.
99. Hnik P, Wasan EK, Wasan KM. Safety, tolerability, and pharmacokinetics of a novel oral amphotericin B formulation (iCo-019) following single-dose administration to healthy human subjects: an alternative approach to parenteral amphotericin B administration. Antimicrob Agents Chemother. 2020;64:e01450-20.
100. Kontogiannidou E, Meikopoulos T, Virgiliou C, Bouropoulos N, Gika H, Vizirianakis IS, et al. Towards the development of self-nano-emulsifying drug delivery systems (SNEDDS) containing trimethyl chitosan for the oral delivery of amphotericin B: in vitro assessment and cytocompatibility studies. J Drug Deliv Sci Technol. 2020;56:101524.

5-Flucytosine

19

Introduction

5-Flucytosine (5-FC) is a synthetic antimycotic compound synthesized first in 1957 as a potential anti-tumour agent [1]. However, it was not sufficiently effective against tumours [2]. In 1961, 5-FC demonstrated activity against experimental cryptococcosis in mice [3] and 7 years later it was utilized in treating human candidiasis and cryptococcosis [4]. In addition to its antifungal properties against *Candida* spp. and *Cryptococcus neoformans*, 5-FC is effective against chromoblastomycosis [5]. Though 5-FC has antifungal properties, monotherapy with this agent is limited owing to frequent development of resistance.

Mechanism of Action

5-FC by itself has no antifungal activity. It needs to get converted to 5-fluorouracil (5-FU) to exhibit its antimycotic properties in susceptible fungal cells. Details of the mechanism of action of 5-FC are elucidated in Fig. 19.1 [5–13].

A. K. Bubna, *Therapeutics in Dermatology - Essentials for Clinical Practice*, https://doi.org/10.1007/978-981-95-3791-4_19

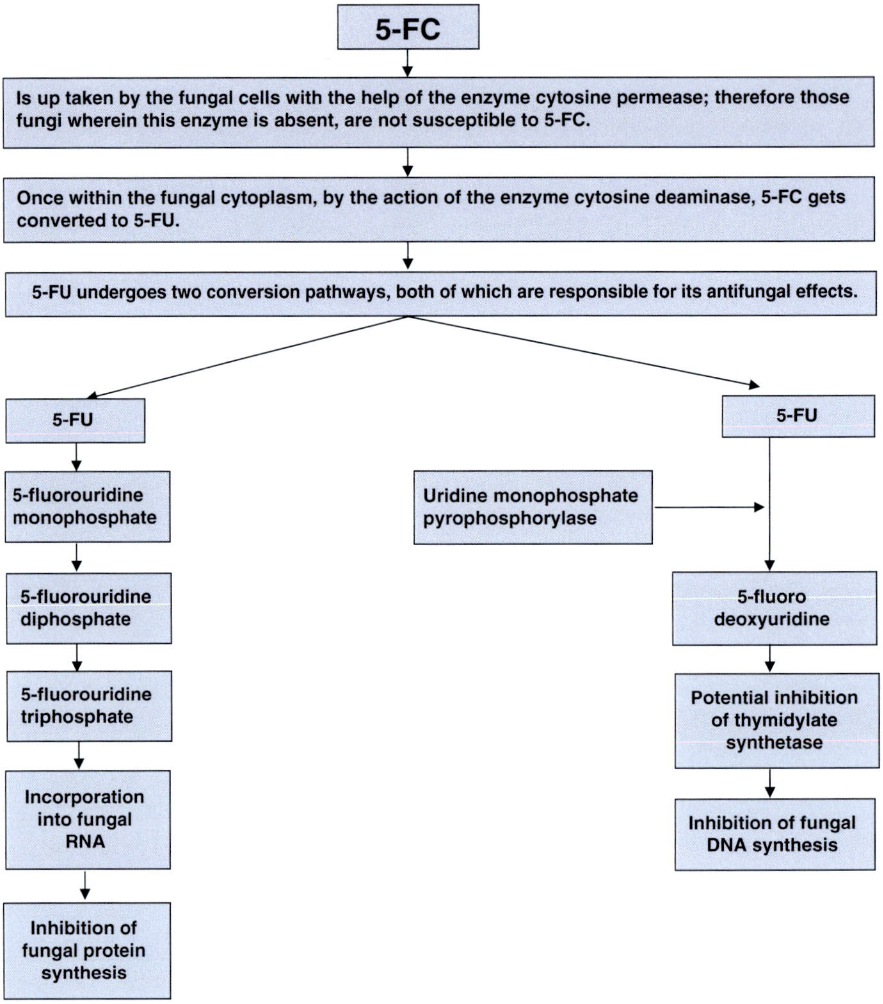

Fig. 19.1 Mechanism of action of 5-flucytosine

Pharmacokinetics

After oral administration, 5-FC is very rapidly and almost completely absorbed with a bioavailability of 76–89% [14]. 5-FC efficiently penetrates into most body sites, including cerebrospinal, vitreous and peritoneal fluids, and into inflamed joints, as 5-FC is a small molecule and is highly water soluble and not bound to serum proteins to a great extent [15]. The $t_{1/2}$ of 5-FC is 3–4 h in patients with normal renal function but can extend up to 85 h in patients with severe renal insufficiency [14]. 5-FC is only minimally metabolized in the liver. Elimination occurs via glomerular filtration in the kidneys [14].

Table 19.1 Dosing guidelines for 5-flucytosine

Criteria	Dosing of 5-flucytosine
Patients with creatinine clearance >40 mL/min	37.5 mg/kg Q6H
Patients with creatinine clearance between 20 and 40 mL/min	37.5 mg/kg Q12H
Patients with creatinine clearance <20 mL/min	37.5 mg/kg once daily
Patients with creatinine clearance <10 mL/min	Frequent determination of 5-FC concentrations should be used as a guidance for dosing frequency

Dosing

The dosing of 5-FC is suggested based on the following guidelines and is elucidated in Table 19.1.

Clinical Uses

Cryptococcosis

5-FC (150 mg/kg/day) combined with amphotericin B (AMB) (0.3 mg/kg/day) administered for 6 weeks has demonstrated efficacy in cryptococcal meningitis with greater superiority compared with AMB alone in non-HIV-infected patients [16]. Some authors have suggested that in non-HIV patients with cryptococcal meningitis, if cerebrospinal fluid (CSF) antigen titre becomes <1:8 along with other favourable prognostic signs, then treatment duration with 5-FC can be shortened to 4 weeks [17].

Van der Horst et al. [18] demonstrated an increased rate of CSF sterilization and reduced mortality 2 weeks following treatment with 5-FC (100 mg/kg/day) in patients with first-episode HIV-associated cryptococcal meningitis who had been earlier treated with high dose of AMB (0.7 mg/kg/day).

Furthermore, combination of 5-FC with fluconazole benefits HIV-infected patients with cryptococcal meningitis [19].

Even so, combination of 5-FC with AMB is found to be effective against large cryptococcal intracerebral masses (cryptococcomas) [20].

Candidiasis

Though monotherapy with 5-FC has been utilized in cases of systemic and disseminated candidiasis in adults, as well as neonates and premature infants, resistance to 5-FC in *Candida* spp. is not rare, and therefore monotherapy of such infections with 5-FC is not recommended [21]. Thus, combination therapy of 5-FC with AMB is preferred, especially for the following types of invasive candidiasis:

- Meningitis
- Hepatosplenic candidiasis
- Endophthalmitis
- Endocarditis
- Peritonitis

Organisms susceptible to this combination include *Candida tropicalis*, *C. parapsilosis*, *C. krusei* and *C. guilliermondii* [21].

Future developments utilizing 5-FC in the treatment of candidiasis lie in its combination with fluconazole and itraconazole. In murine models, 5-FC and itraconazole have demonstrated synergistic effects [22]. Besides, fluconazole and itraconazole combination with 5-FC is equally effective [23].

It is seen that in surgical patients with deep-seated *Candida* mycoses, combination of AMB and 5-FC eliminates fungal organisms more rapidly than fluconazole alone, although cure rates of both groups are similar [24]. However, in patients with *Candida* peritonitis, combination of AMB and 5-FC is more effective in eradicating the infecting yeast [25].

Aspergillosis

In those cases of invasive aspergillosis recalcitrant to AMB, addition of 5-FC to the treatment regimen is often helpful [26]. Pulmonary aspergillosis has been effectively treated with 5-FC monotherapy. However, large comparative trials are lacking.

Chromoblastomycosis

In a small series from the USA and a larger series from Brazil, 5-FC monotherapy has been effective in chromoblastomycosis [26]. Further combination of topical and oral 5-FC demonstrated clinical cure in a patient with chromoblastomycosis by Morison et al. [27]. Another effective combination for chromoblastomycosis includes systemic ketoconazole and 5-FC [28].

Other Mycoses

5-FC has demonstrated efficacy in blastomycosis, coccidioidomycosis, histoplasmosis and sporotrichosis.

Cancer Therapy

5-FC is effective particularly in colorectal cancer. One of the new and promising therapeutic approaches that takes advantage of the effectiveness of 5-FC and minimizes its systemic toxicity is the use of an enzyme/prodrug combination in which 5-FC is combined with *Escherichia coli* gene that encodes the enzyme cytosine deaminase [29]. It is considered that this combination delivers high concentrations of 5-fluorouracil at the tumour site.

Adverse Effects

Gastrointestinal

- Nausea
- Vomiting
- Diarrhoea
- Diffuse abdominal pain

Hepatic

- Elevation of hepatic transaminases

Bone Marrow

- Life-threatening leucopoenia and thrombocytopenia and/or pancytopenia

Pregnancy prescribing status: category 'C'

Drug Interactions

- Cytarabine: completely inhibits the antimycotic activity of 5-FC, so therapy with cytarabine is contraindicated in patients receiving 5-FC [30].
- Zidovudine: as it has myelosuppressive effects, it needs to be used with caution along with 5-FC [31].
- AMB: AMB is highly nephrotoxic and combining with 5-FC can lead to increased 5-FC serum concentrations and $t_{1/2}$ of 5-FC.

Monitoring Guidelines

- Baseline: blood examination to rule out cytopenias and elevated hepatic transaminases.
- Follow-up: blood tests are repeated at monthly intervals till the therapy is on.

If AMB is combined with 5-FC, renal parameters need periodic evaluation also.

Conclusion

5-FC has proven to be a valuable adjunct to AMB in managing a number of systemic mycoses. In this way, it helps reduce the dose of AMB, thereby diminishing its adverse effects.

However, the major limiting factor with 5-FC is its scarce availability in countries with the highest incidence of cryptococcosis. This is highly unfortunate as its availability can play a potential role in reducing mortality rates associated with systemic cryptococcosis.

References

1. Duschinsky K, Pleven E, Heidelberger C. The synthesis of 5-Fluoropyrimidines. J Am Chem Soc. 1957;79:4559–60.
2. Heidelberger C, Griesbach L, Montag BJ, et al. Studies on fluorinated pyrimidines II. Effects on transplanted tumors. Cancer Res. 1958;18:305–17.
3. Grunberg E, Titsworth E, Bennet M. Chemotherapeutic activity of 5-Fluorocytosine. Antimicrob Agent Chemother. 1963;3:566–8.
4. Tassel D, Madoff MA. Treatment of Candida sepsis and Cryptococcus meningitis with 5-Fluorocytosine. A new antifungal agent. JAMA J Am Med Assoc. 1968;206:830–2.
5. Benson JM, Nahata MC. Clinical use of systemic antifungal agents. Clin Pharm. 1988;7:424–38.
6. Bennet JE. Flucytosine. Ann Int Med. 1977;86:319–21.
7. Polak A, Scholer HJ. Mode of action of 5-fluorocytosine. Revue de I' Institute Pasteur de Lyon. 1980;13:233–44.
8. Polak A, Grenson M. Evidence for a common transport system for cytosine, adenine and hypoxanthine in Saccharomyces cerevisiae and Candida albicans. Eur J Biochem. 1973;32:276–82.
9. Polak A, Scholer HJ. Mode of action of 5-Fluorocytosine and mechanisms of resistance. Chemotherapy. 1975;21:113–30.
10. Polak A. 5-fluorocytosine—current status with special reference to mode of action and drug resistance. Contrib Microbiol Immunol. 1977;4:158–67.
11. Bennet JE. Antifungal agents. In: Hardman JG, Limbird LE, Molinoff PB, Ruddon RW, Goodman Gilman A, editors. Goodman and Gilman's the pharmacological basis of therapeutics. 9th ed. New York: McGraw Hill; 1996. p. 1175–90.
12. Scholer HJ. Flucytosine. In: Speller DCE, editor. Antifungal chemotherapy. Chichester: Wiley; 1980. p. 35–106.
13. Waldorf AR, Polak A. Mechanism of action of 5-fluorocytosine. Antimicrob Agent Chemother. 1983;23:79–85.
14. Cutler RE, Blair AD, Kelly MR. Flucytosine kinetics in subjects with normal and impaired renal function. Clin Pharmacol Ther. 1978;24:333–42.
15. Daneshmend TK, Warnock DW. Clinical pharmacokinetics of systemic antifungal drugs. Clin Pharmacokinet. 1983;8:17–42.
16. Bennet JE, Dismukes WE, Duma RJ, et al. A comparison of amphotericin B alone and combined with flucytosine in the treatment of cryptococcal meningitis. New Eng J Med. 1979;301:126–31.
17. Dismukes WE, Cloud G, Gallis HA, et al. Treatment of cryptococcal meningitis with combination of amphotericin B and flucytosine for four as compared to six weeks. New Engl J Med. 1987;317:334–41.
18. van der Horst CM, Saag MS, Cloud GA, et al. Treatment of cryptococcal meningitis associated with the acquired immunodeficiency syndrome. National Institute of Allergy and Infectious Diseases, Mycoses Study Group. New Engl J Med. 1997;337:15–21.

19. Larsen RA, Bozzette SA, Jones BE, et al. Fluconazole combined with flucytosine for the treatment of cryptococcal meningitis in patients with AIDS. Clin Infect Dis. 1994;19:741–5.
20. Lyman CA, Walsh TJ. Systemically administered antifungal agents. A review of their clinical pharmacology and therapeutic applications. Drugs. 1992;44:9–35.
21. Francis P, Walsh TJ. Evolving role of flucytosine in immunocompromised patients: new insights into safety, pharmacokinetics and antifungal therapy. Clin Infect Dis. 1992;15:1003–18.
22. Polak A. combination therapy of experimental candidiasis, crytococcosis, aspergillosis and wangiellosis in mice. Chemotherapy. 1987;33:381–95.
23. Barbaro G, Barbarini G, Di Lorenzo G. Fluconazole vs itraconazole-flucytosine association in the treatment of esophageal candidiasis in AIDS patients. A double-blind multicenter placebo-controlled study. Chest. 1996;110:1507–14.
24. Kujath P, Lerch K, Kochendorfer P, et al. Comparative study of the efficacy of fluconazole versus amphotericin B/flucytosine in surgical patients with systemic mycoses. Infection. 1993;21:376–82.
25. Abele-Horn M, Kopp A, Sternberg U, et al. A randomized study comparing fluconazole with amphotericin B/5-flucytosine for the treatment of systemic candida infections in intensive care patients. Infection. 1996;24:426–32.
26. Patel R. Antifungal agents. Part I. Amphotericin B preparations and flucytosine. Mayo Clin Proc. 1998;73:1205–25.
27. Morison WL, Connor B, Clayton Y. Successful treatment of chromoblastomycosis with 5-fluorocytosine. Br J Dermatol. 1974;90:445–9.
28. Silber JG, Gombert ME, Green KM, et al. Treatment of chromomycosis with ketoconazole and 5-fluorocytosine. J Am Acad Dermatol. 1983;8:236–8.
29. Deonarain MP, Spooner RA, Epenetos AA. Genetic delivery of enzymes for cancer therapy. Gene Ther. 1995;2:235–44.
30. Holt RJ. Clinical problems with 5-fluorocytosine. Mykosen. 1978;21:363–9.
31. Albengres E, Le Louet H, Tillement JP. Systemic antifungal agents. Drug interactions of clinical significance. Drug Saf. 1998;18:83–97.

Echinocandins

20

Introduction

There has been a dramatic increase in fungal infections in the past two decades. Though conventional antifungals were used even in serious infections earlier, many were vulnerable to resistance (like azoles), and others like amphotericin B (AMB) did not demonstrate a favourable toxicity profile.

Echinocandins (ECNs) are a newer and valuable option for managing serious fungal infections, and with their favourable adverse effect profile, a new avenue has opened for treating potentially threatening fungal infections. The drugs in this class include caspofungin (CAS), micafungin (MIF) and anidulafungin (AF).

Mechanism of Action

ECNs affect fungal cell wall biosynthesis through non-competitive inhibition of β 1,3 glucan synthase [1, 2]. In this way, the fungi are unable to synthesize β 1,3 glucan, an important component of fungal cell walls, leading to osmotic instability and ultimately cell death [3].

Pharmacokinetics

All echinocandins have a poor oral bioavailability and therefore require intravenous administration.

A. K. Bubna, *Therapeutics in Dermatology - Essentials for Clinical Practice*, https://doi.org/10.1007/978-981-95-3791-4_20

Caspofungin

CAS is 97% bound to plasma albumin, with a $t_{1/2}$ of 9–11 h. The metabolism of CAS occurs in the liver by peptide hydrolysis and N-acetylation to inactive metabolites [4]. Excretion occurs mainly via the bile, with less than 2% of the drug getting eliminated by the kidneys. The dosage of CAS therefore need not be adjusted in renal insufficiency [4].

Micafungin

More than 99% of MIF is bound to plasma albumin. MIF has a $t_{1/2}$ of 21–22 h. The metabolism of MIF occurs in the liver. Excretion is via the faecal route [5].

Anidulafungin

AF is 84% bound to plasma proteins. The $t_{1/2}$ ranges from 40 to 50 h. Hepatic metabolism has not been observed in AF. Rather, AF undergoes slow chemical degradation at physiologic temperature and pH to a ring-opened peptide that lacks antifungal activity. In vivo it is observed that the opened ring product gets converted to peptide-degraded products and is subsequently eliminated via the faeces [6].

Indications and Dosing Schedule for Echinocandins

The US FDA-approved indications of echinocandins, along with dosing schedule, are elaborated in Table 20.1.

Table 20.1 US FDA-approved and dosing schedule of echinocandins

Drug	Indication	Dosing	Duration
Caspofungin [7]	Oesophageal candidiasis	50 mg intravenously daily	7–21 days
	Candidemia and invasive candidiasis	50 mg intravenously daily	Continue till 14 days after the last positive culture
	Febrile neutropenia	70 mg intravenous loading dose on day 1, followed by 50 mg intravenously daily	Continue till resolution of neutropenia. If fungal infection occurs, then a minimum duration of 14 days is mandatory, with the drug being continued for at least 7 days after resolution of symptoms
	Invasive aspergillosis	70 mg intravenous loading dose on day 1, followed by 50 mg intravenously daily	Based on the severity of the underlying disease
Micafungin [8]	Oesophageal candidiasis	150 mg intravenously daily	10–30 days
	Prophylaxis of haematopoietic stem cell transplant patients	50 mg intravenously daily	6–51 days
	Candidemia	100 mg intravenously daily	10–47 days
	Disseminated candidiasis	100 mg intravenously daily	10–47 days
	Candida peritonitis and abscess	100 mg intravenously daily	10–47 days
Anidulafungin [6]	Oesophageal candidiasis	100 mg intravenous loading dose on day 1, followed by 50 mg intravenously daily	Minimum of 14 days and for at least 7 days following resolution of symptoms
	Candidemia and invasive candidiasis	200 mg intravenous loading dose on day 1, followed by 100 mg intravenously daily	14 days after the last positive culture

Contraindications

Absolute

- Hypersensitivity to the drug.
- Pregnancy: all echinocandins have embryotoxic potential and should be used in pregnancy only if the potential benefit to the mother outweighs the risk to the foetus.

Relative

- Patients developing abnormal liver function tests while on micafungin should be evaluated for the risk/benefit ratio of continued treatment with micafungin [7].

Pregnancy prescribing status: category 'C'.

Adverse Effects

Caspofungin

- Histamine-type reactions like fever and rash
- Infusion-related reactions like phlebitis
- Transient elevations of hepatic transaminase levels
- Headache, nausea and anaemia
- Pulmonary infiltrates and hypercalcemia are two serious drug-related adverse effects that have been reported [4, 9]

Micafungin [10]

- Nausea
- Headache
- Diarrhoea
- Leucopoenia
- Eosinophilia
- Hyperbilirubinemia
- Local thrombophlebitis at the injection site has been reported
- Possible histamine-mediated symptoms and isolated haemolysis and anaphylaxis have been described

Anidulafungin [11]

- Headache
- Flushing
- Nausea
- Dyspnoea

Drug Interactions

Caspofungin

- Co-administration with cyclosporine increases plasma levels of CAS by 35% and can cause transient hepatic transaminase abnormalities [4].
- Concurrent treatment with efavirenz, nelfinavir, phenytoin, dexamethasone, rifampicin and carbamazepine may require an increase in the dose of CAS [4].

Micafungin

- MIF is a mild inhibitor of cyclosporine metabolism; therefore, monitoring cyclosporine levels are prudent when both drugs are simultaneously administered.
- In the presence of steady-state levels of MIF in the circulation, serum concentrations of sirolimus and nifedipine increase by 21% and 18%, respectively. Therefore, in patients receiving sirolimus or nifedipine, together with MIF appropriate, monitoring to detect toxicity secondary to sirolimus and nifedipine is warranted [12, 13].

Anidulafungin

- No significant interactions are seen with AF [14].

Conclusion

Though echinocandins have a broad spectrum of antifungal activity against *Aspergillus* spp. and *Candida* spp., the drug has little or no activity against *Cryptococcus neoformans* or *Mucor* spp. [15] Further, given the high cost of these drugs in comparison to azoles, echinocandins remain more of a reserve drug for most invasive candidal infections and a salvage therapy in azole-resistant invasive aspergillosis.

References

1. Maligie MA, Selitrennikoff CP. Cryptococcus neoformans resistance to echinocandins: (1-3)-β glucan synthase activity is sensitive to echinocandins. Antimicrob Agents Chemother. 2005;49:2851–6.
2. Denning DW. Echinocandin antifungal drugs. Lancet. 2003;362:1142–51.
3. Odds FC, Brown AJ, Gow NA. Antifungal agents: mechanism of action. Trends Microbiol. 2003;11:272–9.
4. Keating GM, Jarvis B. Caspofungin. Drugs. 2001;61:1121–9.
5. Undre N, Pretorius B, Stevenson P. Pharmacokinetics of micafungin in subjects with severe hepatic dysfunction. Eur J Drug Metab Pharmacokinet. 2015;40:285–93.
6. Anidulafungin prescribing information. Pfizer Inc. New York; 2006 February. Available from: www.pfizer.com/pfizer/download/uspi_eraxis.pdf. Accessed on 15 Oct 2007.
7. Caspofungin prescribing information whitehouse station. Merck and Co. Available from: http://www.cancidas.com/caspofungin_acetate/cancidas/hcp/product_information/pi/index.jsp. Accessed on 15 Oct 2007.
8. Micafungin prescribing information. Astellas Pharma US; April 2005. Available from: http://www.mycamine.com/pi.php. Accessed on 15 Oct 2007.
9. Sable CA, Nguyen BY, Chodakewitz JA, et al. Safety and tolerability of caspofungin acetate in the treatment of fungal infections. Transpl Infest Dis. 2002;4:25–30.
10. Chandrasekar PH, Sobel JD. Micafungin: a new echinocandin. Clin Infect Dis. 2006;42:1171–8.
11. Reboli AC, Rostein C, Pappas PG, et al. Anidulafungin study group: anidulafungin versus fluconazole for invasive candidiasis. New Engl J Med. 2007;356:2472–82.
12. Hebert MF, Townsend RW, Austin S, et al. Concomitant cyclosporine and micafungin pharmacokinetics in healthy volunteers. J Clin Pharmacol. 2005;45:954–60.
13. Micafungin(mycamine) for fungal infections. Deerfield: Astellas; 2005.
14. Dowell JA, Stogniew M, Krause D, et al. Assessment of the safety of pharmacokinetics of anidulafungin when administered with cyclosporine. J Clin Pharmacol. 2005;45:227–33.
15. Krishnarao TV, Galgiani JN. Comparison of the in vitro activities of echinocandin LY303366, the pneumocandin MK-0991 and fluconazole against candida species and Cryptococcus neoformans. Antimicrob Agents Chemother. 1997;41:1957–60.

Nikkomycin Z

21

Introduction

Nikkomycin Z (Nik Z) represents a novel class of antifungal drugs derived from *Streptomyces tendae*. This agent has demonstrated activity in mouse models against coccidioidomycosis, histoplasmosis and blastomycosis after oral administration. Compared to conventional antifungal agents (like fluconazole and AMB), Nik Z demonstrates greater killing of *Coccidioides* spp., with the ability to sterilize lung lesions in seven out of eight mice dosed with 50 mg/kg/day for 6 days. Conventional agents, on the other hand, were unable to sterilize lung lesions in all the cases [1–4]. Currently, Nik Z is under development as an orphan product for the treatment of coccidioidomycosis.

Mechanism of Action

Nik Z inhibits the enzyme chitin synthase, an enzyme, present in fungal cell walls responsible for catalyzing the synthesis of chitin. Owing to this blockage, chitin, an essential component of fungal cell walls, is not produced, culminating in fungal cell death [5, 6].

Pharmacokinetics

Nik Z is well absorbed after oral administration, with a median T_{max} ranging from 2 to 4 h. Bioavailability of Nik Z has been found to be dose dependant. The mean terminal half-life for Nik Z ranges from 2 to 2.5 h. Nik Z exhibits linear pharmacokinetics. Elimination of Nik Z is via the kidney [7].

A. K. Bubna, *Therapeutics in Dermatology - Essentials for Clinical Practice*,
https://doi.org/10.1007/978-981-95-3791-4_21

Special Consideration

Recently, Nik Z received orphan drug status for its development as a treatment for coccidioidomycosis. In the past, this drug showed promise against thermally dimorphic fungi, including *Coccidioides immitis, Histoplasma capsulatum* and *Blastomyces dermatitidis* [4]. However, clinical development of this drug was terminated due to difficulties in production. The drug was relicensed to the University of Arizona, allowing for re-institution of clinical development. Nik Z is currently being tested in phase 1 and 2 clinical trials for the treatment of coccidioidomycosis.

Adverse Effects [7]

- Headache
- Dizziness
- Upper respiratory tract infections
- Vasodilation
- Haematoma
- Tooth ache
- Ear ache

Conclusion

Renewed interest in Nik Z reflects momentum exploring fungal cell walls as an antifungal target in general. This fungal-specific cellular feature makes for an ideal target for less toxic antifungal drug development [8].

References

1. Clemons KV, Stevens DA. Efficacy of nikkomycin Z against experimental pulmonary blastomycosis. Antimicrob Agents Chemother. 1997;41:2026–8.
2. Goldberg JP, Connolly C, Schnizlein-Bick M, et al. Comparison of nikkomycin Z with amphotericin B and itraconazole treatment of histoplasmosis in a murine model. Antimicrob Agents Chemother. 2000;44:1624–9.
3. Graybill JR, Najvar LK, Bocanegra R, et al. Efficacy of nikkomycin Z in the treatment of murine histoplasmosis. Antimicrob Agents Chemother. 1998;42:2371–4.
4. Hector RF, Zimmer BL, Pappagianis D. Evaluation of nikkomycin X and Z in murine models of coccidioidomycosis, histoplasmosis and blastomycosis. Antimicrob Agents Chemother. 1990;34:587–93.
5. Obi K, Uda J, Iwase K, et al. Novel nikkomycin analogues: inhibitors of the fungal cell wall biosynthesis enzyme chitin synthase. Bioorg Med Chem Lett. 2000;10:1451–4.
6. Ruiz-Herrera J, San-Blas G. Chitin synthesis as a target for antifungal drugs. Curr Drug Targets Infect Disord. 2003;3:77–91.

7. Nix DE, Swezey RR, Hector R, et al. Pharmacokinetics of nikkomycin Z after single rising oral doses. Antimicrob Agents Chemother. 2009;53:2517–21.
8. Pianalto KM, Alspaugh JA. New horizons in antifungal therapy. J Fungi. 2016;2:26.

Part IV

Systemic Steroids

Systemic Steroids 22

Introduction

The 1951 report by Sulzberger et al. [1] that described the utility of cortisone and Adrenocorticotropic hormone (ACTH) in a variety of inflammatory dermatoses radically changed the therapeutic approach in managing a number of steroid-responsive dermatoses. Today, various corticosteroid molecules form the cornerstone in treating numerous dermatologic disorders, and their significance in the dermatologic armamentarium is immense. Yet, despite its advantages in dermatologic therapeutics, a number of adverse effects encountered make it imperative for the treating dermatologist to be familiar with these events and be able to appropriately tackle them. Structurally, the basic unit of any steroid molecule consists of the cyclo-pentano-perhydro-phenanthrene nucleus. Changes in the side chains give rise to different corticosteroid (CS) molecules.

Classification

Systemic corticosteroids (SCs) are classified based on their duration of action, namely short acting, intermediate acting and long acting. Details of this are elaborated in Table 22.1 [2–4].

A. K. Bubna, *Therapeutics in Dermatology - Essentials for Clinical Practice*, https://doi.org/10.1007/978-981-95-3791-4_22

Table 22.1 Classification of systemic corticosteroids

Corticosteroid molecule	Equivalent dose (mg)	Glucocorticoid potency	Mineralocorticoid potency	Plasma half-life (min)	Biologic half-life (h)
Short acting					
Cortisone	25	0.8	2+	30–90	8–12
Hydrocortisone	20	1	2+	60–120	8–12
Intermediate acting					
Prednisone	5	4	1+	60	24–36
Prednisolone	5	4	1+	115–212	24–36
Methyl prednisolone	4	5	0	180	24–36
Triamcinolone	4	5	0	78–188	24–36
Long acting					
Dexamethasone	0.75	20–30	0	100–300	36–54
Betamethasone	0.6–0.75	20–30	0	100–300	36–54

Mechanism of Action

Various mechanisms of SCs are documented. Prior to producing its effects, all steroid molecules bind to glucocorticoid receptors (GCRs) and bring about conformational changes, following which various effects are produced, as highlighted in Fig. 22.1.

Effect on Transcription Factors

Nuclear Factor κB

Nuclear factor κB (NFκB) is a biologically inactive compound as long as it is bound to IκB (inhibitor κB). If IκB is degraded, then NFκB gets released and induces transcription of various inflammatory cytokines like IL-1β, IL-2, IL-8, TNFα and adhesion molecules like ICAM-1 and E-selectin.

The SC-GCR complex can directly bind to NFκB and inhibit its activity. Further, the SC-GCR complex increases levels of IκB, thereby preventing elevation of free levels of NFκB [5, 6].

Activator Protein 1

SCs inhibit activator protein (AP)-1 activation and DNA binding, facilitating reduction in the expression of various inflammatory cytokines similar to the ones released by NFκB [7].

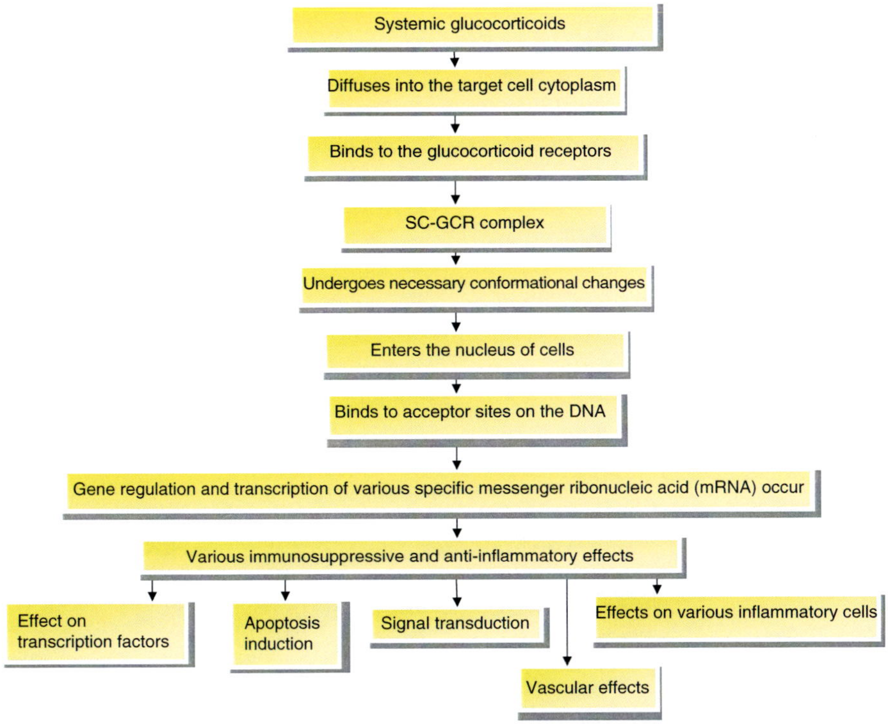

Fig. 22.1 Initial steps of corticosteroid molecules in the cells to ultimately promote their therapeutic effects

Induction of Apoptosis

Apoptosis is an orderly process of programmed cell death that occurs within an intact plasma membrane despite nuclear fragmentation. SCs can bring about this process in lymphocytes and eosinophils [8].

For lymphocytes, apoptosis is brought about in auto-reactive T cells (for autoimmune diseases) and neoplastic T cells (for lymphomas). This may be a direct process or an indirect one via down-regulation of CD3 molecules expressed on T lymphocytes [9]. For eosinophils, it is likely that SCs act by suppression of cytokines essential for cellular survival, and this has potential implications regarding allergic disorders [8].

Signal Transduction

SCs via an indirect effect on lipocortin-1 inhibit phospholipase A2. As a result of this antagonism, production of various prostaglandins, leukotrienes, 12-HETE and 15-HETE inflammatory mediators is reduced. Also, SCs inhibit cyclo-oxygenase 2.

Vascular Effects

SCs reduce angiogenesis in wound healing as reported with proliferative lesions like haemangiomas.

This occurs secondary to vasoconstriction and potentiation of responses to circulatory catecholamines. Further, SCs decrease vascular smooth muscle responses to histamine and bradykinin, reducing vascular permeability.

Effects on Various Inflammatory Cells

- B cells: reduced production of immunoglobulins.
- T cells: reduced IL-2 production and resultant reduced amplification effects.
- Reduced natural killer (NK) cell activity.
- Reduced antibody-dependent cellular cytotoxicity mediated by NK cells.
- Neutrophils: reduced margination and chemotaxis.
- Mast cells: inhibition of degranulation with resultant reduction of release of histamine, kinins and other inflammatory mediators.
- Langerhans cells: impairment of antigen processing and presentation.
- Monocytes and macrophages: reduced access to inflammatory sites and diminution of release of IL-1 and IFN γ from these cells.
- Fibroblasts: decreased production of collagen, ground substance, fibronectin and collagenase.

Pharmacokinetics

Exogenous corticosteroids are absorbed in the upper jejunum [10]. Their affinity to bind to cortisol-binding globulin (CBG) is minimal, allowing a greater free fraction of exogenous corticosteroids to be available. Compared to other synthetic corticosteroids, prednisolone has the greatest affinity towards CBG, with resultant potential for displacement of endogenous cortisol from protein-binding sites.

In conditions like hypothyroidism, liver disease, renal disease and obesity where there is a reduction in CBG, an increased amount of both endogenous and synthetic corticosteroids free fraction results [11], Also, when high-dose and prolonged SCs are used, there typically occur an increase in the free fraction of corticosteroids. Further, in conditions like pregnancy, hyperthyroidism and where oestrogen therapy is administered, CBG increases with reduction in free fractions of both endogenous and exogenous corticosteroids.

Corticosteroids are distributed widely in most body tissues, including foetal tissue, except for prednisone, which does not reach the foetal tissue. The metabolism of corticosteroids occurs in the liver as well as extrahepatic sites. The double bond at the 4,5 position of the steroid nucleus is reduced both hepatically and extrahepatically, resulting in an inactive product [12]. Reduction of the 3-ketone substituent to form tetrahydro cortisol, however, occurs only in the liver [12]. The metabolites produced are water soluble and undergo renal excretion.

It needs to be noted that cortisone gets converted to hydrocortisone and prednisone to prednisolone in the liver by the action of 11β hydroxy dehydrogenase enzyme, and severe hepatic impairment may compromise this conversion. Therefore, administering prednisolone in this setting will be appropriate. Further, liver disease is associated with reduced serum albumin, which leads to an increase in the available free fraction of corticosteroids.

Clinical Uses

Pemphigus Vulgaris

The best studied purely dermatologic indication for SC therapy is pemphigus vulgaris (PV) and is approved by the US FDA for this indication. SCs are appropriate at the start of therapy for any relatively severe case of PV that has no absolute contraindications for their use.

Currently, management of PV includes prednisolone not more than 2 mg/kg/day in divided doses. Usually, in these cases, it is best to start with prednisolone 1 mg/kg/day and increase to 2 mg/kg/day in selective cases of more severe PV. Control of disease is noticed by 1–2 months. Once the disease is adequately controlled, steroids need to be tapered gradually. Steroid-sparing immunosuppressive drugs can be added at the start of therapy or when steroid tapering begins. For more severe cases, it is best to introduce steroid-sparing immunosuppressive agents at the start of treatment [13–15]. Currently, at many centres in India, pulse therapy with methylprednisolone or dexamethasone, along with cyclophosphamide, is being used to treat PV. Details of this are elaborated in the chapter on steroid pulses in dermatology.

Bullous Pemphigoid

Management of bullous pemphigoid (BP) with SCs is approved by the US FDA in those cases that present with widespread involvement. The initiating dose of prednisolone in BP ranges from 0.5 to 1 mg/kg/day [16].

However, as the nature of the disease is heterogeneous, doses need to be individualized for cases presenting with generalized blisters in BP. Once the disease activity is controlled (which generally takes 2–4 weeks), tapering of SCs can be started. By 1–2 months, a physiologic dose range of SCs can be achieved. Treatment with SCs may need continuation for 3–6 months or less. If BP persists beyond this point, then non-steroidal immunosuppressive agents become the major mode of therapy.

Special care must be taken while managing BP in the elderly population. A thorough search to rule out an internal malignancy is essential. Besides, an increased risk of sepsis using high-dose steroids needs to be kept in mind while dealing with these patients, and utilizing alternative therapeutic agents can help in reducing this complication [17].

Cicatricial Pemphigoid

Overall, cicatricial pemphigoid (CP) is less responsive to SCs than BP [16]. In general, 1–1.5 mg/kg/day of prednisolone is required for initially controlling moderate to severe cases.

Consultation with an ophthalmologist is necessary in every case with ocular involvement. Aggressive management is important for ocular involvement, owing to significant potential for blindness. Early diagnosis, moderately aggressive therapy and subsequent mucous membrane grafting by an experienced oculoplastic surgeon are key elements in treating CP. Immunosuppression needs to be carried out at least 3 months prior to the grafting procedure; otherwise, results can be deleterious [18]. Combination of cyclophosphamide with SCs is of particular value in patients with sight-threatening ocular involvement [19].

Lupus Erythematosus

Despite SCs showing rapid and distinctive effects in lupus erythematosus (LE), its use should be limited to patients with cutaneous LE who have highly acute and severe skin lesions.

Some of the indications of SCs in cutaneous LE include (a) LE patients with cutaneous vasculitis, (b) bullous LE and (c) widespread disfiguring discoid LE [20, 21]. In addition, SCs can be administered along with antimalarials because of the delayed onset of action associated with hydroxychloroquine and chloroquine.

The usual dose of SCs in LE is 0.5–1 mg/kg/day over 2–4 weeks followed by dose tapering. Another treatment schedule utilized is the 3-day intravenous (IV) pulse utilizing 1gm of methylprednisolone. In refractory cases of subacute cutaneous LE, lesions have demonstrated clearance within 1–2 weeks of a single IV pulse with methylprednisolone, with the effect being sustained for 3 months [22].

In LE panniculitis, SCs are initially administered with antimalarials to prevent lipoatrophy.

Long-term therapy with SCs in CLE should however be avoided [23].

Dermatomyositis

Although the efficacy of SCs in dermatomyositis (DM) is not established in controlled trials, they are generally accepted as the initial treatment of choice in DM. Around 90% of patients respond to prednisolone at a dose of 1–1.5 mg/kg/day. The dose is adjusted based on the levels of muscle enzymes and quality of muscle strength.

Co-management with either a rheumatologist or a neurologist is appropriate when there is significant muscle disease. When indicated, SCs are often successful as monotherapy [24, 25]. Here, SCs are tapered gradually as improvement in the disease process begins to set in. Frequently, adjunctive therapy with azathioprine (AZA) and methotrexate (MTX) is found to be beneficial in DM.

Vasculitis

In most cases of cutaneous leukocytoclastic vasculitis (LCV), treatment with dapsone and colchicine is sufficient to bring about remission. In cases where response is not witnessed, low-dose prednisolone (10 mg/day) can be added as a second-line drug which can help in alleviating symptoms [26].

However, in certain situations, SCs may need to be started as a first-line agent and include (a) LCV associated with severe ulceration/necrotic cutaneous lesions, (b) gastrointestinal bleeding, (c) acute glomerulonephritis and (d) peripheral neuropathy with impending palsy. In these situations, initiating treatment with high-dose prednisolone (60–80 mg/day) tapered over several weeks is recommended [27].

In children with Henoch–Schönlein purpura (HCP), if SCs are administered at presentation, the risk of developing nephritis is prevented. Further, if SCs are combined with other immunosuppressive drugs, the outcome of existing nephritis improves [28].

In patients with cutaneous polyarteritis nodosa (PAN), high-dose SCs are often required along with aspirin/non-steroidal anti-inflammatory drugs (NSAIDs) to bring about disease control. Once adequate response is obtained, SCs are then gradually tapered [29].

In classic PAN, SCs with or without cyclophosphamide are useful in bringing about disease control. However, in those cases where hepatitis B virus is the proposed aetiologic agent, then therapy with SCs should be short term to prevent risk of viral replication [30].

Short-term SCs (0.5–1.5 mg/kg/day) are also used to treat renal and central nervous system (CNS) manifestations of HCV-associated cutaneous vasculitis [31].

In Wegener's granulomatosis (WG), microscopic polyangiitis and Churg–Strauss syndrome, high dose of prednisolone (1 mg/kg/day) is the initial therapeutic option. Also, IV pulse therapy with methylprednisolone (1 g/day for 3 days) can be administered to patients with life-threatening organ involvement [32].

In Kawasaki's disease, however, SCs are relatively contraindicated to avoid the risk of coronary artery aneurysm formation [32].

Pyoderma Gangrenosum

Prednisolone at a dose of 1 mg/kg/day is useful in quickly attaining disease control in pyoderma gangrenosum (PG), following which dapsone is utilized for long-term maintenance therapy. For unusually severe cases of PG, IV pulse methylprednisolone has been shown to be of benefit [33, 34]. In less severe cases, however, bursts of moderate doses of prednisolone are effective [35]. In general, 40–60 mg of daily prednisolone tapered over 1 month to low-dose alternate-day therapy is successful as initial therapy. In children, prednisolone is frequently utilized for a relatively brief period [36].

Lichen Planus

Prednisolone given at 40–60 mg daily and tapered over 4–6 weeks consistently eradicates or reduces the intensity of generalized lichen planus (LP). Ideally, the regimen should reach a physiologic dose range within 3–4 weeks. For severe oral erosive LP, low-to-moderate-dose SC therapy is mandated [37, 38]. As oral LP is notorious for its chronicity, low doses of SCs may need to be continued for a longer time period. LP is an appropriate indication for even briefer bursts of SC therapy [39].

Acute Dermatitis

Severe acute contact dermatitis due to poison ivy/poison oak is a classic situation in which a 2–3-week burst of SC therapy is usually successful at minimal risk to the patient [40]. Cases with widespread cutaneous involvement, including the face, treated early in their course. Typically respond rapidly. Doses up to 1 mg/kg/day (generally 40–60 mg/day) of prednisolone, tapered over 2–3 weeks yield adequate improvement with a minimal risk of rebound flare after cessation of therapy. A single approach that is easy to follow involves 5 days each of 60, 40 and 20 mg of prednisolone. Acute flares of chronic atopic eczema, nummular dermatitis or contact dermatitis can be managed in a similar fashion [41, 42]. Maintenance SCs are best avoided in these settings.

Sarcoidosis

SCs are indicated in cases of ulcerative sarcoidosis and in those cases where sarcoidosis presents with aggressive facial involvement as seen in lupus pernio [43, 44]. Otherwise, use of SCs in cutaneous sarcoidosis alone is rarely justified. Children with cutaneous features in addition to systemic findings predictably respond to SC therapy [45].

Androgen Excess Syndrome

For hirsutism and recalcitrant acne vulgaris secondary to elevated adrenal androgens (most commonly mild DHEA-S elevations), a suppressive night-time therapy with dexamethasone (0.125–0.375 mg) or prednisolone (5 mg) can be advocated. This timing is important as it suppresses the early morning peak of ACTH which stimulates production of adrenal androgens.

A reasonable approach will be to start dexamethasone 0.125 mg nightly with a repeat laboratory testing of adrenal androgens 2 months later. If the test result has not normalized, dose of dexamethasone can be increased up to a maximum dose of 0.375 mg. Laboratory testing is once again repeated after 2 months of the dose increment [46, 47].

Steven–Johnson Syndrome and Toxic Epidermal Necrolysis

Traditionally, SCs have remained the mainstay of therapy of Steven–Johnson syndrome (SJS) and toxic epidermal necrolysis (TEN) in most centres. The rationale for use is that both conditions are immune-mediated processes and corticosteroids suppress the intensity of inflammation, prevent/decrease skin necrolysis, reduce fever and discomfort, as well as prevents damage to internal organs, when given at an early stage in sufficiently high dosage [48–53].

Most authors agree that SCs are useful when started at an early stage of the disease. SCs are effective in controlling the disease process as well as recovery if started preferably within 3 days (maximum up to 7 days) from the onset of TEN in resource-poor settings [54]. Further, SCs in the initial phase of disease continue to be lifesaving drugs in developing countries like India.

However, if administration of SCs is delayed beyond 7 days, then instead of its beneficial effects, it can impair wound healing and promote sepsis. Therefore, after this duration it is best to avoid usage of SCs. This makes timing with regard to SCs administration in TEN very important [55]. The dosing, duration and route of administration of SCs in SJS/TEN still remain an open debate. Tapering SCs over 7–10 days to as long as 4 weeks is the regimen usually followed [56, 57]. Advocates of SCs recommend administration of a high dose (regardless of route) early in the course of the disease for a short period of time [58].

Table 22.2 elucidates various studies employing the usage of SCs in SJS/TEN [54, 55, 59–65].

Erythema Multiforme Minor

SCs is employed in recurrent oral erythema multiforme (EM) minor [66]. Painful oral erosions respond promptly to prednisolone in doses up to 1 mg/kg/day, rapidly tapered over 2–3 weeks. For recurrent cases, clinicians should also consider acyclovir, valacyclovir and famciclovir on a long-term daily basis, particularly if herpes simplex virus is proved or is strongly suspected to be the causative agent of recurrent EM.

Table 22.2 Summary of corticosteroid studies in Steven–Johnson syndrome and toxic epidermal necrolysis

Author(s)	Type of study	Patients receiving corticosteroids	Dose of corticosteroids	Mortality	Level of evidence	Remarks
Schulz et al. [59]	Retrospective non-controlled case series	(TEN)—34	Not clearly mentioned	13/34	II	Steroid exposure not associated with an increase in mortality
Tripathi et al. [60]	Retrospective non-controlled case series	(SJS)—67	Methylprednisolone 160–240 mg daily; tapered when clinical response seen (no mean duration given)	1/67 (mortality was not related to SJS)	II	All patients had a favourable outcome and there was no mortality or permanent sequelae related to SJS
Kim et al. [61]	Retrospective non-controlled case series	TEN—21	Methylprednisolone 250–1000 mg daily; later switched to oral prednisolone	6/21	III	The authors concluded that the low mortality rate compared with previous studies may be a result of the high rates of steroid use and therefore suggested that steroid therapy should be used early
Kardaun and Jonkman [55]	Retrospective non-controlled case series	SJS—1 SJS-TEN overlap—4 TEN—7	First four patients: IV dexamethasone 100 mg once daily for 3 days +500 mg cyclophosphamide Subsequent patients: 1.5 mg/kg IV dexamethasone for 3 days	1/12	III	The authors concluded that short-term dexamethasone pulse therapy given at an early stage of the disease may contribute to a reduced mortality rate in SJS/TEN without increasing healing time
Schneck et al. [62]	Retrospective multicentre non-controlled case series	SJS—57 SJS-TEN overlap—44 TEN—18	Maximum steroid dose 250 mg prednisolone equivalent given for a median of 4 days (2–12 days)	21/119	II	The authors concluded that there was inadequate evidence that any specific treatment is established as effective for patients with SJS or TEN with only corticosteroids showing a trend for possible benefit

Hirahara et al. [63]	Retrospective non-controlled case series	SJS—3 SJS-TEN overlap—2 TEN—3	1000 mg IV methylprednisolone for 3 days	0/8	III	There was no mortality in spite of the SCORTEN-predicted mortality being 1.6 A decrease in proinflammatory cytokines was also noted
Pasricha et al. [64]	Retrospective non-controlled case series	TEN—5	IV dexamethasone 16–24 mg/day, tapered and withdrawn within 7–10 days	0/5	III	The authors concluded that corticosteroids used in appropriate doses ensure early recovery
Das et al. [54]	Prospective non-controlled case series	TEN—18	Injection dexamethasone (1 mg/kg/day till erythema subsided) tapered and withdrawn within 5 days after subsidence of erythema	0/18	II	Two other patients were given IVIG in a total dose of 2 g/kg (0.4 g/kg/day for 5 consecutive days), both of whom survived The authors opined that systemic corticosteroids in the initial phase of TEN are lifesaving drugs
Rai and Srinivas [65]	Retrospective non-controlled case series	TEN—3	Injection dexamethasone 100 mg for 2 days (two patients) or 4 days (one patient) followed by cyclosporine 2 mg/kg/day (tapered 50 mg every third day and stopped after 2 weeks)	0/3	III	The authors concluded that the combination of initial high dose of steroids and subsequent cyclosporine is a safe alternative

IV intravenous, *IVIG* intravenous immunoglobulin, *SCORTEN* severity of illness score for toxic epidermal necrolysis, *SJS* Stevens–Johnson syndrome, *TEN* toxic epidermal necrolysis

Post-herpetic Neuralgia

Prevention of post-herpetic neuralgia (PHN) is a controversial area of SC therapy. An early study by Eaglstein did suggest that moderate-dose therapy with SCs minimizes the risk of PHN [67]. However, recent evidence suggests that SCs may have a better role in treating acute pain of herpes zoster, rather than preventing PHN [68].

Other Indications

- Epidermolysis bullosa acquisita
- Linear IgA bullous dermatosis
- Herpes gestationis
- Behcet's disease
- Sweet's syndrome
- Severe urticaria (short-term therapy)

Contraindications

Absolute

- Systemic fungal infection
- Herpes simplex keratitis
- Hypersensitivity (primarily occurs with ACTH, occasionally noted with IV preparations)

Relative

- Cardiovascular: hypertension and congestive cardiac failure.
- Neurologic: severe psychosis and depression.
- Gastrointestinal: active peptic ulcer disease, recent anastomosis and active diverticulitis.
- Infections: active tuberculosis and positive tuberculin skin test.
- Metabolic: diabetes mellitus.
- Musculoskeletal: osteoporosis.
- Ocular: cataracts and glaucoma.

Pregnancy prescribing status: category 'C'.

Adverse Effects

Potentially Fatal Complications

When SCs are prescribed for dermatologic indications, it is unusual to have fatal complications. Drug-induced fatalities in older studies using SCs (with or without other immunosuppressive agents) for PV are a noteworthy exception of historical significance and include

- Adrenal crisis (Addisonian crisis): In the current era, this complication is extraordinarily rare. When in doubt, err on the side of prescribing stress CS dose when indicated [69, 70].
- Bowel perforation: Tremendous caution needs to be exercised with prescribing SCs after recent bowel anastomoses and for patients with active diverticulitis [71, 72].
- Peptic ulcer perforation: This complication is most likely with adjunctive non-steroidal anti-inflammatory drugs (NSAIDs) and in patients who have a history of peptic ulcer disease (PUD) [73].
- Pancreatitis: This complication has been documented in patients with triglycerides >800 mg/dL. The clinician needs to promptly intervene with any report of severe abdominal pain in patients who are on SCs [74].
- Severe hyperglycaemia (diabetic ketoacidosis or hyperosmolar non-ketotic coma): This complication is generally associated with pre-existing diabetes mellitus, although it can occur occasionally de novo [75].
- Opportunistic infections: These infections are distinctly uncommon with SCs used for dermatologic indications and occur primarily with multidrug immunosuppression regimens for systemic autoimmune disorders and organ transplantation [76, 77].
- Immunosuppressive malignancies: These include Kaposi's sarcoma, non-Hodgkin's lymphoma and squamous cell carcinoma which are more commonly encountered in organ transplantation patients administered SCs, rather than in patients given SCs for purely cutaneous indications [78, 79].

Adverse Effects with Potential Serious Morbidity

Glucocorticoid-Induced Osteoporosis

Glucocorticoid-induced osteoporosis (GIOP) is the most common cause of secondary osteoporosis and is associated with substantial morbidity [80, 81]. It is estimated that 30% of all patients treated with glucocorticoids for 6 months or more will develop osteoporosis [82]. In patients receiving long-term SCs, fractures are often the presenting manifestation of GIOP [82].

The World Health Organization (WHO) has described a computer-based algorithm called Fracture Risk Assessment Tool (FRAX®) that provides models for the assessment of fracture probability in postmenopausal women and men aged >40 years [83, 84].

Patient information required for FRAX® calculation is stated in Table 22.3 [83, 84].

The FRAX® model is country-specific according to life expectancy and fracture incidence. As FRAX® assesses glucocorticoid treatment, based on whether the patient does or does not take glucocorticoids, it underestimates the risk of fractures that relate to current and cumulative doses of glucocorticoids and duration of therapy. Estimation of risk should therefore be adjusted according to these parameters [85].

Based on current literature, Dodiuk-Gad et al. [86] have bone protection recommendations and medical guidelines for patients treated with systemic steroids, and these are elaborated in Tables 22.4 and 22.5, respectively [86, 87].

Table 22.3 Patient information required for FRAX® calculation

Parameters	Variables
Clinical	Age Gender Weight and height Rheumatoid arthritis: clinical or laboratory evidence to support the diagnosis Oral glucocorticoids: current or previous exposure to oral glucocorticoids for >3 months at a dose equivalent to prednisolone ≥5 mg/day
Metabolic bone status	Bone mineral density (BMD): the site and reference technology is dual X-ray absorptiometry (DXA) at the femoral neck. T-scores are based on the National Health and nutrition examination survey (NHANES) reference values for women aged 20–29 years. The same absolute values are used in men Previous fracture in adult life occurring spontaneously and arising from trauma, which in a healthy individual, would not have resulted in a fracture Parent's hip fracture: history of hip fracture in the patient's mother or father Secondary osteoporosis: having a disorder strongly associated with osteoporosis: Type 1 (insulin dependent) diabetes; osteogenesis imperfecta in adults; untreated longstanding hyperthyroidism; hypogonadism or premature menopause (<45 years); chronic malnutrition or malabsorption; and chronic liver disease
Habits	Alcohol consumption: ≥3 units of alcohol per day (a unit is equivalent to a medium-sized glass of wine) Smoking

Table 22.4 Bone protection recommendations for patients treated with systemic glucocorticoids

Parameters	Premenopausal women and men aged <50 years	Postmenopausal women and men aged >50 years
Lifestyle modifications	Weight-bearing activities Smoking cessation Avoidance of excessive alcohol intake	–
Nutritional supplements	Calcium intake 1200–1500 mg/day Vitamin D 800–1000 IU/day	–
Guidelines to pharmacologic treatment according to ACR 2010 guidelines [87]	Prevalent fragility fracture: NO: inadequate data for treatment recommendation YES[a]: (i) Prednisone >3 months: bisphosphonate[b] or teriparatide (ii) Prednisone 1–3 months: (a) Bisphosphonate[c] in men or women without childbearing potential (b) No consensus in women with childbearing potential	FRAX®[d] risk[e] for major osteoporotic fracture per 10 years: (i) <10%, low risk[f]: treatment with bisphosphonate[g] only if prednisone ≥7.5 mg/day (ii) 10–20%, medium risk[f]: bisphosphonate[g] (iii) 20%, high risk: bisphosphonate[g] or teriparatide
Other pharmacologic treatment to consider	Denosumab: monoclonal antibody against RANKL	–
Drugs	Bisphosphonates: (i) Alendronate: oral, 10 mg/day or 70 mg/week (ii) Risedronate: oral, 5 mg/day or 35 mg/week (iii) Zoledronic acid: IV 5 mg/year Teriparatide: SC 20 μg/day for 2 years Denosumab: SC 60 mg every 6 months	–

(continued)

Table 22.4 (continued)

Parameters	Premenopausal women and men aged <50 years	Postmenopausal women and men aged >50 years
Issues to discuss	*Clinical guidelines for safebisphosphonate usage*: Take first thing in the morning on an empty stomach Swallow the tablet with 240 mL water Do not eat, drink or take any other medications or supplements for 30–60 min after taking the medication Stay upright for 30–60 min *Side effects ofbisphosphonates and other drugs* Yearly BMD testing Duration of treatment: continued treatment re-evaluated periodically	–

[a]Treatment decision is based on childbearing potential and dosage and duration of glucocorticoid treatment

[b]Treatment with alendronate or risedronate. In women with childbearing potential, treatment is recommended only if the prednisone dose is ≥7.5 mg/day. Zoledronic acid is recommended only in women without childbearing potential

[c]Treatment with alendronate or risedronate if prednisone ≥5 mg/day or zoledronic acid if prednisolone ≥7.5 mg/day

[d]Fracture Risk Assessment Tool: see Table 22.3

[e]If the presence of the following, consider a shift to higher fracture risk category (low-medium or medium-high): high daily dose of glucocorticoid, high cumulative glucocorticoid dose, declining BMD or serial DEXA

[f]For low- and medium-risk patients, recommendations are for anticipated or prevalent duration of glucocorticoid treatment ≥3 months

[g]Treatment with alendronate, risedronate or zolendronic acid. Medium-risk group: if glucocorticoid dose is <7.5 mg/day, zolendronic acid is not indicated. High-risk group: if glucocorticoid ≥5 mg/day for ≤1 month or at any dose of glucocorticoid for >1 month, teriparatide is also a treatment option

ACR American College of Rheumatology, *BMD* bone mineral density, *DXA* dual X-ray absorptiometry, *SC* subcutaneous

Growth Impairment in Children

This rarely is an issue for dermatologic indications. Even when SCs are used for transplantation and serious systemic autoimmune conditions in children, catch-up growth is possible as SCs are decreased to physiologic levels or below.

Table 22.5 Medical guidelines for patients treated with systemic glucocorticoids

Assessment	Physical examination Blood pressure Weight and height (in children, plotted on a growth curve) Ophthalmoscopic examination for cataracts (slit lamp) and glaucoma Blood work Baseline: HBV and HCV screening, complete blood count, fasting glucose, lipid profile, electrolytes, serum 25-hydroxyvitamin D, calcium, renal and liver function For steroid-sparing treatment: TPMT genotyping, G6PD, HIV screening Radiology Chest X-ray BMD testing Others Tuberculosis skin test, fall risk assessment FRAX® (Table 22.3)
Preventive treatment	Lifestyle modifications, nutritional supplements and anti-osteoporotic therapy (Table 22.4) Consider H2 blockers/proton pump inhibitors for peptic ulcer prophylaxis Consider PCP prophylaxis Recommended adult immunization schedule prior to treatment
Patient education	Side effects Preventive treatment Precautions[a]
follow-up	Thorough history at each visit for adverse effects Consider further evaluation and treatment according to medical assessment on follow-up

[a]Physicians should educate patients on glucocorticoid withdrawal syndrome and the need for stress dose adjustments, including perioperative steroid coverage. Consider recommending wearing medication identification jewellery

BMD bone mineral density, *HBV* hepatitis B virus, *HCV* hepatitis C virus, *HIV* human immunodeficiency virus, *PCP* pneumocystis pneumonia, *TPMT* thiopurine methyltransferase

Other Side Effects

Cutaneous [88]

- Non-healing wounds and ulcers.
- Striae, atrophy and telangiectasias.

→ Due to reduced ground substance and collagen and reduced epithelialization and angiogenesis

- Steroid acne and rosacea secondary to androgenicity.
- Purpura due to catabolic effects on vascular smooth muscle.
- Hirsutism and telogen effluvium.
- Staphylococcal and herpes virus infections.

Metabolic [89]

- Hyperglycaemia
- Hypocalcaemia
- Hypokalaemia

Ophthalmologic [90]

- Cataracts
- Glaucoma
- Infection
- Haemorrhage
- Exophthalmos
- Refraction changes

Gastrointestinal [89]

- Nausea
- Vomiting
- Oesophagitis
- Fatty liver changes

Cardiovascular [91]

- Hypertension
- Atherosclerosis
- Oedema

Psychiatric and Neurologic [92]

- Mood changes
- Psychiatric disorders
- Sleep disturbances
- Pseudotumor cerebri
- Peripheral neuropathy
- Seizures

Endocrine [91]

- HPA axis suppression
- Adrenal crisis
- Withdrawal syndrome
- Menstrual irregularities

Haematologic and Cellular [89]

- Leucocytosis
- Lymphopenia
- Eosinopenia
- Immunosuppression
- Infections

Pregnancy and Systemic Corticosteroids

Multiple studies in humans concerning patients with SCs-dependent systemic conditions like SLE, severe asthma and organ transplantation during pregnancy have demonstrated no significantly increased risk of congenital malformations in humans [93–96]. Nevertheless, as with any drug in pregnancy, SCs should only be used when the drug is clearly indicated and if the potential benefit far exceeds the potential risk to the mother and foetus. Foetal HPA axis suppression is important to consider particularly when SCs are used near the time of delivery. There may be an increased risk of stillbirths and spontaneous abortions [88].

Tapering Principles with Systemic Glucocorticoids

- A rough guideline for tapering intermediate to chronic duration SC therapy (greater than 1 month) would be to reduce the dose by 20–30% every 1–2 weeks as disease activity allows.
- More serious conditions like vesiculobullous dermatoses may demand gradual steroid tapers over monthly intervals or more.
- Significant disease flare during the tapering process requires the corticosteroid dose to bc escalated once again.
- When the daily corticosteroid dose exceeds physiologic levels for more than 4 weeks, clinicians should consider alternate-day therapy.
- In alternate-day corticosteroid therapy, during the off day, cell-mediated immunity, white blood cells subset levels and potassium excretion all are essentially normalized.
- Alternate-day corticosteroid therapy should be used to maintain disease activity suppression once adequate control of the disease has been obtained using daily corticosteroid therapy. Here, patients need to be counselled that complete suppression of disease activity on the off day may not be possible.
- Nearing the end of long-term high-dose corticosteroid therapy, basal HPA function can be determined through morning cortisol levels. A cortisol value above 10 μm/dl ensures adequate basal HPA function.

Drug Interactions

- Erythromycin, clarithromycin and itraconazole (potent CYP 3A4 inhibitors): increase corticosteroid levels.
- Rifampicin, phenytoin and phenobarbital (CYP 3A4 inducers): decrease corticosteroid levels.
- Isoniazid: reduce corticosteroid levels.
- Cyclosporine: corticosteroid increase cyclosporine levels, thereby potentiating cyclosporine toxicity.

- Fluoroquinolones: theoretically, there is an increase in the risk of tendon rupture when used along with corticosteroids.
- Loop and thiazide diuretics: augment corticosteroid-induced hypokalaemia.
- NSAIDS: increased risk of gastrointestinal bleeding with corticosteroids.

Monitoring Guidelines

Baseline (When Anticipating Long-Term Corticosteroid Therapy)

Examination

- Blood pressure
- Height and weight plotted against a growth curve (for children)
- Ophthalmologic examination for cataracts (at or near start of corticosteroid therapy)

Laboratory

- Tuberculosis screening (strongly consider in high-risk patients): tuberculin test and chest X-ray.
- Fasting glucose and triglycerides.
- Potassium levels.

Follow-Up (with Long-Term Corticosteroid Therapy Above Physiologic Dose Levels)

Examination (at 1 Month and Then at Least Every 2–3 Months)

- Blood pressure
- Height and weight plotted against a growth curve (for children)
- Thorough history each visit for adverse effects (as mentioned in the adverse effects section)

At Least Every 6 Months Initially, Then Once Every 12 Months Long Term

- Ophthalmologic examination for cataracts and glaucoma

Laboratory

(at 1 month and then at least every 3–4 months while on pharmacologic dose of corticosteroid)

- Potassium levels
- Fasting glucose
- Fasting triglycerides

Near Time of Cessation of Long-Term Pharmacologic Dose Corticosteroid Therapy (Optional)

- AM cortisol level

Conclusion

SCs are indispensable for numerous dermatologic disorders. Though it happens to be an extremely valuable drug, its usage needs to be carefully employed with appropriate monitoring guidelines to avoid adverse effects associated with long-term use of systemic corticosteroids.

References

1. Sulzberger MB, Witten VH, Yaffe SN. Cortisone acetate administered orally in dermatologic therapy. Arch Dermatol Syphilol. 1951;64:573–8.
2. Schimmer BP, Parker KL. Adrenocortical steroids and their synthetic analogues. In: Hardman JG, Limbird LE, Molinoff PB, et al., editors. Goodman and Gilman's the pharmacologic basis of therapeutics. 9th ed. New York: McGraw Hill; 1996. p. 1459–86.
3. Axelrod L. Glucocorticoid therapy. Medicine. 1976;55:39–65.
4. Fauci AS, Dale DC, Balow JE. Glucocorticoid therapy: mechanism of action and clinical consideration. Ann Intern Med. 1976;84:304–15.
5. Barnes PJ, Karin M. Nuclear factor-kappaB: a pivotal transcription factor in chronic inflammatory diseases. N Engl J Med. 1997;336:1066–171.
6. Scheinman RI, Cogswell PC, Lofquist AK, et al. Role of transcriptional activation of I kappa B alpha in mediation of immunosuppression by glucocorticoids. Science. 1995;270:283–6.
7. Karin M, Liu ZG, Zandi E. AP-1 function and regulation. Curr Opin Cell Biol. 1997;9:240–6.
8. Ohta K, Yamashita N. Apoptosis of eosinophils and lymphocytes in allergic inflammation. J Allergy Clin Immunol. 1999;104:14–21.
9. Scudeletti M, Lanza L, Monaco E, et al. Immune regulatory properties of corticosteroids: prednisone induces apoptosis of human T lymphocytes following CD3 down regulation. Ann N Y Acad Sci. 1999;86:164–79.
10. Lester RS. Corticosteroids. Clin Dermatol. 1989;7:80–97.
11. Wand GS, Ney RL. Disorder of hypothalamo-pituitary adrenal axis. Clin Endocrinol Metabol. 1985;14:33–53.
12. Ziment I. Steroids. Clin Chest Med. 1986;7:341–54.
13. Mourellou O, Chaidemenos GC, Koussidou T, et al. The treatment of pemphigus vulgaris. Experience with 48 patients seen over an 11 year period. Br J Dermatol. 1995;133:83–7.
14. Bystryn JC, Rudolph JL. Pemphigus. Lancet. 2005;366:61–73.
15. Mahajan VK, Sharma NL, Sharma RC, et al. Twelve year clinico-therapeutic experience in pemphigus: a retrospective study of 54 cases. Int J Dermatol. 2005;44:821–7.
16. Anhalt GJ, Morrison LH. Pemphigoid: bullous, gestational and cicatricial. Curr Probl Dermatol. 1989;1:128–56.
17. Roujeau JC, Lok C, Bastuji-Garin S, et al. High risk death in elderly patients with extensive bullous pemphigoid. Arch Dermatol. 1998;134:465–9.
18. Heiligenhaus A, Shore JW, Rubin PA, et al. Long term results of mucous membrane grafting in ocular cicatricial pemphigoid. Implications for patient selection and surgical considerations. Ophthalmology. 1993;100:1283–8.

19. Sacher C, Hunzelman N. Cicatricial pemphigoid (mucous membrane pemphigoid): current emerging therapeutic approaches. Am J Clin Dermatol. 2005;6:93–103.
20. Lee LA, David KM. Cutaneous lupus erythematosus. Curr Probl Dermatol. 1989;1:165–200.
21. Callen JP, Klein J. Subacute cutaneous lupus erythematosus. Arthritis Rheum. 1988;31:1007–13.
22. Goldberg JW, Lidsky MD. Pulse methylprednisolone therapy for persistent subacute cutaneous lupus. Arthritis Rheum. 1984;27:837–8.
23. Kuhn A, Ruland V, Bonsmann G. Cutaneous lupus erythematosus: update of therapeutic options—part I. J Am Acad Dermatol. 2011;65:e179–93.
24. Callen JP. Dermatomyositis. Lancet. 2000;355:53–7.
25. Dawkins MA, Jorizzo JL, Walker FO, et al. Dermatomyositis: a dermatology-based case series. J Am Acad Dermatol. 1998;38:397–404.
26. Callen JP. Cutaneous vasculitis. What have we learned in the past 20 years. Arch Dermatol. 1998;134:355–7.
27. Palit A, Inamadar A. Vasculitis: approach to diagnosis and therapy. Indian J Dermatol Venereol Leprol. 2006;72:334–45.
28. Mollica F, Li Volti S, Garozzo R, et al. Effectiveness of early prednisone treatment in preventing the development of nephropathy in anaphylactoid purpura. Eur J Pediatr. 1992;151:140–4.
29. Sheth AP, Olsen JC, Esterly NB. Cutaneous polyarteritis nodosa of childhood. J Am Acad Dermatol. 1994;31:561–6.
30. Guillevin L, Lhote F, Cohen P, et al. Polyarteritis nodosa related to hepatitis B virus. A prospective study with long term observation of 41 patients. Medicine (Baltimore). 1995;74:238–53.
31. Fiorentino DF. Cutaneous vasculitis. J Am Acad Dermatol. 2003;48:311–40.
32. Roane DW, Griger DR. An approach to diagnosis and initial management of systemic vasculitis. Am Fam Physician. 1999;60:1421–30.
33. Johnson RB, Lazarus GS. Pulse therapy: therapeutic efficacy in the treatment of pyoderma gangrenosum. Arch Dermatol. 1982;118:76–84.
34. Prystowsky JH, Kahn SN, Lazarus GS. Present status of pyoderma gangrenosum. Review of 21 cases. Arch Dermatol. 1989;125:57–74.
35. Chow RK, Ho VC. Treatment of pyoderma gangrenosum. J Am Acad Dermatol. 1996;34:1047–60.
36. Graham JA, Hansen KK, Rabinowitz LG, et al. Pyoderma gangrenosum in infants and children. Pediatr Dermatol. 1994;11:10–7.
37. Lozada-Nur F, Miranda C. Oral lichen planus: topical and systemic therapy. Semin Cutan Med Surg. 1997;16:295–300.
38. Silverman S Jr, Bahl S. Oral lichen planus update: clinical characteristics, treatment responses and malignant transformation. Am J Dent. 1997;10:259–63.
39. Edwards L, Friedrich EG. Desquamative gingivitis: lichen planus in disguise. Obstet Gynecol. 1988;71:832–6.
40. Baer RL. Poison ivy dermatitis. Cutis. 1990;46:34–6.
41. Raimer SS. Managing pediatric atopic dermatitis. Clin Pediatr. 2000;391:1–14.
42. Tay YK, Khoo BP, Goh CL. The profile of atopic dermatitis in a tertiary dermatology out patient clinic in Singapore. Int J Dermatol. 1999;38:689–92.
43. Albertini JG, Tyler W, Miller OF. Ulcerative sarcoidosis. Case report and review of literature. Arch Dermatol. 1997;133:215–9.
44. Muthiah MM, Macfarlane JT. Current concepts in the management of sarcoidois. Drugs. 1990;40:231–7.
45. Milman N, Hoffman AL, Byg KE. Sarcoidosis in children. Epidemiology in Danes, clinical features, diagnosis, treatment and prognosis. Acta Pediatr. 1998;87:871–8.
46. Redmond GP, Gidwani GP, Gupta MK, et al. Treatment of androgenic disorders with dexamethasone: dose-response relationship for suppression of dehydroepiandrosterone sulfate. J Am Acad Dermatol. 1990;22:91–3.
47. Lucky AW. Hormonal correlatyes of acne and hirsutism. Am J Med. 1995;98:89S–94S.
48. Bjornberg A. Fifteen cases of toxic epidermal necrolysis (Lyell). Acta Derm Venereol. 1973;53:149–52.

49. Ohlenschlaeger K. Toxic epidermal necrolysis and Steven Johnson disease. Acta Derm Venereol. 1966;46:204–9.
50. Sherertz EF, Jegasothy BV, Lazarus GS. Phenytoin hypersensitivity reaction presenting with toxic epidermal necrolysis and severe hepatitis. Report in a patient treated with corticosteroid pulse therapy. J Am Acad Dermatol. 1985;12(1 Pt 2):178–81.
51. Prediville JS, Hebert AA, Greenwald MJ, et al. Management of Steven-Johnson syndrome and toxic epidermal necrolysis in children. J Pediatr. 1989;115:881–7.
52. Cheriyan S, Patterson R, Greenberger PA, et al. The outcome of Steven-Johnson syndrome treated with corticosteroids. Allergy Proc. 1995;16:151–5.
53. Patterson R, Grammer LC, Greenberger PA, et al. Steven-Johnson syndrome (SJS): effectiveness of corticosteroids in management and recurrent SJS. Allergy Proc. 1992;13:89–95.
54. Das S, Roy AK, Biswas I. A six month prospective study to find out the treatment outcomes, prognosis and offending drugs in toxic epidermal necrolysis from an urban institution in Kolkata. Indian J Dermatol. 2013;58:191–3.
55. Kardaun SH, Jonkman MF. Dexamethasone pulse therapy for Steven-Johnson syndrome/toxic epidermal necrolysis. Acta Derm Venereol. 2007;87:144–8.
56. Patterson R, Miller M, Kaplan M, et al. Effectiveness of early therapy with corticosteroids in Steven Johnson syndrome: a total series of 67 cases. Allergy Asthma Proc. 2000;21:101–5.
57. Chorousous GP. Adrenocorticosteroids and adrenocortical antagonists. In: Katzung BG, editor. Basic and clinical pharmacology. 9th ed. New York: Lange Medical Books/McGraw Hill; 2004. p. 641–60.
58. Gupta LK, Martin AM, Agarwal N, et al. Guidelines for the management of Steven's Johnson syndrome/toxic epidermal necrolysis. An Indian perspective. Indian J Dermatol Venereol Leprol. 2016;82:603–25.
59. Schultz JT, Sheridan RL, Ryan CM, et al. A 10-year-old experience with toxic epidermal necrolysis. J Burn Care Rehabil. 2000;21:199–204.
60. Tripathi A, Ditto AM, Grammer LC, et al. Corticosteroid therapy in an additional 13 cases of Steven-Johnson syndrome: a total series of 67 cases. Allergy Asthma Proc. 2000;21:101–5.
61. Kim KJ, Lee DP, Suh HS, et al. Toxic epidermal necrolysis: analysis of clinical course and SCORTEN-based comparison of mortality rate and treatment modalities in Korean patients. Acta Derm Venereol. 2005;85:497–502.
62. Schneck J, Fagot TP, Sekula P, et al. Effects of treatments on the mortality of Stevens-Johnson syndrome and toxic epidermal necrolysis: a retrospective study on patients included in the prospective EuroSCAR study. J Am Acad Dermatol. 2008;58:33–40.
63. Hirahara K, Kano Y, Sato Y, et al. Methylprednisolone pulse therapy for Stevens-Johnson's syndrome/toxic epidermal necrolysis: clinical evaluation and analysis of biomarkers. J Am Acad Dermatol. 2013;69:496–8.
64. Pasricha JS, Khaitan BK, Shantharaman R, et al. Toxic epidermal necrolysis. Int J Dermatol. 1996;35:523–7.
65. Rai R, Srinivas CR. Suprapharmacologic doses of intravenous dexamethasone followed by cyclosporine in the treatment of toxic epidermal necrolysis. Indian J Dermatol Venereol Leprol. 2008;74:263–5.
66. Bean SF. Diagnosis and management of chronic oral mucosal bullous diseases. Dermatol Clin. 1987;5:751–60.
67. Eaglstein WH, Katz R, Brown JA. The effects of early corticosteroid therapy on the skin eruption and pain of herpes zoster. JAMA. 1970;211:1681–3.
68. Santee JA. Corticosteroids for herpes zoster: what do they accomplish? Am J Clin Dermatol. 2002;3:517–24.
69. Allanby KD. Deaths associated with steroid hormone therapy. Lancet. 1957;1:1104–10.
70. Christy N. Clinical significance of pituitary adrenal suppression by exogenous corticosteroids. J Chronic Dis. 1973;26:261–4.
71. Lauber JS, Abrams HL, Ray MC. Silent bowel perforation occurring during corticosteroid treatment for pemphigus vulgaris. Cutis. 1989;43:27–8.

72. Weiner HL, Rezai AR, Cooper PR. Sigmoid diverticular perforation in neurosurgical patients receiving high dose corticosteroids. Neurosurgery. 1993;33:40–3.
73. Dayton MT, Kleckner SC, Brown DK. Peptic ulcer perforation associated with steroid use. Arch Surg. 1987;122:376–80.
74. Keefe M, Munro F. Acute pancreatitis: a fatal complication of treatment of bullous pemphigoid with systemic corticosteroids. Dermatologica. 1989;179:73–5.
75. Yang JY, Cui XL, He XJ. Non ketotic hyperosmolar coma complicating steroid treatment in childhood nephrosis. Pediatr Nephrol. 1995;9:621–2.
76. Wiest PM, Flanigan T, Salata RA, et al. Serious infectious complications of corticosteroid therapy for COPD. Chest. 1989;95:1180–4.
77. Hellmann DB, Petri M, et al. Fatal infections in systemic lupus erythematosus: the role of opportunistic organisms. Medicine. 1987;66:341–8.
78. Wolverton SE. Major adverse effects from systemic drugs: defining the risks. Cur Probl Dermatol. 1995;7:1–40.
79. Qian XC, Huang YZ, Huang RK. Kaposi's sarcoma after steroid therapy for pemphigus foliaceous. Chin Med J. 1989;102:647–9.
80. Weinstein RS. Clinical practice. Glucocorticoid induced bone disease. N Engl J Med. 2011;365:62–70.
81. Clarke BL. Corticosteroid induced osteoporosis: an update for dermatologists. Am J Clin Dermatol. 2012;13:167–90.
82. Bultink IE, Baden M, Lems WF. Glucocorticoid induced osteoporosis: an update on current pharmacotherapy and future directions. Expert Opin Pharmacother. 2013;14:185–97.
83. Kanis JA, Oden A, Johansson H, et al. FRAX® and its applications in clinical practice. Bone. 2009;44:734–43.
84. World Health Organization collaborating Centre for Metabolic Diseases. University of Scheffield. FRAX® WHO Fracture risk assessment tool. http://www.shef.ac.uk/FRAX. Accessed on 25 Sept 2013.
85. Kanis JA, Hans D, Cooper C. Task force of the FRAX initiative. Interpretation and use of FRAX in clinical practice. Osteoporosis Int. 2011;22:2395–411.
86. Dodiuk-Gad RP, Ish-Shalom S, Shear NH. Systemic glucocorticoids: important issues and practical guidelines for the dermatologist. Int J Dermatol. 2015;54:723–9.
87. Grossman JM, Gordon R, Ranganath VK, et al. American College of Rheumatology 2010 recommendations for the prevention and treatment of glucocorticoid induced osteoporosis. Arthritis Care Res (Hoboken). 2010;62:1515–26.
88. Gallant C, Kenny P. Oral glucocorticoids and their complications: a review. J Am Acad Dermatol. 1986;14:161–77.
89. Jackson S, Gilchrist H, Nesbitt LT. Update on the dermatologic use of systemic glucocorticoids. Dermatol Ther. 2007;20:187–205.
90. Carnahan MC, Goldstein DA. Ocular complications of topical, peri-ocular and systemic corticosteroids. Curr Opin Ophthalmol. 2000;11:478–83.
91. Fardet L, Kassar A, Cabane J, et al. Corticosteroid induced severe adverse events in adults: frequency, screening and prevention. Drug Saf. 2007;30:861–81.
92. Warrington TP, Bostwick JM. Psychiatric adverse effects of corticosteroids. Mayo Clin Proc. 2006;81:1361–7.
93. Fraser FC, Sajoo A. Teratogenic potential of corticosteroids in humans. Teratology. 1995;51:45–6.
94. Wong KM, Bailey RR, Lynn KL, et al. Pregnancy in renal transplant recipients: the Christchurch experience. N Z Med J. 1995;108:190–2.
95. Stenius Aarniale B, Hedman J, Teramo KA. Acute asthma during pregnancy. Thorax. 1996;51:411–4.
96. Buchanan NM, Khamashta MA, Morton KE, et al. A study of 100 high risk lupus pregnancies. Am J Reprod Immunol. 1992;28:192–4.

Steroid Pulses in Dermatology

23

Introduction

Pulse therapy refers to the administration of supra-pharmacological doses of drugs in an intermittent manner to obtain heightened therapeutic benefits, along with reduction in the adverse effect profile [1]. Kountz and Cohn were the pioneers of administering pulse corticosteroids (in 1973) to prevent rejection of a renal graft [2]. Further, in 1976, steroid pulse therapy was utilized to treat a recalcitrant case of lupus nephritis [3].

In India, it was Pasricha and Srivastava who introduced dexamethasone cyclophosphamide pulse (DCP) therapy in 1981 to treat pemphigus vulgaris and its allied disorders. Today apart from pemphigus, there are a number of dermatoses where steroid pulses are of value.

Mechanism of Action

Glucocorticoids exert their beneficial activity owing to immunosuppressive, anti-inflammatory and anti-allergic properties. These drugs function in three modules utilizing both genomic and non-genomic methods [4] based on the amount concentrated within cells and include (a) genomic event-mediated activities in case the concentration of the drug is low [5], (b) both genomic and non-genomic intracellular function and activation of cross membrane signal transduction, with medium intracellular drug levels, [5] and (c) mainly genomic effects when very large concentrations of steroids are employed as this produces greater stability to cellular membranes [5].

A. K. Bubna, *Therapeutics in Dermatology - Essentials for Clinical Practice*,
https://doi.org/10.1007/978-981-95-3791-4_23

Genomic Effects

These effects are mediated mainly via two mechanisms: transactivation [5] and trans expression [6].

In transactivation, induction of transcription occurs following activation of glucocorticoid response elements after interaction with the glucocorticoid-cytosolic glucocorticoid receptor complex (GCR) in cells, which in turn downregulates inflammatory mediators, adhesion molecules and inflammatory enzymes [5].

In trans expression, monomers of glucocorticoid-GCR complex directly or indirectly interact with transcription factors and reduce the amount of the pro-inflammatory transcription factor NF-κB, thus reducing levels of cytokines like IL-1, IL-6 and TNFα [6].

These effects, though, are not exhibited immediately and manifest after a few hours or days.

Non-genomic Effects

Non-genomic effects occur following three mechanisms: (a) cGCR-mediated effects, (b) physiochemical interactions with plasma membrane at high glucocorticoid concentrations and (c) effects mediated by membrane-bound glucocorticoid receptors [5, 6].

These effects are characterized by reduced calcium and sodium cycling across plasma membranes of immune cells, which is thought to contribute to rapid immunosuppression and subsequent reduction of inflammatory processes.

Indications

Commonly Employed

- Pemphigus vulgaris
- Bullous dermatitis herpetiformis
- Alopecia totalis

Infrequently Used

- Pyoderma gangrenosum (PG)
- Rapidly progressive vitiligo
- Systemic lupus erythematosus (SLE)
- Systemic sclerosis
- Dermatomyositis
- Lichen planus (LP)
- Alopecia areata (AA)

- Sarcoidosis
- Systemic vasculitis

Contraindications

- Known hypersensitivity
- Systemic infections
- Fungal sepsis
- Uncontrolled hypertension

Clinical Uses

Pemphigus

Pemphigus is a blistering disorder which is associated with high morbidity and mortality. Systemic steroids and other immunosuppressive drugs have remained the cornerstone of pemphigus management.

DCP therapy was designed in 1981 by Pasricha et al. The aim for its introduction was to reduce corticosteroid toxicity and achieve better therapeutic results. This therapy is widely used in the Indian subcontinent, with complete remission of pemphigus also being reported [7, 8].

It consists of four phases:

Phase I

- Dexamethasone 100 mg in 5% dextrose is administered as a slow intravenous (IV) infusion over 2 h for three consecutive days, along with cyclophosphamide 500 mg with the infusion on any one of the 3 days, usually the second day. The reason why 5% dextrose is utilised instead of normal saline is because steroids can cause hypernatremia and hypokalemia.
- DCP is repeated every 28 days until no new lesions are identifiable between pulses.
- On the remaining days, 50 mg of cyclophosphamide is continued via the oral route.
- If recurrences are observed between DCPs, oral steroids maybe required in between pulses at lower dosages to achieve quicker clinical recovery without compromising patient safety. In most cases, oral betamethasone (1–2 mg/day) suffices [9].
- Once the skin and mucus membrane lesions have completely subsided with no recurrences between pulses, the patient is considered to have entered phase II.

Phase II

- This is a phase of remission while on therapy.
- DCP is administered for another 9 months.

Phase III

- Monthly pulses are stopped completely in this phase.
- Oral cyclophosphamide 50 mg/day is continued daily for another 9 months.

Phase IV

- Treatment is completely stopped.
- Patient is regularly followed up for the next 10 years.

Pre-pulse Evaluation Indices

- Detailed clinical history and examination.
- Evaluation for any existing comorbidity.
- Blood investigations: haemogram, total and differential blood counts, platelet count, erythrocyte sedimentation rate, sugars, hepatic and renal profiles, electrolytes.
- Urinalysis.
- Chest X-ray.
- Electrocardiogram.

Special Scenario Patients

- In diabetic patients receiving DCP, 10 units of soluble insulin are administered for every 500 mL bottle of 5% dextrose, dissolved in the same drip [10].
- In addition, regular anti-diabetic drugs are continued [10].
- In patients with hypertension and tuberculosis, DCP can be administered, provided patients are receiving concomitant treatment for the respective disorders.
- If there happens to be a serious infection, then the pulse maybe deferred for 7–14 days and restarted once infection is controlled [11]. Besides, if the clinician feels that the pulse therapy can be continued along with antibiotics and antifungals, then that can be considered as well [9].

Paediatric Consideration

- In children below 12 years, the dose of DCP needs to be reduced to half.
- Otherwise, its usage in this group is not associated with significant risks [12].

Unmarried Patients and Those Who Have Not Completed Their Families

- As cyclophosphamide is associated with oligo/azoospermia and amenorrhoea, it is replaced with azathioprine (50 mg/day) during the first three phases of pulse therapy [13].
- The other possibility would be to use dexamethasone pulse alone.

While treating patients using DCP therapy, it is observed that [9]

- Thorough cleaning of the skin, scalp and oral cavity even with the presence of erosions helps in faster remission.
- Use of oral antibiotics and anti-candida drugs predictably enables clearing and healing of lesions by preventing super-added infections that can impair wound healing.
- Simultaneous use of oral steroids also hastens healing of skin lesions, potentiating psychological benefit to patients.
- By using the above standards, it is observed that phase I of DCP therapy can be reduced to a duration of as little as 3–4 months.

Duration of phase II and III is fixed at 9 months each, with the total duration of treatment being approximately 2 years.

Out of these 2 years, it is seen that the patient suffers from clinical lesions for only the first 2–3 months after which the patient is quite normal and can attend his/her normal duties and responsibilities. Completing treatment during phase II and III serves to prevent relapses in the future. The major causes of relapses are linked to incomplete/irregular treatment and the use of either cyclophosphamide or dexamethasone alone rather than in combination [9].

Lichen Planus

LP is a chronic inflammatory disease involving the skin and the mucosa. Oral mini pulse (OMP) with betamethasone is found to be of value in both oral and cutaneous LP.

Here, betamethasone (5 mg on two consecutive days per week) is administered for a period of around 6 weeks, which generally results in considerable improvement in various parameters like burning pain (in oral lesions), pruritus (for cutaneous lesions), as well as flattening of cutaneous plaques and healing of oral erosions [14, 15]. Further, betamethasone OMP is found to be superior to triamcinolone 0.1% orabase in oral LP, resulting in quicker and more sustained levels of efficacy [16]. In a case report of eruptive LP treated with betamethasone OMP (5 mg on two consecutive days per week), improvement was observed within 3 weeks of initiation of therapy [17]. In another case of generalized bullous LP using the same treatment protocol, improvement was witnessed as early as 2 weeks [18].

Table 23.1 Various studies where oral steroid pulses have been utilized in vitiligo

Author(s)	Study details	Remarks
Pasricha et al. [19]	Oral betamethasone pulse (5 mg for two consecutive days per week) was utilized in patients having extensive and fast spreading vitiligo	In 89% patients, by 1–3 months, disease progression was halted By 2–4 months, in 80% patients, re-pigmentation was appreciated
Kanwar et al. [20]	Oral dexamethasone pulse at doses ranging from 5 to 25 mg on two consecutive days per week was administered to patients with unstable vitiligo	In 43.8% of patients, disease progression stopped and mild-to-moderate re-pigmentation was observed In the remaining 56.2% patients, no re-pigmentation was observed
Rath et al. [21]	Study was done to evaluate combination of betamethasone oral mini pulse (0.1 mg/kg on two consecutive days/week) with phototherapy for vitiligo	Combination of NB-UVB enabled better re-pigmentation in 18% of patients compared to 8% patients on phototherapy alone
Radakovic-Fijan et al. [22]	Here, 10 mg of dexamethasone was administered on two consecutive days per week	Though progression of vitiligo was arrested in 88% of patients, re-pigmentation was achieved in only 17.2% cases
Majid et al. [23]	In 400 children with progressive vitiligo, methylprednisolone (0.8 mg/kg with a maximum dose of 32 mg) was given on two consecutive days/week for 6 months	Disease progression was halted in >90% of patients, with moderate re-pigmentation being observed in 65.5% of patients

Vitiligo

Vitiligo is a disorder characterized by depigmented macules that usually is progressive in quality. Various steroid pulses are utilized for the treatment of vitiligo and are elucidated in Table 23.1 [19–23].

Alopecia Areata

AA is an autoimmune disease characterized by patches of non-scarring alopecia. Similar to vitiligo, OMP has been utilized for treating AA. Various reports incorporating the same are summarized in Table 23.2 [24–26]. Further, even 100 mg of IV methylprednisolone pulse on three consecutive days at monthly intervals has been utilized in AA, with good efficacy [27].

Psoriasis

Topical pulse steroids are effective in psoriasis. This consists of intermittent use of super-potent corticosteroids. Clobetasol propionate (0.05%) ointment applied at 12 hourly intervals (with a total of three applications) is utilized in psoriasis in the maintenance phase of therapy [28]. During other days, vitamin D3 analogues, topical retinoids or emollients are used. This schedule helps in reducing side effects like cutaneous atrophy, telangiectasia, hypothalamo-pituitary axis suppression and

Table 23.2 Utility of oral mini pulse in alopecia areata: various reports

Author(s)	Study details	Remarks
Pasricha and Kumrah [24]	Betamethasone 5 mg on two consecutive days/ week for 3 months in an 8-year-old girl with alopecia areata (AA)	Regrowth of hair on the entire scalp was observed
Sharma and Gupta [25]	Betamethasone 5 mg on two consecutive days/ week was given to 30 patients with extensive AA for 12 weeks	In 63.3% of patients, complete to excellent hair regrowth was observed In 20% patients, no hair regrowth was seen
Bajaj et al [26]	Administration of oral prednisolone 30 mg on three consecutive days per week for 6 months	In 63.3% of cases, complete regrowth was observed In 27.3% patients, good to average regrowth of hair was witnessed

tachyphylaxis associated with prolonged topical steroid application. Further, intermittent application of topical steroids also helps in maintaining remission, preventing a relapse that can otherwise occur with abrupt cessation of therapy.

Urticaria

In a study of 10 patients with severe chronic urticaria, methylprednisolone (16 mg) administered twice weekly for 2 months resulted in significant improvement of wheal diameters and pruritus [29].

Haemangioma

Around 90% improvement of haemangioma after administration of 2 mg betamethasone twice weekly for 12 weeks was observed in a 1-month-old infant with periocular haemangioma [30].

Adverse Effects

Related to Pulse Therapy

- Hiccups [31]
- Facial flushing [32]
- Joint and muscle pain [33]
- Weakness
- Diarrhoea
- Generalized swelling and weight gain
- Arrhythmias
- Shock

Other Side Effects [34]

- Abnormal behaviour
- Mood alteration
- Hyperactivity
- Psychosis
- Disorientation
- Sleep disturbances
- Hyperglycaemia
- Hypokalaemia
- Higher risk of infection (when cumulative doses of methyl prednisolone is >5 g) [35]

Serious Side Effects

- Increase in blood pressure in already hypertensive patients during and after infusion
- Seizures, particularly in systemic lupus erythematosus, which may be related to rapid flux in electrolytes
- Anaphylactic shock even after one prior infusion, usually associated with the succinate ester of methyl prednisolone [36]

Monitoring

Baseline

- Haemogram
- Serum electrolytes
- Liver function tests
- Renal function tests
- Blood sugars
- HbA1C
- Chest X-ray
- Electrocardiogram
- Pregnancy testing
- Urine—routine and microscopy
- Blood pressure
- Body weight

At Each Visit

- Blood sugar
- Serum electrolytes

- Urine—routine and microscopy
- Blood pressure
- Body weight

Conclusion

Steroids given intermittently are found to be safer compared to daily administrations. In dermatology, DCP therapy is an extremely valuable tool for managing pemphigus with minimal incidence of steroid-induced side effects.

References

1. Bell PR, Briggs JD, Calman KC, et al. Reversal of acute clinical and experimental organ rejection using large doses of intravenous prednisolone. Lancet. 1971;1:876–80.
2. Kountz SL, Cohn R. Initial treatment of renal allografts with large intravenous doses of immunosuppressive drugs. Lancet. 1969;1:338–40.
3. Cathcart ES, Idelson BA, Scheinberg MA, Couser WG. Beneficial effects of methyl prednisolone pulse therapy in diffuse proliferative lupus nephritis. Lancet. 1976;1:163–6.
4. Schimmer BP, Parker KL. Adrenocorticotropic hormones; adrenocortical steroids and their synthetic analogs; inhibitors of synthesis and actions of adrenocortical hormones. In: Brunton LL, Lazo JS, Parker KL, editors. Goodman and Gilman's the pharmacological basis of therapeutics. 11th ed. New York: McGraw Hill Professional; 2006. p. 1587–612.
5. Buttgereit F, Saag KG, Cutolo M, da Silva JA, Bijilsma JW. The molecular basis for effectiveness, toxicity and resistance to glucocorticoids: focus on the treatment of rheumatoid arthritis. Scand J Rheumatol. 2005;34:14–2.
6. Stahn C, Lowenberg M, Hommes DW, Buttergeit F. Molecular mechanisms of glucocorticoid action and selective glucocorticoid receptor agonists. Mol Cell Endocrinol. 2007;275:71–8.
7. Kaur S, Kanwar AJ. Dexamethasone cyclophosphamide pulse therapy in pemphigus. Int J Dermatol. 1990;29:371–4.
8. Thappa DM, Karthikeyan K, Jeevankumar B. Dexamethasone cyclophosphamide pulse therapy in pemphigus: an appraisal of its outcome in a tertiary health care center in South India. Indian J Dermatol. 2004;49:9–13.
9. Pasricha JS, Poonam. Current regimen of pulse therapy for pemphigus. Minor modifications, improved results. Indian J Dermatol Venereol Leprol. 2008;74:217–21.
10. Mittal R, Sudha R, Murugan S, Adikrishnan S, Shobana S, Anandan S. Pulse therapy in dermatology. Sri Ramachandra J Med. 2007;1:44–6.
11. Sinha A, Bagga A. Pulse steroid therapy. Indian J Pediatr. 2008;75:1057–66.
12. Pasricha JS. Pulse therapy as a cure for autoimmune diseases. Indian J Dermatol Venereol Leprol. 2003;69:323–8.
13. Rao PN, Lakshmi TS. Pulse therapy and its modifications in pemphigus. A six-year study. Indian J Dermatol Venereol Leprol. 2003;69:329–33.
14. Ramesh M, Balachnadran C, Shenoi SD, et al. Efficacy of steroid oral mini pulse therapy in lichen planus. An open trial in 35 patients. Indian J Dermatol Venereol Leprol. 2006;72:156–7.
15. Mittal R, Manchanda Y. Lichen planus treated with dexamethasone oral mini pulse therapy. Indian J Dermatol Venereol Leprol. 2000;66:34–5.
16. Malhotra AK, Khaitan BK, Sethuraman G, et al. Betamethasone oral mini pulse therapy compared with topical triamcinolone acetonide (0.1%) paste in oral lichen planus. A randomized comparative study. J Am Acad Dermatol. 2008;58:596–602.
17. Al-Mutairi N, Joshi A, Zaki A, et al. Acute generalized lichen planus treated with weekly betamethasone 5 mg oral mini pulse. J Drugs Dermatol. 2005;4:218–20.

18. Joshi A, Khaitan BK, Verma KK, et al. Generalized and bullous lichen planus treated successfully with oral mini pulse therapy. Indian J Dermatol Venereol Leprol. 1999;65:303–4.
19. Pasricha JS, Khaitan BK. Oral mini pulse therapy with betamethasone in vitiligo patients having extensive or fast spreading disease. Int J Dermatol. 1993;32:753–7.
20. Kanwar AJ, Dhar S, Dawn G. Oral mini pulse therapy in vitiligo. Dermatology. 1995;190:251–2.
21. Rath N, Kar HK, Sabhnani S. An open labeled, comparative clinical study on efficacy and tolerability of oral mini pulse of steroid (OMP) alone, OMP with PUVA and broad/narrow band UVB phototherapy in progressive vitiligo. Indian J Dermatol Venereol Leprol. 2008;74:357–60.
22. Radakovic-Fijan S, Furnsinn-Friedl AM, Honigsman H, et al. Oral dexamethasone pulse treatment for vitiligo. J Am Acad Dermatol. 2001;44:814–7.
23. Majid I, Masood Q, Hassan I, et al. Childhood vitiligo: response to methylprednisolone oral mini pulse therapy and topical fluticasone combination. Indian J Dermatol. 2009;54:124–7.
24. Pasricha JS, Kumrah L. Alopecia totalis treated with oral mini pulse (OMP) therapy with betamethasone. Indian J Dermatol Venereol Leprol. 1996;62:106–9.
25. Sharma VK, Gupta S. Twice weekly 5 mg dexamethasone oral pulse in the treatment of extensive alopecia areata. J Dermatol. 1999;26:562–5.
26. Bajaj DR, Devrajani BR, Shah SZA, et al. Treatment of extensive alopecia areata with oral prednisolone mini pulse regimen. J Pak Assoc Dermatol. 2008;18:226–31.
27. Efentaki P, Altenburg A, Haerting J, et al. Medium dose of prednisolone pulse therapy in alopecia areata. Dermatoendocrinol. 2009;1:310–3.
28. Minocha YC, Sood VK, Singh D, et al. Topical corticosteroid pulse therapy in psoriasis. Indian J Dermatol Venereol Leprol. 1991;57:307–8.
29. Godse KV. Severe chronic urticaria treated with oral mini pulse steroid therapy. Indian J Dermatol. 2010;55:402–3.
30. Verma K, Verma KK. Infantile hemangioma treated with two days in a week betamethasone oral mini pulse therapy. Indian J Pediatr. 2001;68:355–6.
31. Kanwar AJ, Kaur S, Dhar S, et al. Hiccup—a side effect of pulse therapy. Dermatology. 1993;187:279.
32. Dhar S, Kanwar AJ. Facial flushing—a side effect of pulse therapy. Dermatology. 1994;188:332.
33. Appelhans M, Bonsmann G, Orge C, et al. Dexamethasone-cyclophosphamide pulse therapy in bullous autoimmune dermatoses. Hautarzt. 1993;44:143–7.
34. Klein-Gitelman MS, Pachman LM. Intravenous corticosteroids: adverse reactions are more variable than expected in children. J Rheumatol. 1998;25:1995–2002.
35. Kang I, Park SH. Infectious complications in SLE after immunosuppressive therapies. Curr Opin Rhematol. 2003;15:528–34.
36. Baethge BA, Lidsky MD, Goldberg JW. A study of adverse effects of high dose intravenous (pulse) methylprednisolone therapy in patients with rheumatic disease. Ann Pharmacother. 1992;26:316–20.

Part V

Immunosuppressive Drugs

Cyclophosphamide

24

Introduction

Cyclophosphamide (CPE) (an alkylating agent) is synthesized primarily as a derivative of nitrogen mustard. Apart from its use in malignancies, CPE is utilized in treating a number of autoimmune diseases. Besides, CPE possesses the greatest therapeutic index, with regard to other nitrogen mustards.

Figure 24.1 depicts the mechanism of action of CPE.

The toxicity of CPE involves all phases of the cell cycle, making it cell cycle specific, and not phase specific [1]. Although CPE reduces the function of both B and T cells, its action against B cells is more pronounced. Further, superior activity of CPE is observed if it is given prior to antigen presentation. Additionally, the effect of CPE on suppressor T cells is notable [2].

A. K. Bubna, *Therapeutics in Dermatology - Essentials for Clinical Practice*,
https://doi.org/10.1007/978-981-95-3791-4_24

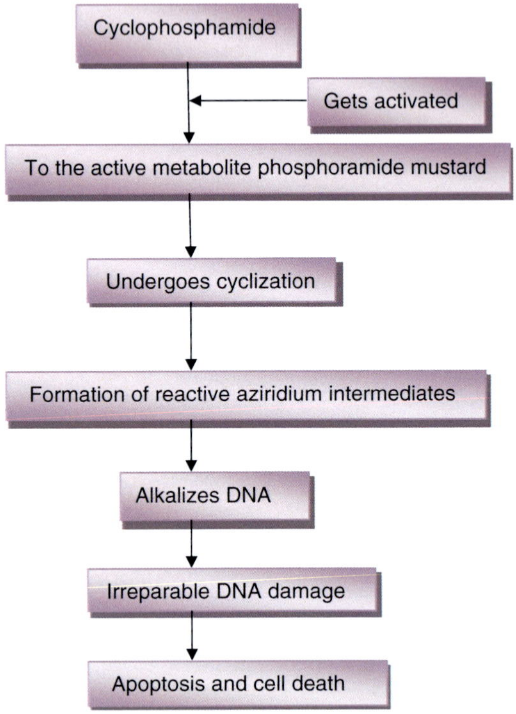

Fig. 24.1 Mechanism of action of cyclophosphamide

Pharmacokinetics

Peak plasma levels of CPE are observed after an hour of oral administration. CPE elaborates a bioavailability of 74%, with a $t_{1/2}$ ranging from 2 to 10 h. Following hepatic metabolism, it breaks down into 4-hydroxycyclophosphamide and chloro-acetaldehyde. The former delineates anti-neoplastic effects, and the latter demonstrates immunosuppressive effects. Excretion of CPE occurs via the kidney. Besides, 13% of the drug is bound to plasma proteins [3].

Indications

FDA-Approved

- Advanced mycosis fungoides.

Off-Label

Vasculitis

- Wegener's granulomatosis (WG).
- Lymphomatoid granulomatosis (LG).
- Leukocytoclastic vasculitis (LCV).
- Polyarteritis nodosa (PAN).
- Cryoglobulinemia.

Bullous Dermatoses

- Pemphigus vulgaris/foliaceous.
- Bullous pemphigoid (BP).
- Paraneoplastic pemphigus.

Neutrophilic Dermatoses

- Pyoderma gangrenosum (PG).
- Behcet's disease (BD).
- Erythema elevatum diutinum (EED).

Autoimmune Connective Tissue Diseases

- Dermatomyositis (DM).
- Lupus erythematosus (LE).
- Systemic sclerosis (SS).
- Relapsing polychondritis.

Neoplasms

- Langerhans cell histiocytosis.

Infiltrative Diseases

- Lichen myxedematosus.
- Scleromyxedema.

Miscellaneous

- Psoriatic arthropathy.
- Severe eczematous dermatitis.
- Severe non-responsive bullous erythema multiforme.
- Multicentric reticulohistiocytosis.
- Cytophagic histiocytic panniculitis.
- Ichthyosis linearis circumflexa.

Contraindications

Absolute

- Pregnancy.
- Lactation.
- Hypersensitivity to CPE.
- Decreased bone marrow function.

Relative

- Infections.
- Deranged renal and hepatic function.

Pregnancy prescribing status: category 'D'.

Dosing

The dose of CPE ranges from 1 to 3 mg/kg/day or 0.5 to 1gm/m^2 of body surface area as a once-monthly intravenous pulse dose for most dermatologic disorders. For daily dosing, CPE is given as 50–100 mg/day as a single oral dose in the morning. Doses greater than 200 mg/day are associated with a high risk of myelosuppression.

Following administration of pulse CPE, the lowest drop of leukocytes takes place after 10–12 days. As rebound proliferation of lymphocytes occurs within 2 weeks, therefore, pulsing is mandated every 3–4 weeks. In this way, the cytotoxic effects of CPE can be claimed when proliferation of B cells is endangered most. Clinical responses with pulse CPE are evident within 4–6 weeks of therapy [1, 4–6].

For proteinuric lupus nephropathy and severe lupus vasculitis, intravenous boluses of CPE (5–9 mg/kg/day over 7–15 days) have demonstrated efficacy. Further, co-administration of sodium 2-mercaptoethane sulfonate (MESNA) is essential in these patients to reduce bladder toxicity.

Clinical Uses

Pemphigus

As per a Cochrane analysis and latest systematic appraisals, the cornerstone of treating pemphigus vulgaris (PV) and pemphigus foliaceous (PF) is high-dose glucocorticoid monotherapy or in coalition with steroid-sparing drugs [7–9]. Azathioprine and mycophenolate mofetil are the first-line steroid-sparing agents, while CPE is customarily second line [10]. Precedence of one steroid-sparing drug over another is yet to be established by clinical trials [8]. A retrospective publication involving 101 patients with moderate-to-severe mucocutaneous PV studied the end result of four treatment schedules:

- Prednisolone (1.1–1.5 mg/kg/day) alone.
- Prednisolone combined with oral azathioprine (1.1–1.5 mg/kg/day).
- Prednisolone combined with oral cyclosporine (2.5–3 mg/kg/day).
- Prednisolone combined with oral CPE (1.1–1.5 mg/kg/day).

It was deduced that the average time for clinical abeyance (defined by the absence of mucocutaneous lesions for at least 6 weeks) was remarkably shorter for the CPE group. Further, usage of oral CPE as an adjunct corresponded with the lowest accumulative dose of prednisolone. Besides, on juxtaposing prednisolone combined with CPE to prednisolone monotherapy, it was observed that the time for immunologic remission had reduced significantly with CPE addition. Also, this concoction elucidated the lowest 5-year clinical relapse, with CPE not exceeding 15gms as the cumulative dose. Besides, in these patients haemorrhagic cystitis was not encountered, neither was bladder cancer diagnosed at 5–18 years follow-up [11]. Other regimens, including CPE for pemphigus, include

- CPE pulse therapy along with prednisolone.
- Dexamethasone CPE pulse (DCP) therapy.

Cyclophosphamide Pulse Therapy with Prednisolone

Though there exists anecdotal supportive evidence regarding the efficacy of CPE pulse therapy, randomized controlled trials (RCT) have not inveterated the same because data on remission induction, relapses and time to disease control have been indeterminate and statistically inconsequential due to small sample sizes.

In 2013, Sharma and Khandpur [12] compared prednisolone monotherapy with prednisolone and monthly CPE (15 mg/kg) in 60 PV patients for a period of 1 year. They concluded superior remission induction rates (88% for prednisolone and CPE pulse therapy group versus 73% for the prednisolone monotherapy group), faster time to disease control and abrogation (8.1 weeks in prednisolone plus CPE pulse therapy group versus 9.5 weeks in the prednisolone monotherapy group) and curtailed relapse rate per cent for the prednisolone and CPE pulse therapy group (during treatment: 52% for prednisolone and pulse CPE group versus 71% for the prednisolone monotherapy group, following treatment (42% for prednisolone and pulse CPE group versus 60% for the prednisolone monotherapy group). Also, the side effect profile in both groups was synonymous.

In another RCT conducted on 28 patients, dexamethasone cyclophosphamide pulse (DCP), along with oral CPE 50 mg/day between pulses and prednisolone combined with monthly CPE (15 mg/kg) for 12–15 months, was compared and outlined similar induction rates in each group (60% each). Also, the duration taken for disease control was swifter in the group receiving prednisolone and monthly CPE (3.16 weeks) in comparison to the group receiving DCP and daily CPE (50 mg/

day between pulses) (7.33 weeks). Besides, the time for disease remission was condensed in the prednisolone and monthly CPE group (8.4 ± 3.2 weeks) when collated with DCP and oral CPE group (13 ± 9.2 weeks). However, relapse rates were experienced more in the prednisolone and combined monthly CPE group, both during therapy and following remission [13].

Dexamethasone Cyclophosphamide Pulse Therapy

In India, DCP is widely utilized for pemphigus therapy [14, 15].

DCP has delineated efficacy in restraining disease activity and keeping down adverse effects induced by corticosteroids. Pasricha et al. [14] introduced DCP for the treatment of pemphigus vulgaris. Treatment protocol comprises administering 100 mg of dexamethasone in 500 ml of 5% dextrose on days 1, 2 and 3 and 500 mg of intravenous CPE on day 2 along with dexamethasone infusion. This schedule is rerun once every 28 days, with 50 mg of oral CPE given each day.

DCP consists of four phases:

Phase I: In this phase, the above therapeutic regimen is administered to the patient till the achievement of remission.

Phase II: Here, DCP therapy is conferred for 9 more months following achievement of clinical remission.

Phase III: Here, DCP is discontinued. However, CPE (per oral 50 mg/day) is continued for 1 year.

Phase IV: All drugs are pulled out in this phase, with the patient being on regular follow-up.

DCP therapy is a substantially safe treatment and can even be given to the paediatric population. However, in children <12 years, the dose is decreased to half [15].

Bullous Pemphigoid (BP)

CPE has a plausible role in moderate-to-severe BP, unresponsive to azathioprine and mycophenolate. In a series of 20 patients, Gual et al. [16] outlined systemic glucocorticoids along with CPE (PO 50 mg/day, with dose escalation to 100 mg/day in 5 patients) to be effective in achieving complete remission (defined as no lesions and treatment able to be tapered) in 58% patients and partial improvement (defined as no new lesions but treatment unable to be tapered) in 21% patients. Further, leucopoenia and anaemia were the adverse effects commonly observed.

Mucous Membrane Pemphigoid (MMP)

Prednisolone, along with CPE (1–2 mg/kg/day), is considered the benchmark treatment for high-risk MMP (i.e. ocular, nasopharyngeal, laryngeal, oesophageal and genital involvement) [17]. In most studies in ocular MMP, CPE is utilized as a second-line agent after failure of mycophenolate mofetil [18–20]. In a report studying 13 patients with extra MMP, the authors delineated CPE (2 mg/kg/day) to be highly effective in critical, progressive and recalcitrant cases [21]. Besides, it is identified that ocular inflammation regresses faster than extraocular lesions of MMP.

Pemphigoid Gestationis

CPE was highly efficient in bringing about abeyance of severe postpartum pemphigoid gestationis in a patient recalcitrant to high-dose CS after receiving three cycles of 0.75gm/m^2 of CPE [22].

Systemic Hypocomplementemic Urticarial Vasculitis

Worm et al. [23] elaborated propitious outcomes of systemic hypocomplementemic urticarial vasculitis in two patients following 2–4 weekly DCP therapy, with administration of oral CPE (50 mg/day) betwixt pulses, who were unresponsive to other immunosuppressants. Remission was ascertained post administration of the tenth pulse.

Eosinophilic Granulomatosis with Polyangiitis (EGPA) and Polyarteritis Nodosa (PAN)

In severe EGPA delineating poor prognostic indicators, CPE is a valuable adjuvant [24].

In a long-term follow-up report involving 278 patients with PAN, microscopic polyangiitis and EGPA, Gayraud et al. elucidated statistically significant prolongation of survival in seriously ill patients who were given corticosteroids, as well as either pulse CPE or quotidian CPE [25]. On the other hand, in the RCT performed on 13 patients by Ribi and colleagues, the superiority of CPE over azathioprine in PAN that was resistant to systemic glucocorticoids and had a relapsing nature was not described [26].

Wegener's Granulomatosis

Relying on several RCTs, high-dose corticosteroids, along with adjuvant CPE, are regarded as a first-line treatment for critical WG [27]. Earlier, in spite of profitable outcomes using high-dose CPE (2 mg/kg/day) and high-dose prednisolone in WG, noteworthy relapse rates and adverse effects were the greatest limitation [28]. Recently, in antineutrophilic cytoplasmic antibody (ANCA)-associated vasculitis, pulse CPE (15 mg/kg once in 2 or 3 weeks for 6 months) was outlined to be productive and safe when collated with daily administration of oral CPE [29].

Cutaneous Lupus Erythematosus

Though strong evidence exists regarding the value of CPE in the treatment of severe systemic lupus erythematosus (SLE), corroboration for CPE in the therapy of cutaneous LE is restricted.

In 14 patients with refractory SLE, Petri and colleagues delineated solo high-dose CPE pulse therapy (50 mg/kg/day for 4 days along with MESNA) to be effective in promoting resolution of all cutaneous lesions. Further, in two patients with concurrent pyoderma gangrenosum, complete rectification of lesions was outlined with CPE [30].

In another evaluation of six patients with cutaneous LE, resistant to other systemic therapies (systemic CS, antimalarials and azathioprine), complete lesional correction was seen in four patients and partial improvement was observed in two patients following 7–12 months of treatment with monthly methylprednisolone and CPE pulse, along with low-dose prednisolone between cycles [31].

Dermatomyositis

The level of evidence regarding the efficacy of CPE for severe/refractory DM in children and adults is low.

Nonetheless, in the exposition by Riley et al. [32], in 12 patients with refractory juvenile DM, pulse CPE (1gm/m^2 monthly) outlined improvement in cutaneous, musculoskeletal, as well as systemic features of DM. To note, in this sequence, 2 of 12 patients, who were on mechanical ventilation, expired before CPE could demonstrate its beneficial effects [32].

Further, Tsujimura et al. [33] elaborated complete resolution of refractory DM in an adult patient with concomitant cutaneous vasculitis, with repeated cycles of intravenous CPE pulse (15 mg/kg each pulse).

Systemic Sclerosis (SS)

Though CPE is advocated in SS with interstitial lung disease, CPE also demonstrates some amelioration in skin changes linked with SS.

Tashkin et al. demonstrated CPE ($\leq$ 2 mg/kg/day for 6–12 months) to be of value in significantly reducing skin thickness in 85 of 158 patients with SS, also having interstitial lung disease. Interestingly, this benefit was observed only in those patients who had diffuse skin involvement and not in patients with SS having limited cutaneous involvement [34]. Besides, in a follow-up survey of the same patients at 2 years, although there was curtailment in whole skin thickness during the first 1 year, these effects diminished from 1 to 2 years [35]. In another randomized clinical trial on 13 patients with early diffuse SS, similar findings were iterated. In this study, CPE (per oral 2–2.5 mg/kg/day), along with methylprednisolone (30 mg/every other day), was employed for 12 months [36].

Relapsing Polychondritis

In corticosteroid-resistant relapsing polychondritis associated with glomerulonephritis, CPE (per oral 150 mg/day) or monthly intravenous CPE pulse (750 mg/month) demonstrates propitious outcomes for renal involvement [37, 38].

Primary Cutaneous T Cell Lymphoma

High-dose CPE constituting chemotherapeutic regimens is reserved for refractory, relapsed and rapidly progressive cutaneous T cell lymphoma, including advanced mycosis fungoides (MF) and Sezary syndrome [39]. Though previously CPE monotherapy was utilized for MF, today multidrug regimens like CHOP [CPE, doxorubicin, vincristine (oncovin) and prednisolone] are being used [40]. For refractory or progressive Sezary syndrome, combination of CPE and fludarabine is recommended as second-line treatment [40].

Behcet's Disease

The use of CPE in BD is confined to those cases manifesting with life-threatening ocular, neurologic and large vessel involvement [41, 42].

Pyoderma Gangrenosum

For the treatment of PG, CPE is dispensed both orally and intravenously [43]. In a sequence of nine patients, 100% ulcer healing was observed in seven patients and partial remission in one patient, following treatment with intravenous CPE pulse (500 mg/m^2 monthly) for 6 months [44].

Sweet's Syndrome (SS)

Evans et al. outlined CPE to be effective in a patient with SS associated with myelodysplasia [45].

Chronic Urticaria

A favourable response to CPE in chronic idiopathic urticaria has been delineated in two publications [46, 47].

Steven–Johnson Syndrome and Toxic Epidermal Necrolysis

Affirmation of CPE for use in Steven–Johnson syndrome (SJS) and toxic epidermal necrolysis (TEN) is restricted and inconsistent. Early reports have shown improvement in SJS and TEN with CPE, including those cases recalcitrant to systemic steroids [48, 49].

In one study, eight patients received CPE (300 mg/day initially, tapering to 100–150 mg/day for up to 6 days) monotherapy, following which there was halting of bulla formation [49].

However, as per recent reports, CPE is not in general use anymore for TEN, with cyclosporine being a superior drug in achieving re-epithelialization, halting disease progression and reducing mortality [50].

Interestingly, rapid control of erythema multiforme major has been reported with prednisolone and low-dose CPE [51].

Generalized Eruptive Keratoacanthoma of Grzybowski (GEKG)

In two case reports of GEKG where methotrexate and acitretin had failed, remission was acquired with oral CPE (100–200 mg/day for 3–15 months) [52, 53].

Further, among three patients with GEKG, two reported remission following six cycles of CPE pulse therapy with monthly 1gm of CPE. In all patients, the disease had been present for 5–7 years and was recalcitrant to methotrexate therapy [54].

Severe Eczematous Dermatitis

Interestingly, CPE has been used for treating eczemas. Within an average duration of 3.25 months, satisfactory responses are noted. However, high relapse rates are accounted following stoppage of treatment [55].

Scleromyxedema

CPE (100–200 mg/day) was productive in bringing about clinical amelioration in three patients with scleromyxedema. [56–58] Further, Kuldeep et al [59] reported three cycles of DCP therapy to be effectual in promoting clinical attenuation of skin lesions, with near-total skin softening after 24 cycles of DCP.

Multicentric Reticulohistiocytosis (MR)

In MR, improvement in dermatologic, rheumatologic and systemic symptoms has been documented with CPE (per oral 1–2 mg/kg/day) monotherapy as well as combination therapy with glucocorticoids and methotrexate [60–62]. Besides, pulse therapy with CPE (750–1000 mg intravenously) as a monthly schedule has also elaborated propitious outcomes in MR. [63]

Langerhans Cell Histiocytosis

Complete remission of LCH with oral CPE monotherapy (50 mg/day) within 60 days of initiating treatment was documented by Nakajima and colleagues [64]. Further, treatment was continued for a total period of 6 months and was then stopped. Besides, the disease did not recur.

Xanthoma Disseminatum

Seaton et al. [65] reported dramatic resolution of extensive and refractory lesions of xanthoma disseminatum involving the skin, eyes, larynx, pituitary and nervous system with oral CPE (50–100 mg/day) for a period of one-and-a-half years.

Cutaneous Nodular Amyloidosis

A case report of primary localized nodular amyloidosis associated with Sjogren's syndrome and CREST syndrome, previously unresponsive to multiple immunosuppressants, demonstrated stabilization of existing nodules with no new deposits within 2 months of treatment with prednisolone and oral CPE [66].

Others

Case reports regarding the effectiveness of CPE in necrobiotic xanthogranuloma and cytophagic histiocytic panniculitis have been delineated in various reports [67, 68].

Adverse Effects

Haematologic

- Myelosuppression, with leucopoenia, is the most important dose-limiting adverse effect, occurring usually 8–12 days following initiation of CPE treatment.
- Thrombocytopenia (less common).
- Anaemia (less commonly seen).
- The above effects are observed with high doses of CPE and are usually reversible.

Urologic [69]

- Increased frequency of urination.
- Dysuria.
- Urgency.
- Microscopic haematuria.
- Bladder fibrosis.
- Vesicoureteral reflux.
- Haemorrhagic cystitis (HC):
  - This adverse effect is dose related.
  - It occurs due to acrolein, a toxic metabolite of CPE.
  - Patients with HC express an increased risk of bladder carcinoma.
  - Risk of HC is 5–10% in doses employed for dermatologic disorders.
  - MESNA is simultaneously given when high-dose CPE is dispensed to alleviate the toxic effect of HC.

Gastrointestinal

- Anorexia.
- Nausea.
- Vomiting.
- Diarrhoea.
- Stomatitis.
- In high doses: hepatotoxicity and haemorrhagic colitis.

Gonadal

- Azoospermia: characterized by testicular germ cell depletion.
- Premature ovarian failure: characterized by the disappearance of primordial ovarian follicles.
- Reversibility of gonadal damage is unpredictable.

Cutaneous [70, 71]

- Anagen effluvium (which could be irreversible).
- Irreversible pigmented band on the teeth.
- Diffuse skin hyperpigmentation.
- Transverse nail ridging.
- Steven–Johnson syndrome (this is a therapeutic paradox).
- Rarely mucosal ulceration and urticaria.

Carcinogenicity [72]

- Increased risk of transitional cell cancer of the urinary bladder.
- Acute myeloid leukaemia.
- Squamous cell carcinoma.
- Non-Hodgkin's lymphoma.

Others

- Cardiomyopathy.
- Pneumonitis.
- Opportunistic infections.
- Pulmonary fibrosis.
- Syndrome of inappropriate antidiuretic hormone secretion (SIADH).
- Seizures.
- Progressive muscular paralysis.
- Cholinergic effects.

Monitoring Guidelines

Baseline

- Detailed physical examination.
- WBC count: should be more than 5000/mm^3.
- Urine analysis: to rule out microscopic haematuria.
- Chest X-ray PA view.
- Pregnancy test.
- Liver function tests.
- Renal function tests.

Follow-Up

- In the first 3 months: WBC counts, platelet count and urinalysis should be done every 2–3 weeks.
- After that: the above tests, along with chest X-ray, lymph node screening and serum chemistry profile, need to be performed once a month.

Indications for Discontinuing Therapy

- WBC count <3000/mm^3.
- Platelet count <100,000/mm^3.
- RBC in urine.

Conclusion

CPE is a boon for the treatment of autoimmune blistering disorders, especially in developing countries like India. However, the utility of CPE still remains widely unused for many other dermatoses.

References

1. Ho V, Zloty D. Immunosuppressive agents in dermatology. Dermatol Clin. 1993;11:73–85.
2. Rapini RP. Cytotoxic drugs in the treatment of skin disease. Int J Dermatol. 1991;30:313–21.
3. Ahmed AR, Hombal SM. Cyclophosphamide: a review on relevant pharmacology and clinical uses. J Am Acad Dermatol. 1984;11:1115–26.
4. Ghate J. Immunosuppressive therapies in dermatology: cyclophosphamide. Curr Probl Dermatol. 2000;12:265–7.
5. Silvis NG. Antimetabolites and cytotoxic drugs. Dermatol Clin. 2001;19:105–18.
6. Pandya A, Sontheimer R. Treatment of pemphigus with pulse intravenous cyclophosphamide. Arch Dermatol. 1992;128:1626–30.
7. Kasper Kiewicz M, Schmidt E, Zillikens D. Current therapy of the pemphigus group. Clin Dermatol. 2012;30:84–94.
8. Zhao CY, Murrell DF. Pemphigus vulgaris: an evidence based treatment update. Drugs. 2015;75:271–84.
9. Martin LK, Werth V, Villanueva E, et al. Interventions for pemphigus vulgaris and pemphigus foliaceous. Cochrane Database Syst Rev. 2009;1:CD006263.
10. Atzmony L, Hodak E, Gdalevich M, et al. Treatment of pemphigus vulgaris and pemphigus foliaceous: a systematic review and meta analysis. Am J Clin Dermatol. 2014;15:503–15.
11. Oleszewska M, Kolacinka-Strasz Z, Sulej J, et al. Efficacy and safety of cyclophosphamide, azathioprine and cyclosporine as adjuvant drugs in pemphigus vulgaris. Am J Clin Dermatol. 2007;8:85–92.
12. Sharma VK, Khandpur S. Evaluation of cyclophosphamide pulse therapy as an adjuvant to oral corticosteroid in the management of pemphigus vulgaris. Clin Exp Dermatol. 2013;38:659–64.
13. Sethy PK, Khandpur S, Sharma VK. Randomized open comparative trial of dexamethasone cyclophosphamide pulse and daily oral cyclophosphamide versus cyclophosphamide pulse and daily oral prednisolone in pemphigus vulgaris. Indian J Dermatol Venereol Leprol. 2009;75:476–82.
14. Pasricha JS, Thanzama J, Khan U. Intermittent high dose dexamethasone cyclophosphamide therapy for pemphigus. Br J Dermatol. 1988;119:73–7.
15. Pasricha JS. Pulse therapy as a cure for autoimmune diseases. Indian J Dermatol Venereol Leprol. 2003;69:323–8.
16. Gual A, Iranzo P, Mascaro JM Jr. Treatment of bullous pemphigoid with low dose oral cyclophosphamide: a case series of 20 patients. J Eur Acad Dermato, Venereol. 2014;28:814–8.
17. Chan LS, Ahmed AR, Anhalt GJ, et al. The first international consensus on mucous membrane pemphigoid: definition, diagnostic criteria, pathogenic factors, medical treatment and prognostic indicators. Arch Dermatol. 2002;138:370–9.
18. Friedman J, Marcovich AL, Kleinmann G, et al. Low dose pulsed intravenous cyclophosphamide for severe ocular cicatricial pemphigoid in elderly patients. Cornea. 2014;33:1066–70.
19. Yesudian PO, Armstrong S, Cawood JI, et al. mucous membrane pemphigoid: management of advanced ocular disease with intravenous cyclophosphamide and amniotic membrane transplantation. Br J Dermatol. 2005;153:692–4.
20. Gibbons A, Johnson TE, Wester ST, et al. Management of patients with confirmed and oresumed mucous membrane pemphigoid undergoing entropion repair. Am J Ophthalmol. 2015;159:846–52.

21. Munyangango EM, Le Roux-Villet C, Doan S, et al. Oral cyclophosphamide without corticosteroids to treat mucous membrane pemphigoid. Br J Dermatol. 2013;168:381–90.
22. Castle SP, Mather-Mondrey M, Bennion S, et al. Chronic herpes gestationis and antiphospholipid syndrome successfully treated with cyclophosphamide. J Am Acad Dermatol. 1996;34:333–6.
23. Worm M, Muche M, Schulze P, et al. Hypocomplemententemic urticarial vasculitis: successful treatment with cyclophosphamide-dexamethasone pulse therapy. Br J Dermatol. 1998;139:704–7.
24. Lally L, Spiera R. Current landscape of antineutrophilic cytoplasmic antibody associated vasculitis: classification, diagnosis and treatment. Rheum Dis Clin N Am. 2015;41:1–19.
25. Gayraud M, Guillevin L, Le Toumelin P, et al. Long-term follow up of polyarteritis nodosa, microscopic polyangiitis and Churg Strauss syndrome: analysis of four prospective trials including 278 patients. Arthritis Rheum. 2001;44:666–75.
26. Ribi C, Cohen P, Pagnoux C, et al. Treatment of polyarteritis nodosa and microscopic polyangiitis without poor prognostic factors: a prospective randomized study of 124 patients. Arthritis Rheum. 2010;62:1186–97.
27. Langford CA. Cyclophosphamide as induction therapy for Wegener's granulomatosis and microscopic polyangiitis. Clin Exp Immunol. 2011;164:31–4.
28. Fauci AS, Haynes BF, Katz P, et al. Wegener's granulomatosis: prospective trial and therapeutic experience with 85 patients for 21 years. Ann Intern Med. 1983;98:76–85.
29. de Groot K, Harper L, Jayne DR, et al. Pulse versus daily oral cyclophosphamide for induction of remission in antineutrophil cytoplasmic antibody associated vasculitis: a randomized trial. Ann Intern Med. 2009;150:670–80.
30. Petri M, Jones RJ, Brodsky RA. High dose cyclophosphamide without stem cell transplantation in systemic lupus erythematosus. Arthritis Rheum. 2003;48:166–73.
31. Raptopoulou A, Linardakis C, Sidiropoulos P, et al. Pulse cyclophosphamide treatment for severe refractory cutaneous lupus erythematosus. Lupus. 2010;19:744–7.
32. Riley P, Maillard SM, Wedderburn LR, et al. Intravenous cyclophosphamide pulse therapy in juvenile dermatomyositis. A review of efficacy and safety. Rheumatology. 2004;43:491–6.
33. Tsujimura S, Saito K, Tanaka Y. Complete resolution of dermatomyositis with refractory cutaneous vasculitis by intravenous cyclophosphamide pulse therapy. Intern Med. 2008;47:1935–40.
34. Tashkin DP, Elashoff R, Clements PJ, et al. Cyclophosphamide versus placebo in scleroderma lung disease. N Engl J Med. 2006;354:2655–66.
35. Tashkin DP, Elashoff R, Clements PJ, et al. Effects of 1 year treatment with cyclophosphamide on outcomes at 2 years in scleroderma lung disease. Am J Respir Crit Care Med. 2007;176:1026–34.
36. Van Laar JM, Farge D, Sont JK, et al. Autologous hematopoietic stem cell transplantation versus intravenous pulse cyclophosphamide in diffuse cutaneous systemic sclerosis: a randomized clinical trial. JAMA. 2014;311:2490–8.
37. Ruhlen JL, Hutson KA, Wood WG. Relapsing polychondritis with glomerulonephritis. Improvement with prednisolone and cyclophosphamide. JAMA. 1981;245:847–8.
38. Stewart KA, Mazanne DJ. Pulse intravenous cyclophosphamide for kidney disease in relapsing polychondritis. J Rheumatol. 1992;19:498–500.
39. Jawed SI, Myskowski PL, Horwitz S, et al. Primary cutaneous T cell lymphoma (mycosis fungoides and Sezary syndrome): part II. Prognosis, management and future directions. J Am Acad Dermatol. 2014;70:223.e1–17.
40. Oslen EA, Rook AH, Zic J, et al. Sezary syndrome: immunopathogenesis, literature review of therapeutic options, and recommendations for therapy by United States lymphoma consortium (USCLE). J Am Acad Dermatol. 2011;64:352–404.
41. Alpsoy E. New evidence-based treatment approach in Behcet's disease. Pathol Res Int. 2012;2012:871019.
42. Saleh Z, Arayssi T. Update on therapy of Behcet's disease. Ther Adv Chronic Dis. 2014;5:112–34.

43. Reichrath J, Bens G, Benowitz A, et al. Treatment recommendations for pyoderma gangrenosum: an evidence-based review of literature based on more than 350 patients. J Am Acad Dermatol. 2005;53:273–83.
44. Reynosi-von Drateln C, Perla-Navarro AV, Gamez-Nava JI, et al. Intravenous cyclophosphamide pulses in pyoderma gangrenosum: an open trial. J Rheumatol. 1997;24:689–93.
45. Evans AV, Sabroe RA, Liddel K, et al. Lymphocytic infiltrates as a presenting feature of sweet's syndrome with myelodysplasia and response to cyclophosphamide. Br J Dermatol. 2002;146:1087–90.
46. Bernstein JA, Garramone SM, Lower EG. Successful treatment of autoimmune idiopathic urticaria with intravenous cyclophosphamide. Ann Allergy Asthma Immunol. 2002;89:212–4.
47. Donaldson VH, Berstein DI, Wagner CJ, et al. Angioneurotic edema with acquired C1-inhibitor deficiency and autoantibody to C1 inhibitor: response to plasmapheresis and cytotoxic therapy. J Lab Clin Med. 1992;119:397–406.
48. Heng MC, Allen SG. Efficacy of cyclophosphamide in toxic epidermal necrolysis. Clinical and pathophysiologic aspects. J Am Acad Dermatol. 1991;25:778–86.
49. Trautmann A, Klein CE, Kampgen E, et al. Severe bullous drug reactions treated successfully with cyclophosphamide. Br J Dermatol. 1998;139:1127–8.
50. Arevalo JM, Lorente JA, Gonsalez-Herrada C, et al. Treatment of toxic epidermal necrolysis with cyclosporine a. J Trauma. 2000;48:473–8.
51. Eastham JH, Segal JL, Gomez MF, et al. Reversal of erythema multiforme major with cyclophosphamide and prednisolone. Ann Pharmacother. 1996;30:606–7.
52. Oakley A, Ng S. Grzybowski's generalized eruptive keratoacanthoma: remission with cyclophosphamide. Australas J Dermatol. 2005;46:118–23.
53. Grine RC, Hendrix JD, Greer KE. Generalized eruptive keratoacanthoma of Grzybowski: response to cyclophosphamide. J Am Acad Dermatol. 1997;36:786–7.
54. Nofal A, Assaf M, Ghonemy S, et al. Generalized eruptive keratoacanthoma: a diagnostic and therapeutic challenge. Int J Dermatol. 2015;54:160–7.
55. Morrison JG, Schulz EJ. Treatment of eczema with cyclophosphamide and azathioprine. Br J Dermatol. 1978;98:203–7.
56. Craig NM, Putterman AM, Roenignk RK, et al. Multiple periorbital cutaneous myxomas progressing to scleromyxedema. J Am Acad Dermatol. 1996;34:928–30.
57. Howsden SM, Herndon JH Jr, Freeman RG. Lichen myxedematous: a dermal infiltrative disorder responsive to cyclophosphamide therapy. Arch Dermatol. 1975;111:1325–30.
58. Jessen RT, Straight M, Becker LE. Lichen myxedematous. Treatment with cyclophosphamide. Int J Dermatol. 1978;17:833–9.
59. Kuldeep CM, Mittal AK, Gupta LK, et al. Successful treatment of scleromyxedema with dexamethasone cyclophosphamide pulse therapy. Indian J Dermatol Venereol Leprol. 2005;71:44–5.
60. Lui YH, Fang K. Multicentric reticulohistiocytosis with generalized systemic involvement. Clin Exp Dermatol. 2004;29:373–6.
61. Liang GC, Granston AS. Complete remission of multicentric reticulohistiocytosis with combination therapy of steroid, cyclophosphamide and low dose pulse methotrexate. Case report, review of literature and proposal for treatment. Arthritis Rheum. 1996;39:171–4.
62. Ginsburg WW, Duffy JO, Morris JL, et al. Multicentric reticulohistiocytosis: response to alkylating agents in six patients. Ann Intern Med. 1989;111:384–8.
63. Blanco JJ, Hernandez FJ, Cerezo JG, et al. Multicentric reticulohistiocytosis. The long course of a rare disease. Scand J Rheumatol. 2002;31:107–9.
64. Nakajama K, Morisawa R, Kodama H, et al. Successful treatment with cyclophosphamide of Langerhans cell histiocytosis involving the skin and lymph nodes in an adult patient. Clin Exp Dermatol. 2010;35:791–2.
65. Seaton ED, Pillai GJ, Chu AC. Treatment of xanthoma disseminatum with cyclophosphamide. Br J Dermatol. 2004;150:346–9.
66. Tong PL, Walker WA, Glancy RJ, et al. Primary localized cutaneous nodular amyloidosis successfully treated with cyclophosphamide. Australas J Dermatol. 2013;54:e12–5.
67. Spicknall KE, Mehregan DA. Necrobiotic xanthogranuloma. Int J Dermatol. 2009;48:1–10.

68. Petterson T, Kariniemi AL, Tervonen S, et al. Cytopathic histiocytic panniculitis: a report of four cases. Br J Dermatol. 1992;127:635–40.
69. Brock N, Pohl J, Stekar J. Studies on the urotoxicity of oxazaphosphorine cytostatics and its prevention I. Experimental studies on the urotoxicity of alkylating agents. Eur J Cancer Clin Oncol. 1981;17:596–607.
70. Bronner AK, Hood AF. Cutaneous complications of chemotherapeutic agents. J Am Acad Dermatol. 1983;9:645–63.
71. Assier-Bonnet H, Aractingi S, Cadranel J, et al. Steven Johnson syndrome induced by cyclophosphamide. Report of 2 cases. Br J Dermatol. 1996;135:864–6.
72. Baker GL, Kahl LE, Zee BC. Malignancy following treatment of rheumatoid arthritis with cyclophosphamide. Am J Med. 1987;83:1–9.

Cyclosporine

25

Introduction

Cyclosporine A (CsA) is an immunosuppressive drug derived primarily from the soil fungus *Tolypocladium inflatum gams* and *Cylindrocarpon lucidum* [1]. Structurally, CsA is a neutral cyclic peptide composed of 11 amino acids. As CsA is not cytotoxic, it does not repress the bone marrow. Besides, CsA does not harm the foetus.

Mechanism of Action

The mechanism of action of CsA is not completely understood. However, it is observed that there are a variety of actions responsible for the immunosuppressive effects of CsA as elaborated in Fig. 25.1 [2, 3].

A. K. Bubna, *Therapeutics in Dermatology - Essentials for Clinical Practice*, https://doi.org/10.1007/978-981-95-3791-4_25

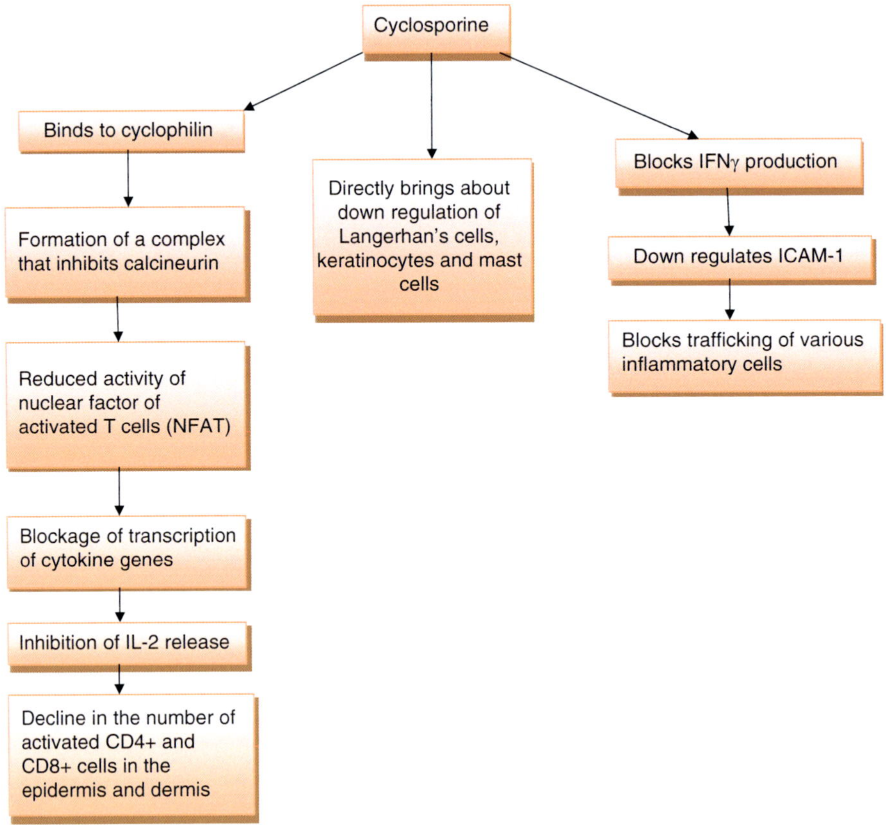

Fig. 25.1 Mechanism of action of cyclosporine

Pharmacokinetics

The bioavailability of ingested CsA is 25–35%. Peak plasma levels occur from 1.5 to 4 h after oral administration. CsA is metabolized by the cytochrome P450 enzyme system in the liver. Hepatic insufficiency may prolong the $t_{1/2}$ of CsA, and therefore requires adjustments. Excretion is via the bile through faeces. Only 6% of the drug is eliminated via the urine.

Indications

FDA-Approved

- Psoriasis: severe psoriasis, recalcitrant and treatment-resistant psoriasis, and disabling psoriasis (including localized versions like hand and foot psoriasis).

Off-Label

Eczemas

- Atopic dermatitis (AD).

Papulosquamous Disorders

- Lichen planus (LP).

Bullous Dermatoses

- Pemphigus.
- Bullous pemphigoid (BP).
- Epidermolysis bullosa acquisita (EBA).
- Linear IgA bullous dermatosis (LABD).

Autoimmune Connective Tissue Disorders

- Dermatomyositis (DM).
- Lupus erythematosus (LE).
- Systemic sclerosis (SS).

Neutrophilic Dermatoses

- Behcet's disease (BD).
- Pyoderma gangrenosum (PG).

Alopecia

- Lichen planopilaris (LPP).
- Alopecia areata (AA).

Granulomatous Dermatoses

- Granuloma annulare (GA).
- Sarcoidosis.

Photosensitivity Dermatosis

- Chronic actinic dermatitis (CAD).

Urticaria

- Chronic idiopathic urticaria.
- Cold urticaria.
- Solar urticaria.

Others

- Steven–Johnson syndrome (SJS).
- Toxic epidermal necrolysis (TEN).
- Eosinophilic cellulitis.
- Kimura's disease.
- Morphoea.

- Prurigo nodularis.
- Papuloerythroderma of Ofuji.
- Reiter's syndrome.
- Persistent papular acantholytic dermatosis.

Contraindications

Absolute

- Significantly reduced renal function.
- Uncontrolled hypertension.
- Hypersensitivity to CsA or any ingredient in the formulation.
- Cutaneous T cell lymphoma.
- Clinically cured or persistent malignancy (except non-melanoma skin cancers).

Relative

- Age < 18 years or > 64 years.
- Controlled hypertension.
- Planning to receive a live-attenuated vaccine.
- On medications that potentiate renal dysfunction or interfere with CsA metabolism.
- Active infection.
- Evidence of immune-deficiency.
- Concomitantly receiving phototherapy.
- Pregnancy and lactation.
- Unreliable patients.

Pregnancy prescribing status: category 'C'.

Clinical Uses

Psoriasis

CsA in psoriasis is used in patients:

- With severe flare-ups.
- With severe disabling psoriasis who cannot tolerate, have contraindications to or have failed other systemic therapies.
- Who have a major life incident (such as a wedding) coming up, where substantial clearing is important.

In these scenarios, intermittent short-term therapy with CsA is employed with an initiating dose of 5 mg/kg/day [4]. Here, treatment generally lasts for 12–16 weeks, during which significant improvement is noticeable. In case of relapse, treatment with CsA is reinstituted at the same dose [5].

On the other hand, for patients with generalized but relatively stable plaque-type psoriasis, a dose of 2.5–3 mg/kg/day can be used. If improvement is not seen at the end of 1 month, the dose of CsA needs to be escalated by 0.5–1 mg/kg/day every 2 weeks but never to exceed more than 5 mg/kg/day. If there is an inadequate response with 5 mg/kg/day of CsA after 3 months of therapy, CsA needs to be discontinued. While discontinuing CsA, it should be gradually tapered, with simultaneous introduction of another anti-psoriatic agent. Sudden stoppage of CsA can result in pustular flares [6, 7].

Sequential Therapy in Psoriasis with Cyclosporine

The idea behind administering sequential therapy is that clinicians can use specific medications in a deliberate sequence to optimize the strength of each drug, while minimizing their weaknesses. This is in contrast to the usual approach where psoriasis patients are given one main therapeutic agent with the expectation that if it works well it will be continued and if it does not it will be replaced with another drug.

The rationale for sequential therapy include

- Some medications are ideal for quick fixes, while others are ideal for maintenance therapy.
- Systemic therapy in psoriasis elaborates strengths as well as weaknesses for each patient.
- Maximizing the strength and minimizing the weaknesses of each therapeutic agent involved.

This therapy is of particular value in the treatment of erythrodermic, sub-erythrodermic and generalized pustular forms of psoriasis.

Sequential therapy has three stages:

- Phase I (clearing phase).
- Phase II (transition phase).
- Phases III A and B (maintenance phase).

Phase I

Here, CsA alone is used at the maximum dermatologic dose of 5 mg/kg/day.

Phase II

Here, the dose of CsA is reduced to 4 mg/kg/day, and then gradually reduced by 1 mg/kg/day every month till the 3 mg/kg/day dose is obtained.

Now drugs like acitretin (25 mg/day)/methotrexate (7.5–10 mg/week) are introduced. Their doses may need escalation to achieve appropriate clinical remission as CsA is being tapered.

Phase IIIA

Maintenance of treatment with acitretin/methotrexate, without CsA.

Phase IIIB

Maintenance of treatment with acitretin and UVB or PUVA (Re-UVB or Re-PUVA) or methotrexate alone.

Used in combination with CsA, acitretin is effective in clearing severe psoriasis, along with safely maintaining clearance on a long-term basis.

Long-Term Therapy

In majority of psoriasis patients, efficacy has been maintained with long-term CsA therapy. Besides, the aim of maintenance is to attain significant improvement rather than complete clinical clearance. The maintenance dose of CsA employed is 3–3.2 mg/kg/day [8].

In a comparative study evaluating 36 months intermittent therapy versus continuous therapy with CsA (average dose of 3.06 mg/kg/day), it was observed that the continuous dosed group maintained remission for 69% of the time compared to 32% for the intermittently dosed group [9].

In another study, comparing intermittent 12-week courses to continuous therapy with CsA for 1 year, it was seen that 62% of the intermittent group (mean dose, 3 mg/kg/day) achieved a 75% reduction in the Psoriasis Area and Severity Index (PASI) score compared with 92% of the continuous group (mean dose, 1.8 mg/kg/day) [10].

The Current American Academy of Dermatology (AAD) guidelines suggest intermittent therapy to be preferable to long-term therapy, and treatment regimens need to be tailored as per individual patient needs. Besides, the duration of continuous therapy with CsA needs to be kept below 1 year whenever possible.

Combination Therapy

CsA can be combined with topical therapies like corticosteroids [11], anthralin [12] or vitamin D3 analogues [13] for an improved response. Systemic drugs like methotrexate, fumaric acid esters, mycophenolate mofetil and acitretin have been safely used in combination with CsA, allowing for dose reduction of CsA, thereby minimizing toxicity [14–17].

Psoriatic Arthropathy

The most widely employed disease-modifying antirheumatic drugs (DMARDs) for psoriatic arthropathy (PsA) include methotrexate, sulfasalazine and CsA [18]. These drugs are introduced only if the disease is resistant to NSAIDs or if the disease is progressive. Various studies have documented the efficacy of CSA, either alone or in combination with methotrexate in PsA. Some of them are elaborated in Table 25.1 [18–22].

Table 25.1 Studies highlighting the utility of cyclosporine in psoriatic arthropathy

Authors	Study details	Remarks
Gupta et al [19]	Six patients with psoriatic arthropathy (PsA) who were treated with cyclosporine 6 mg/kg/day for 8 weeks	Significant improvement in joint strength, mean grip strength and activity level was noted However, within 2 weeks of discontinuing treatment, joint pain and swelling recurred
Steinsson et al [20]	Open-label prospective study Seven patients with PsA treated with cyclosporine (3.5 mg/kg/day) for 6 months	All patients had improvement in joint pain and swelling Time to relapse was not documented in this study
Salvarani et al [21]	A series of 12 patients who had failed second-line PsA treatment All were treated with cyclosporine (3 mg/kg/day) for 6 months	At the end of treatment, seven patients had greater than 50% reduction in joint tenderness and swelling In four patients, the disease had stabilized One patient had to withdraw from the study owing to significant nephrotoxicity
Spadaro et al [22]	Prospective controlled trial with 35 PsA patients Conducted to compare the effectiveness and toxicity of cyclosporine (3 mg/kg/day) versus low-dose methotrexate (7.5–15 mg/week)	At the end of 6 and 12 months of treatment, number of painful joints, swollen joints, Ritchie index, duration of morning stiffness, grip strength and C-reactive protein levels were reduced equally in both treatment groups However, toxicity profile was more in the cyclosporine group with more patients withdrawing from the cyclosporine group (41.2%) compared to the methotrexate group (27.8%)
Fraser et al [18]	A 12-month randomized, multicentre, double-blind placebo-controlled trial to study the efficacy and safety of combining cyclosporine with methotrexate in patients with PsA who had previous incomplete response to methotrexate monotherapy Out of 72 patients recruited, 38 were randomized to receive cyclosporine in addition to methotrexate (15 mg/week) and the remaining 34 were given a placebo along with methotrexate in the same dose Cyclosporine was started at a dose of 2.5 mg/kg/day, with increments at weeks 4, 8 and 12, increasing by 0.5 mg/kg till a maximum dose of 4 mg/kg/day was obtained (if tolerated by the patient)	Significant improvement in the following parameters was observed in the group receiving cyclosporine along with methotrexate compared to the group receiving methotrexate alone respectively Improvement in swollen joint count (11.7% versus 6.5%) C-reactive protein (17.4% versus 12.7%) Synovitis (33% versus 6%) However, significant difference in pain and quality of life was not detected in this study

Atopic Dermatitis

Cyclosporine is the only immunosuppressant approved in Europe and the United Kingdom for short-term treatment of severe AD, recalcitrant to topical therapy. Though not formally approved by the FDA for this indication [23], it is recommended by the American Academy of Dermatologists (AAD) Guidelines of Care Committee as being effective for the treatment of AD, unresponsive to conventional treatment, with no statement to the recommended dosage [24]. In treating refractory cases of AD, a commencing dose of CsA (5 mg/kg/day) for 2 weeks with gradual tapering as dictated by the clinical response over the ensuing 3 months, to a dose of 1.5 mg/kg/day where possible, is suggested. [25–28]

In a study by Zonneveld et al on 78 patients with severe AD, two long-term CsA dosing schedules were employed. One group initially received CsA 5 mg/kg/day, being gradually reduced to 3 mg/kg/day as needed. The other group obtained 3 mg/kg/day of CsA initially, with the dose escalated to 5 mg/kg/day as needed. Once optimal dosage was reached, treatment continued for 10 months. After 1 year when both groups were evaluated, it was found that the safety profile and tolerability to treatment were indistinguishable in both groups. However, efficacy was slightly better in the group started with 5 mg/kg/day of cyclosporine [29].

Regimens involving dose reduction of CsA after an inceptive dose of 5 mg/kg/day (and decreasing the daily dose by 1 mg/kg/day every fortnight), as well as schedules characterized by prolonging the dose interval (with the 5 mg/kg/day dose being administered by expanding the duration between doses by 1 day every 2 weeks), were found to be equally effective [30].

Further, for maintenance therapy, it is suggested to utilize the lowest productive dose of CsA [28].

There are mixed reports regarding disease relapse following cessation of CsA. Relapse generally occurs after 6–9 months of therapy cessation. However, the extent of AD and symptom scores remains improved compared to baseline, elucidating a plausible remission in some patients [31, 32].

However, according to Schmitt et al [33] and Naeyaert et al [34], there is no evidence of a rebound occurrence following CsA withdrawal.

Steven–Johnson Syndrome and Toxic Epidermal Necrolysis

Of late, CsA has gained recognition in the therapy of SJS/TEN. As T-lymphocytes contribute to the pathogenesis of TEN, use of CsA for this indication is suggested. CsA suppresses IL-2 production from helper T cells, and in this way impedes the activation of CD4+ and CD8+ (cytotoxic T cells) in the epidermis. Some studies have even suggested superiority of CsA over other therapies, including intravenous immunoglobulins (IVIG), corticosteroids, cyclophosphamide and supportive care alone.

CsA is used in a dose of 3–5 mg/kg/day as an oral capsule or solution in divided doses. However, there apparently is no agreement on the exact duration of therapy.

Most authors employ it for a month or till remission of skin lesions and re-epithelialization. It is proposed that prolonged therapy with CsA is perhaps not required, as disease progression usually halts before the tenth day of CsA administration. Hence, CsA treatment for short term (7–10 days) is apt in this setting.

Singh et al [35] treated 11 patients with CsA at a dose of 3 mg/kg/day for 7 days, gradually tapering over the next 7 days; compared with nine patients treated with systemic corticosteroids, it demonstrated CsA to significantly reduce the time to arrest progression of SJS/TEN, total re-epithelialization time, as well as hospital stay compared to corticosteroids.

In the exposition by Kirchhof et al. [36], where CsA and IVIG in SJS/TEN were compared, the expected mortality rate based on SCORTEN in 17 patients treated with CsA was 14.1%. The observed mortality rate, however, was 5.9%. Similarly in the 37 patients who received IVIG, the expected mortality rate calculated was 20.8%, with the observed mortality rate being 29.7% (even higher), thereby concluding CsA to be a better agent than IVIG. Further, even the calculated standardized mortality ratio propounded survival benefit to CsA use.

In a retrospective non-controlled case series of 29 patients (SJS, SJS-TEN overlap, TEN) who received CSA at a dose of 1.5 mg/kg Q12H, 1 mg/kg Q12H and 0.5 mg/kg Q12H for 10 days each, in a tapering fashion, demonstrated no deaths in any of the 29 patients despite SCORTEN predicting 2.8 deaths in this study, concluding positively with regard to the efficacy of CsA in SJS and TEN [37].

Nevertheless, while using short-term therapy with CsA, septic complications and severe leucopoenia (< 1000 cells/mm^3) should be kept in mind.

Chronic Urticaria

CsA is advocated in those patients with chronic idiopathic urticaria/chronic-inducible urticaria who do not respond even following fourfold dose intensification of second-generation antihistamines.

Although the T cell-arbitrated action of CsA is widely recognised in immunosuppression, blockade of basophil activity and mast cell degranulation is also demonstrated. [38] Further, CsA reduces serum levels of inflammatory cytokines like IL-2R, IL-5 and TNFα, which is elevated in patients with chronic idiopathic urticaria [39]. Long-term use of CsA, however, is not endorsed. [40]

In an RCT conducted by Vena et al, comparing CsA to placebo, CsA was a propitious treatment option for chronic idiopathic urticaria (CIU). In this study, CsA was started at 5 mg/kg/day for 13 days, and then decreased to 4 mg/kg/day from day 14 to 27, followed by a dose of 3 mg/kg/day from day 28 to the end of the study (either 8 weeks or 16 weeks). All participants in the study also were given cetirizine (10 mg) every day. Reduction in the severity score and symptoms was statistically significant compared to placebo after 2 months and 4 months of CsA therapy. However, there was no statistical difference when evaluated at 6 months. Also, patients completing 4 months of CsA therapy required lower amount of rescue medication than those who completed 2 months of treatment or placebo [41].

Another comparative study of chronic urticaria managed with CsA (4 mg/kg/day) for 1 month (n = 10) or 3 months (n = 10) demonstrated dramatic clinical improvement in the first month of treatment in both groups. At 3 months, however, there was no drastic change between patients who remained on CsA for 3 months when collated to those receiving CsA for 1 month [42].

Among 30 patients with CIU, who were autologous serum skin test positive, the efficacy of low-dose CsA (1.5-2 mg/kg/day) over 5 months was found to be promising. After 1 year of follow-up, 20 out of 23 patients were under complete remission and 3 relapsed [43].

A patient with Schnitzler's syndrome (a rare condition associated with chronic urticaria, intermittent fever and monoclonal IgM gammopathy) not responding to antihistamines and systemic corticosteroids obtained complete amelioration of fever, malaise and partial reduction of urticaria following 4 months of low-dose CsA (2.5 mg/kg/day) [44].

Another patient with Schnitzler's syndrome refractory to other therapies demonstrated clearance of urticaria after 1 month of cyclosporine (5 mg/kg/day). The patient was maintained on cyclosporine (2.6 mg/kg/day) with no lesions at 6 months of follow-up [45].

For cases of CIU resistant to conventional therapy, CsA should be started at 3 mg/kg/day (administered as two divided doses) for 6 weeks, followed by 2 mg/kg/day for 3 weeks and then 1 mg/kg/day for another 3 weeks before discontinuing it [46].

Dyshidrotic Eczema

Cyclosporine can be employed in the treatment of severe recalcitrant dyshidrotic eczema. Dramatic improvement in severe chronic vesicular hand dermatitis was reported in a patient within 2 weeks of high-dose CsA therapy (5 mg/kg/day). The patient remained disease free while on CsA (2.5 mg/kg/day). However, when the drug was discontinued (because of elevated blood pressure in the patient), hand eczema rapidly returned. [47]

Chronic Hand Dermatitis

In seven patients with chronic hand dermatitis treated with CsA, no improvement was seen at a starting dose of 1.25 mg/kg/day. However, when the dose of CsA was escalated to 2.5 mg/kg/day, five of the seven patients demonstrated improvement [48].

Pyoderma Gangrenosum

CsA at a dose of 5 mg/kg/day or less with or without corticosteroids is recommended as first-line treatment for PG (grade of recommendation, B), with rapid responses and dramatic improvement observed within 1–3 weeks [25]. However, high relapse rates occur on drug discontinuation, with long-term treatment becoming necessary in most patients.

PG on the thigh of an 8-month-old infant demonstrated excellent healing following the addition of CsA (5 mg/kg/day) and 1% silver sulfadiazine to the existing regimen of oral prednisolone (3 mg/kg/day), to which lesions were not responding. Within the first 3 days of adding CsA, clinical improvement was observed and after 7 days granulation tissue and re-epithelialization were seen [49].

Reich et al. [50] reported a case of recalcitrant periungual PG that responded within 6 weeks of CsA (5 mg/kg/day) and resolved after 6 months of treatment. The patient was subsequently maintained on 3 mg/kg/day of CsA for a total of 24 months.

Behcet's Disease

CsA monotherapy is an effective treatment for BD. It is valuable especially in managing ocular, arthritic and mucocutaneous components of BD [51].

Masuda et al. [52], in a randomized double-blind trial comparing CsA (10 mg/kg/day) with colchicine (1 mg/day) in 96 patients with BD with ocular and mucocutaneous disease, demonstrated CsA to be superior in treating oral and genital aphthae. However, adverse effects were more in the CsA group (because of the high dose employed).

In an open-label study with CsA (5 mg/kg/day, then reduced to 2.5 mg/kg/day if serum creatinine increased by 33%) for a period of 6 months in BD, depicted considerable improvement in oral and genital aphthae, ocular and arthritic components associated with BD [53].

In a case report with cutaneous polyarteritis nodosa-like lesions in BD (a rare cutaneous manifestation), CsA (3 mg/kg/day) given for 2 weeks was effective in clearing these lesions. Moreover, the patient was in clinical remission after 4 months in the follow-up period [54].

Though ocular, mucocutaneous and joint manifestations of BD show good results with CsA, response to neurologic manifestations is less effective. In these cases, drugs like IFNα and azathioprine are better alternatives. In a retrospective review of 117 patients, it was reported that the incidence of new-onset neurological involvement was significantly higher with cyclosporine compared to other immunosuppressive drugs [55].

Dermatomyositis

In DM, CsA is proposed as a second-line agent both for adult and juvenile forms of the disease in those unresponsive to immunosuppressive agents like methotrexate and azathioprine [56]. CsA, along with systemic corticosteroids, is valuable in the management of pulmonary and oesophageal involvement associated with DM.

CsA (1 mg/kg/day) combined with prednisolone for 1 month demonstrated control of oesophageal involvement in DM in a report by Mii et al. [57] Further, owing to its steroid-sparing property, CsA allows gradual tapering of prednisolone [57].

To note, interstitial lung disease and pneumomediastinum associated with DM have demonstrated improvement with CsA (1.8 mg/kg/day) and prednisolone (40 mg/day) after 2 months of treatment [58]. In those patients with DM associated with subacute interstitial pneumonia, if CsA (at doses ≥200 mg/day) is initiated within 15 days of diagnosis, disease prognosis substantially improves [59].

Pemphigus Vulgaris

According to the British Association of Dermatology guidelines for the management of pemphigus, cyclosporine is not recommended as an adjuvant drug for this indication. This is based on a randomized controlled trial (RCT) which showed no additional benefit and more side effects with CsA compared to methylprednisolone alone [60].

Despite a few reports showing CsA to be of some value in pemphigus vulgaris (PV), other immunosuppressives are preferable over CsA.

In a study by Olszewska et al [61], prednisolone alone and in combination with azathioprine, cyclophosphamide and cyclosporine was compared in 101 patients with PV. Though the safety profiles were similar in all four groups, cyclophosphamide (1.1–1.5 mg/kg/day) was found to be slightly better compared to other combinations.

Mobini et al. [62] demonstrated CsA (1–3 mg/kg/day) to be effective in controlling acute disease in six patients with moderate-to-severe PV uncontrolled with other conventional therapies. Within 8–10 weeks of therapy with CsA, lesions began to heal without the occurrence of any new lesions. Once the patient's disease cleared and was in remission for 3–4 months, CsA was gradually tapered over 8–12 months and then completely stopped. Besides, no recurrence after 3 years of follow-up was noted.

Epidermolysis Bullosa Acquisita

A report combining CsA (4 mg/kg/day) and prednisolone (80 mg/day) demonstrated improvement in EBA that had previously failed to respond to prednisolone and dapsone. However, after 2 months of treatment, there was a disease flare. This was tackled by increasing the dose of CsA to 5 mg/kg/day for 6 months. At 19-month follow-up, the patient was maintained on CsA (4 mg/kg/day) and prednisolone (10 mg/day) with one identifiable bulla and no adverse effects [63].

Maize and Cohen highlighted CsA (4 mg/kg/day) along with prednisolone (60 mg/day) to be effective in treating a patient with EBA and acquired factor VIII deficiency, who had been unresponsive to previous therapies (prednisolone, colchicine and cyclophosphamide). Within 3 weeks of therapy, significant improvement in both diseases was noted. The patient was later maintained on CsA (4 mg/kg/day) for 11 months with slow tapering and discontinuation of prednisolone. Later still, the patient was maintained on CsA (1.5 mg/kg/day) for 2 years without there being a relapse of either of the two diseases, and no evidence of any significant adverse effects [64].

Lichen Planus

CsA is considered to be the treatment of choice for generalized LP recalcitrant to systemic corticosteroids and retinoids [65]. On average, within 2 weeks improvement in pruritus is observed, and clearing of lesions occurs by 6 weeks [65].

Patrone et al demonstrated CsA to be useful in a case of plantar erosive LP. Within 1 month of CsA (4.5 mg/kg/day) use, rapid improvement in lesions was observed. Following this, the dose was reduced to 3 mg/kg/day and continued for 1 year. However, once CsA was discontinued, lesions resurfaced. [66] For this, a repeat course of CsA was administered, followed by a split-thickness graft. After the graft was placed, the patient was continued on CsA (3 mg/kg/day) for another 8 months. At 10 months of follow-up despite discontinuing CsA, the foot had healed and become pain free [66].

A case report of palmoplantar LP with umbilicated papules recalcitrant to topical steroids demonstrated improvement with CsA (3.5 mg/kg/day) [67]. Within 2 weeks of therapy, there was a reduction in pruritus, and skin lesions began showing improvement after 1 month of treatment, following which the dose of CsA was gradually tapered and discontinued at 8 weeks.

Gallo et al. [68] demonstrated CsA (3 mg/kg/day) to be successful in treating a patient with actinic LP for 3 months who had been unresponsive to other therapeutic modalities.

Lichen Planopilaris

There are several reports suggesting CsA to be effective in the initial stages of LPP before the commencement of severe follicular damage.

Lane et al demonstrated beneficial effects of CsA in a patient with LPP who had coexistent psoriasis. CsA (3 mg/kg/day) was given along with topical betamethasone valerate 0.12% foam twice daily to the patient and was effective in reducing perifollicular erythema and pruritus within 2 weeks of initiation of therapy [69].

In a series of three patients with LPP, CsA (3–5 mg/kg/day) proved successful in halting the disease progress. Maximal clinical response with improvement in pruritus, pain and burning, along with cessation in disease progression, was seen within 3–5 months of starting CsA therapy. However, within 1–4 months of stopping CsA, hair growth reversed. [70]

Bianchi et al demonstrated CsA (4 mg/kg/day) to be effective in a patient with Graham–Little–Piccardi–Lasseuer syndrome. After 3 months of therapy with CsA, perifollicular erythema and follicular hyperkeratotic papules reduced. Also, areas of hair regrowth in scarred patches and consistent improvement in follicular papules were noticed after another 3 months. [71]

Alopecia Areata

Although CsA is effective in AA, withdrawal of the drug is heralded with a significant loss of hair that had regrown with CsA [72].

Studies have demonstrated the efficacy of CsA in AA. Some of them are summarized in Table 25.2 [73–76].

However, guidelines on the treatment of AA conclude that cosmetically worthwhile response rates to be very low to justify the risks associated with CsA treatment (strength of recommendation D, quality of evidence III) [77].

Pityriasis Rubra Pilaris

Recent case reports have concluded CsA to be a viable treatment option for the erythrodermic variant of PRP. A report of a 4-year-old boy with erythrodermic juvenile PRP documented significant regression of the disease within 5 weeks of starting treatment with CsA (3 mg/kg/day). The dose of CsA was gradually tapered and then stopped, with no recurrence after 8 months of therapy cessation [78].

Further, in a series of three adult patients with erythrodermic PRP, CsA demonstrated value. Here, CsA was started at a dose of 5 mg/kg/day, with improvements being discernible as early as 2–4 weeks of drug initiation. Once the disease was under control, all patients were maintained on CsA (2 mg/kg/day) for 6 months, 3 years and 4 years, respectively [79].

Prurigo Nodularis

CsA may be considered a second-line agent in PN. Dosage ranging from 3.5 to 4 mg/kg/day for 24–36 weeks has been shown to significantly bring about improvement in lesions along with reduction in pruritus [80].

Table 25.2 Studies on cyclosporine for alopecia areata

Author(s)	Study details	Remarks
Ferrando et al [73]	15 patients with alopecia areata were treated with cyclosporine (5 mg/kg/day) for 6–12 months	One patient discontinued the treatment because of hypertension Vellus hair regrowth was seen in 12 of 14 patients by 1–3 months of treatment Of these, five patients had cosmetically acceptable partial hair growth and two had complete hair growth Of the two with complete hair growth, one had recurrence of alopecia areata 2 months after cessation of cyclosporine; in the other patient, there was no evidence of disease after 4 years of follow-up
Schepis et al [74]	A down's syndrome child with alopecia areata treated with cyclosporine (3 mg/kg/day) for 6 months	At the end of treatment, the patient demonstrated hair regrowth However, after 3 months of stopping treatment, there was a relapse
Kim et al [75]	46 patients were treated with combination of cyclosporine (200 mg Q12H) and methylprednisolone (24 mg Q12H for men, 20 mg Q12H for women and 12 mg Q12H for children) The dose of methylprednisolone was reduced by 4 mg/day every week and cyclosporine was reduced by 50 mg/day weekly or biweekly once methylprednisolone was totally withdrawn The total duration of treatment was 7–14 weeks	3 patients discontinued treatment because of side effects 38 patients had significant hair growth 5 patients failed to respond to treatment During the 12-month observation period, 9 of 38 patients demonstrated a disease relapse
Shaheedi-Dadra et al [76]	6 patients with alopecia totalis and 12 patients with alopecia universalis were treated with monthly intravenous methylprednisolone in doses of 500 mg for 3 days and oral cyclosporine (2.5 mg/kg/day) for 5–8 months	Hair growth >70% (an adequate treatment response) in the affected area was seen in six patients (three patients with alopecia totalis and three patients with alopecia universalis) At 8 months post treatment, no relapses were seen in the six patients who demonstrated an adequate treatment response

Hailey–Hailey Disease

Usmani et al reported rapid improvement in a recalcitrant case of Hailey–Hailey disease (HHD) using a combination of CsA (1.2 mg/kg/day) and acitretin (10 mg/day), with the patient maintaining clinical remission at 8 months [81].

In another report, CsA (2.8–3.4 mg/kg/day) was useful in improving HHD with responses maintained for 24 weeks. However, gradual deterioration of the disease was seen following discontinuation of CsA therapy [82].

Eosinophilic Pustular Folliculitis of Ofuji

CsA is considered a third-line drug for eosinophilic pustular folliculitis of Ofuji [83]. Fukamachi et al. [84], in a series of six patients, reported CsA (100–150 mg/day) for 2–12 weeks to be effective in all patients treated. However, long-term follow-up was not performed.

Hidradenitis Suppurativa

There have been reports stating the beneficial role of CsA in HS and are elucidated in Table 25.3 [85, 86].

Table 25.3 Report of CsA use for hidradenitis suppurativa

Authors	Case report	Remarks
Buckley and Rogers [85]	A patient with pyoderma gangrenosum and perianal hidradenitis suppurativa, treated with cyclosporine (4.5 mg/kg/day) and broad-spectrum antibiotics	After 8 months of treatment, healing of discharging sinuses and diminished pain was noted After 15 months of treatment, the patient was noted to have stable disease Improvement in patient's quality of life was noted No adverse effects were reported
Rose et al [86]	Cyclosporine (4 mg/kg/day) was started in a patient with 20 years history of hidradenitis suppurativa previously treated with minocycline, clindamycin, clarithromycin, oral steroids, intravenous steroids, intralesional steroids and surgical excision	After 3 months of treatment with cyclosporine, flares were prevented At 7 months of follow-up, the dose of cyclosporine was reduced to 2 mg/kg/day No significant episodes of inflammation were encountered after initiation of treatment with cyclosporine

Solar Urticaria

A case of treatment-resistant solar urticaria (SU) improved with CsA (4.5 mg/kg/day). However, relapse of SU was encountered once the drug was withdrawn [87].

Polymorphous Light Eruption

CsA is generally used in polymorphous light eruption (PMLE) as a prophylactic agent. The dose of CsA in PMLE ranges from 3 to 4 mg/kg/day. CsA is started 1 week prior to travel to a sunny climate, with discontinuation of treatment upon return. This helps in preventing flares of PMLE, as well as avoiding long-term adverse effects associated with CsA [88].

Chronic Actinic Dermatitis

Cases of CAD unresponsive to systemic corticosteroids [89] and beta-carotene [89] demonstrate response with CsA (4–4.5 mg/kg/day), within 1–3 months of therapy initiation.

Scleroderma

Morton et al. [90] and Zachariae et al. [91] reported significant skin softening and resolution of digital infarcts in some patients with scleroderma following CsA therapy. However, despite these anecdotal reports, extreme caution needs to be exercised while using CsA for this indication, owing to its ability to potentially worsen hypertension and renal disease associated with systemic sclerosis.

Further, the European League Against Rheumatism (EULAR) Scleroderma Trials Research Group recently published a set of recommendations for the treatment of scleroderma and suggests the need for further evaluation of CsA regarding this indication [92].

Adverse Effects

Renal

- Renal dysfunction requires monitoring of serum creatinine levels while administering CsA and is elaborated in Fig. 25.2 [93].

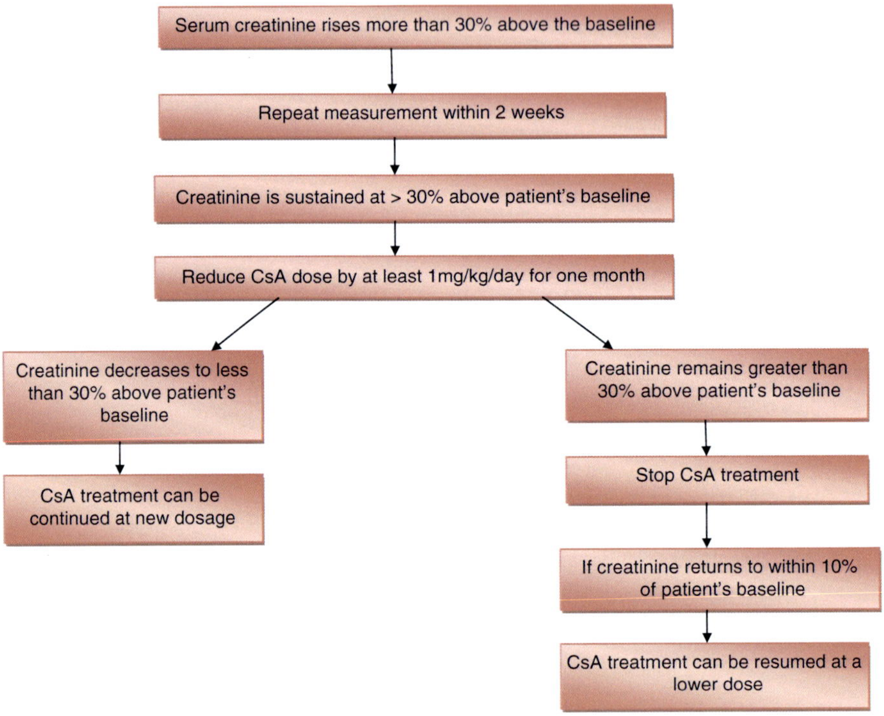

Fig. 25.2 Monitoring of serum creatinine in patients on treatment with cyclosporine A

Cardiovascular

- Hypertension.

Neurologic

- Tremors.
- Headache.
- Paraesthesias.
- Hyperesthesia.

Mucocutaneous

- Hypertrichosis (reversible).
- Gingival hyperplasia.
- Follicular keratosis.

- Sebaceous hyperplasia.
- Epidermal inclusion cysts.
- Acneiform eruptions.

Gastrointestinal

- Nausea.
- Vomiting.
- Abdominal discomfort.

Musculoskeletal

- Myalgia.
- Lethargy.
- Arthralgia.

Metabolic

- Hyperkalaemia.
- Hyperuricemia.
- Hypomagnesemia.
- Hyperlipidaemia.

Malignancy Risk

- Lymphoma.
- Non-melanoma skin cancer.
- Kaposi's sarcoma.
- Melanoma.

Drug Interactions

- Drugs increasing CsA serum levels: amiodarone, erythromycin, ciprofloxacin, cephalosporins, doxycycline, itraconazole, grapefruit juice, dexamethasone, thiazides and allopurinol.
- Drugs decreasing CsA serum levels: nafcillin, rifampicin, griseofulvin, bexarotene and phenytoin.
- Drugs increasing renal toxicity in combination with CsA: gentamycin, co-trimoxazole, vancomycin, amphotericin-B and NSAIDs.

Monitoring Guidelines

Baseline

Examination

- Complete history and physical examination (to rule out active infections or tumours).
- At least two baseline blood pressures.

Laboratory

- Serum creatinine levels (some authors suggest two baseline serum creatinine levels).
- Blood urea nitrogen.
- Urinalysis with microscopy.
- Complete blood count.
- Hepatic transaminase estimation.
- Fasting lipid profile.
- Magnesium.
- Potassium.
- Uric acid.

Follow-Up

- Re-evaluate the patient, including laboratory parameters, every 2 weeks for the first 1–2 months, and then monthly while on CsA.
- Blood pressure needs to be checked at each visit.

Tests Indicated Infrequently in High-Risk Patients

- Serum CsA levels.
- Creatinine clearance (if therapy has been ongoing for more than 6 months, then this needs to be considered).
- Rarely renal biopsy.

Conclusion and Future Direction

CsA is very effective in controlling flares in psoriasis and AD. However, owing to its side effect profile, long-term usage of CsA is not recommended.

Voclosporine is a novel calcineurin inhibitor with a better safety profile than CsA. Given at 1.5 mg/kg/day, it is able to bring about good therapeutic responses without much change in blood pressure and serum lipid profile. Further, its efficacy is superior compared to CsA, thereby making it a promising therapy for psoriasis in the near future [93, 94].

References

1. Borel JF, Feurer C, Gubler HU. Biological effects of cyclosporine a: a new antilymphocyte agent. Agents Act. 1976;6:468–75.
2. Schreiber SL, Crabtree GR. The mechanism of action of cyclosporine and FK506. Immunol Today. 1992;13:136–42.
3. Furue M, Gaspari AH, Katz SI. Effect of cyclosporine a on epiderma cells II. Cyclosporine a inhibits proliferation of normal and transformed keratinocytes. J Invest Dermatol. 1988;90:796–800.
4. Shupack J, Abel E, Bauer E, et al. Cyclosporine as maintenance therapy in patients with severe psoriasis. J Am Acad Dermatol. 1997;36:423–32.
5. Lebowhl M, Ellis C, Gottlieb A, et al. Cyclosporine consensus conference. With emphasis on the treatment of psoriasis. J Am Acad Dermatol. 1998;39:464–75.
6. Cacoub P, Artru L, Canesi M, et al. Life-threatening psoriasis relapse on withdrawal of cyclosporine. Lancet. 1988;2:219–20.
7. Heidenheim M, Oxholm A, Da Cunha BF. Generalized pustular psoriasis in relation to withdrawal of Cycosporin a. Br J Dermatol. 1990;122:719.
8. Griffiths CE, Clark CM, Chambers RJ, et al. A systematic review of treatments for severe psoriasis. Health Technol Assess. 2000;4:1–125.
9. Ozawa A, Sugai J, Ohkido M, et al. Cyclosporine in psoriasis: continuous monotherpy versus intermittent long term therapy. Eur J Dermatol. 1999;9:218–23.
10. Chaidemenos GC, Mourellou O, Avgoustinaki N, et al. Intermittent versus continuous 1 year cyclosporine uses in chronic plaque psoriasis. J Eur Acad Dermatol Venereol. 2007;21:1203–8.
11. Griffiths CEM, Powles AV, McFadden J, et al. Long term cyclosporine for psoriasis. Br J Dermatol. 1989;120:256–66.
12. Gottlieb SL, Hefter NS, Gilleaudeau P, et al. Short contact with anthralin treatments augments therapeutic efficacy of cyclosporine in psoriasis: a clinical and pathologic study. J Am Acad Dermatol. 1995;33:637–45.
13. Grossman RM, Thivolet J, Claudy A, et al. A novel therapeutic approach to psoriasis with combination calcipotriol ointment and very low dose of cyclosporine: results of a multicentre placebo controlled study. J Am Acad Dermatol. 1994;31:68–74.
14. Amen M, Smith HR, Barker JN. Combined mycophenolate mofetil and cyclosporine therapy for severe recalcitrant psoriasis. Clin Exp Dermatol. 2001;26:480–3.
15. Balasubramaniam P, Stevenson O, Berth-Jones J. Fumaric acid esters in severe psoriasis, including experience of use in combination with other systemic modalities. Br J Dermatol. 2004;150:741–6.
16. Roenigk HH. Acitretin combination therapy. J Am Acad Dermatol. 1994;41(3 Pt 2):S18–21.
17. Clark CM, Kirby B, Morris AD, et al. Combination treatment with methotrexate and cyclosporine for severe recalcitrant psoriasis. Br J Dermatol. 1999;141:279–82.
18. Fraser AD, van Kuijk AW, Westhovens R, et al. A randomized, double blind placebo controlled multicentre trial of combination therapy with methotrexate plus cyclosporine in patients with active psoriatic arthritis. Ann Rheum Dis. 2005;64:859–64.
19. Gupta AK, Matteson EL, Ellis CN, et al. Cyclosporine in the treatment of psoriatic arthritis. Arch Dermatol. 1989;125:507–10.
20. Steinsson K, Jonsdottir I, Valdimarrson H. Cyclosporine a in psoriatic arthritis: an open label study. Ann Rheum Dis. 1990;49:603–6.

21. Salvarani C, Macchioni P, Boiardi L, et al. Low dose cyclosporine a in psoriatic arthritis: relation between soluble interleukin 2 receptors and response to therapy. J Rheumatol. 1992;19:74–9.
22. Spadaro A, Riccieri V, Sili-Scavalli A, et al. Comparison of cyclosporine a and methotrexate in the treatment of psoriatic arthritis: a one-year prospective study. Clin Exp Rheumatol. 1995;13:589–93.
23. BuBmann C, Bieber T, Novak N. Systemic therapeutic options for severe atopic dermatitis. J Dtsch Dermatol Ges. 2009;7:205–19.
24. Hanifin JM, Cooper KD, Ho VC, et al. Guidelines for the care of atopic dermatitis. J Am Acad Dermatol. 2004;50:391–400.
25. Griffiths CE, Katsambas A, Dykmans BA, et al. Update on the use of cyclosporine in immune mediated dermatoses. Br J Dermatol. 2006;155:1–16.
26. Schmitt J, Schakel K, Schmitt N, et al. Systemic treatment of severe atopic eczema. A systematic review. Acta Derm Venereol. 2007;87:100–11.
27. Harper JI, et al. cyclosporine for atopic dermatitis in children. Dermatology. 2001;203:3–6.
28. Camp RD, Reitamo S, Friedmann PS, et al. Cyclosporine a in severe, therapy resistant atopic dermatitis: a report of an international workshop, April 1993. Br J Dermatol. 1993;129:217–20.
29. Zonneveld IM, de Rie MA, Beljaards RC, et al. The long-term safety and efficacy of cyclosporine in severe refractory atopic dermatitis: a comparison of two dosage regimens. Br J Dermatol. 1996;135:15–20.
30. Munro CS, Levell NJ, Shuster S, et al. Maintenance treatment with cyclosporine in atopic eczema. Br J Dermatol. 1994;130:376–80.
31. Sepp N, Fritsch PO. Can cyclosporine a induce permanent remission of atopic dermatitis? Br J Dermatol. 1993;128:213–6.
32. Salek MS, Finlay AY, Luscombe DK, et al. Cyclosporine greatly improves the quality of life in adults with severe atopic dermatitis. A randomized, double blind, placebo-controlled trial. Br J Dermatol. 1993;129:422–30.
33. Schmitt J, Schmitt N, Meurer M. Cyclosporine in the treatment of patients with atopic dermatitis – a systematic review and meta-analysis. J Eur Acad Dermatol Venereol. 2007;21:606–19.
34. Naeyaert JM, Lachapelle JM, Degreef H, et al. Cyclosporine in atopic dermatitis: review of the literature and outline of a Belgian consensus. Dermatology. 1999;198:145–52.
35. Singh GK, Chatterjee M, Verma R. Cyclosporine in Steven-Johnson syndrome and toxic epidermal necrolysis and retrospective comparison with systemic corticosteroids. Indian J Dermatol Venereol Leprol. 2013;79:686–92.
36. Kirchhof MG, Miliszewski MA, Sikora S, et al. Retrospective review of Steven-Johnson syndrome/toxic epidermal necrolysis treatment comparing intravenous immunoglobulin with cyclosporine. J Am Acad Dermatol. 2014;71:941–7.
37. Valeyrie-Allanore L, Wolkenstein P, Brochard L, et al. Open trial of cyclosporine treatment for Steven-Johnson syndrome and toxic epidermal necrolysis. Br J Dermatol. 2010;163:847–53.
38. Godse K, De A, Zawar V, et al. Consensus statement for the diagnosis and treatment of urticaria. A 2017 update. Indian J Dermatol. 2018;63:2–15.
39. Serhat Inaloz H, Ozturk S, Akcali C, et al. Low dose and short-term cyclosporine treatment in patients with chronic idiopathic urticaria: a clinical and immunological evaluation. J Dermatol. 2008;35:276–82.
40. Lebwohl M, Ellis C, Gottleib A, et al. Cyclosporine consensus conference: with emphasis on the treatment of psoriasis. J Am Acad Dermatol. 1998;39:464–75.
41. Vena GA, Cassano N, Colombo D, et al. Cyclosporine in chronic idiopathic urticaria: a double blind, randomized, placebo-controlled trial. J Am Acad Dermatol. 2006;55:705–9.
42. Baskean EB, Tunali S, Turker T, et al. Comparison of short- and long-term cyclosporine a therapy in chronic idiopathic urticaria. J Dermatolog Treat. 2004;15:164–8.
43. Boubouka CD, et al. Treatment of autoimmune urticaria with low dose cyclosporine a: a one year follow up. Acta Derm Venereol. 2011;91:50–4.
44. Carbone J, Paravisini A, Sarmiento E, et al. Partial response to cyclosporine in a patient with Schnitzler's syndrome. Allergol Immunopathol (Madr). 2007;35:71–3.

45. Pascual-Lopez M, Hernandez-Nunez A, Sanchez-Perez J, et al. Schnitzler's syndrome with monoclonal IgG kappa gammopathy: good response to cyclosporine. J Eur Acad Dermatol Venereol. 2002;16:267–70.
46. Galindo Bouilla PA, Borja Segade J, Gomez Torrijos E, et al. Urticaria and cyclosporine. Allergy. 2002;57:650–1.
47. Peterson CS, Menne T. Cyclosporine a responsive chronic severe vesicular hand eczema. Acta Derm Venereol. 1992;72:436–7.
48. Reitamo S, Granlund H. Cyclosporine a in the treatment of chronic dermatitis of the hands. Br J Dermatol. 1994;130:75–8.
49. McAleer MA, Powell FC, Devaney D, et al. Infantile pyoderma gangrenosum. J Am Acad Dermatol. 2008;58(2 Suppl):S23–8.
50. Reich A, Maj J, Cislo M, et al. Periungual lesions in pyoderma gamgrenosum. Clin Exp Dermatol. 2009;34:e81–4.
51. Mendes D, Correia M, Barbedo M, et al. Behcet's disease – a contemporary review. J Autoimmun. 2009;32:178–88.
52. Masuda K, Nakayama A, Urayama A, et al. Double masked trial of cyclosporine versus colchicine and long-term open study of cyclosporine in Behcet's disease. Lancet. 1989;1:1093–5.
53. Avci O, Gurler N, Gunes AT. Efficacy of cyclosporine on mucocutaneous manifestations of Behcet's disease. J Am Acad Dermatol. 1997;36:796–7.
54. Vikas A, Atul S, Singh R, et al. Behcet's disease with relapsing cutaneous polyarteritis nodosa like lesions, responsive to oral cyclosporine therapy. Dermatol Online J. 2003;9:9.
55. Kotter I, Gunaydin I, Batra M, et al. CNS involvement occurs more frequently in patients with Behcet's disease inder cyclosporine a than under other medications: results of a retrospective analysis of 117 cases. Clin Rheumatol. 2006;25:482–6.
56. Maeda K, Kimura R, et al. Cyclosporine treatment for polymyositis/dermatomyositis: is it possible to rescue the deteriorating cases with interstitial pneumonitis. Scand J Rheumatol. 1997;2:24–9.
57. Mii S, Niiyama S, Kusunoki M, et al. Cyclosporine a as treatment of esophageal involvement in dermatomyositis. Rheumatol Int. 2006;27:183–5.
58. Terao M, Ozawa K, Inui S, et al. A case of dermatomyositis complicated with pneumomediastinum. Mod Rheumatol. 2007;17:156–9.
59. Kotani T, Makino S, Takeuchi T, et al. Early intervention with corticosteroids and cyclosporine a and 2-hour post dose blood concentration monitoring improves the prognosis of acute/subacute interstitial pneumonia in dermatomyositis. J Rheumatol. 2008;35:254–9.
60. Ionnides D, Chrysomallis F, Bystryn JC. Ineffectiveness of cyclosporine as an adjuvant to corticosteroids in the treatment of pemphigus. Arch Dermatol. 2000;136:868–72.
61. Olszewska M, Kolacinska-Strasz Z, Sulej J, et al. Efficacy and safety of cyclophosphamide, azathioprine and cyclosporine as adjuvant drugs in pemphigus vulgaris. Am J Clin Dermatol. 2007;8:85–92.
62. Mobini N, Padilla T Jr, Ahmed AR. Long term remission in selected patients with pemphigus vulgaris treated with cyclosporine. J Am Acad Dermatol. 1997;36:264–6.
63. Khatri ML, Benghazeil M, Shafi M. Epidermolysis bullosa acquisita responsive to cyclosporine therapy. J Eur Acad Dermatol Venereol. 2001;15:182–4.
64. Maize JC Jr, Cohen JB. Cyclosporine controls epidermolysis bullosa acquisita co-occuring with acquired factor VII deficiency. Int J Dermatol. 2005;44:692–4.
65. Cribier B, Frances C, Chosidow O. Treatment of lichen planus: an evidence-based medicine analysis of efficacy. Arch Dermatol. 1998;134:1521–30.
66. Patrone P, Stinco G, La Pia E, et al. Surgery and cyclosporine a in the treatment of erosive lichen planus of the feet. Eur J Dermatol. 1998;8:243–4.
67. Karakatsanis G, Patsati A, Kastoridou C, et al. Palmoplantar lesions of lichen planus with umbilicated papules: an atypical case with rapid response to cyclosporine. J Eur Acad Dermatol Venereol. 2007;21:1006–7.
68. Gallo L, Ayala F, Ayala F. Relapsing lichen actinicus successfully treated with cyclosporine. J Eur Acad Dermatol Venereol. 2008;22:370–1.

69. Lane TK, Kamino H, Walters RF, et al. Lichen planopilaris with psoriasis. Dermatol Online J. 2008;14:4.
70. Mirmirani P, Willey A, Price VH. Short course of oral cyclosporine in lichen planopilaris. J Am Acad Dermatol. 2003;49:667–71.
71. Bianchi L, Paro Vidolin A, Piemonte P, et al. Graham little Piccardi Lassueue syndrome: effective treatment with cyclosporine. Clin Exp Dermatol. 2001;26:518–20.
72. Gupta AK, Ellis CN, Cooper KD, et al. Oral cyclosporine for the treatment of alopecia areata. J Am Acad Dermatol. 1990;22:242–50.
73. Ferrando J, Grimalt R. Partial response of sever alopecia areata to cyclosporine a. Dermatology. 1999;199:67–9.
74. Schepis C, Barone C, Lazzaro Danzuso GC, et al. Alopecia areata in down's syndrome: a clinical evaluation. J Eur Acad Dermatol Venereol. 2005;19:769–70.
75. Kim BJ, Min S, Park KY, et al. Combination therapy of cyclosporine and methylprednisolone on severe alopecia areata. J Dermatolog Treat. 2008;19:216–20.
76. Shaheedi-Dadras M, Karami A, Mollaei F, et al. the effect of methylprednisolone pulse therapy plus oral cyclosporine in the treatment of alopecia totalis and universalis. Arch Iran Med. 2008;11:90–3.
77. McDonald Hull SP, Wood ML, Hutchinson PE, et al. Guidelines for the management of alopecia areata. Br J Dermatol. 2003;149:692–9.
78. Wetzig T, Sticherling M. Juvenile pityriasis rubra pilaris: successful treatment with cyclosporine. Br J Dermatol. 2003;149:202–3.
79. Usuki K, Sekiyama M, Shimada T, et al. Three cases of pityriasis rubra pilaris successfully treated with cyclosporine a. Dermatology. 2000;200:997–9.
80. Lee MR, Shumack S. Prurigo nodularis: a review. Australas J Dermatol. 2005;46:211–8.
81. Usmani N, Wilson C. A novel treatment for recalcitrant benign familial pemphigus. J Eur Acad Dermatol Venereol. 2007;21:264–6.
82. Berth-Jones J, Smith SG, Graham-Brown RA. Benign familial chronic pemphigus (Hailey-Hailey disease) responds to cyclosporine. Clin Exp Dermatol. 1995;20:70–2.
83. Ellis E, Scheinfeld N. Eosinophilic pustular folliculitis: a comprehensive review and treatment options. Am J Clin Dermatol. 2004;5:189–97.
84. Fukamachi S, Kabashima K, Sugita K, et al. Therapeutic effectiveness of various treatments for eosinophilic pustular folliculitis. Acta Derm Venereol. 2009;89:155–9.
85. Buckley DA, Rogers S. Cyclosporine responsive hidradenitis suppurativa. J R Soc Med. 1995;88:289–90.
86. Rose RF, Goodfield MJ, Clark SM. Treatment of recalcitrant hidradenitis suppurativa with oral ciclosporin. Clin Exp Dermatol. 2006;31:154–5.
87. Eldstorm DW, Ros AM. Cyclosporine a therapy for severe solar urticaria. Photodermatol Photoimmunol Photomed. 1997;13:61–3.
88. Lasa O, Trebol I, Gardeazabal J, et al. Prophylactic short-term use of cyclosporine in refractory polymorphous light eruption. J Eur Acad Dermatol Venereol. 2004;18:747–8.
89. Paquet P, Pierard GE. Severe chronic actinic dermatitis treated with cyclosporine: 2 cases. Ann Dermatol Venereol. 2001;128:42–8.
90. Morton SJ, Powell RJ. Cyclosporine and tacrolimus: their use in a routine clinical setting of scleroderma. Rheumatology. 2000;39:365–9.
91. Zachariae H, Halkier-Sorensen L, Heickendorff L, et al. Cyclosporine treatment of systemic sclerosis. Br J Dermatol. 1990;122:677–81.
92. Kowal-Bielecka O, Landewe R, Avouac J, et al. EULAR recommendations for the treatment of systemic sclerosis: a report from the EULAR scleroderma trials and research group (EUSTAR). Ann Rheum Dis. 2009;68:620–8.
93. Bissonnette R, Papp K, Poulin Y, et al. A randomized multicentre double-blind placebo controlled phase 2 trial of ISA247 in patients with chronic plaque psoriasis. J Am Acad Dermatol. 2006;54:472–8.
94. Papp K, Bissonnette R, Rosoph L, et al. Efficacy of ISA247 in plaque psoriasis: a randomized multicentre double-blind placebo controlled phase III study. Lancet. 2008;371:1337–42.

Methotrexate 26

Introduction

Methotrexate (MTX) was the first effective systemic drug used in the treatment of psoriasis and continues to be the standard therapy for psoriasis, against which other drugs are compared [1]. Edmondson and Guy in 1958 evaluated the effectiveness of MTX in the treatment of psoriasis and since then MTX has replaced aminopterin as a more stable and clinically manageable drug in treating psoriasis [2].

Mechanism of Action

MTX has multifaceted actions elaborating its therapeutic effects and are broadly divided into:

- Anti-proliferative action,
- Immunosuppressive action, and.
- Anti-inflammatory action.

Anti-proliferative Action

MTX competitively inhibits the enzyme dihydrofolate reductase (DHFR), thereby preventing conversion of folic acid to tetrahydrofolate (THF). THF is a co-factor necessary for the production of 1-carbon units critical for the synthesis of purine nucleotides. This blockade prevents purine synthesis, thereby clamping RNA and DNA synthesis [3]. Now as DNA synthesis is impaired, cell division gets arrested in the S phase of the normal cell cycle [3].

A. K. Bubna, *Therapeutics in Dermatology - Essentials for Clinical Practice*,
https://doi.org/10.1007/978-981-95-3791-4_26

Immunosuppressive Action

By targeting DNA synthesis in immunologically competent cells, MTX brings about suppression of both primary and secondary antibody responses [4, 5].

Anti-inflammatory Effects

- MTX reduces expression of T cells in the endothelial cells of blood vessels, thereby blocking T cell migration to effected tissues [6].
- MTX inhibits the enzyme aminoimidocarboxyamido ribonucleotide transformylase. This blockade increases local tissue concentrations of adenosine, a potent anti-inflammatory mediator [7].
- MTX inhibits methionine synthetase. This blockade reduces levels of S-adenosyl methionine, a potent pro-inflammatory mediator, thus reducing inflammation [7].
- MTX suppresses the inflammatory mediator LB_4, as well as reduces inflammation caused by C5a [8].

Pharmacokinetics

MTX can be given orally, intravenously, intramuscularly, subcutaneously and intrathecally. Given orally, it is rapidly absorbed from the intestine. Though oral absorption is incomplete, it provides a more reliable blood level than parenteral administration. In adults, food does not interfere with MTX absorption. However, in children milk containing meals may decrease the drug's bioavailability [9, 10]. Once absorbed, MTX has a triphasic reduction in the plasma.

First phase: This occurs 45 min after its intake and represents the distribution of MTX throughout the body.
Second phase: This occurs 2–4 h later and represents renal excretion.
Third phase: This portrays the $t_{1/2}$ of the drug, which is around 10–27 h and represents release of MTX primarily bound to DHFR from tissues.

The metabolism of MTX occurs in the liver to polyglutamated forms, which may account for its toxicity. The elimination is via glomerular filtration and tubular secretion [11, 12].

Indications

FDA Approved

- Psoriasis.
- Sezary syndrome.

Off Label

Proliferative Dermatoses

- Pityriasis rubra pilaris (PRP).
- Pityriasis lichenoides *et* varioliformis acuta (PLEVA).
- Reiter's disease.
- Lichen planus (LP).

Immunobullous Disorders

- Pemphigus vulgaris.
- Bullous pemphigoid (BP).
- Cicatricial pemphigoid.
- Epidermolysis bullosa acquisita.

Autoimmune Connective Tissue Disorders

- Dermatomyositis.
- Subacute cutaneous lupus erythematosus (SCLE).
- Systemic lupus erythematosus (SLE).
- Scleroderma.
- Morphoea.

Vasculitis

- Leukocytoclastic vasculitis (LCV).
- Cutaneous polyarteritis nodosa (PAN).
- Kawasaki's disease.

Neutrophilic Dermatoses

- Sweet's syndrome.
- Pyoderma gangrenosum (PG).

Dermatitis

- Atopic dermatitis (AD).

Others

- Sarcoidosis.
- Keloids.
- Lymphomatoid papulosis.
- Keratoacanthoma.
- Mycosis fungoides.
- Chronic idiopathic urticaria.
- Cutaneous Crohn's disease.

Contraindications

Absolute

- Pregnancy.
- Lactation.

Relative

- Unrealistic expectations.
- Alcohol intake in excess.
- Diminished renal function.
- Diabetes mellitus.
- Obesity.
- Hepatic disease: abnormal liver function tests, active hepatitis, cirrhosis, history of liver disease.
- Severe hematologic abnormalities.
- Tuberculosis/HIV.
- Man or woman contemplating conception (3 months off the drug for men and one ovulatory cycle in females).

Pregnancy prescribing status: Category 'X'.

Clinical Uses

Psoriasis

In psoriasis, MTX is administered in the following scenarios:

- Psoriasis involving >20% body surface area (BSA),
- Erythrodermic psoriasis,
- Psoriatic arthropathy,
- Psoriasis adversely affecting the ability to maintain employment, and.
- Failure of topical treatment or PUVA.

In 70–80% of cases, within 4 weeks a favourable response is noticeable, and by 12 weeks a significant response is attained in those patients who are responsive to MTX. During the first month, clearing of scales is evident. By the second month, erythema decreases with breakage of plaques, and by the third month, islands of normal skin are obtained.

In cases where the extent and clinical profile of patients are on the poorer side, such as in generalized pustular psoriasis (GPP), MTX can be combined with drugs such as cyclosporine and biological agents, which can rapidly help in clearing severe disease following which MTX treatment as monotherapy can continue.

Combining MTX with cyclosporine is a good combination for GPP, where the principle of sequential therapy is employed. Sequential therapy usually consists of three phases.

Phase 1: Clearing phase,
Phase 2: Transition phase, and.
Phase 3: Maintenance phase.

The rationale of sequential therapy of MTX with cyclosporine is based on the following properties:

- Cyclosporine is more ideal for a quick fix, whereas MTX proves to be better drug for maintenance.
- This combination helps to prevent cyclosporine toxicity, as cyclosporine's prolonged usage is halted.

Clearing Phase

Here, cyclosporine is used at the maximum dermatologic dose (5 mg/kg/day) till a favourable response is obtained, which usually takes 4–6 weeks.

Transition Phase

Here, MTX is introduced, and cyclosporine is tapered gradually, no faster than 1 mg/kg/month and is stopped once the dose has come to 2 mg/kg/day. This means cyclosporine needs to be continued for almost 3 months, though there may be variations amongst patients and treatment may thus need to be individualized.

MTX is either given as a single weekly dose, or in three divided doses over a 12-h period each week (Weinstein Frost Regimen). The initial dose of MTX should be fairly conservative to prevent myelosuppression. Usually a test dose of 5–10 mg of MTX is administered, with a complete blood count and liver function tests being repeated after a week of MTX administration. If no toxicity is noticeable, dose of MTX is gradually escalated by 2.5–5 mg/week to a level where reasonable benefit is achieved without encountering side effects. In general, doses ranging from 10 to 15 mg/week are sufficient enough to provide beneficial effects. Rarely does the weekly dose of MTX exceed 30 mg. When maximal benefit is reached, MTX can be tapered by 2.5 mg/week till the lowest possible dose is obtained to maintain disease control.

Maintenance Phase

Here, patients are maintained on MTX alone. As disease improves, it is always prudent to taper MTX gradually prior to stopping it rather than an abrupt halt, as there is a high chance of relapse with sudden cessation of the drug [13].

Use of Methotrexate with Biological Agents

The combination of MTX with infliximab is indicated in cases of unstable psoriasis or very severe psoriasis as per the British association of dermatologists guidelines [14]. In these cases, the dose of MTX is <12.5 mg/week [15].

The American Academy of Dermatologists, however, does not recommend concomitant administration of low dose MTX, although some clinicians do so to reduce formation of autoantibodies [16].

As infliximab is a human chimeric monoclonal antibody, it can incite neutralizing antibodies, which can account for loss of efficacy with subsequent infusions [17]. Further, infusion reactions are 2–3 times more common in patients who develop antibodies. Concomitant use of MTX may prevent development of these antibodies and reduce frequency of infusion reactions [18].

Besides, MTX in conjunction with etanercept is approved by the US FDA for psoriatic arthropathy.

Pityriasis Rubra Pilaris

Although utilized in the treatment of pityriasis rubra pilaris (PRP), the response of MTX is not as good, as that observed for psoriasis [19]. This can be explained by the fact that in PRP, the epidermal turnover time is substantially slower when compared to that of psoriasis, and MTX primarily acts here by its anti-inflammatory effects, rather than its anti-proliferative action [20]. Moreover, in PRP, treatment efficacy cannot be appropriately deciphered, owing to the propensity of spontaneous clearing in up to 80% of cases, after an average period of 3 years. Nevertheless, MTX has shown to be effective in a number of reports [21].

Currently, there is no official statement regarding the dose of MTX for PRP. Based on available data, it is suggested to utilize a dose of 15–25 mg/week, and escalating the dose as per individual patient requirement. Further, once clinical improvement is obtained, the dose of MTX can be gradually tapered to obtain the lowest effective dose for maintenance, and then accordingly stopped [21].

Overall though, MTX can be considered a first-line therapeutic option for PRP, which also means taking into account the financial limitations associated with biologic drugs [21].

Pityriasis Lichenoides et Varioliformis Acuta

Reports have demonstrated MTX to be effective in the treatment of PLEVA. MTX, 7.5–20 mg/week, is generally utilized for this indication, and within a few weeks, improvement is noticeable. However, MTX is a second-line drug for PLEVA, reserved for patients in whom first-line therapy with systemic antibiotics and phototherapy have failed. Besides, relapses during MTX taper have commonly been reported [22–24].

Bullous Pemphigoid

MTX is a very good drug for bullous pemphigoid (BP). It is primarily used for its steroid sparing status. Dose utilized in BP ranges from 7.5 to 12.5 mg/week. In elderly patients, dose may require reduction, owing to diminished renal function [25].

Dermatomyositis

MTX is extremely useful for dermatomyositis, especially to control muscle disease and pulmonary involvement. Dosing ranges from 30 to 35 mg/week, with an average dose of 25 mg/week. Clinicians can objectively measure clinical response after MTX treatment by detecting muscle strength and levels of muscle enzymes. MTX is started as an empiric weekly dose, along with systemic corticosteroids. Onset of noticeable improvement is by 4–8 weeks [26, 27].

Morphoea

Both childhood and adult morphoea benefit with MTX. However, MTX is of value in the early inflammatory phase of the disease. For linear morphoea, MTX is the first-line treatment along with systemic steroids. In generalized morphoea, MTX is used as a second-line treatment with systemic steroids, if no improvement is seen following phototherapy.

Urticaria

Urticaria is characterized by the development of recurrent wheals, which if extends more than 6 weeks is labelled as chronic urticaria (CU).

Although antihistamines are effective in most cases, a subset of patients are refractory even after dose escalation (up to 4 times). Based on the EAACI/GA^{2}LEN/EuroGuiDerm/APAAACI guidelines, for the management of CU, if antihistamines fail, omalizumab is the next line of therapy, followed by cyclosporine, in cases unresponsive to omalizumab [28]. These drugs, however, are expensive, due to which their utility is limited to settings with adequate resources, making it imperative for dermatologists to explore the efficacy of other drugs for the same.

It is observed that MTX is effective in those cases of CU refractory to antihistamines, and can be used as a second-line drug especially in resource-poor settings. Besides, Indian guidelines still recommend MTX for CU, despite the scarcity of quality evidence, owing to its applicability with regard to economics, availability, dosing programme and acceptance [29].

MTX dosing in CU ranges from 10 to 25 mg/week. In children, a dose of 0.2 mg/kg/week is given. Oral administration is the route of choice, with subcutaneous administration being reserved for those patients delineating gastrointestinal side effects [30–38]. Interestingly, in reports by Weiner [37], Godse [38] and Mora et al. [35], MTX was given 2–3 days per week, without encountering any adverse effects. Moreover, combining MTX with antihistamines in CU is preferable to MTX monotherapy [30, 32–34, 38].

Besides, the propitious role of MTX has been outlined in steroid-dependant patients with CU, with outcomes ranging from complete response to considerable/some benefit, thereby enabling reduction in the dose of systemic steroids [33, 34].

In most patients receiving MTX, the onset of effect occurs by 3–5 weeks and is maintained for 2–15 months [39].

The beneficial effects of MTX in urticaria is attributed to its immunomodulatory and anti-inflammatory effects [40].

Atopic Dermatitis

MTX is prescribed as an off-label drug to control symptoms related to atopic dermatitis (AD). Based on previous research, MTX is widely prescribed as a first-line treatment for AD [41, 42] and most commonly used as a second-line therapeutic agent in the Netherlands [42] and the United Kingdom [41].

Reasons behind the wide applicability of MTX in AD include:

- Long history of use by dermatologists and rheumatologists for various disorders,
- Affordability, and.
- Efficacy.

Although cyclosporine is considered the initial conventional choice for AD, in two randomized control trials (RCTs), MTX elucidated comparable efficacy to cyclosporine, with conclusively lower adverse effects [43, 44]. Further, the drug survival of MTX is significantly prolonged in comparison to cyclosporine, which again is an added advantage [45].

With regard to azathioprine, improvements of SCORAD are almost similar to MTX. Nevertheless, given the once weekly schedule of MTX and its wide applicability, it has a better acceptance [46].

MTX in AD acts by its anti-inflammatory action mediated by adenosine pathways and repression of T cell activation, following blockade of DNA/RNA synthesis [47]. Additionally, another mechanism outlining the immunomodulatory/anti-inflammatory effects of MTX in AD involves suppression of the JAK/STAT pathway [48].

MTX helps prevent disease flares of AD and controls eczema symptoms, thereby improving the quality of life of patients.

In adults, the suggested dose of MTX in AD is 5–15 mg/week, with the maximum dose not exceeding 25 mg/week. In children, the starting dose is 10–15 mg/m^2/week. Both oral and subcutaneous routes have been employed for MTX in AD. Dose escalation is done at 5 mg/week in case of inadequate response to the lower dose [49]. Folic acid (5 mg) supplementation in adults can either be done once weekly, the day after MTX intake, or it can be given daily, except on the day of MTX use [49]. In children the dose of folic acid is 400 mcg/week [49].

Response to MTX in AD can be seen as early as 2 weeks, but in some individuals it may take longer, based on different immunological backgrounds, thereby warranting dose adjustments as per the therapeutic response to MTX [50].

Lichen Planus (LP)

The propitious role of MTX in generalized LP has been propounded in various studies [51–53]. Doses ranging from 10 to 20 mg/week are effective in treating LP. Improvement of mucocutaneous lesions become visible as early as 4 weeks following treatment initiation, with complete resolution occurring generally by 3–4 months of therapy [51–53].

Interestingly, the efficacy of MTX in LP can be compared to that or oral steroids. Hazra and scholars delineated no significant disparity in their exposition comparing oral betamethasone pulse (5 mg twice weekly), with MTX (10 mg/week) in the treatment of generalized LP in 44 patients [54]. Another report further reiterated that treatment with oral steroids (40 mg/day) was not superior to MTX (10 mg/week) for generalized LP [55].

After discontinuation of MTX therapy in LP, proper follow up is essential, owing to a tendency to relapse, which tends to occur generally after a mean duration of one and a half years [53].

Owing to its profound effects on T lymphocytes, MTX is considered a good choice for treating LP [48]. Further, by suppressing Th1 cell lines, and simultaneously increasing differentiation of regulatory T cells, MTX reduces the ongoing inflammation and therefore helps alleviating lesions in LP [56]. Also, MTX downregulates CXCL10, a major mediator of chronic inflammation, further augmenting its therapeutic effects [57].

Lichen Planopilaris (LPP)

MTX can be given as a second-line therapy in LPP [58]. Based on its antagonistic T cell effects, MTX is utilized for treating LPP [59].

The dose of MTX in LPP generally does not exceed 15 mg/week. Within 6 months of treatment, statistically significant reduction in the lichen planopilaris activity index is noted in those patients responding to MTX treatment [60].

Further, MTX is superior to hydroxychloroquine in treating LPP, and synonymous to cyclosporine for the same [61, 62]. It is therefore suggested to prescribe MTX first, because of its wider applicability, weekly dosing schedule and better toxicity profile. Also, in severely inflamed cases, MTX serves as a valuable steroid sparing agent, enabling maintenance of efficacy following steroid taper [63].

Cutaneous Lupus Erythematosus (CLE)

MTX (up to 25 mg/week) is considered a valid second-line treatment for CLE cases refractory to antimalarials. It is preferable to administer MTX subcutaneously in these cases, along with antimalarials [64]. Though inferior to thalidomide in CLE, owing to its favourable toxicity profile, it remains a valuable option [65].

MTX is particularly effective in subacute cutaneous lupus erythematosus and in patients with hypocomplementemia [66]. In discoid lupus erythematosus, better responses are outlined in patients with localized disease [66].

MTX can also be combined with cyclosporine in CLE with profitable outcomes, also facilitating cyclosporine dose reduction [67].

The effects of MTX in LE is usually evident by 4–6 weeks and as treatment continues, improvement is progressive [64].

However, while administering MTX in LE, a close watch on the hematologic and hepatic parameters need attention, in order to avoid any toxic effects.

Adverse Effects

Hepatotoxicity

Acute or chronic hepatotoxicity may develop during the course of MTX treatment. Psoriatic patients have 2.5–5-fold increased risk of developing liver fibrosis and cirrhosis from treatment with MTX, compared to rheumatoid arthritis patients treated with the same dose. Patients who are at an increased risk of developing MTX-induced hepatotoxicity include those with:

- Diabetes mellitus,
- Obesity,
- Renal insufficiency,
- History of liver disease, and.
- Alcoholism.

In the presence of liver damage, there is a possibility of liver function tests being normal, therefore it becomes imperative to examine the histological appearance of the liver and detect any abnormality, if the patient has been on long-term treatment with MTX [3].

Further, the risk of liver damage is low in patients whose cumulative MTX dose is <1.5 g [5].

Recent studies with more careful patient selection demonstrate liver fibrosis and cirrhosis to be less even at cumulative doses of 4 g.

According to Roenigk et al., liver damage is classified into four grades as shown in Table 26.1 [68].

Cirrhosis induced by MTX, however, is often non-aggressive. A patient with an abnormal liver biopsy may with time experience a reversal of findings, while off

Table 26.1 Grades of liver damage as classified by Roenigk et al

Grades of liver damage	Features
Grade I	Liver essentially normal Mild fatty infiltration Mild nuclear variability Mild portal tract inflammation
Grade II	Moderate fatty infiltration Moderate to severe nuclear variability and portal tract inflammation
Grade IIIA	Mild fibrosis
Grade IIIB	Moderate to severe fibrosis
Grade IV	Cirrhosis

MTX treatment, and it is possible to resume MTX after a significant period of time off the drug [69].

To detect MTX-induced hepatic fibrosis and cirrhosis, USG-guided liver biopsy is the gold standard method employed for accurate diagnosis. Other non-invasive tests employed include radionucleotide scan, USG and estimation of serum amino terminal of type III procollagen peptide (PIIINP). However, none of these are diagnostic. USG fails to distinguish fat from fibrosis [70], and PIIINP assessments fail to identify in which organ the underlying fibrosis is occurring. Further, it is unreliable in patients with significant psoriatic arthritis [71].

Hematologic

Predisposing factors for patients on MTX to develop hematologic toxicity include:

- Elderly patients,
- Patients on concomitant drugs such as NSAIDs and co-trimoxazole,
- No co-prescription of folic acid,
- Patients on a daily dose of MTX,
- Albumin <3 g/dL,
- Major surgery in the past, and.
- Bleeding episodes.

Frequent complete blood counts may help in monitoring bone marrow toxicity [72]. Should significant myelosuppression develop, the patient should promptly be treated with folinic acid (leucovorin rescue), which can bypass the enzyme DHFR and allow normal cell division to resume.

Pulmonary

- Acute pneumonitis.

- Insidious pulmonary fibrosis: This occurs owing to an idiosyncratic response. It is commoner in patients with rheumatoid arthritis and is life-threatening, requiring immediate cessation of MTX therapy. Other postulates regarding the occurrence of pulmonary toxicity with MTX include a direct toxic reaction, hypersensitivity reaction, immunologic reaction and folate deficiency [73–75].

Secondary Malignancy

The use of MTX in collagen vascular diseases is associated with lymphoma development. However, it is rarely seen in psoriatic patients. In many of these patients, an association with Epstein–Barr virus is documented. It is still not clearly understood why some patients develop lymphoma, and there is no specific clinical scenario that is suggested stating a unique risk for lymphoma development [76, 77].

Gastrointestinal

- Nausea.
- Vomiting.
- Ulcerative stomatitis.

Gastrointestinal side effects of MTX can be minimized by incorporating folic acid in the treatment regimen, without compromising the efficacy of MTX [78].

Reproductive

- Teratogenic.
- Abortifacient.

Renal

High dose therapy (50–250 mg/m^2 via the intravenous route) may lead to renal toxicity secondary to precipitation of MTX in renal tubules. Usually in doses administered for psoriasis this is not encountered.

Cutaneous

- Folliculitis.
- Mild alopecia.
- Recent sunburn recalled or previously irradiated skin develops a toxic reaction on administration of MTX (photo recall).

- Acral erythema.
- Papular eruption in patients with rheumatic disease.
- Epidermal necrosis.
- Cutaneous ulceration.

Others

- Osteopathy.
- Rarely stress fracture.

Drug Interactions

- Drugs that increase methotrexate levels: doxycycline, minocycline, tetracycline, phenytoin, phenothiazines, sulfonamides, NSAIDS, chloramphenicol.
- Drugs that decrease methotrexate levels: ciprofloxacin, penicillin, amiodarone, dipyridamole.
- Methotrexate increases serum levels of theophylline.
- Methotrexate reduces serum levels of digoxin.
- Drugs increasing risk of hematologic toxicity with MTX: dapsone, sulfonamides.

Monitoring Guidelines

Baseline

- Careful history and physical examination.
- Identification of any risk factors for toxicity.
- Recording any concomitant medicines that can interact with MTX.
- Complete blood count with platelets.
- Liver function test/renal function tests.
- Hepatitis A, B, C serology.
- HIV testing in patients at risk for AIDS.

Follow-Up

- Complete blood count with platelets, liver function tests: done once every 2 weeks for the first month, and then repeated once every 3–4 months.
- Renal function tests: done once or twice yearly.

Liver Biopsy

- Done after 1.5–2 g of total MTX for low-risk patients.
- Done after a total of 1 g of MTX for high-risk patients.
- Done every 6 months for patients with grade IIIA liver biopsy changes.

Conclusion

MTX still remains the cornerstone in the management of psoriasis. Despite introduction of numerous newer agents, MTX is considered the first choice in managing psoriasis until there happens to be a contraindication for its use.

References

1. Silvis NG. Antimetabolites and cytotoxic drugs. Dermatol Clin. 2001;19:105–18.
2. Edmundson WF, Guy WB. Treatment of psoriasis with folic acid antagonists. Arch Dermatol. 1958;78:200–3.
3. Callen PJ, Kulp Shorten CL, Wolverton SE. Methotrexate. In: Wolverton SE, editor. Comprehensive dermatologic drug therapy. 1st ed. London: WB Saunders Company; 2001. p. 147–64.
4. Hersh EM, Carbone PP, Wond VG, et al. Inhibition of primary immune response in man by antimetabolites. Cancer Res. 1965;25:1997–2001.
5. Mitchelle MS, Wade ME, Decenti RC, et al. Immune suppressive effects of cytosine arabinoside and methotrexate in man. Ann Intern Med. 1969;70:535–47.
6. Sigmundsdottir H, Johnston A, Gudjonsson JE, et al. Methotrexate markedly reduces the expression of vascular E-selectin, cutaneous lymphocyte associated antigen and the numbers of mononuclear leucocytes in psoriatic skin. Exp Dermatol. 2004;13:426–34.
7. Cronstein BN. The mechanism of action of methotrexate. Rheum Dis Clin N Am. 1997;23:739–55.
8. Kuhn A, Specker C, Ruzika T, et al. Methotrexate treatment for refractory subacute cutaneous lupus erythematosus. J Am Acad Dermatol. 2002;46:600–3.
9. Balis FM, Savitch JL, Bleyer WA. Pharmacokinetics of oral methotrexate in children. Cancer Res. 1983;43:2242–5.
10. Dupuis LL, Koren G, Silevrman ED, et al. Influence of food on the bioavailability of oral methotrexate in children. J Rheumatol. 1995;22:1570–3.
11. Galivan J, Pupons A, Rhee M. Hepatic parenchymal cell glutamylation of methotrexate studied on monolayer culture. Cancer Res. 1986;46:670–5.
12. Kamen BA, Nylen PA, Camitta DM, et al. Methotrexate accumulation in the cells as a possible mechanism of chronic toxicity to the drug. Br J Haematol. 1981;49:355–60.
13. Singh SK, Rai T. Relapse in psoriasis with two different tapering regimens of methotrexate: a randomized open label-controlled study. Indian J Dermatol Venereol Leprol. 2015;81:144–7.
14. Smith CH, Anstey AV, Barker JN, et al. British association of dermatologists guidelines for biologic interventions for psoriasis 2009. Br J Dermatol. 2009;161:987–1019.
15. Colman RJ, Rubin DT. Optimal doses of methotrexate combined with anti-TNF therapy to maintain clinical remission of inflammatory bowel disease. J Crohns Colitis. 2015:312–7.
16. Menter A, Gottlieb A, Feldman SR, et al. Guidelines of care for management of psoriasis and psoriatic arthritis: section 1. Overview of psoriasis and psoriatic arthritis: section 1. Overview

of psoriasis and guidelines of care for the treatment of psoriasis with biologics. J Am Acad Dermatol. 2008;58:826–50.
17. Rott S, Mrowietz U. Recent developments in the use of biologics in psoriasis and autoimmune disorders. The role of autoantibodies. BMJ. 2005;330:716–20.
18. Thappa DM, Laxmisha C. Immunomodulators in the treatment of psoriasis. Indian J Dermatol Venereol Leprol. 2004;70:1–9.
19. Brown J, Perry HO. Pityriasis rubra pilaris. Treatment with folic acid antagonists. Arch Dermatol. 1966;94:636–8.
20. Cutolo M, Sulli A, Pizzorni C, et al. Anti-inflammatory mechanisms of methotrexate in rheumatoid arthritis. Ann Rheum Dis. 2001;60:729–35.
21. Koch L, Schoffl C, Aberer W, et al. Methotrexate for the treatment of pityriasis rubra pilaris: a case series and literature review. Acta Derm Venereol. 2018;98:501–5.
22. Lynch PJ, Saied NK. Methotrexate treatment for pityriasis lichenoides and lymphomatoid papulosis. Cutis. 1979;23:634.
23. Cornelison RL Jr, Everett MA. Methotrexate for the treatment of Mucha-Habermann disease. Arch Dermatol. 1972;106:507.
24. Lazaridou E, Fotiadou C, Tsorovac C, et al. Resistant pityriasis lichenoid et varioliformis acuta in a 3 year old boy: successful treatment with methotrexate. Int J Dermatol. 2010;49:215.
25. Bara C, Maillard H, Briand N, et al. Methotrexate for bullous pemphigoid: preliminary study. Arch Dermatol. 2003;139:1506–7.
26. Zeiglscmid-Adams ME, Pandya AG, Cohen SB, et al. Treatment of dermatomyositis with methotrexate. J Am Acad Dermatol. 1995;32:754–7.
27. Zipitis CS, Baildam EM, Ramanan AV. Treatment approaches to juvenile dermatomyositis. Expert Opin Rheumatol. 2004;5:1509–15.
28. Zuberbier T, Latif AHA, Abuzakouk M, et al. The international EAACI/GA2LEN/EuroGuiDerm/APAAACI guideline for the definition, classification, diagnosis and management of urticaria. Allergy. 2022;77:734–66.
29. Godse K, De A, Zawar V, et al. Consensus statement for the diagnosis and treatment of urticaria: a 2017 update. Indian J Dermatol. 2018;63:2–15.
30. Leducq S, Samimi M, Bernier C, et al. Efficacy and safety of methotrexate versus placebo as add-on therapy to H1 antihistamines for patients with difficult-to-treat chronic spontaneous urticaria. A randomized controlled trial. J Am Acad Dermatol. 2020;82:240–3.
31. Yadav S, Jain D. Effectiveness, safety and tolerability of methotrexate in chronic urticaria at a tertiary care Centre. Int J Contemp Med Res. 2017;4:1952–5.
32. Sharma V, Singh S, Ramam M, et al. A randomized placebo controlled double blind pilot study of methotrexate in the treatment of H1 antihistamines-resistant chronic spontaneous urticaria. Indian J Dermatol Venereol Leprol. 2014;80:122–8.
33. Sagi L, Solomon M, Baum S, et al. Evidence for methotrexate as a useful treatment for steroid dependant chronic urticaria. Acta Derm Venereol. 2011;91:303–6.
34. Perez A, Woods A, Grattan CE. Methotrexate: a useful steroid-sparing agent in chronic urticaria. Br J Dermatol. 2010;162:191–4.
35. Mora PM, Perez Mdel CG, Arvizu VA, et al. Urticaria autoimmunitaria Tratamiento con metotrxato [Autoimmune urticaria: treatment with methotrexate]. Rev Allerg Mex. 2004;51:167–72.
36. Gach JE, Sabroe RA, Greaves MW, et al. Methotrexate responsive chronic idiopathic urticaria. A report of two cases. Br J Dermatol. 2001;145:340–3.
37. Weiner MJ. Methotrexate in corticosteroid resistant urticaria. Ann Intern Med. 1989;1110:848.
38. Godse K. Methotrexate in autoimmune urticaria. Indian J Dermatol Venereol Leprol. 2004;70:377.
39. Yadav AK. Study of effectiveness of methotrexate oral pulse in refractory chronic urticaria. Indian J Skin Allergy. 2024;3:66–70.
40. Cronstein BBN, Naime D, Ostad E. The anti-inflammatory mechanism of methotrexate. Increased adenosine release at inflamed sited diminishes leukocyte accumulation in an in vivo model of inflammation. J Clin Invest. 1993;92:2675–82.

41. Eckert L, Amand C, Gadkari A, et al. Treatment patterns in UK adult patients with atopic dermatitis treated with systemic immunosuppressants: data from the health improvement network (THIN). J Dermatolog Treat. 2019;31:815–20.
42. Garristen FM, van den Heuvel JM, Bruijnzeel-Koomen C, et al. Use of oral immunosuppressive drugs in atopic dermatitis in The Netherlands. J Eur Acad Dermatol Venereol. 2018;32:1336–42.
43. El-Khalawany MA, Hassan H, Shaaban D, et al. Methotrexate versus cyclosporine in the treatment of severe atopic dermatitis in children: a multicentre experience from Egypt [Comparative study, multicentre study, randomized controlled trial]. Eur J Pediatr. 2013;172:351–6.
44. Goujon C, Viguer M, Staumont-Salle D, et al. Methotrexate versus cyclosporine in adults with moderate to severe atopic dermatitis: a phase III randomized non-inferiority trial [Clinical trial, phase III, multicentre study, randomized controlled trial, research support, non-US]. J Allergy Clin Immunol Pract. 2018;6:562.e3–9.e3.
45. Law Ping Man S, Bouzille G, Beneton N, et al. Drug survival and post drug survival of first line immunosuppressive treatments for atopic dermatitis: comparison between methotrexate and cyclosporine [comparative study]. J Eur Acad Dermatol Venereol. 2018;32:1327–35.
46. Roekevisch E, Schram ME, Leeflang MMG, et al. Methotrexate versus azathioprine in patients with atopic dermatitis: 2 year follow up data. J Allergy Clin Immunol. 2018;141:825–7.
47. Chan ES, Cronstein BN. Molecular action of methotrexate in inflammatory diseases. Arthritis Res. 2002;4:266–73.
48. Thomas S, Fisher KH, Snowden JA, et al. Methotrexate is a JAK/STAT pathway inhibitor. PLoS One. 2015;10:e0130078.
49. Caron AGM, Bloem M, El Khattali H, et al. The wide variety of methotrexate dosing regimens for the treatment of atopic dermatitis: a systematic review. J Dermatol Treat. 2024;35:2292962.
50. Lee JH, Yun SJ, Lee JB, et al. Therapeutic efficacy and safety of methotrexate in moderate to severe atopic dermatitis: a retrospective study of Korean patients at a tertiary referral hospital. Ann Dermatol. 2020;32:402–8.
51. Kanwar AJ, De D. Methotrexate for the treatment of lichen planus. Old drug, new indication. J Eur Acad Dermatol Venereol. 2013;27:e410–3.
52. Turan H, Baskan EB, Tunali S, et al. Methotrexate for the treatment of generalized lichen planus. J Am Acad Dermatol. 2009;60:164–6.
53. Khurana A, Sharath S, Sardana K. Efficacy and safety of low dose methotrexate in generalized and recalcitrant lichen planus. A retrospective study at a tertiary care Centre. Dermatol Pract Concept. 2024;14:e2024220.
54. Hazra SC, Choudhury AM, Khondker L, et al. Comparative efficacy of methotrexate and mini pulse betamethasone in the treatment of lichen planus. Mymensingh Med J. 2013;22:787–97.
55. Bakhtiar R, Noor SM, Paracha MM. Effectiveness of oral methotrexate therapy versus systemic corticosteroid therapy in treatment of generalized lichen planus. J Coll Physicians Surg Pak. 2018;28:505–8.
56. Vicic M, Hlaca N, Kastelon M, et al. Comprehensive insight into lichen planus immunopathogenesis. Int J Mol Sci. 2023;24:3038.
57. Di Lernia V. Targeting the IFN gamma/CXCL10 pathway in lichen planus. Med Hypothesis. 2016;92:60–1.
58. Errichetti E, Figini M, Croatto M, et al. Therapeutic management of classic lichen planopilaris: a systematic review. Clin Cosmet Investig Dermatol. 2018;11:91–102.
59. Raimondi MV, Randazzo O, La Franca M, et al. DHFR inhibitors: reading the past for discovering novel anticancer agents. Molecules. 2019;24:1140.
60. Fatemi F, Esfahanian F, Asilian A, et al. Comparative efficacy study combination of oral methotrexate and prednisolone versus oral methotrexate in patients with lichen planopilaris. Dermatol Res Pract. 2022;2022:3792489.
61. Naeini FF, Saber M, Asilian A, et al. Clinical efficacy and safety of methotrexate versus hydroxychloroquine in preventing lichen planopilaris progress: a randomized clinical trial. Int J Prev Med. 2017;8:37.

62. Naeini FF, Mohaghegh F, Jelvan M, et al. Cyclosporine or methotrexate, which one is more promising in the treatment of lichen planopilaris. Int Immunopharmacol. 2020;86:106765.
63. Manousaridis I, Manousaridis K, Peetsch WK, et al. Individualising treatment and choice of medication in lichen planus: a step by step approach. J Dtsch Dermatol Ges. 2013;11:981–91.
64. Verdelli A, Corra A, Marioth EB, et al. An update on the management of refractory cutaneous lupus erythematosus. Front Med. 2022;9:941003.
65. Fruchtec R, Kurtzman DJB, Patel M, et al. Characteristics and alternative treatment outcomes of antimalarial refractory cutaneous lupus erythematosus. JAMA Dermatol. 2017;153:937–9.
66. Wenzel J, Brahler S, Bauer R, et al. Efficacy and safety of methotrexate in recalcitrant cutaneous lupus erythematosus: results of a retrospective study in 43 patients. Br J Dermatol. 2005;153:157–62.
67. Klein A, Vogt T, Wenzel SM, et al. Cyclosporine combined with methotrexate in two patients with recalcitrant subacute cutaneous lupus erythematosus. Australas J Dermatol. 2011;52:43–7.
68. Aithal GP, Haugk B, Das S, et al. Monitoring methotrexate-induced hepatic fibrosis in patients with psoriasis: are serial liver biopsies justified? Aliment Pharmacol Ther. 2004;19:391–9.
69. Zachariae H, Sogaard H. Methotrexate induced liver cirrhosis: a follow up. Dermatologica. 1987;175:178–82.
70. Coulson HH, et al. A comparison of liver ultrasound with liver biopsy histology in psoriatics receiving long term methotrexate therapy. Br J Dermatol. 1987;116:491–5.
71. Zachariae H, Aslam HM, Bjerring P, et al. Serum amino terminal propeptide of type III procollagen in psoriasis and psoriatic arthritis: relation to liver fibrosis and arthritis. J Am Acad Dermatol. 1991;25:50–3.
72. Roenigk HH, Auerbach R, Maibach HI, et al. Methotrexate in psoriasis: revised guidelines. J Am Acad Dermatol. 1998;38:478–85.
73. Bedrossian CWM, Miller WC, et al. Methotrexate induced diffuse interstitial pulmonary fibrosis. South Med J. 1979;72:313–8.
74. Akoun GM, Gauthier Rahman S, Maynaud CM, et al. Leukocyte migration inhibition in methotrexate induced pneumonitis. Evidence for an immunologic cell mediated mechanism. Chest. 1987;91:96–7.
75. Barrera P, Laon RFJM, Van Reil PLCM, et al. Methotrexate related pulmonary complications in rheumatoid arthritis. Ann Rheum Dis. 1994;53:434–9.
76. Bleyer WA. Methotrexate induced lymphoma. J Rheumatol. 1998;25:404–8.
77. Kamel OW. Lymphomas during long term methotrexate therapy. Arch Dermatol. 1997;133:907–8.
78. Duhra P. Treatment of gastrointestinal symptoms associated with methotrexate therapy for psoriasis. J Am Acad Dermatol. 1993;28:466–9.

Azathioprine

27

Introduction

Azathioprine (AZE) made its clinical debut in 1961, as an immunosuppressant for renal transplantation. It is synthesized from 6-mercaptopurine (6-MP) and is less toxic than 6-MP for an equivalent degree of immunosuppression [1].

AZE is a prodrug for mercaptopurine, with an imidazole group attached to the SH group of mercaptopurine. In tissues, AZE is non-enzymatically converted to mercaptopurine [2].

Mechanism of Action

AZE:

- Decreases both B and T cell function,
- Inhibits cell division,
- Decrease the number of Langerhans cells (thereby reducing its antigen-presenting ability),
- Diminishes production of prostaglandins, and.
- Reduces antibody production by B cells [3, 4].

Pharmacokinetics

Given orally, >88% of AZE is absorbed from the gut [1]. AZE crosses the placenta, but does not penetrate the blood–brain barrier. AZE is metabolized in the liver to the active metabolite 6-thioguanine. This accumulates in tissues and provides maximal clinical immunosuppression by 8–12 weeks [5]. Its $t_{1/2}$ is 5 h. The metabolism of AZE is schematically represented in Fig. 27.1.

A. K. Bubna, *Therapeutics in Dermatology - Essentials for Clinical Practice*,
https://doi.org/10.1007/978-981-95-3791-4_27

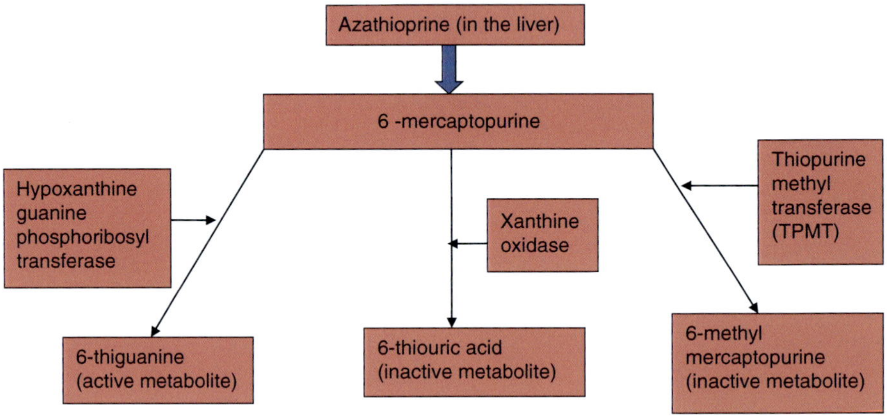

Fig. 27.1 Metabolism of azathioprine

Patients with low thiopurine methyl transferase (TPMT) activity can cause increased accumulation of the active metabolite, 6-thioguanine, which can produce fatal myelosuppression. Therefore, it is best to avoid AZE in these patients. In patients with increased TPMT activity, the dosing of AZE needs to be accordingly escalated [6]. AZE is virtually completely metabolized. Negligible unmetabolized AZE is excreted via the kidneys.

Indications

FDA Approved

- Organ transplantation.
- Severe rheumatoid arthritis.

Off Label

Immunobullous Disorders

- Bullous pemphigoid (BP).
- Pemphigus vulgaris (PV).
- Cicatricial pemphigoid (CP).

Vasculitis

- Leukocytoclastic vasculitis (LCV).
- Wegener's granulomatosis (WG).
- Polyarteritis nodosa (PAN).

Neutrophilic Dermatoses

- Behcet's disease (BD).
- Pyoderma gangrenosum (PG).

Autoimmune Connective Tissue Diseases

- Systemic lupus erythematosus (SLE).
- Discoid lupus erythematosus (DLE).
- Dermatomyositis/polymyositis.
- Relapsing polychondritis (RP).

Papulosquamous Disorders

- Psoriasis.
- Lichen planus (LP).

Eczemas

- Atopic dermatitis (AD).
- Contact dermatitis (CD).

Photo Dermatoses

- Chronic actinic dermatitis (CAD).
- Polymorphous light eruption (PMLE).
- Persistent light reactors.

Others

- Sarcoidosis.
- Persistent erythema multiforme.
- Chronic graft versus host disease.

Contraindications

Absolute

- Pregnancy.
- Hypersensitivity to the drug.
- Active/clinically significant infections.

Relative

- Alopurinol use.
- Prior use of alkylating agents (increases the risk of malignancy).

Pregnancy prescribing status: Category 'D'.

General Guidelines for the Use of Azathioprine in Dermatology

- Disease should be life threatening.
- Disease should be reversible or controllable.
- Disease is unresponsive to less potentially risky therapies.
- Disease should have measurable clinical or laboratory measures of improvement.
- Risks and adverse effects should be carefully discussed with the patient.
- Alternative therapies should be discussed with the patient.
- Patient should be compliant with various laboratory monitoring tests.

Clinical Uses

Immunobullous Disorders

AZE, for the above indication, is usually utilized in combination with systemic steroids. Initiating dose of AZE is 2–3 mg/kg/day, which is then tapered to 1–2 mg/kg/day when 50% improvement is ascertained [7]. The main role of AZE in vesiculobullous disorders is that of a steroid sparing agent. Besides, in mild cases of BP, AZE can be used along with potent topical corticosteroids with favourable outcomes [8]. In PV, apart from the conventional dosing of AZE, pulse therapy with AZE is administered to patients in whom cyclophosphamide is contraindicated. Dose of dexamethasone is similar as used for the dexamethasone cyclophosphamide pulse, and AZE is dosed at 50 mg/day. This is referred to as the dexamethasone azathioprine pulse (DAP). No bolus dose of AZE is required for DAP therapy. Further, AZE (100mg/day) along with 40mg of alternate day prednisolone is another pulse therapy followed in PV (referred to as Lever mini therapy), with efficacious results.

Vasculitis

In LCV related to rheumatoid arthritis, AZE is effective in combination with prednisolone [9]. Advantages noted with AZE include lower incidence of vascular relapse, fewer serious complications and a relatively lower mortality. In WG, both renal and pulmonary disease demonstrate improvement with combination of AZE and systemic steroids [10]. In PAN, renal disease in particular shows improvement with AZE [11].

Neutrophilic Dermatoses

In BD, AZE is helpful in reducing ocular abnormalities such as hypopyon and emergent blindness. Further, AZE is beneficial in decreasing complications such as arthritis, genital and oral ulcers in BD [12, 13].

AZE has only occasionally been utilized in PG, with variable success [14, 15].

Connective Tissue Disorders

In SLE, AZE is used particularly for lupus nephritis [16]. Besides, AZE demonstrates benefit in treating extensive discoid skin lesions with palmoplantar involvement [17].

In RP, AZE is particularly useful for treating ocular symptoms [18].

In systemic sclerosis, AZE is not effective as monotherapy, but may be beneficial for systemic sclerosis-associated interstitial lung disease as well as cutaneous manifestations, as follow-up maintenance therapy after cyclophosphamide induction.

In dermatomyositis, AZE proves helpful more for respiratory and muscle symptoms, rather than cutaneous lesions [19].

The dose of AZE in connective tissue disorders is 2–3 mg/day, with gradual taper once clinical improvement becomes noticeable. It is usually administered in combination with systemic glucocorticoids as a steroid sparing agent for this indication.

Atopic Dermatitis

AZE is used in severe treatment resistant cases of AD. AZE is used as a 100 mg daily dose in adults and 2–3.5 mg/kg/day in children [20]. AZE provides a cheaper alternative to cyclosporine for AD. Response to therapy is evident within 8–10 weeks. Besides, duration of remission seen with AZE is much longer when compared to cyclosporine following drug cessation.

Lichen Planus

AZE has been particularly useful in generalized LP [21] and erosive LP [22], with responses being obtained even with monotherapy.

Psoriasis

AZE is not a prime treatment option for psoriasis, as other drugs are available for this indication. However, it can be used as a last resort where other treatments have failed [23].

Photo Dermatoses

In CAD, AZE (100 mg/day) has shown value. Improvement in lesions is evident by 6 months. Remission is usually sustained [24]. In PMLE, AZE is reserved for severe and recalcitrant cases [25].

Sarcoidosis

Lung disease in sarcoidosis demonstrates responsiveness to AZE, with less predictable benefit for dermatologic lesions [26].

Adverse Effects

Hematologic

- Myelosuppression (most frequent and serious side effect and correlates with low TPMT activity).
- Neutropenia.
- Agranulocytosis.
- Pancytopenia (AZE treatment needs to be stopped when WBC count lies between 4000–4500 cells/mm^3, platelets <100,000 cells/mm^3 and Hb <10 g/dL).

Carcinogenesis

- Lymphomas.
- Squamous cell carcinoma (as AZE is an immunosuppressant, it reduces the host's ability of immune surveillance).

Opportunistic Infections

- Herpes simplex.
- Human papilloma virus.
- Scabies.

Gastrointestinal

- Nausea.
- Vomiting.
- Diarrhoea.
- Gastritis.
- Pancreatitis.
- Rarely, hepatotoxicity (taking the drug with food, reducing the dose or dividing the dose reduces these symptoms).

Teratogenicity

- Bilateral hip dislocation.
- Bilateral talipes equinivarus.
- Preaxial polydactyly.
- Myelomeningocele.

Hypersensitivity syndrome that resembles anticonvulsant hypersensitivity syndrome and is characterized by:

- Cardiovascular collapse.
- Gastrointestinal: Nausea, hepatotoxicity and pancreatitis.
- Cutaneous: Macular erythema, maculopapular rash, purpura, petechiae, erythema multiforme, urticaria, angioedema and erythema nodosum.
- Arthralgia, myalgia.
- Respiratory: Cough, pneumonitis.

These features develop within 1-4 weeks of initiation of therapy with AZE in susceptible patients

Drug Interactions

Drugs such as ACE inhibitors, allopurinol and methotrexate (MTX) that increase the potential of myelosuppression with AZE are best avoided.

However, in certain difficult-to-treat dermatomes, MTX and AZE can be used in combination with careful monitoring. MTX provides rapid improvement, while AZE requires at least 4–6 weeks for it to demonstrate its effect [27]. Moreover, MTX and AZE have synergistic effects. MTX blocks xanthine oxidase and therefore increases the number of 6-thioguanine nucleotides, which are now available for better immunosuppression. Although no severe side effects have been observed with this combination, reports of increased liver enzymes and an acute febrile toxic reaction were observed in one study, characterized by fever, myalgia, joint pains and a generalized erythematous rash [28].

In a study from North India, the combination of MTX and AZE was given to patients with atopic dermatitis, CAD, phytophotodermatitis and pyoderma gangrenosum with LCV, which were recalcitrant to standard treatment with systemic glucocorticoids. In these patients, MTX and AZE combination was continued for 40 weeks, with no adverse effects being encountered. Therefore, this strategy can be of value in treating patients not responding to standard therapy. However, an extreme cautious approach with monitoring of appropriate hematologic and hepatic parameters needs to be exercised [29].

Monitoring Guidelines

Baseline

Baseline monitoring guidelines are summarized in Table 27.1.

Follow-Up

- Clinical evaluation to rule out development of lymphoma or squamous cell carcinoma.
- Same laboratory parameters done at baseline to be repeated once in 2 weeks for 2 months, and then once every 3 months.

Table 27.1 Baseline monitoring guidelines of azathioprine

Clinical evaluation	Laboratory parameters
Discuss the risk–benefit profile and the likely toxic effects of the drug	Pregnancy test in females of child bearing age
Discuss the need for multiple blood tests	Complete blood count with platelets
Discuss alternative modalities available	Blood biochemistry
Discuss the teratogenic properties of azathioprine and the precautions required	Urinalysis
Find out any history of usage of allopurinol, ACE inhibitors and other immunosuppressive agents	
Careful examination of the skin and the lymphoreticular system	

Table 27.2 Dosing guidelines of azathioprine based on the activity of thiopurine methyltransferase

Thiopurine methyltransferase activity	Dose of azathioprine (AZE)
<5, U/m	AZE not recommended
>5 and < 15 U/mL	0.5 mg/kg/day
15 and < 20 U/mL	1.5 mg/kg/day
>20 and < 30 U/mL	2.5 mg/kg/day

Dosing

A new recommendation for dosing has been proposed by Snow and Gibson [6] based on the activity of TPMT in erythrocytes and is summarized in Table 27.2.

However, in most set ups in India where the facility of estimating levels of TPMT is non-existent, it is prudent to start AZE at 1 mg/kg/day and gradually step it up to the required dose, with careful monitoring of parameters stated in the monitoring guidelines.

Conclusion

AZE is an economically valuable drug with a number of dermatologic indications. However, the major drawback of AZE is the delayed time taken for it to show its response. It is therefore recommended that AZE always be utilized along with other faster acting drugs in the initial phase, before it begins to manifest its effects.

References

1. Chan GLC, Canafax DM, Johnson CA. The therapeutic use of azathioprine in renal transplantation. Pharmacotherapy. 1987;7:165–77.
2. El-Azhary RA. Azathioprine. Current status and future consideration. Int J Dermatol. 2003;42:335–41.
3. Lin H, Wong C. In vitro immunosuppressive effects of methotrexate and azathioprine on Langerhans cells. Arch Dermatol Res. 1997;289:94–7.
4. Younger IR, Harris DWS, Clover CB. Azathioprine in dermatology. J Am Acad Dermatol. 1991;25:281–8.
5. Anstey AV, Walkelin S, Reynolds NJ. Guidelines for prescribing azathioprine in dermatology. Br J Dermatol. 2004;151:1123–32.
6. Snow JL, Gibson LE. The role of genetic variation in thiopurine methyltransferase activity and the efficacy and/or side effects of azathioprine therapy in dermatologic patients. Arch Dermatol. 1995;131:193–7.
7. Aberer W, Wolff-Schreiner EC, Stingl G. Azathioprine in the treatment of pemphigus vulgaris: a long term follow up. J Am Acad Dermatol. 1987;16:527–33.

8. Tan BB, Lear JT, Gawkrodger DJ, English JSC. Azathioprine in dermatology: a survey of current practice in the UK. Br J Dermatol. 1997;136:351–5.
9. Heurkens AH, Westedt ML, Breedveld FC. Prednisolone plus azathioprine treatment in patients with rheumatoid arthritis complicated by vasculitis. Arch Int Med. 1991;151:2249–54.
10. Wishart JM. Wegener's granulomatosis – controlled by azathioprine and corticosteroids. Br J Dermatol. 1975;92:471–7.
11. Brock PG, Richard P. Reversal of rapidly progressive renal failure associated with polyarteritis. Proc Roy Soc Med. 1973;66:656–7.
12. Yazici H, Pazarli H, Barnes CG, et al. A controlled trial of azathioprine in Behcet's syndrome. N Engl J Med. 1990;322:281–5.
13. Hamuryudan V, Ozyazgan Y, Hizli N, et al. Azathioprine in Behcet's syndrome: effects on long term prognosis. Arthritis Rheum. 1997;40:769–74.
14. Duffill MB. Cyclosporine, azathioprine and local therapy for pyoderma gangrenosum. Australas J Dermatol. 1994;35:15–8.
15. Wollina U. Clinical management of pyoderma gangrenosum. Am J Clin Dermatol. 2002;3:149–58.
16. Swaak AJ, Statius van Eps LW, Aarden LA, et al. Azathioprine in the treatment of systemic lupus erythematosus: a three-year prospective study. Clin Rheumatol. 1984:285–91.
17. Ashinoff R, Werth VP, Franks AG Jr. Resistant discoid lupus erythematosus of palms and soles: successful treatment with azathioprine. J Am Acad Dermatol. 1988;19:961–5.
18. Hoang Xuan T, Foster CS, Rice BA. Scleritis in relapsing polychondritis: response to therapy. Ophthalmology. 1990;97:892–8.
19. Lever WF. Dermatomyositis. Arch Dermatol. 1972;105:771–2.
20. Lear JT, English JS, Smith AG. Retrospective review of the use of azathioprine in severe atopic dermatitis. J Am Acad Dermatol. 1996;35:642–3.
21. Lear JT, English JS. Erosive and generalized lichen planus responsive to azathioprine. Clin Exp Dermatol. 1996;21:56–7.
22. Klein LR, Callen JP. Azathioprine: effective steroid sparing therapy for generalized lichen planus. South Med J. 1992;82:198–201.
23. Hacker SM, Ramos Caro FA, Ford MJ, et al. Azathioprine: a forgotten alternative for the treatment of severe psoriasis. Int J Dermatol. 1992;31:873–4.
24. Kingston J, Lowe N, Sofen H, et al. Actinic reticuloid in a black man: successful therapy with azathioprine. J Am Acad Dermatol. 1987;16:1079–83.
25. Norris P, Hawk J. Successful treatment of severe polymorphous light eruption with azathioprine. Arch Dermatol. 1989;125:1377–9.
26. Pacheco Y, Marechal C, Marchal F, et al. Azathioprine treatment of chronic pulmonary sarcoidosis. Sarcoidosis. 1985;2:107–13.
27. Balis FM, Holcenburg JS, Zimm S, et al. The effect of methotrexate on the bioavailability of oral 6-mercaptopurine. Clin Pharmacol. 1987;41:384–7.
28. Innocenti F, Danesi R, Di Paolo A, et al. Clinical and experimental pharmacokinetic interaction between 6-mercaptopurine and methotrexate. Cancer Chemother Pharmacol. 1996;37:409–14.
29. Agarwal P, Agarwal US, Meena RS, et al. A combination of oral azathioprine and methotrexate in difficult to treat dermatoses. Indian J Dermatol Venereol Leprol. 2017;83:389–92.

Mycophenolate Mofetil 28

Introduction

Mycophenolate mofetil (MMF) is an immunosuppressant used in a variety of dermatologic disorders. It was originally obtained as a fermentation product from fungal cultures of *Penicillium stoloniferum*. MMF is a prodrug of the active compound mycophenolic acid (MPA) [1].

Mechanism of Action

On ingestion, MMF is acted upon by plasma esterases, which converts it to the active metabolite MPA. MPA is a potent immunosuppressive agent. It acts on the enzyme inosine monophosphate dehydrogenase and inhibits it in a non-competitive manner, thereby preventing conversion of inosine monophosphate to xanthine monophosphate and guanosine monophosphate. The latter two nucleotides are essential for DNA synthesis in both T and B lymphocytes, and when there is unavailability of these substrates, arrest in the replication of lymphocytes in the S phase occurs. Because of this, immunoglobulin levels plummet along with reduction in delayed type hypersensitivity responses [2, 3]. Apart from this, MMF also inhibits chemotaxis, hinders presentation of antigens, and brings about immune tolerance by preventing glycosylation of glycoproteins associated with lymphocytes and monocytes, which are associated with endothelial cell adhesion [4].

Pharmacokinetics

Following oral administration, MMF has a mean bioavailability of 94%. As food reduces bioavailability of MMF, it is best administered on an empty stomach. It is metabolized in the liver and undergoes glucuronide conjugation to form an inactive

A. K. Bubna, *Therapeutics in Dermatology - Essentials for Clinical Practice*,
https://doi.org/10.1007/978-981-95-3791-4_28

compound referred to as mycophenolic acid glucuronide (MPAG) [5]. Two peak levels in the plasma are recorded following MMF intake. The first occurs after an hour of drug ingestion, signifying initial drug distribution and the second peak is demonstrable after 8 h, which occurs owing to enterohepatic recycling of MPAG, that is hydrolysed back to MPA in the gastrointestinal tract by the enzyme beta glucuronidase. The $t_{1/2}$ of MPA is around 18 h. Excretion is mainly by the kidneys with a meagre amount of MMF being cleared through the faeces [6].

Indications

The only US FDA approved indication of MMF is as a prophylactic agent to prevent rejection of organ transplant, usually in conjunction with corticosteroids and cyclosporine [7]. In dermatology, all indications are off-label and are enumerated in Table 28.1.

Table 28.1 Dermatological indications of mycophenolate mofetil

Indications in dermatology	
Psoriasis	
Vesiculobullous disorders	
Pemphigus group	Pemphigus vulgaris
	Pemphigus foliaceous
	Paraneoplastic pemphigus
Pemphigoid group	Bullous pemphigoid
	Cicatricial pemphigoid
	Linear IgA bullous disease
	Epidermolysis bullosa acquisita
Connective tissue disorders	Systemic lupus erythematosus (SLE)
	Subacute cutaneous lupus erythematosus (SCLE)
	Discoid lupus erythematosus (DLE)
	Systemic sclerosis and morphea
	Dermatomyositis
Eczemas	Atopic eczema
	Pompholyx
	Chronic actinic dermatitis
Vasculitis	Urticarial vasculitis
	Takayasu's arteritis
	Polyarteritis nodosa
	Wegner's granulomatosis
Miscellaneous	Lichen planus
	Pyoderma gangrenosum
	Recurrent erythema multiforme
	Sarcoidosis
	Chronic idiopathic urticaria
	Weber–Christian disease

Clinical Uses

Psoriasis

MMF is effective in patients with moderate to severe psoriasis vulgaris, erythrodermic psoriasis, refractory psoriasis and psoriatic arthropathy. MMF, however, is never utilized as a first-line drug for this indication. However, in patients intolerant to conventional anti-psoriatic treatments, introduction of MMF can be a viable alternative [8–11].

Vesiculobullous Disorders

The role of MMF as a steroid sparing agent in these disorders cannot be underestimated. Reports regarding the beneficial role in vesicobullous disorders have been well documented [12–17]. In pemphigus vulgaris, MMF and azathioprine are considered the first line steroid sparing drugs for its management.

Connective Tissue Disorders

In systemic lupus erythematosus (SLE), MMF is particularly useful in diffuse proliferative lupus nephritis [18], neuropsychiatric manifestations in SLE [19] and immune thrombocytopenia associated with SLE [20]. In SCLE and DLE where the response is not satisfactory with systemic steroids and other immunosuppressive agents, MMF demonstrates successful outcomes [21, 22]. In patients with diffuse scleroderma with clinically apparent alveolitis, early institution of MMF in the therapeutic protocol can prove an effective and safe alternative therapy [23]. For dermatomyositis, MMF as monotherapy in combination with intravenous immunoglobulins (IVIGs) has shown lasting remission, along with avoiding long-term toxic effects of systemic steroids [24].

Vasculitis

In both large and small vessel vasculitis, MMF has been used, though not as a first-line drug. It usually is combined with systemic corticosteroids as a steroid sparing agent [25, 26].

Contraindications

Absolute

- Hypersensitivity to the drug
- Pregnancy

Relative

- Peptic ulcer disease
- Cardiopulmonary disease
- Hepatic disease
- Renal disease

Pregnancy prescribing status: Category 'C'.

Dosage and Monitoring

MMF is available as 250 mg capsules, 500 mg tablets and a powder for oral suspension (200 mg/mL). It also has an intravenous preparation containing 500 mg MMF as a hydrochloride salt. In adults the dose ranges from 1.25 to 2 g/day. As skin lesions improve, MMF can be tapered to 1 g/day in divided doses. In children the dose is 600 mg/m^2 every 12 hourly with a maximum of 2 g/day. In patients with renal impairment, dose reduction needs contemplation. Enteric coated tablets of mycophenolate sodium is also available as slow releasing tablets containing 180 or 360 mg of MPA, and is extremely valuable in patients with MMF-induced gastrointestinal (GI) side effects [27, 28]. Complete physical examination should be carried out at each visit or every 6–12 months to look for any opportunistic infections and malignancy. Complete blood counts should be performed at baseline and biweekly during the first 2–3 months and then monthly through the first year. LFT and RFT should be performed at baseline and serum transaminases should be repeated after 1 month and then quarterly. During follow-up, treatment should be discontinued if the leukocyte count is <3500–4000 cells/mm^3 [3–5, 9].

Drug Interactions

The drug interactions of mycophenolate mofetil is summarized in Table 28.2.

Table 28.2 Drug interactions of mycophenolate mofetil

Drugs inhibiting tubular secretion of MMF, thereby increasing its levels in the plasma
Acyclovir, ganciclovir, probenecid
Drugs decreasing the absorption and bioavailability of MMF
Antacids containing magnesium and aluminium, ferrous sulfate, metronidazole, fluoroquinolones
Drug inhibiting enterohepatic circulation of MMF and reducing its level
Cholestyramine
Drugs increasing MMF elimination by competing with the plasma albumin binding site
Salicylates, frusemide
Drugs blocking purine synthesis by the same pathway as MMF and therefore to avoid such a combination
Azathioprine

Adverse Effects

Gastrointestinal

- Nausea
- Diarrhoea
- Constipation
- Soft stools
- Abdominal cramps
- Anorexia

Genitourinary

- Urgency
- Frequency
- Dysuria
- Haematuria
- Sterile pyuria

Infections

- Increased risk of bacterial, fungal and viral infections.

Carcinogenicity

- Increased risk of lymphomas.

Blood

- Anaemia
- Neutropenia
- Thrombocytopenia

Neurologic

- Tinnitus
- Headache
- Insomnia

Cutaneous

- Exanthematous eruptions
- Onycholysis

Metabolic

- Hypercholesterolemia
- Hyperglycaemia
- Hypophosphatemia
- Hypo/hyperkalaemia

Conclusion

MMF is beneficial both as monotherapy and in combination with systemic glucocorticoids as a steroid sparing drug for a number of dermatologic indications. MMF is of value in those patients with hepatic and renal dysfunction where other immunosuppressive drugs cannot be given [29].

References

1. Surjushe A, Saple DG. Mycophenolate mofetil. Indian J Dermatol Venereol Leprol. 2008;74:180–4.
2. Carr SF, Papp E, Wu JC, Natsumeda Y. Characterization of human type 1 and type 2 IMP dehydrogenases. J Biol Chem. 1993;268:272–86.
3. Sliverman KJE, Pomeinanz MK, Pak G, Washenik K, Schupack JL. Rediscovering mycophenolic acid: a review of its mechanism, side effects and potential uses. J Am Acad Dermatol. 1997;37:445.
4. Mehling A, Grabbe S, Voskort M, Schwarz T, Luger TA, Biessert S. Mycophenolate mofetil impairs the maturation and function of murine dendritic cells. J Immunol. 2000;165:2374.
5. Nousari HC, Grant JA. Immunosuppressive and immunomodulatory drugs. In: Freedberg IM, Eisen AZ, Wolff K, editors. Fitzpatrick's dermatology in general medicine. 5th ed. Philadelphia: McGraw Hill; 1999. p. 2680.
6. Bullingham RE, Nicholls AJ, Kamm BR. Clinical pharmacokinetics of mycophenolate mofetil. Clin Pharmacokinet. 1998;34:429.
7. European Mycophenolate Mofetil Study Group. Placebo controlled study of mycophenolate mofetil combined with cyclosporine and corticosteroids for prevention of acute rejection. Lancet. 1995;345:1321.
8. Tong DW, Walder BK. Widespread plaque psoriasis responsive to mycophenolate mofetil. Australas J Dermatol. 1999;40:135.
9. Haufs MG, Biessert S, Grabbe S, Schutte B, Luger TA. Psoriasis vulgaris treated successfully with mycophenolate mofetil. Br J Dermatol. 1998;138:179.
10. Geilen CC, Tebble B, Garcia Bartels C, Krengel S, Orfanos CE. Successful treatment of erythrodermic psoriasis with mycophenolate mofetil. Br J Dermatol. 1998;138:1101.

11. Grundmann-Kollmann M, Mooser G, Schrader P, Zollner T, Kaskel P, Ochsendorf F, et al. Treatment of chronic plaque stage psoriasis and psoriatic arthritis with mycophenolate mofetil. J Am Acad Dermatol. 2000;42:835.
12. Mimouni D, Anhalt GJ, Cummins DL, Kouba DJ, Thorne JE, Nousary HC. Treatment of pemphigus vulgaris and pemphigus foliaceous with mycophenolate mofetil. Arch Dermatol. 2003;139:739.
13. Nousari HC, Griffith WA, Anhalt GJ. Successful therapy of bullous pemphigoid with mycophenolate mofetil. J Am Acad Dermatol. 1998;39:497.
14. Williams JV, Marks JG Jr, Billingsley EM. Use of mycophenlate mofetil in the treatment of paraneoplastic pemphigus. Br J Dermatol. 2000;142:506.
15. Megahed M, Schmiedeberg S, Becker J, Ruzicka T. Treatment of cicatricial pemphigoid with mycophenolate mofetil as a steroid sparing agent. J Am Acad Dermatol. 2001;45:256.
16. Farley-Li J, Macini AJ. Treatment of linear IgA bullous dermatosis of childhood with mycophenolate mofetil. Arch Dermatol. 2003;139:1121.
17. Kowalzick L, Suckow S, Zeigler H, Waldmann T, Ponnighaus J, Glaser V. Mycophenolate mofetil in epidermolysis bullosa acquistica. Dermatology. 2003;207:332.
18. Chan TM, Li FK, Tang CS, Wong RW, Fang GX, Ji YL, et al. Efficacy of mycophenolate mofetil in patients with diffuse proliferative lupus nephritis. N Engl J Med. 2000;343:1156.
19. Jose J, Paulose BK, Vasuki Z, Danda D. Mycophenolate mofetil in neuropsychiatric systemic lupus erythematosus. Indian J Med Sci. 2005;59:353.
20. Vasso S, Thumboo J, Fong KY. Refractory immune thrombocytopenia in systemic lupus erythematosus: response to mycophenolate mofetil. Lupus. 2003;12:630–2.
21. Schaanz S, Ulmer A, Rassner G, Fierlbeck G. Successful treatment of subacute cutaneous lupus erythematosus with mycophenolate mofetil. Br J Dermatol. 2002;147:174.
22. Goyal S, Nousari HC. Treatment of resistant discoid lupus erythematosus of the palms and soles with mycophenolate mofetil. J Am Acad Dermatol. 2001;45:142.
23. Liossis SN, Bounas A, Andonopoulous AP. Mycophenolate mofetil as first line treatment improves clinically evident early scleroderma lung disease. Rheumatology. 2006;45:1005.
24. Ann-Kathrin T, Michael M. Mycophenolate mofetil for dermatomyositis. Dermatology. 2001;202:341.
25. Daina E, Schieppati A, Remuzzi G. Mycophenolate mofetil for the treatment of Takayasu arteritis. Report of three cases. Am Intern Med. 1999;130:422.
26. Russell JP, Le G. Primary cutaneous small vessel vasculitis: approach to diagnosis and treatment. Int J Dermatol. 2006;45:3.
27. Perlis C, Pan TD, McDonald CJ. Cytotoxic agents. In: Wolverton S, editor. Comprehensive dermatologic drug therapy. 2nd ed. Philadelphia: WB Saunders; 2000. p. 197–217.
28. Assmann T, Ruzicka T. New immunosuppressive drugs in dermatology (mycophenolate mofetil, tacrolimus): unapproved uses, dosages and indications. Clin Dermatol. 2002;20:505.
29. Khopkar U, Pande S, Nischal KC, editors. Non-steroidal immunosuppressive drugs. In: Handbook of dermatological drug therapy, 1st ed. New Delhi: Elsevier; 2007. p. 127–38.

Hydroxyurea

29

Introduction

Hydroxyurea (HU) is a small molecule with the chemical structure of urea along with an attached hydroxyl group. HU is used for various dermatologic disorders only when other treatments have failed or are contraindicated. As it lacks the hepatotoxic potential of methotrexate, nephrotoxic potential of cyclosporine, HU proves advantageous in these scenarios.

Mechanism of Action

HU acts primarily by inhibiting the enzyme ribonucleotide reductase (RR), a rate limiting step in DNA synthesis [1, 2]. RR is made of two subunits, a regulatory M1 protein and a catalytic M2 protein. The detailed mechanism of action of HU is depicted in Fig. 29.1 [3–5].

Further, HU acts as a radiation sensitizer and causes increase in gene transcription by hypomethylation of the foetal Hb gene. This hypomethylation results in foetal Hb induction, promotion of differentiation and normalization of psoriatic skin, and induction of other genes as episomes [5].

A. K. Bubna, *Therapeutics in Dermatology - Essentials for Clinical Practice*, https://doi.org/10.1007/978-981-95-3791-4_29

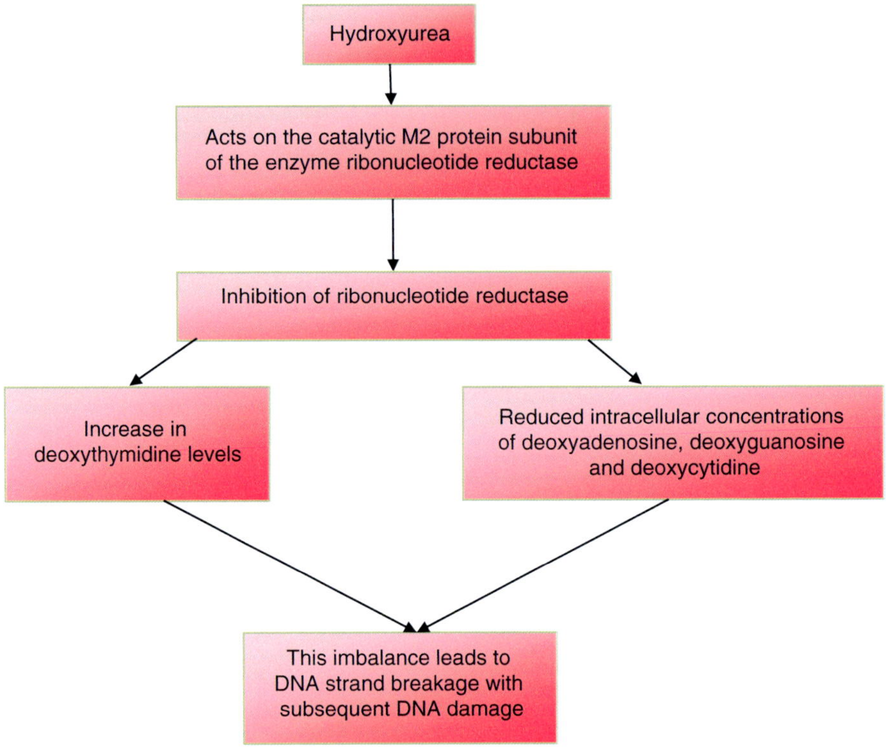

Fig. 29.1 Mechanism of action of hydroxyurea

Pharmacokinetics

HU has good oral absorption, attaining peak plasma levels within 2 h [6]. The onset of action HU begins within 5–8 h, with the $t_{1/2}$ being around 5 h. The majority of the drug remains free in the serum, but a fraction of it is bound to plasma fibrinogen. However, the complete metabolic pathway of HU is not clearly understood and is suggested that it gets metabolized to acetohydroxamic acid. Renal excretion is the main route of elimination [7–9].

Indications

FDA Approved

- Squamous cell carcinoma of head and neck
- Metastatic melanoma
- Gastrointestinal melanoma

Off-Label

- Sweet's syndrome (particularly when associated with an underlying haematologic malignancy)
- Psoriasis
- Sickle cell anaemia (HU helps by increasing the production of fetal haemoglobin. This dilutes the sickled haemoglobin, thereby making red cells less likely to become sickle shaped)
- Hyper eosinophilic syndrome (HU is a second line treatment here, and helps lowering the white blood cell count, particularly when steroids are insufficient or ineffective)
- Polycythaemia rubra vera (HU slows down the production of new cells in the bone marrow, including red blood cells, white blood cells and platelets)
- Chronic granulocytic leukaemia cutis (HU is an effective treatment for this indication, particularly when other treatments like busulphan fail. Treatment with HU is followed by marked reduction in spleen size, a decrease in white cell count and healing of skin lesions.)

Contraindications

Absolute

- Hypersensitivity to the drug
- Pregnancy
- Lactation

Relative

- Blood dyscrasias
- Endocrine dysfunction
- Hepatic disease
- Renal disease
- Cardiopulmonary disease

Pregnancy prescribing status: Category 'X'.

Clinical Use

Psoriasis

HU is used in psoriasis refractory to other forms of treatment. The dose of HU ranges from 1 to 2 g/day. The effects are usually noticeable by 6–8 weeks [10, 11]. Besides, HU can be combined with methotrexate and gradually tapered off once desired clinical improvement is obtained [12]. HU is particularly valuable in treating those patients of psoriasis who are HIV positive.

Adverse Effects

Hematologic

- Megaloblastic anaemia
- Thrombocytopenia
- Leucopoenia (as a result of myelosuppression)

Gastrointestinal

- Elevated liver enzymes

Cutaneous

- Flu like syndrome
- Lichenoid eruption
- Dermatomyositis like reactions
- Radiation recall
- Leg ulcers
- Fixed drug eruptions
- Urticaria
- Erythema multiforme

Drug Interactions

HU does not have significant interactions with drugs used in dermatologic practice. However, as a rule, HU should not be used with other myelosuppressive agents as the risk of toxicity can substantially increase.

Monitoring Guidelines

Baseline

- Complete physical examination
- Complete blood count
- Platelet count
- Liver function tests
- Renal function tests
- Urinalysis
- Cardiopulmonary workup

Follow-Up

- Complete physical examination at least once a year.
- All the above-mentioned laboratory parameters to be done monthly initially for the first 6 months, and then once every 3 monthly.

Indications for Discontinuing Therapy

- Reduction in Hb by 3 g/dL or more
- Total leucocyte count <4000 cells/mm^3
- Platelet count <100,000 cells/mm^3
- Lack of efficacy after 2 months of treatment
- Presence of infection or other organ involvement
- Flu like syndrome

Conclusion

HU is not a very commonly used drug by most dermatologists. However, the author considers it to be an excellent standby drug in those conditions where conventional therapy has failed.

References

1. Krakoff IH, Brown NC, Reichard P. Inhibition of ribonucleoside diphosphate reductase by hydroxyurea. Cancer Res. 1968;28:1559–65.
2. Thalander L, Reichard P. Reduction of ribonucleoside. Annu Rev Biochem. 1979;48:133–58.
3. Francis AA, Blevins RD, Carrier WL, et al. Inhibition of DNA repair in ultraviolet irradiated human cells by hydroxyurea. Biochem Biophys Acta. 1979;563:385–92.
4. Donehower RC. An overview of the clinical experience with hydroxyurea. Semin Oncol. 1992;19:11–9.
5. Christen RD, Shalinsky DR, Howell SB. Enhancement of the loss of multiple drug resistance by hydroxyurea. Semin Oncol. 1992;19:94–100.
6. McDonald CJ. Uses of systemic chemotherapeutic agents in psoriasis. Pharmacol Ther. 1981;14:1–24.
7. McDonald CJ. Cytotoxic agents for use in dermatology. J Am Acad Dermatol. 1985;12:753–75.
8. Yarbo JW. Mechanism of action of hydroxyurea. Semin Oncol. 1992;19:1–10.
9. Fishbein WN, Carbone PP. Hydroxyurea: mechanism of action. Science. 1963;142:1069–70.
10. Rosten M. Hydroxyurea: a new antimetabolite in the treatment of psoriasis. Br J Dermatol. 1971;85:177–81.
11. Hunter GA, Simmons IJ, Thomas BM. A clinical trial of hydroxyurea for psoriasis. Australas J Dermatol. 1972;13:93–9.
12. Sauer GC. Combined methotrexate and hydroxyurea therapy for psoriasis. Arch Dermatol. 1973;107:369–70.

Part VI

Oral Retinoids

Isotretinoin

30

Introduction

Isotretinoin (ISO) is a non-aromatic, synthetic first-generation retinoid and is obtained following substitution of the polyene side chain and polar groups of vitamin A. In 1982, ISO was approved by the US FDA for the treatment of nodulocystic acne, and even after 43 years, ISO remains the most effective treatment for acne. Besides, ISO has proven to be effective for a number of other cutaneous disorders as well.

Mechanism of Action

Figure 30.1 describes the mechanism of action of isotretinoin. [1–7]

A. K. Bubna, *Therapeutics in Dermatology - Essentials for Clinical Practice*, https://doi.org/10.1007/978-981-95-3791-4_30

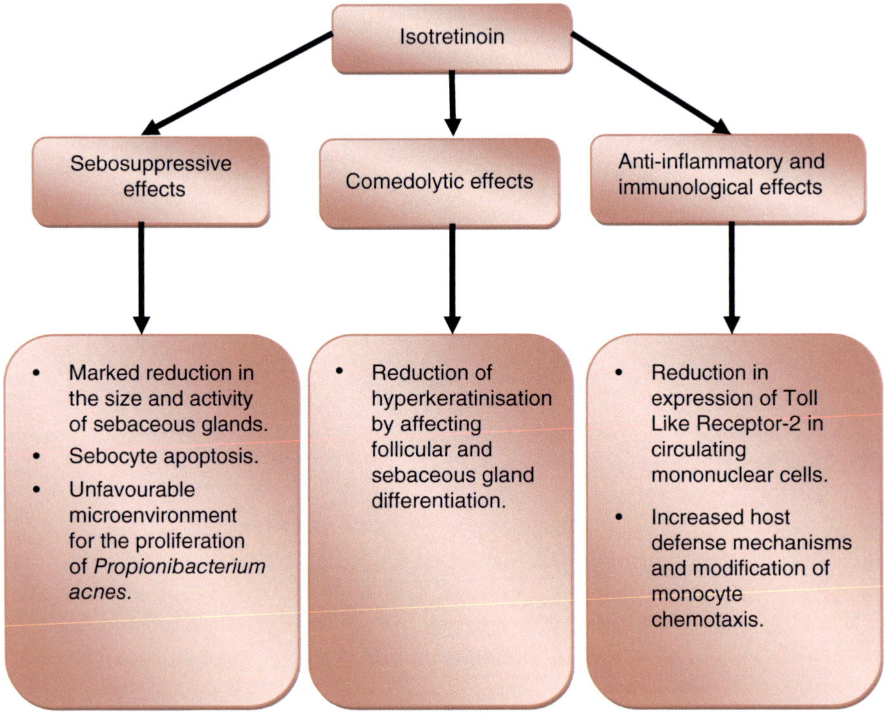

Fig. 30.1 Mechanism of action of isotretinoin

Pharmacokinetics

ISO attains peak plasma levels after 3 h of oral administration. It is best to give ISO following a fat-rich meal, because it gets easily dissolved in dietary fat, and in this way the absorption of ISO is enhanced [8]. The $t_{1/2}$ of ISO varies from 10 to 20 h, with 99% of the drug being bound to plasma albumin. ISO is metabolized in the liver and eliminated via the renal route [9].

Indications

FDA Approved

- Nodulocystic acne.

Off-Label

- Hidradenitis suppurativa (HS).
- Acanthosis nigricans (AN).
- Rosacea.
- Pityriasis rubra pilaris (PRP).
- Psoriasis.
- Darier's disease (DD).
- Ichthyosis.
- Disseminate and recurrent infundibulofolliculitis (DRIF).
- Photoaging.
- Lupus erythematosus (LE).
- Granuloma annulare (GA).
- Lichen planus (LP).
- Non melanoma skin cancer prophylaxis.
- Condyloma accuminata (CA).

Contraindications

Absolute

- Pregnancy.

Relative

- Abnormal hepatic profile.
- Abnormal lipid profile.
- Impaired renal function.

Pregnancy prescribing status: Category 'X'.

Clinical Uses

Acne

ISO still remains the linchpin for the management of nodulocystic acne, ever since it was approved by the US FDA. Though ISO is prescribed essentially for severe nodular/inflammatory acne, it is now conceded that ISO comprises an exceedingly successful alternative in the following contexts as well:

- Recalcitrant inflammatory acne: not manifesting as multiple nodules but having a high propensity for acne scarring.

Table 30.1 Acne vulgaris management guidelines on recommendations for the use of isotretinoin

Source	Details
European evidence-based guidelines for treatment of acne [10]	ISO is not recommended for comedonal acne ISO is not generally recommended for non-nodular inflammatory(papulopustular) acne
Acne guidelines (global Alliance to improve outcomes in acne) [11]	ISO is recognized as the most effective anti-acne treatment, but should be reserved for severe cases, moderate but unresponsive cases and acne with psychological distress
Consensus on evidence-based practice in acne (Asian working group) [12]	ISO is recommended as primary therapy for severe acne and second tier treatment for moderate acne that is poorly responsive to other treatments, and suggests a target cumulative dose of 120–150 mg/kg to be reached over the treatment course
Guidelines for acne vulgaris management (American Academy of Dermatology) [13]	It is unanimously agreed that ISO is also useful for lesser degrees of acne that resist treatment or produce physical or psychological scarring
Evidence-based recommendations for paediatric acne (American acne and rosacea society and American Academy of Pediatrics) [14]	ISO is recommended starting at 0.5 mg/kg/day for the first 4 weeks, then increasing to 1 mg/kg /day Recommended uses include severe nodular acne, acne with scarring and/or refractory inflammatory acne Extensive counselling is suggested particularly with respect to pregnancy prevention in girls

- Non-nodular acne: in cases where rectification of lesions is <50% even post 6 months of antibiotic therapy and there exists noteworthy acne scarring, or if there is corresponding psychological anguish.

Guidelines advocating isotretinoin in acne is summed up in Table 30.1.

Dosing for Isotretinoin

The standard approved dose of ISO is 0.5–1 mg/kg/day, ranging from 16 to 32 weeks with the highest accumulative dose not exceeding 120–150 mg/kg [15–17]. However, other dosing regimens of ISO are also utilized in dermatologic practice, as discussed below.

Traditional Dosing

The ideal proposed initiating dose of ISO is 0.5 mg/kg/day, which is carried on for 1 month, ensuing that the dose is increased to 1 mg/kg/day, which is sustained over the treatment course unless adverse laboratory values and clinical effects require dose modification [1, 2, 18]. Treatment with ISO is pursued till the aggregate dose of 120–150 mg/kg is achieved. The dosing frequency for ISO approved by the FDA is twice daily. Further, there are no pharmacokinetic studies that have replaced this endorsement with regard to efficacy and safety [19, 20]. Moreover, it is observed that twice daily ISO dosing encourages steady levels of the drug in the serum [21, 22]. However, many dermatologists favour once daily dosing of ISO owing to concerns regarding the frequency of missing the second dose of the drug [23].

Following 1.5–2 months of ISO therapy, satisfactory amelioration of lesions is visible. However, if dosing is started with ≥1 mg/kg/day, initial flaring of acne may be encountered, in the form of multiple deep inflammatory papules and nodules. Though these can be treated without affecting completion of ISO therapy, initiating ISO at a dose of 0.5 mg/kg/day helps prevent these initial flares, without compromising the therapeutic efficacy.

Once the target cumulative dose of ISO is obtained, the prospect of securing long-term remission is boosted. In patients experiencing annoying side effects such as xerosis, muscle aches, cheilitis and dry eyes, a lower dosing regimen with ISO can be incorporated with the goal of achieving a cumulative dose of 120–150 mg/kg, which in this situation may take an extended time to be attained. (However, administering the entire course of treatment within 20 weeks is suggested, without renouncing the target cumulative dose.)

Other Dosing Schedules with Isotretinoin

High Dose Schedule

It is proposed that using enhanced daily doses of ISO (>1 mg/kg/day), and getting a higher total cumulative dose of ISO than what is advocated, promotes a lesser risk of acne recurrence. Besides, even while utilizing higher dosing of ISO (mean daily dosing of 1.6 mg/kg/day), duration of treatment is not abridged even after obtaining the standard cumulative dose, but is carried on for 5–6 months, so that a total cumulative dose of 290 mg/kg is secured at the conclusion of therapy [24]. Besides, at this cumulative dose, ISO therapy is documented to be well tolerated, not requiring treatment discontinuation.

Further, Blasiak et al. in their publication iterated a cumulative dose of ISO >220 mg/kg to be remarkably higher ranking than a cumulative dose of ISO <220 mg/kg in preventing relapse. Even so, the probability of major side effects with ISO are not considered significant in this scenario, thereby furnishing an added edge [25].

Retinoid dermatitis has been commonly observed in patients where the cumulative dose is greater than 220 mg/kg. Other features such as xerosis and cheilitis have also observed. However, none of them called for cessation of ISO therapy.

Low Dose Isotretinoin Therapy

Many scholars have used ISO at a dose lower than the routine dose for acne vulgaris. Dosages have varied from 0.14 to 0.75 mg/kg/day and have been prescribed either as a daily dose [26, 27], as discontinuous schedules [28–30], alternately every 2 days, [31] or as progressive dose increments [32].

However, in this schedule, often there is recurrence of acne, following an initial abrogation, making retreatment compulsory. It therefore becomes essential to recompense for the lower dose of ISO, by expanding the course of therapy in order to perfect the cumulative exposure of ISO over the treatment course [33].

White et al. [34] found that the chances of acne resurgence was eight-fold pronounced in patients treated with a cumulative dose of ISO <100 mg/kg when juxtaposed with patients who received a cumulative dose >100 mg/kg. Moreover, acne reappearance was recorded in 92% of patients treated with a cumulative total ISO dose of <90 mg/kg, and in 40–50% of patients who received a cumulative dose of ISO ≥110 mg/kg. Besides, in their survey, they noted that out of 61% of patients receiving ISO retreatment for acne, 22.9% needed at least one extra sequence of ISO.

In the publication by Stainforth et al. [35], 69% of patients treated with ISO (0.1 mg/kg/day), for a period of 4 months reported recurrence of acne. Besides, in these patients, 88% of patients, required more than two courses of ISO, in contrast to 9.5% of the cases who were on treatment with 1 mg/kg/day of ISO.

It therefore needs to be reckoned that dose modifications of ISO should only be employed if adverse effects related to ISO become unacceptable. Moreover, if the dose of ISO is lowered, then treatment span needs to be expanded to attain the cumulative dose, thus increasing the duration of exposure to systemic retinoids and elevating chances of encountering idiosyncratic adverse reactions. Besides, in women with child-bearing potential, the long duration of ISO treatment proves a limitation, mandating avoidance of conception for a longer duration.

Although low dose ISO therapy controls the initial flare of acne, there is a high likelihood of relapse following stoppage of therapy if the cumulative dose is not achieved. Besides, when weighing brief gains against sustained control, it becomes obvious that dosing of ISO at 1 mg/kg/day is more helpful for long-term success. Interestingly, repeated courses of ISO do not compromise its therapeutic efficacy. [36, 37]

Conditions where 1 mg/kg/day of ISO or even higher dosing may become necessary include [38]:

- History of acne in the family.
- Acne with an early onset.
- Hyperseborrhoea.
- Truncal acne.
- Acne having a tendency to scar.
- Psychological difficulties.
- Persistent/late-onset acne.
- Acne in males.
- Sinus tracts.
- Macrocomedones.
- Androgen excess (e.g. polycystic ovarian syndrome [PCOS]).

Responses to Isotretinoin

Generally, the beneficial effects of ISO are demonstrable by 1–2 months. However, the responsiveness may be slow in certain cases. In these cases, macrocomedones are recognized in 70% of cases, although hyperandrogenism may also contribute to resistance with ISO therapy [39]. Further, in 25% of patients, poor responses to ISO is linked with differences in receptor sensitivity, colonization with *Staphylococcus aureus* and atypical variants of acne. In the remaining 5%, the cause of poor response to ISO is unspecified [39].

Therefore, macrocomedones need to be ascertained before starting treatment with ISO. In most cases, these macrocomedones are indistinct and need identification after extending the skin under appropriate light. Their identification is crucial because if not traced and managed, the likelihood of precipitating an acute flare of acne is high, following administration of ISO. Light cautery or hyfrecation is the treatment adopted for these macrocomedones [40]. The procedure is first carried out on a test area of 10 cm^2 and if there is no scarring/dyspigmentation, then the procedure is executed on all lesions [40].

In cases where an acute burst of acne follows ISO therapy due to some other reason, antibiotics such as azithromycin 1 g daily, or trimethoprim 200–300 mg twice daily, can be availed accordingly [41]. Besides, short courses of oral glucocorticoids maybe advantageous in patients with extremely inflammatory acne along with ISO.

In some patients the metabolism of ISO may not be as convincing as others and therefore higher doses of the drug may be needed. Mucocutaneous side effects especially cheilitis generally delineate good drug absorption. In atypical variants of acne, particularly in women with PCOS, apart from ISO, auxiliary treatment with hormonal preparations such as cyproterone acetate, ethinyl oestradiol and drospirenone may become necessary.

For acne relapses, further courses of ISO exceedingly benefit the patient without encountering tachyphylaxis.

Patient Adherence to Treatment

As ISO therapy for acne is long standing, patient compliance to therapy becomes essential. At times patients delineate flawed adherence like not being able to take ISO with a high fat (HF)/high calorie (HC) meal. This comes to a very practical musing about how realistic would it be to ingest a HF/HC meal with ISO throughout the therapeutic schedule as many dermatologists feel that the diet endorsed is not very healthy for such an extended duration [8]. Further, if ISO is taken on an empty stomach, there is a striking reduction of the drug's bioavailability by approximately 60%. Interestingly, the bioavailability of ISO following intake of meals with low fat and calorie content is not accurately known. So, the question arises regarding the exact amount of fat and calorie intake for acquiring sufficient blood levels of ISO. Unfortunately, the answer to this question remains unresolved [8].

It is observed that the amount of calories and fat prescribed in most diets is clearly lower than the required amount, when analysed using pharmacokinetic study protocols with ISO. Therefore, realistically, it may not be feasible to adhere to these specific dietary directions elucidated with reference to ISO ingestion. The best possible perspective thus would be to take ISO after consuming meals well balanced in both macronutrients and micronutrients.

iPLEDGE Program

This program was implemented in the year 2006 and is an FDA-assigned computer-based risk management program providing chronicled, traceable links to prescribers, pharmacists, patients and manufacturers [42]. All patients prescribed ISO are expected to engage in this program including men, as well as women who are not of child-bearing potential. Besides, in women belonging to the child-bearing age group, a negative pregnancy test before and during ISO therapy and at uniform intervals is required, only then can they obtain ISO. The iPLEDGE program requires one negative pregnancy test 30 days before commencing prescription of ISO and another negative pregnancy test during a 7-day window during which time the drug is given to the patient. Thus, two negative pregnancy tests are required to begin treatment with ISO. If the drug is not provided in the 7-day window, the patient is locked out and must delay another 12 days to offer a new negative pregnancy test and open a new 7-day window period. This feature of the program, however has been arraigned as being an additional encumbrance for the health care system and unprofitable for patient therapy. Nonetheless, there remains a responsibility on the patient to be compliant to this program [43].

Additionally, apart from conducting regular pregnancy tests and overseeing prescriptions, iPLEDGE also renders monthly education to the patient regarding:

- Not sharing of medications,
- Not donating blood, and.
- Different forms of birth control.

Besides, women with child-bearing potential need to use two forms of contraception acknowledged on the list assigned in the iPLEDGE birth control workbook [44].

Rosacea

Although oral ISO is particularly effective in treating papulopustular rosacea (PPR), propitious properties of ISO have also been documented for erythematelengiectatic rosacea (ETR) and phymatous rosacea [45, 46]. In rosacea, ISO diminishes cutaneous blood flow and reduces the size and number of sebaceous glands in the pre-fibrotic stage [47]. Apart from facial rosacea, ISO is used for the treatment of extra-facial rosacea (excluding ocular rosacea) [48]. The most effective dose of ISO for rosacea is 20 mg/day or 0.3 mg/kg/day.

In the publication by Uslu et al. [49], 20 mg of ISO was employed for rosacea patients for 16 weeks and then steadily attenuated over the next 24 weeks till an end dose of 20 mg/week was attained. This dosing regimen delineated outstanding improvement within the first 4 weeks of treatment for both the papulopustular and erythematous components of rosacea.

Similarly, in the report by Gollnick et al. [50], favourable effects were outlined with ISO (0.3 mg/kg/day) for rosacea, over a 3-month period, equalling the efficacy of doxycycline.

Besides, another dosing schedule for rosacea has been propounded. Here, continuous microdoses of ISO (mean of 34.2 mg/week for 33 months) are generally employed after obtaining adequate control of rosacea [51].

At higher doses (≥0.5 mg/kg/day) for rosacea, ISO often precipitates dermatitis facialis and therefore should be eschewed.

Besides, in rare variants of rosacea, e.g. rosacea fulminans (pyoderma faciale), ISO has shown value. Rosen et al. [52] elucidated ISO to be the only consistent treatment outlining successful outputs in rosacea fulminans. In this setting before giving ISO, prednisolone (40–60 mg/day for a fortnight with gradual taper) is administered to the patient after which ISO is gradually introduced to the therapeutic schedule at 0.2–0.5 mg/kg/day, with the dose progressively elevated to 0.5–1 mg/kg/day. Treatment with ISO needs to go on for 3–4 months or longer till the cumulative dose of 150 mg/kg is obtained or till lesions abate [52–55].

Extrafacial Rosacea

Though extrafacial rosacea (EFR) is onerous to diagnose, there are multiple reports in literature [56–58]. EFR is principally seen in males and affects photo-exposed surfaces of the skin. ISO monotherapy (10–20 mg/day) or in coalition with oral glucocorticoids (Deflazacort 30 mg for 3 weeks) and azithromycin 500 mg for 3 days/week for 1 month has delineated efficacy for the same [48, 56].

Pityriasis Rubra Pilaris

In pityriasis rubra pilaris (PRP), responses with ISO have been mixed. Based on the publications by Dicken [59] and Allison et al. [60], ISO can be given as a first-line drug for PRP, and demonstrates superior outcomes than UVB + tar, topical calcipotriol, keratolytics, azathioprine, methotrexate and cyclosporine. Further, there are no precise dosing schedules of ISO for PRP. In the report by Dicken [59], the dose of ISO varied from 1 to 1.5 mg/kg/day, and Allison et al. [60] applied a dose of 20 and 40 mg/day for children and adults, respectively, with both outlining efficacious results. Besides, in another study, 0.5 mg/kg/day of ISO was employed for PRP and was associated with complete lesional clearance in 25% of patients, and 50% amelioration in the remaining 75% patients [61]. Treatment duration of PRP with ISO ranges from 16 to 24 weeks. Responses with ISO in PRP is evident by 14–16 weeks [61]. Other supportive care like adequate emollient use needs to be implemented along with ISO therapy. In erythrodermic PRP, however, prednisolone 40 mg/day and hospital admission may be needed [62].

Psoriasis

In psoriasis, ISO can be regarded as a therapeutic option in females belonging to the child-bearing age group, and wish to evade long-term use of contraceptives (almost 2–3 years) following acitretin use, because of its shorter half-life. As ISO regulates inflammatory cells and keratinocyte hyperproliferation and differentiation, it is of value in psoriasis [63]. The best outcomes with ISO have been observed in pustular psoriasis. In children, a dose of 40 mg/day is given, and in adults the dose ranges 1.5–2 mg/kg/day, with good responses [64]. Additionally, while combining ISO with NBUVB, the dose of ISO can be reduced to 0.5 mg/kg/day and is found to be exhibit equally effective [65]. In plaque-type psoriasis, however, the efficacy of ISO is not satisfactory [63].

Hidradenitis Suppurativa

Hidradenitis suppurativa (HS) is characterized by painful deep-seated nodules/abscesses involving the axillary, inguinal and anogenital regions associated with profound disability, with a negative impact on the quality of life of patients [66]. Follicular occlusion and apocrine gland dysfunction are considered etiological factors for the occurrence of HS [67]. Besides, although ISO is not mentioned in the treatment guideline of HS, reports have emphasized its utility in HS.

Reasons for the usage of ISO in HS include [6, 7, 68, 69]:

- ISO promotes reduction of ductal obstruction and hypercornification,
- Sebocyte apoptosis is induced by ISO,
- ISO assists in modulating the rate of sebum excretion,
- ISO helps regulating apocrine function,
- ISO outlines immunomodulatory as well as anti-inflammatory characteristics, and.
- ISO precludes infundibular plugging and decreases the function of sebaceous and apocrine glands.

Interestingly, there are certain patient characteristics that influence good therapeutic responses to ISO in HS and are stated as follows [70]:

- Younger patients,
- Women,
- Lower body weight,
- Personal history of acne, and.
- Hurley grade I and II HS.

Reports elaborating the efficacy of ISO in HS are mixed. Boer and Van Gemert [71] used ISO at 0.5–0.8 mg/kg/day for 4–6 months in HS and reported complete responsiveness in 24% of their patients, with lesser improvement in 37%.

Soria et al. [72] delineated the outcomes of ISO in 88 HS patients who were treated with ISO (20–140 mg/day for a mean duration of 7–8 months). Improvement was witnessed in 16% of their subjects, with 77% elaborating no rectification, and in the lingering 7%, the disease deteriorated. Interestingly, in patients where disease improved, Hurley stage I disease was identified.

Generalized Granuloma Annulare

Generalized granuloma annulare (GA) presents as widespread annular papules, plaques and nodules that generally is unresponsive to most treatments. Many individual reports have propounded ISO to be of benefit in generalized GA. The dose utilized for GA is 0.5 mg/kg/day, and in those patients where the dermatosis responds to ISO, remission is noticeable by 2–6 months and persists for 6–12 months after treatment completion [73–77].

Further, in some cases it is seen that if appropriate responses with ISO are not outlined at a dose of 0.5 mg/kg/day, then elevating the dose to 1 mg/kg/day may prove beneficial [78, 79]. In those exhibiting relapses, post-treatment with ISO utilizing a low sustaining dose for another 3 months to 1 year can be productive [80, 81].

Darier's Disease

Darier's disease (DD) is an autosomal dominant disease involving seborrheic areas, and manifesting generally before 30 years of age [82]. In cases with severe symptoms, a trial of ISO is explainable. Several reports have delineated the propitious effects of ISO in DD [83–86]. Usually a dose of 0.5–1 mg/kg/day is used for this indication. However, many authors employ a lower initial dose of 0.2 mg/kg/day, which is then slowly increased as treatment advances to curtail side effects accompanying ISO. Within 2–4 weeks responses following treatment with ISO are visible. Besides, in some cases, a low supportive dosing protocol can be utilized [82]. Although a cumulative dose of 1075 mg/kg of ISO is not connected with skeletal abnormalities, care needs to be practiced with methodical monitoring when patients are receiving long-term treatment with ISO for DD [87].

Cutaneous Lupus Erythematosus

It is observed that ISO and acitretin are effectual in treating those patients of subacute cutaneous lupus erythematosus (SCLE), discoid lupus erythematosus (DLE) and chronic cutaneous lupus erythematosus (CCLE) that are recalcitrant to traditional treatments.

Vena et al. [88] in a 4-month trial with ISO for cutaneous LE (0.15 mg/kg/day and then escalated to 0.5 mg/kg/day) outlined both clinical and microscopic improvement of lesions in 86.9% of the 24 patients treated.

Shornick et al. [89] in their series of six patients with CCLE delineated swift responses with 1 mg/kg/day of ISO. However, there was a relapse in all patients following stoppage of ISO.

D'Erme et al. [90] demonstrated remarkable response with ISO (40 mg/day) in a 26-year-old woman with cutaneous LE refractory to routine therapies.

However, following cessation of ISO therapy, rapid and more severe recurrence of cutaneous LE has been encountered. This is tackled by using lower maintenance dosage of ISO [91]. Other drawbacks of ISO include its cost and avoidance in those cases of cutaneous LE with Sjogren's syndrome, because of keratoconjunctivitis sicca. Nonetheless, retinoid therapy is of value in CLE. Dosage ranges from 0.2 to 1 mg/kg/day with effects being visible by 2–6 weeks.

Condylomata Accuminata

ISO has been utilized both as monotherapy and in coalition with interferon α (IFNα) for condylomata accuminata (CA). ISO induces regression of CA in line with its immunomodulatory effects. Studies on ISO monotherapy as well as combination therapy with IFNα for CA are delineated in Tables 30.2 and 30.3, respectively [92–96].

It is observed that IFNα is best used as an adjunct to other modalities of therapy including 5-FU, laser ablation and surgical excision, and its combined utility has led to lower recurrence rates.

Till date, very few studies exist that delineate the efficacy of combining IFNα and ISO for CA, following traditional destructive therapies. This can be a valuable zone for exploration in the near future.

Table 30.2 Studies on ISO monotherapy for condylomata accuminata

Authors	Dose of ISO utilized	Results
Georgala et al. [92]	0.5 mg/kg/day for 12 weeks	Out of 28 patients, 9 achieved complete clearing, 11 had partial response, with 8 showing no response
Tsambaos et al. [93]	1 mg/kg/day for 12 weeks	Out of 53 patients, 21 patients achieved complete clearing, 7 had partial response, and 25 had no response
Oslen et al. [94]	1 mg/kg/day	No objective response was seen in the 7 patients treated

Table 30.3 Studies on combination therapy with ISO and IFNα for condylomata accuminata

Authors	Dose of the drugs utilized	Remarks
Cardamakis et al. [95]	ISO: 1 mg/kg/day IFNα 2a: 3×10^5 U s/c three times per week (treatment continued not more than 8 weeks)	Effective treatment modality with a lower recurrence rate and shorter duration of treatment than ISO alone
Yildrim et al. [96]	ISO: 0.5 mg/kg/day IFNα 2a: 3×10^5 U s/c three times per week	Effective in treating CA

Disseminate and Recurrent Infundibulofolliculitis (DRIF)

Hundreds of skin-coloured follicular papules resembling goose bumps characterize DRIF. They last for months to years and can be associated with pruritis. ISO (0.5 mg/kg/day) for 4 months has been used for DRIF, but evidence for its efficacy is anecdotal.

Acanthosis Nigricans (AN)

AN is a cutaneous manifestation characterized by coarse, velvety and thick skin, which may be idiopathic or linked with an underlying endocrinopathy. Katz [97] reported solo therapy with ISO to be effective in a 33-year-old woman with AN, involving the angles of the mouth, axilla, antecubital fossa, groins, dorsa of the hands and inferior segments of the breast and neck. She was started with ISO (0.5 mg/kg/day), but as all lesions did not respond, weekly increments, by 0.5 mg/kg/day, was done till a maximum dose of 3 mg/kg/day was administered. This dose enabled resolution of AN. However, owing to hypertriglyceridemia and mucocutaneous side effects of ISO, the dose was reduced to 2 mg/kg/day and after 16 weeks of therapy, owing to complete resolution of lesions, the drug was stopped. However, after 2 months of cessation of ISO, AN relapsed to the level of pre-treatment severity. Patient was then started with a maintenance dosing of 2 mg/kg/day with a satisfactory clinical response and minimal side effects.

Walling et al. [98] combined ISO with metformin for AN, demonstrating propitious outcomes.

Lichen Planus (LP)

Handler [99] utilized ISO for the treatment oral and cutaneous LP. The initial dose employed was 0.25 mg/kg/day, not exceeding 20 mg/day. Treatment duration did not surpass 2 months and results observed were good to excellent (without relapses).

Woo reported systemic ISO (0.5 mg/kg/day) to be useful in severe LP with oral and cutaneous manifestations in two patients [100].

However, according to Camisa and Allen [101], propitious effects with ISO (10–60 mg daily for 8 weeks) in oral erosive LP were not obtained in their series of six patients. Improvement witnessed was minimal with relapse to the pre-treatment status following 2 months of treatment discontinuation. Moreover, as side effects were troublesome, patients refused ISO retreatment.

Photoaging

Though topical tretinoin is generally accepted as a cosmetically beneficial medication for photo-damaged skin, oral ISO is not.

However, Perez et al. [102] elucidated notable cosmetic improvement with ISO administered at 10–20 mg 3 times a week over 2 months in combined rejuvenation cosmetic procedures when compared to individual usage of both treatments. Parameters that delineated improvement included:

- Wrinkles,
- Skin colour and thickness,
- Elasticity of skin,
- Pore size, and.
- Decrease in mottled pigmentation.

Correspondingly, the above discovery was restated by Rabello-Fonseca et al. [103]

Precancerous Cutaneous Conditions

Actinic Keratosis

ISO (20 mg/day), in combination with topical 5-FU, assists in largely decreasing the number of existing lesions of actinic keratosis (AK), along with averting the development of new lesions. Besides, beneficial effects of ISO pertaining to mending of photo-damaged skin is also noticed [104].

Combining ISO with topical 5-FU is specifically useful in patients with severe actinic damage, where solo therapy with 5-FU is insufficient. It is further highlighted that this combination amplifies cellular apoptosis and significantly blocks expansion of oral squamous cell carcinoma cell lines [105].

Leukoplakia

Clinical improvement of leukoplakia is reported with ISO (1–2 mg/kg/day) following usage for 3 months. However, after stopping treatment, high relapse rates have been described [106].

Further, ISO is advantageous in achieving better relapse free states in oral carcinogenesis with dose adjustments (first at 1.5 mg/kg/day for 3 months, succeeded by a lower continuation dose of 0.5 mg/kg/day for 9 months). [107]

Topical ISO (0.18%) cream has also been employed for leukoplakia with favourable outcomes [108].

However, despite short-term effectiveness, retinoids do not prevent recurrence of lesions, with no remarkable increase of cancer-free survival.

Cutaneous Malignancies

Cutaneous T Cell Lymphoma

Duvic et al. demonstrated 82% response rates in patients with stage I and stage II cutaneous T cell lymphoma, using combination of ISO (1 mg/kg/day) and INFα. [109]

Squamous Cell Carcinoma

Combining ISO and IFNα proves advantageous in squamous cell carcinoma (SCC) of the skin with remission rates varying from 17% to 68% [110, 111]. Also, ISO (1 mg/kg/day), when combined with daily radiotherapy, potentiates rapid trimming of tumour size [112]. ISO can therefore be a reasonable adjuvant with other methods of treatment in advanced SCC.

Chemoprevention in High-Risk Populations

Xeroderma Pigmentosum

Kraemer et al. outlined the profitable usage of ISO in averting skin cancer in xeroderma pigmentosum. Dose of ISO administered was 2 mg/kg/day initially, followed by a maintenance dose of 0.5–1 mg/kg/day. [113]

Muir–Torre Syndrome

ISO (50 mg/day) along with IFNα-2a (3×10^6 U s/c) thrice a week with topical ISO elucidated pronounced tumour regression in Muir–Torre syndrome [114].

Resistant Dermatophytosis

ISO (20 mg/day), combined with itraconazole (200 mg/day) and topical sertaconazole for 30 days, highlighted effectiveness in a 23-year-old male patient with resistant dermatophytosis, secondary to *Trichophyton rubrum*. Besides, patient maintained remission even at 6 months of follow-up [115].

Erythema Dyschromicum Perstans

Erythema dyschromicum perstans (EDP) is a pigmentary dermatosis presenting as asymptomatic, symmetrically distributed ashy grey patches. Unfortunately, most treatments for EDP have been unsatisfactory. Wang et al. [116] outlined the profitability of ISO for EDP. In their case report of a 41-year-old patient with EDP, ISO was started at a dose of 20 mg/day for 4 months, following which there was 90%

improvement of the condition. However, when treatment was stopped, there was a relapse. Owing to this, patient was again started on ISO but at a lower dose of 10 mg (on an intermittent basis), which the patient consumed for almost 7 years. During this period, apart from dryness of the face, no adverse effect was encountered, thereby suggesting long-term, low-dose systemic treatment with ISO to be effective and safe for EDP. The plausible mechanism of ISO suggested for EDP is based on its anti-inflammatory and immunomodulatory properties.

Other Conditions

Anecdotal reports have suggested the beneficial role of ISO for Kyrle's disease, ulerythema ophryogens, Ofuji's disease and scleromyxedema [117–120].

Adverse Effects

Cutaneous

- Acne flare.
- Xerosis.
- Retinoid dermatitis.
- Skin fragility.
- *S. aureus* infection.
- Pyogenic granuloma.
- Stickiness involving the palms and soles.
- Urticaria.
- Vasculitis.

Mucosal

- Cheilitis.
- Soreness of mouth and tongue.
- Epistaxis.
- Dryness of nose and mouth.

Hair

- Telogen effluvium.
- Abnormal hair structure.

Nails

- Onycholysis.
- Paronychia.
- Nail softening.

Ocular

- Dry eyes.
- Blepheroconjunctivitis.
- Photophobia.
- Pterygium.

Bone

- Diffuse idiopathic skeletal hyperostosis (DISH).
- Osteoporosis.

Gastrointestinal

- Nausea.
- Diarrhoea.
- Abdominal pain.

Neurologic

- Depression.
- Mild headache.
- Suicidal ideation.

Musculoskeletal

- Arthralgia.
- Myalgia.
- Achilles tendonitis.

Metabolic

- Elevated hepatic transaminases.
- Hypercholesterolemia.
- Hypertriglyceridemia.

Retinoid Embryopathy

- *Craniofacial*: microcephaly, cleft palate, microphthalmia, facial asymmetry.
- *Central nervous system*: hydrocephalus, cortical agenesis, mental retardation.
- *Cardiovascular*: Fallot's tetralogy, hypoplastic aorta, transposition of great vessels.
- *Others*: limb abnormalities, anal and vaginal atresia.

Drug Interactions

Tetracyclines

- Increased risk of pseudotumour cerebri with concomitant ISO administration.
- Symptoms of pseudotumour cerebri include visual disturbances, visual loss, headache, nausea, vomiting and papilledema.
- Symptoms tend to subside when treatment is stopped [121].

Vitamin A

- Co-administration with ISO results in hypervitaminosis.
- Symptoms include gum inflammation, vertigo, pruritus and dry, scaly skin.
- It is therefore prudent to avoid this concoction.

Teriflunomide

- Associated risk of liver toxicity with ISO.

Methotrexate

- Associated risk of liver toxicity with ISO.

Carbamazepine

- When administered concurrently with ISO, plasma levels of carbamazepine reduce and needs to be meticulously monitored [122].

Indomethacin

- Displaces ISO from albumin, culminating in increased unbound concentration of ISO [123].

Monitoring Guidelines

Baseline

- Urine pregnancy test (particularly two tests to be done as described in the iPLEDGE section).
- Liver function tests.
- Fasting lipid profile.
- X-ray ankles, wrist and spine in case of long-term therapy.

Once Every 2 Monthly

Hepatic and lipid profile [123].

Conclusion

Apart from being indispensable for managing nodulocystic acne, ISO proves to be of value in a number of dermatologic conditions. Like any other drug, ISO is associated with a toxicity profile. Therefore, it is mandatory for all clinicians to be adherent regarding monitoring guidelines related to ISO.

References

1. Gollnick H, Cunliffe W, Berson D, Dreno B, Finlay A, Leyden JJ, et al. Management of acne: a report from the global alliance to improve outcomes in acne. J Am Acad Dermatol. 2003;49(1 Suppl):S1–S37.
2. Ward A, Brogden RN, Heel RC, Speight TM, Avery GS. Isotretinoin: a review of its pharmacologic properties and therapeutic efficacy in acne and other skin disorders. Drugs. 1984;28:6–37.

3. Golstein JA, Socha-Szott A, Thomsen RJ, Pochi PE, Shalita AR, Strauss JS. Comparative effect of isotretinoin on acne and sebaceous gland secretion. J Am Acad Dermatol. 1982;4(4 Pt 2 Suppl):760–5.
4. Dispenza MC, Wolpert EB, Gilliland KL, Dai JP, Cong Z, Nelson AM, et al. Systemic isotretinoin therapy normalizes exaggerated TLR-2 mediated innate immune responses in acne patients. J Invest Dermatol. 2012;132:2198–220.
5. Nelson AM, Zhao W, Gilliland KL, Zaenglein AL, Liu W, Thiboutot DM. Isotretinoin temporarily regulates distinct sets of genes in patient skin. J Invest Dermatol. 2009;129:1038–42.
6. Nelson AM, Gilliland KL, Cong Z, Thiboutot DM. 13 cis retinoic acid induces apoptosis and cell cycle arrest in human SEB-1 sebocytes. J Invest Dermatol. 2006;126:2178–89.
7. Nelson AM, Cong Z, Gilliland KL, Thiboutot DM. TRAIL contributes to the apoptotic effect of 13 cis retinoic acid in human sebaceous gland cells. Br J Dermatol. 2011;165:526–33.
8. Del Rosso JQ. Face to face with oral isotretinoin: a closer look at the spectrum of therapeutic outcomes and why some patients need repeated courses. J Clin Aesthet Dermatol. 2012;5:17–24.
9. Aryal A, Upreti S. A brief review on systemic retinoids. Int J Pharm Sci Res. 2017;8:3630–9.
10. Nast A, Dreno B, Bettoli V, Degitz K, Erdmann R, Finlay AY, et al. European evidence based (S3) guidelines for the treatment of acne. J Eur Acad Dermatol Venereol. 2012;26(Suppl 1):1–29.
11. Sinclair W, Jordan HF. Acne guidelines 2005 update: global alliance to improve outcomes in acne. S Afr Med J. 2005;95(11 Pt 2):881–92.
12. Abad-Casintahan F, Chow SK, Goh CL, Kubba R, Miyachi Y, Noppakun N, et al. Toward evidence based practice in acne: consensus of an Asian working group. J Dermatol. 2011;38:1041–8.
13. Strauss JS, Krowchuk DP, Leyden JJ, Lucky AW, Shalita AR, Siegfried EC, et al. Guidelines of care for acne vulgaris management. J Am Acad Dermatol. 2007;56:651–63.
14. Eichenfield LF, Krakowski AC, Piggott C, Del Rosso J, Baldwin H, Friedlander SF, et al. Evidence based recommendations for the diagnosis and treatment of pediatric acne. Pediatrics. 2013;131(Suppl 3):S163–86.
15. Cunliffe WJ, van de Kerkhof PC, Caputo R, Cavicchini S, Cooper A, Fyrand OL, et al. Roaccutane treatment guidelines; Result of an international survey. Dermatology. 1997;194:351–7.
16. Pochi PE, Shalita AR, Strauss JS, Webster SB, Cunliffe WJ, Katz HI, et al. Report of the consensus conference on acne classification. Washington DC. March 24 and 25.1990. J Am Acad Dermatol. 1991;24:495–500.
17. Dreno B, Bodokh I, Chivot M, Daniel F, Humbert P, Poli F, et al. ECLA grading: a system of acne classification for every day dermatological practice. Ann Dermatol Venereol. 1999;126:136–41.
18. Layton A. The use of isotretinoin in acne. Dermatoendocrinology. 2009;1:162–9.
19. Claravis (isotretinoin capsules) [package insert] North Wales, Pennsylvania: Barr Laboratories; August 2012.
20. Zenetane (isotretinoin capsules USP) [package insert]. Bachupally, India: Dr Reddy's Laboratories Limited; January 2013.
21. Brazzell RK, Vane FM, Ehma M, Colburn WA. Pharmacokinetics of isotretinoin during repetitive dosing to patients. Eur J Clin Pharmacol. 1983;24:695–702.
22. Colburn WA, Vane FM, Shorter HJ. Pharmacokinetics of isotretinoin and its major blood metabolite following a single oral dose to man. Eur J Clin Pharmacol. 1983;24:689–94.
23. Del Rosso JQ. An assessment of isotretinoin dosing regimens used by dermatology practitioners in the United States: survey results. J Clin Aesthet Dermatol. 2014;
24. Cyrulink AA, Viola KV, Gewirtzman AJ, Cohen SR. High dose isotretinoin in acne vulgaris: improved treatment outcomes and quality of life. Int J Dermatol. 2012;51:1123–30.
25. Blasiak RC, Stamey CR, Burkhart CN, Lugo-Somolinos A, Morrell DS. High dose isotretinoin treatment and the rate of retrial, relapse and adverse effects in patients with acne vulgaris. JAMA Dermatol. 2013;149:1392–8.

26. Hermes B, Practel C, Henz BM. Medium dose isotretinoin for the treatment of acne. J Eur Acad Dermatol Venereol. 1998;11:117–21.
27. Stauss JS, Leydon JJ, Lucky AW, Lookingbill DP, Drake LA, Hanifin JM, et al. A randomized trial of the efficacy of a new micronized formulation versus standard formulation of isotretinoin in patients with severe recalcitrant nodular acne. J Am Acad Dermatol. 2001;45:187–95.
28. Goulden V, Clark SM, McGeown C, Cunliffe WJ. Treatment of acne with intermittent isotretinoin. Br J Dermatol. 1997;137:106–8.
29. Kaymak Y, Ilter N. The effectiveness of intermittent isotretinoin treatment in mild to moderate acne. J Eur Acad Dermatol Venereol. 2006;20:1256–60.
30. Akman A, Durusoy C, Senturk M, Koc CK, Soyturk D, Alpsoy E. Treatment of acne with intermittent and conventional isotretinoin. A randomized controlled multicentre study. Arch Dermatol Res. 2007;299:467–73.
31. Sardana K, Garg VK, Sehgal VN, Mahajan S, Bhushan P. Efficacy of fixed low dose isotretinoin (20mg, alternate days) with topical clindamycin gel in moderately severe acne vulgaris. J Eur Acad Dermatol Venereol. 2009;23:556–60.
32. Seukeran DC, Cunliffe WJ. Acne vulgaris in the elderly; the response to low dose isotretinoin. Br J Dermatol. 1998;139:99–101.
33. Patton TJ, Ferris LK. Systemic retinoids. In: Wolverton SE, editor. Comprehensive dermatologic drug therapy. 3rd ed. Edinburg: Elsevier-Saunders; 2013. p. 252–68.
34. White GM, Chen W. Recurrence rates after first course of isotretinoin. Arch Dermatol. 1998;134:376–8.
35. Stainforth JM, Layton AM, Taylor JP, Cunliffe WJ. Isotretinoin for treatment of acne vulgaris: which factors may predict the need for more than one course. Br J Dermatol. 1993;129:297–301.
36. Shahidullah M, Tham SN, Goh CL. Isotretinoin therapy in acne vulgaris: a 10 year retrospective study in Singapore. Int J Dermatol. 1994;33:60–3.
37. Ng PP, Goh CL. Treatment outcome of acne vulgaris with oral isotretinoin in 89 patients. Int J Dermatol. 1999;38:213–6.
38. Layton A. The use of isotretinoin in acne. Dermatoendocrinol. 2009;1:162–9.
39. Clark SM, Cunliffe WJ. Acne flare and isotretinoin – incidence and treatment. Br J Dermatol. 1995;133:26.
40. Pepall LM, Cosgrove MP, Cunliffe WJ. Ablation of whiteheads with cautery under topical anaesthesia. Br J Dermatol. 1991;125:256–9.
41. Clark SM, Goulden V, Cunliffe WJ. The management of acne patients who respond slowly to oral isotretinoin. Br J Dermatol. 1996;135:20.
42. iPledgeprogram.com. iPledge REMS-Public Home Page. [Online] Available at http://www.ipledgeprogram.com/iPledgeUI/home.u. Accessed on 08 Jan 2019 (2019)
43. Thiboutot DM, Cockerell CJ. iPLEDGE: a report from the frontlines of dermatologic practice. Virtual Mentor. 2006;8:524–8.
44. Anon (2019). iPledge (isotretinoin) REMS-FDA [online] Available at: https://www.fda.gov/downloads/Drugs/Drugsafety/PostmarketDrugSafetyInformationforPatientsandProviders/UCM234639.pdf. Accessed on 08 Jan 2019.
45. Baldwin HE. Systemic therapy for rosacea. Skin Therapy Lett. 2007;12:1–5.
46. Erdogan FG, Yurtsever P, Aksoy D, Eskioglu F. Efficacy of low dose isotretinoin in patients with treatment resistant rosacea. Arch Dermatol. 1998;134:884–5.
47. Dalziel K, Barton S, Marks R. The effects of isotretinoin on follicular and sebaceous gland differentiation. Br J Dermatol. 1987;117:317–23.
48. Bostanci O, Borelli C, Schaller M. Treatment of extrafacial rosacea with low dose isotretinoin. Acta Derm Venereol. 2010;90:409–10.
49. Uslu M, Savk E, Karaman G, Sendur N. Rosacea treatment with intermediate dose of isotretinoin: follow up with erythema and sebum measurements. Acta Derm Venereol. 2012;92:73–7.
50. Gollnick H, Blume-Peytavi U, Szabo EL, Meyer KG, Hauptmann P, Popp G, et al. Systemic isotretinoin in the treatment of rosacea-doxycycline-and placebo controlled randomized clinical study. J Dtsch Dermatol Ges. 2010;8:505–15.

51. Hofer T. Continuous microdose isotretinoin in adult recalcitrant rosacea. Clin Exp Dermatol. 2004;29:204–5.
52. Rosen T, Unkefer RP. Treatment of pyoderma faciale with isotretinoin in a patient with ulcerative colitis. Cutis. 1999;64:107–9.
53. Strauss JS. Rosacea fulminans. J Eur Acad Dermatol Venereol. 2001;15:385.
54. Selden S. Pyoderma faciale. J Am Acad Dermatol. 2005;53:1104–5.
55. Firooz A, Firoozabadi MR, Dowlati Y. Rosacea fulminans (pyoderma faciale): successful treatment of a 3-year-old girl with oral isotretinoin. Int J Dermatol. 2001;40:203–5.
56. Periera TM, Vieira AP, Basto AS. Rosacea with extensive extrafacial lesions. Int J Dermatol. 2008;47:52–5.
57. Dupont C. How common is extrafacial rosacea? J Am Acad Dermatol. 1986;14:839.
58. Ayres S Jr. Extrafacial rosacea is rare but does exist. J Am Acad Dermatol. 1987;16:391–2.
59. Dicken CH. Isotretinoin treatment of pityriasis rubra pilaris. J Am Acad Dermatol. 1987;16:297–31.
60. Allison DS, El-Azhary RA, Colobrisi SD, Dicken CH. Pityriasis rubra pilaris in children. J Am Acad Dermatol. 2002;47:386–9.
61. Akyol M, Ozcelik S. Non acne dermatologic indications for systemic isotretinoin. Am J Clin Dermatol. 2005;6:175–84.
62. Sehgal VN, Srivastava G, Sardana K. Erythroderma/exfoliative dermatitis: a synopsis. Int J Dermatol. 2004;43:39–47.
63. Arechalde A, Saurat JH. Management of psoriasis: the position of retinoid drugs. BioDrugs. 2000;13:327–33.
64. Al-Shobaili H, Al-Khenaizan S. Childhood generalized pustular psoriasis successful treatment with isotretinoin. Pediatr Dermatol. 2007;24:563–4.
65. Mortazavi H, Khezri S, Hosseini H, et al. A single blind randomized clinical study: the efficacy of isotretinoin plus narrow band ultraviolet B in the treatment of psoriasis vulgaris. Photoderm Photoimmunol Photomed. 2011;27:159–61.
66. Revuz J. Hidradenitis suppurativa. J Eur Acad Dermatol Venereol. 2009;23:985–98.
67. Slade DEM, Powell BW, Mortimer PS. Hidradenitis suppurativa: pathogenesis and management. Br J Plast Surg. 2003;56:451–61.
68. Monk BE. Fordyce spots responding to isotretinoin therapy. Br J Dermatol. 1993;129:355.
69. Pino-Lagos K, Benson MJ, Noelle RJ. Retinoic acid in the immune system. Ann N Y Acad Sci. 2008;1143:170–87.
70. Huang CM, Kirchhof MG. A new perspective on isotretinoin treatment of hidradenitis suppurativa: a retrospective chart review of patient outcomes. Dermatology. 2017;233:120–5.
71. Boer J, Van Gemert MJ. Long term results of isotretinoin in the treatment of 68 patients with hidradenitis suppurativa. J Am Acad Dermatol. 1999;40:73–6.
72. Soria A, Canoui-Poitrine F, Wolkenstein P, Poli F, Gabison G, Pouget F, et al. Absence of efficacy of oral isotretinoin in hidradenitis suppurativa: a retrospective study based on patient outcome assessment. J Am Acad Dermatol. 2009;218:134–5.
73. Looney M, Smith KM. Isotretinoin in the treatment of granuloma annulare. Ann Pharmacother. 2004;38:494–7.
74. Pasmatzi E, Georgiou S, Mouastirli A, Tsambaos D. Temporary remission of disseminated granuloma annulare under oral isotretinoin therapy. Int J Dermatol. 2005;44:169–71.
75. Tang WY, Chong LY, Lo KK. Resolution of generalized granuloma annulare with isotretinoin therapy. Int J Dermatol. 1996;35:455–6.
76. Schleicher SM, Miltstein HJ, Lim SJM, Stanton CD. Resolution of disseminated granuloma annulare with isotretinoin. Int J Dermatol. 1992;31:371–2.
77. Buendia-Eisman A, Ruiz-Villaverde R, Blasco-Melguizo J, Serrano-Ortega S. Generalized granuloma annulare: response to isotretinoin. Int J Dermatol. 2003;42:321–2.
78. Baskan EB, Turan A, Tunali S. A case of generalized granuloma annulare with myelodysplastic syndrome: successful treatment with systemic isotretinoin and topical pimecrolimus 1% cream combination. J Eur Acad Dermatol Venereol. 2007;21:693–5.

79. Young HS, Coulson IH. Granuloma annulare following waxing induced folliculitis – resolution with isotretinoin. Clin Exp Dermatol. 2000;25:274–6.
80. Ratnavel RC, Norris PG. Perforating granuloma annulare: response to treatment with isotretinoin. J Am Acad Dermatol. 1995;32:126–7.
81. Adams DC, Hogan DJ. Improvement of chronic generalized granuloma annulare with isotretinoin. Arch Dermatol. 2002;138:1518–9.
82. Sehgal VN, Srivastava G. Dariers (Darier – White) disease/keratosis follicularis. Int J Dermatol. 2005;44:184–92.
83. Del Rosso DQ, Horowitz DC. Treatment of Darier's disease with isotretinoin: report of a case. J Am Osteopath Assoc. 1986;86:634–8.
84. Rotunda AM, Cotliar J, Haley JC, Craft N. Unilateral Darier's disease associated with migraine headache responsive to isotretinoin. J Am Acad Dermatol. 2005;52:175–6.
85. Dicken CH, Bauer EA, Hazen PG. Isotretinoin treatment of Darier's disease. J Am Acad Dermatol. 1982;6(4 Pt 2 Suppl):721–6.
86. Bhat RM, Ullal KR, Pinto AC, Sukumar D. Darier White disease in siblings responding to isotretinoin. Indian Dermatol Online J. 2010;1:18–20.
87. Ling TC, Parkin G, Islam J, et al. What is the cumulative effect of long-term low dose of isotretinoin on the development of DISH. Br J Dermatol. 2001;144:630–2.
88. Vena GA, Coviello C, Angelini G. Use of oral isotretinoin in the treatment of cutaneous lupus eruthematosus. G Ital Dermatol Venereol. 1989;124:311–5.
89. Shornick JK, Fornica N, Parke AL. Isotretinoin for refractory lupus erythematosus. J Am Acad Dermatol. 1991;24:49–52.
90. D'Erme AM, Milanesi N, Difonzo EM, et al. Treatment of refractory subacute cutaneous lupus erythematosus with oral isotretinoin: a valid therapeutic option. Dermatol Ther. 2012;25:281–2.
91. Richardson TT, Cohen PR. Subacute cutaneous lupus erythematosus: report of a patient who subsequently developed meningioma and whose skin lesions were treated with isotretinoin. Cutis. 2000;66:183–8.
92. Georgala S, Katoulis AC, Georgala C, Bozi E, Mortakis A. Oral isotretinoin in the treatment of recalcitrant condyloma accuminata of the cervix: a randomized placebo-controlled trial. Sex Transm Infect. 2004;80:216–8.
93. Tsambaos D, Georgiou S, Monastirli A, Sakkis T, Sagriotis A, Goerz G. Treatment of condylomata accuminata with oral isotretinoin. J Urol. 1997;158:1810–2.
94. Oslen EA, Kelly FF, Vollmer RT, Buddin DA, Weck PK. Comparative study of systemic interferon alfa-nl and isotretinoin in the treatment of resistant condyloma accuminata. J Am Acad Dermatol. 1989;20:1023–30.
95. Cardamakis E, Michopoulos J, Kotoulas IG, Stathopoulose E, Relakis K. Comparative study of systemic interferon alfa-2a plus isotretinoin versus isotretinoin in the treatment of recurrent condyloma accuminatum in men. Urology. 1995;45:857–60.
96. Yildrim M, Inaloz HS, Baysal V, Kesici D, Candir O. A case of condyloma accuminatum treated successfully with low dose of isotretinoin and interferon. Int J Clin Pract. 2004;58:889–91.
97. Katz RA. Treatment of acanthosis nigricans with oral isotretinoin. Arch Dermatol. 1980;116:110–1.
98. Walling HW, Messingham M, Myers LM, Mason CL, Strauss JS. Improvement of acanthosis nigricans on isotretinoin and metformin. J Drugs Dermatol. 2003;2:677–81.
99. Handler HL. Isotretinoin for oral lichen planus. J Am Acad Dermatol. 1984;10:674.
100. Woo TY. Systemic isotretinoin treatment of oral and cutaneous lichen planus. Cutis. 1985;35:385–93.
101. Camisa C, Allen CM. Treatment of oral erosive lichen planus with systemic isotretinoin. Oral Surg Oral Med Oral Pathol. 1986;62:393–6.
102. Hernandez-Perez E, Khawaja HA, Alvarez TY. Oral isotretinoin as part of treatment of cutaneous aging. Dermatologic Surg. 2000;26:649–52.

103. Rabello-Fonseca R, Azulay D, Luiz R, Mandarim-de-Lacerda CA, Cuzzi T, Manela-Azulay M. Oral isotretinoin in photoaging: clinical and histopathological evidence of efficacy of an off-label indication. J Eur Acad Dermatol Venereol. 2009;23:115–23.
104. Sander CA, Pfeiffer C, Kligman AM, Plewig G. Chemotherapy for disseminated actinic keratosis with 5-fluorouracil and isotretinoin. J Am Acad Dermatol. 1997;36(2 Pt 1):236–8.
105. Dalirsani Z, Farajnia S, Javadzadeh Y, Mehdipour M, Koozegari S. The effects of 5-fluorouracil alone and in combination with 13-cis retinoic acid and vitamin D3 on human oral squamous cell carcinoma lines. J Contemp Dent Pract. 2012;13:345–50.
106. Hong WK, Endicott J, Itri LM, Doos W, Batsakis JG, Bell R, et al. 13-cis-retinoic acid in the treatment of oral leukoplakia. N Engl J Med. 1986;315:1501–5.
107. Lippman SM, Batsakis JG, Toth BB, Weber RS, Lee JJ, Martin JW, et al. Comparison of low dose isotretinoin with beta carotene to prevent oral carcinogenesis. N Engl J Med. 1993;328:15–20.
108. Scardina GA, Carini F, Maresi E, Valenza V, Messina P. Evaluation of the clinical and histological effectiveness of isotretinoin in the therapy of oral leukoplakia: ten years of experience: is management still up to date and effective? Methods Find Exp Clin Pharmacol. 2006;28:115–9.
109. Duvic M, Lemak NA, Redman JR, Eifel PJ, Tucker SL, Cabanillas FF, et al. Combined modality therapy for cutaneous T cell lymphoma. J Am Acad Dermatol. 1996;35:587.
110. Shin DM, Glisson BS, Khuri FR, Clifford JL, Clayman G, Benner SE, et al. Phase II and biologic study of interferon alfa, retinoic acid and cisplatin in advanced squamous skin cancer. J Clin Oncol. 2002;20:364–70.
111. Lippmann SM, Parkinson DR, Itri LM, Weber RS, Schantz SP, Ota DM, et al. 13-cis retinoic acid and interferon alpha-2a: effective combination therapy for advanced squamous cell carcinoma of the skin. J Natl Cancer Inst. 1992;84:235–41.
112. Danopoulou I, Korfitis C, Koliarakis N, Trafalis DT. Rapid improvement of extensive nonmelanoma skin cancers with combination of 13-cis retinoic acid and radiotherapy: report of three cases. J BOUN. 2009;14:515–7.
113. Kraemer KH, Di Giovanna JJ, Moshell AN, Tarone RE, Peck GL. Prevention of skin cancer in xeroderma pigmentosum with the use of oral isotretinoin. N Engl J Med. 1988;318:1633–7.
114. Graefe T, Wollina U, Schulz H, Burgdorf W. Muir-Torre syndrome treatment with isotretinoin and interferon alpha-2a can prevent tumour development. Dermatology. 2000;200:331–3.
115. Ardeshna KP, Rohatgi S, Jerajani HR. Successful treatment of recurrent dermatophytosis with isotretinoin and itraconazole. Indian J Dermatol Venereol Leprol. 2016;82:579–82.
116. Wang F, Zhao YK, Wang Z, Liu JH, Luo DQ. Erythema dyschromicum perstans response to isotretinoin. JAMA Dermatol. 2016;152:841–2.
117. Saleh HA, Lloyd KM, Fatteh S. Kyrle's disease: effectively treated with isotretinoin. J Fla Med Assoc. 1993;80:395–7.
118. Layton AM, Cunliffe WJ. A case of ulerythema ophryogenes responding to isotretinoin. Br J Dermatol. 1993;129:645–6.
119. Berbis P, Jancovici E, Lebreuil G, Benderitter T, Dubertret L, Privat Y. Eosinophilic pustular folliculitis (Ofuji's disease): efficacy of isotretinoin. Dermatologica. 1989;179:214–6.
120. Serdar ZA, Altunacy IK, Yasar SP, Erfan GT, Gunes P. Generalized papular and sclerodermoid eruption: scleromyxedema. Indian J Dermatol Venereol Leprol. 2010;76:592.
121. Lee AG. Pseudotumor cerebri after treatment with tetracycline and isotretinoin for acne. Cutis. 1995;55:165–8.
122. Marsden JR. Effects of isotretinoin on carbamazepine pharmacokinetics. Br J Dermatol. 1988;119:403–4.
123. Berbis P. Retinoid drug interactions. Ann Dermatol Venereol. 1991;118:271–2.

Acitretin

31

Introduction

Acitretin (ACT) is a synthetic second-generation retinoid that has gradually replaced etretinate in today's dermatologic practice, because of its favourable pharmacokinetics. It is successfully employed both as monotherapy and combination therapy for a number of cutaneous disorders. Acitretin is an aromatic retinoid and a pharmacologic active metabolite of etretinate.

Mechanism of Action

The mechanism of action is described in Fig. 31.1 [1–5].

Anti-keratinizing Effects

- Induction of epidermal differentiation.
- Normalization of accelerated epidermopoeisis in psoriatic skin.

Anti-inflammatory Effects

- Reduction in release of leukotrienes and dihydroeicosatetraenoic acid products.
- Inhibition of vasculoendothelial growth factor (VEGF) production from keratinocytes.
- Inhibition of ornithine decarboxylase, with ultimate inhibition of neutrophilic chemotaxis.

A. K. Bubna, *Therapeutics in Dermatology - Essentials for Clinical Practice*,
https://doi.org/10.1007/978-981-95-3791-4_31

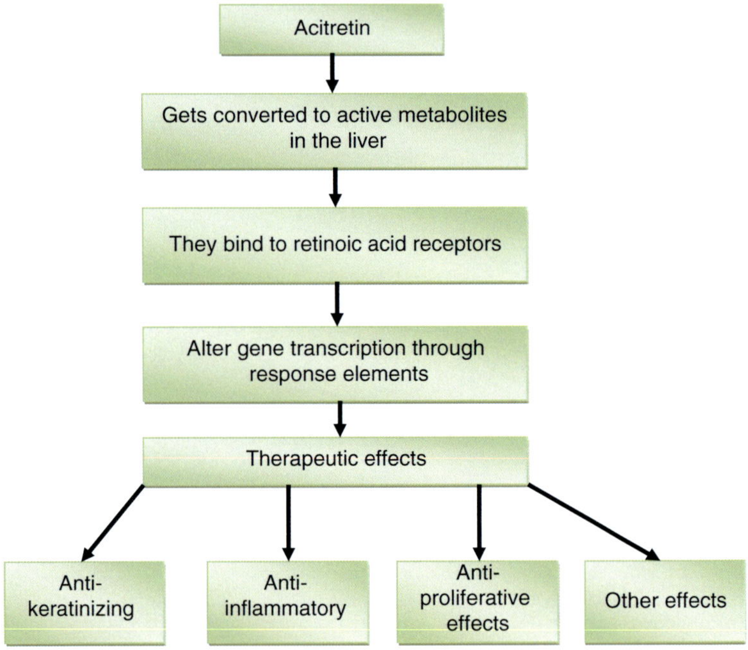

Fig. 31.1 Mechanism of action of acitretin

Anti-proliferative Effects

- Increases growth inhibiting effects of cAMP in fibroblasts.

Other Effects

Antineoplastic Effects

- Inhibits tumour cell angiogenesis.
- Modulates cellular apoptosis.
- Directly downregulates proto-oncogenes.
- Increases intracellular levels of ceramides, possibly inhibiting malignant progression.

Anti-acne and Anti-sebum Effects

- Inhibits sebocyte proliferation.

Wound Healing

- Increases mucopolysaccharides, collagen and fibronectin synthesis.
- Decreases collagenase production, and thereby helps wound healing.

Pharmacokinetics

The bioavailability of ACT (which is 60%) increases following food consumption. Within 4 h of oral intake, peak plasma levels of ACT are attained, with a $t_{1/2}$ of 50 h. The metabolism of ACT occurs in the liver to 13-*cis*-isoacitretin. The drug is 95% bound to plasma albumin. Excretion occurs both via urine and faeces. The consumption of alcohol along with ACT indirectly brings about conversion of ACT to etretinate by a process called reverse esterification. The mechanism of this conversion is not completely clear, and whether other substances apart from alcohol are involved needs further elucidation [6–8].

Indications

FDA Approved

Psoriasis.

Off-Label

Disorders of Keratinization

- Pityriasis rubra pilaris (PRP)
- Ichthyosis
- Keratodermas

Inflammatory Dermatosis

- Lichen planus (LP)

Connective Tissue Disorders

- Lupus erythematosus (LE)
- Lichen sclerosus et atrophicus (LSetA)
- Graft versus host disease (GVHD)

Vesiculobullous Disorders

- IgA pemphigus
- Pemphigus vegetans

Disorders of Skin Appendages

- Hidradenitis suppurativa (HS)
- Pachyonychia congenita
- Erosive pustular dermatosis of the scalp

Mucosal Disorders

- Oral leukoplakia
- Bowenoid papulosis

Infections

- *Viral*: recalcitrant extensive warts, Buschke–Lowenstein tumour
- *Bacterial*: blastomycosis like pyoderma
- *Parasitic*: elephantiasis nostras verrucosa

Others

- Darier's disease (DD)
- Granuloma annulare (GA)
- Hyperkeratotic hand eczema
- Lichen nitidus (LN)
- Lichen amyloidosis
- Langerhans cell histiocytosis (LCH)
- Actinic keratosis (AK)
- Bowen's disease
- Disseminated porokeratosis
- Keratosis lichenoid chronica

Contraindications [9]

Absolute

- Pregnancy
- Lactation
- Women of child-bearing potential who cannot guarantee adequate contraception during and up to 3 years

Relative

- Except under special situations, ACT should never be used when the following medical problems exist:
  1. Allergy to parabens
  2. Hyperlipidaemia, intractable (especially those with diabetes mellitus (DM), obesity, increased alcohol intake or family history)
  3. Pancreatitis or history of hypervitaminosis A or history of hypersensitivity to etretinate, isotretinoin or vitamin A
- Risk benefit should be considered when the following medical problems exist:
  1. DM type 1 or 2
  2. Liver disease
  3. Kidney disease
  4. Alcohol abuse
  5. Concurrent intake of hepatotoxic drugs
  6. Concurrent intake of drugs interfering with ACT metabolism

  Pregnancy prescribing status: Category 'X'.

Clinical Uses

Psoriasis

ACT is found to be useful both as monotherapy and combination therapy for psoriasis. However, efficacy of ACT differs in various forms of psoriasis. Variants of psoriasis where ACT demonstrates better results include generalized pustular psoriasis, palmoplantar pustulosis, erythrodermic psoriasis and psoriasis associated with HIV.

In severe plaque-type psoriasis, efficacy of ACT as solo therapy is less than methotrexate and cyclosporine. However, when combined with topical and systemic therapies (such as topical corticosteroids, topical vitamin D analogues and phototherapy), ACT outlines equal clinical efficacy as methotrexate and cyclosporine [8, 10–12].

Interestingly, the dosing schedule of ACT in psoriasis differ among patients. Further, based on conclusions from various studies, no strict dosing regimen has been postulated for psoriasis.

Ormerod et al. [13] demonstrated ACT given at 50–75 mg/day to be more effective than ACT given at 10–25 mg/day. Similarly, Gollinick and colleagues [11] delineated ACT (50 mg/day) to be superior than ACT (10–25 mg/day) with respect to clinical efficacy. However, according to Dogra et al. [14], ACT dosed at 35 mg/day was more effective than the 25 and 50 mg/day dosing schedules.

Sbidian et al. [15], in their compilation of 44 randomized controlled trials, concluded that 10–25 mg of ACT per day to be the apt starting dose in psoriasis. Further, in patients with inadequate clinical responses, gradual dose escalation enabled achievement of optimal disease clearance (with minimal side effects). The duration of treatment generally lasts for 12–16 weeks.

In nail psoriasis, the dose usually employed is 0.2–0.3 mg/kg/day. Treatment here needs to be continued for 24 weeks [16].

Apart from monotherapy, ACT can be combined with the following therapeutic modalities in psoriasis:

PUVA

When combined with PUVA, the therapy is referred to as Re-PUVA. The advantages with this combination include:

- More effective than PUVA alone (Synergism),
- Reduces the number of PUVA treatments, and
- Reduces risk of malignancies, especially squamous cell carcinoma (SCC) (in association with phototherapy) [13, 17].

Ultraviolet B

Like Re-PUVA, Re-UVB is found to be more efficacious than ACT monotherapy [13].

Calcipotriol Ointment

Combining systemic ACT with calcipotriol ointment has elucidated statistically significant results when compared to ACT therapy alone [18].

Etanercept

ACT (0.4 g/kg/day) can be combined with etanercept (250 mg subcutaneously once a week) for chronic plaque psoriasis. Not only is this combination more effective but also helps in reducing the dose of etanercept to once a week [19].

Methotrexate

Theoretically, ACT and methotrexate combination would alarm the concern of severe hepatotoxic responses. However, in severe cases of psoriasis, recalcitrant to other treatments, this concoction can be considered, provided the patient cooperates for regular and periodic monitoring of the hepatic profile [9, 20].

Cyclosporine

As both drugs are inactivated by the same cytochrome P450 system, it is suggested that this combination can precipitate cyclosporine toxicity [21]. However, while treating patients with generalized pustular psoriasis in the sequential format, the combination of cyclosporine and ACT has shown value. In the initiation phase, only cyclosporine is administered and once substantial clearance of the disease is obtained, the dose of cyclosporine is reduced and ACT is introduced in the continuation phase of treatment, which may last for 1–2 months. Following this in the maintenance phase, cyclosporine is completely stopped and ACT is continued alone.

Pioglitazone

Pioglitazone demonstrates potential anti-psoriatic effects and combining it with ACT elaborates reduction in PASI scores by 64.2%, compared to 51.7% with ACT monotherapy [9].

Lichen Planus

ACT is found to be valuable in treating LP, particularly the hypertrophic variant, owing to its modulating effects on keratinization [22]. In the hypertrophic variant of LP, it may take almost 9 months to witness excellent clinical responses, and therefore treatment needs to be continued for a longer time period. In the classical variant of LP, ACT is effectual at a dose of 30 mg/day [23].

Pityriasis Rubra Pilaris

ACT has been effectively employed in treating PRP. It is particularly beneficial for type I PRP. The dose of ACT here is 0.5-0.75mg/kg/day. Further, combining ACT and UVB/UVA1 exhibits better responses [24]. Moreover, owing to the rarity of the disease and lack of standardized studies for PRP, there is no consistent data regarding the exact duration of ACT therapy, the risk of relapse following treatment cessation and the need for maintenance treatment. In PRP, ACT works by regulating skin proliferation and differentiation, as well as its anti-inflammatory effects.

Darier's Disease

Low doses of ACT (ranging from 10 to 25 mg/day) is beneficial in DD [25].

Lupus Erythematosus

ACT is employed in treating subacute cutaneous lupus erythematosus (LE) with remission of lesions by 2–4 weeks [26]. Also, in verrucous plaques of lupus, ACT is effective owing to its immunomodulatory properties [9]. However, ACT should never be used as a first-line drug in LE.

Lichen Sclerosus

Though reported to be useful in LSetA, ACT should not be routinely employed [27].

Ichthyosis

ACT is useful in lamellar ichthyosis, X linked ichthyosis, bullous and non-bullous ichthyosiform erythroderma and Sjogren's Larsson syndrome. In these trials, marked remission was noticed when patients were on treatment [28–30]. However, ACT must not be used in Netherton's syndrome as it may worsen the condition.

Keratodermas

In a small series, beneficial effects of ACT were observed in Vohwinkel's syndrome, keratitis-ichthyosis-deafness (KID) syndrome, epidermolytic hyperkeratosis, punctuate palmoplantar keratodermas and Papillon–Lefevre syndrome [31–33].

Warts

ACT is effective in recalcitrant warts in a number of case reports [34]. Further, ACT has been used along with imiquimod and excision for treating giant condyloma accuminata [35].

Blastomycosis Like Pyoderma

Beneficial effects of ACT in blastomycosis like pyoderma have been reported. Within 3 months of initiating therapy, propitious effects of ACT were visible, and after 9 months of stopping treatment, no recurrence was observed [36].

Hidradenitis Suppurativa

In hidradenitis suppurativa (HS), ACT targets the infundibular follicular epithelium and abolishes the follicular mass of the keratinocyte–keratin complex [37]. The dose ranges from 25 to 50 mg/day (lasting for 9–12 months), with significant improvement of pain, and decrease in the number of nodules and abscesses following completion of therapy [37].

Chemoprevention, Treatment of Precancerous and Malignant Conditions

ACT is used for preventing cutaneous malignancies in photo-damaged skin and in certain conditions that predispose to skin cancer such as epidermodysplasia verruciformis (EDV), GVHD, xeroderma pigmentosum, keratoacanthoma and Gorlin's syndrome [38–41]. In EDV, ACT can be combined with IFNα-2a.

Further, ACT is considered the drug of selection in the management of keratoacanthomas, SCC and giant basal cell carcinoma (as an adjuvant to surgical removal) in individual case reports [41–43].

Chen et al. [44] demonstrated a significant reduction in the incidence of SCC, basal cell carcinoma and pre-malignant lesions with ACT. Besides, chemoprevention with ACT has helped in reducing the incidence of new primary non-melanoma skin cancers (NMSCs) in immunocompromised post-transplant recipients.

Moreover, ACT is effective in early-stage CTCL [45].

Others

Other conditions where anecdotal reports of the use of ACT exist include porokeratosis, subcorneal pustular dermatosis, erosive pustular dermatosis of the scalp and lichen amyloidosis [46–49].

Dosing

Response to ACT is dose dependent with higher dose capitulating greater and swifter improvements. An initial dosing of 25–30 mg for 1 month, with gradual dose escalation may be required if the dermatosis is unresponsive. In most cases, the optimal dose is 25–50 mg/day. However, in certain cases, a maximum dose of 75–100 mg/day can be given.

In children, dosing is 1 mg/kg/day. In those children on long-term therapy with ACT, growth charting and annual radiographic screening is advisable. In children, while administering ACT, it is advisable to freeze the capsule, cut it into a fraction depending on the dosage and dispense it in a liquid similar to other solid crushed tablets.

Adverse Effects

Teratogenicity

- Retinoid embryopathy
- As it is teratogenic, two forms of effective contraception should be used, beginning 1 month prior to starting ACT, and throughout the duration of treatment, continuing for 2 years in Europe and 3 years in the United States after stopping therapy. Both primary and secondary forms of contraception can be used.

Mucocutaneous

- Epistaxis
- Rhinitis
- Cheilitis
- Dry mouth
- Stomatitis
- Gingivitis
- Taste disturbances
- Thinning and redness of palms and soles
- Hair loss
- Nail fragility
- Paronychia
- Periungual pyogenic granuloma
- Retinoid dermatitis that may resemble unstable psoriasis and can develop in around 25% of patients receiving ACT.

Hepatotoxicity

Hyperlipidaemia

Pancreatitis

Influenza-Like Symptoms

Gastrointestinal

- Constipation
- Diarrhoea

Central Nervous System

- Pseudotumour cerebri especially with concomitant administration of tetracyclines.

Ocular

- Blepharitis
- Conjunctivitis
- Photophobia
- Eye pain
- Recurring stye
- Reduced night vision
- Cortical, nuclear and posterior subcapsular cataract
- Pannus

Others

- Vulvovaginitis
- Delayed wound healing
- Increased insulin sensitivity

Drug Interactions

- *Methotrexate*: Increased chance of hepatotoxicity.
- *Alcohol*: Increased conversion to etretinate, increased risk of hepatotoxicity.
- *Vitamin A*: Hypervitaminosis A, the intake of vitamin A should therefore not exceed the recommended dose of 2400–3000 IU daily.
- *Corticosteroids*: Increased risk of hyperlipidaemia.

Monitoring Guidelines

Baseline

- Liver function tests
- Fasting lipid profile
- Blood sugar in diabetics

  These tests are repeated every 2–4 weeks for the first 2 months and then once every 3 months.

In case of abnormalities in laboratory parameters, the dose of ACT is to be adjusted accordingly.

ACT is to be discontinued if:

- Hepatic transaminases are elevated 3 times their upper normal limit.
- Bilirubin >3 mg/dL.
- Alanine aminotransferase >200 IU/L.

If these abnormalities exist, it also becomes mandatory for the treating dermatologist to refer the patient to a gastroenterologist. If levels are between 2 and 3 times the normal range, ACT is to be discontinued till they normalize and restarted at lower doses [13].

If the elevation is only 2 times, then levels usually resolve even on therapy. However, frequent monitoring is required.

Hypertriglyceridemia >884.96 mg/mL warrants discontinuation of the drug [13].

Newer Topical Preparation of Acitretin

ACT nanostructured lipid carriers (NLCs) are prepared by solvent diffusion technique using 3 (2) fuel factorial design and NLCs incorporated in 1% (w/w) carbopol 934P gel base. They are lyophilized, and crystallinity of NLC is characterized by differential scanning calorimetry (DSC) and powder X-ray diffraction (XRD). This preparation can offer a new ray of hope in topical treatment of psoriasis [50].

Conclusion

ACT has proven valuable in the management of psoriasis, both as monotherapy and when combined with other modalities of treatment. Apart from psoriasis there are a number of other dermatologic indications where ACT is beneficial.

Currently, with a topical preparation of ACT being formulated, it can prove to be an additional boon for managing many more dermatological conditions, along with averting systemic toxicity associated with ACT.

References

1. Wiegand UW, Chou RC. Pharmacokinetics of acitretin and etretinate. J Am Acad Dermatol. 1998;39:S25–33.
2. Pilkigton T, Brogden RN. Acitretin: a review of its pharmacology and therapeutic use. Drugs. 1992;43:597–627.
3. Tong PS, Horoitz NN, Wheeler LA. Trans retinoic acid enhances the growth response of epidermal keratinocytes to epidermal growth factor and transforming growth factor beta. J Invest Dermatol. 1990;94:126–31.
4. Goldfarb MT, Ellis CN, Gupta AK, et al. Acitretin improves psoriasis in a dose dependant fashion. J Am Acad Dermatol. 1988;18:655–62.
5. Koo J, Nguyen Q, Gambla C. Avances in psoriasis therapy. Adv Dermatol. 1997;12:47–72.
6. McNamara PJ, Jewell RC, Jensen BK, et al. Food increases the bioavailability of acitretin. J Clin Pharmacol. 1988;28:1051–5.
7. Aryal A, Upreti S. A brief review on systemic retinoids. Int J Pharm Sci Res. 2017;8:3630–9.
8. Nikam BP, Amladi S, Wadhwa SL. Acitretin. Indian J Dermatol Venereol Leprol. 2006;72:167–72.
9. Sarkar R, Chugh S, Garg VK. Acitretin in dermatology. Indian J Dermatol Venereol Leprol. 2013;79:759–71.
10. Lassus A, Geiger JM. Acitretin and etretinate in the treatment of palmoplantar pustulosis. A double-blind comparative trial. Br J Dermatol. 1984;111:37–44.
11. Gollnick H, Bauer R, Brindley C, et al. Acitretin versus etretinate in psoriasis: clinical and pharmacokinetic results of a German multicenter study. J Am Acad Dermatol. 1988;19:458–69.
12. Geiger J, Saurat JH. Acitretin and etretinate. How and why, they should be used. Dermatol Clin. 1993;11:117–29.
13. Ormerod AD, Campalani E, Godfield MJ. British association of dermatologists guidelines on the efficacy and use of acitretin in dermatology. Br J Dermatol. 2010;162:952–63.
14. Dogra S, Jain A, Kanwar AJ. Efficacy and safety of acitretin in adult patients with severe plaque type psoriasis: a randomized double blind, parallel group, dose ranging study in three fixed doses of 25 mg, 35 mg and 50 mg. J Eur Acad Dermatol Venereol. 2012;27(3):e305–11.
15. Sbidian E, Maza A, Montaudie H, et al. Efficacy and safety of oral retinoids in different psoriasis subtypes. A systematic literature review. J Eur Acad Dermatol Venereol. 2011;25(Suppl 2):S28–33.
16. Tosti A, Ricotti C, Romanelli P, et al. Evaluation of the efficacy of acitretin therapy for nail psoriasis. Arch Dermatol. 2009;145:269–71.
17. Saurat JH, Geiger JM, Amblard P, et al. Randomized double blind multicentre study comparing acitretin-PUVA, etretinate-PUVA and placebo-PUVA in the treatment of severe psoriasis. Dermatologica. 1988;177:218–24.
18. Rim JH, Park JY, Choe YB, et al. The efficacy of calcipotriol plus acitretin combination therapy for psoriasis: comparison with acitretin monotherapy. Am J Clin Dermatol. 2003;4:507–10.
19. Gisondi P, Del Giglio M, Cotena C, et al. Combining etanercept and acitretin in the therapy of chronic plaque psoriasis: a 24 week, randomized, controlled investigator blinded pilot trial. Br J Dermatol. 2008;158:1345–9.
20. Beck HI, Foged EK. Toxic hepatitis due to combination therapy with methotrexate and etretinate in psoriasis. Dermatologica. 1983;167:94–6.
21. Kuijpers AL, van Dooren-Geebe RJ, van de Kerkhof PC. Failure of combination therapy with acitretin and cyclosporine a in three patients with erythrodermic psoriasis. Dermatology. 1997;194:88–90.
22. Jamie TJ, Gauraldi Bde M, Melo DF, et al. Disseminated hypertrophic lichen planus: relevant response to acitretin. An Bras Dermatol. 2011;86:96–9.
23. Laurberg G, Geiger JM, Hjorth N, et al. Treatment of lichen planus with acitretin. A double-blind placebo-controlled study in 65 patients. J Am Acad Dermatol. 1991;24:434–7.

24. Kirby B, Watson R. Pityriasis rubra pilaris treated with acitretin and narrow band ultraviolet B(Re-TL-01). Br J Dermatol. 2002;142:376–7.
25. Van Dooren-Greebe RJ, van de Kerkhof PC, et al. Acitretin monotherapy in Darier's disease. Br J Dermatol. 1989;121:375–9.
26. Ruzicka T, Meurer M, Beiber T. Efficacy of acitretin in the treatment of cutaneous lupus erythematosus. Arch Dermatol. 1988;124:897–902.
27. Bousema MT, Romppanen U, Geiger JM, et al. Acitretin in the treatment of severe lichen sclerosus et atrophicus of the vulva: a double-blind placebo-controlled study. J Am Acad Dermatol. 1994;30:225–31.
28. Lacour M, Mehta-Nikhar B, Atherton DJ, et al. An appraisal of acitretin therapy in children with inherited disorders of keratinisation. Br J Dermatol. 1996;134:1023–9.
29. Happle R, van de Kerkhof PC, Traupe H. Retinoids in disorders of keratinization: their use in adults. Dermatologica. 1987;175(Suppl 1):8107–24.
30. Katugampola RP, Finlay AY. Oral retinoid therapy for disorders of keratinization: single centre retrospective 25 years experience on 23 patients. Br J Dermatol. 2006;154:267–76.
31. Bondeson ML, Nystrom AM, Gunnarsson U, et al. Connexin 26 (GJB2) mutations in two Swedish patients with atypical Vohwinkel (mutilating keratoderma plus deafness) and KID syndrome both extensively treated with acitretin. Acta Derm Venereol (Stockh). 2006;86:533–8.
32. Erkek E, Erdogan S, Tuncez F, et al. Type I hereditary punctate keratoderma associated with widespread lentigo simplex and successfully treated with low dose oral acitretin. Arch Dermatol. 2006;142:1076–7.
33. Lundgren T, Crossner CG, Twetman S, et al. Systemic retinoid medication and periodontal health in patients with papillon-lefevre syndrome. J Clin Periodontol. 1996;23:176–9.
34. Choi YL, Lee KJ, Kim WS, et al. Treatment of extensive and recalcitrant viral warts with acitretin. Int J Dermatol. 2006;45:480–2.
35. Erkek E, Basar H, Bozdogan O, et al. Giant condyloma accuminata of Buschke Lowenstein: successful treatment with a combination of surgical excision, oral acitretin and topical imiquimod. Clin Exp Dermatol. 2009;34:366–8.
36. Lee YS, Jung SW, Sim HS, et al. Blastomycosis like pyoderma with good response to acitretin. Ann Dermatol. 2011;23:365–8.
37. Boer J, Nazary M. Long term results of acitretin therapy hidradenitis suppurativa: is acne inversa also a misnomer? Br J Dermatol. 2011;164:170–5.
38. Anadolu R, Oskay T, Erdem C, et al. Treatment of epidermodysplasia verruciformis with a combination of acitretin and interferon alpha-2a. J Am Acad Dermatol. 2001;45:296–9.
39. Borroni RG, Poddighe D, Zecca M, et al. Efficacy of acitretin for porokeratosis in the child with chronic cutaneous graft versus host disease. Paediatr Dermatol. 2013;30:148–50.
40. Berth-Jones J, Cole J, Lehmann AR, et al. Xeroderma pigmentosum variant: 5 years of tumour suppression by etretinate. J R Soc Med. 1993;86:355–6.
41. Robertson SJ, Bashir SJ, Pichert G, et al. Severe exacerbation of multiple self-healing squamous cell epithelioma (Fergusson Smith disease) with radiotherapy which was successfully treated with acitretin. Clin Exp Dermatol. 2010;35:e100–2.
42. Sanmartin V, Aquavo R, Baradad M, et al. Oral acitretin and topical imiquimod as a neoadjuvant therapy for giant basal cell carcinoma. Actas Dermosifiliogr. 2012;103:149–52.
43. Foxton G, Delaney T. Eruptive keratoacanthoma and squamous cell carcinoma complicating imiquimod therapy: response to oral acitretin. Australas J Dermatol. 2011;52:66–9.
44. Chen K, Craig JC, Shumack S. Oral retinoids for the prevention of skin cancers in solid organ transplant recipients: a systematic review of randomized controlled trials. Br J Dermatol. 2005;152:518–23.
45. Cheely J, Sahn RE, Delong LK, et al. Acitretin for the treatment of cutaneous T cell lymphoma. J Am Acad Dermatol. 2013;68:247–54.
46. Garg T, Ramchandar, Varghese B, et al. Generalized linear porokeratosis: a rare entity with excellent response to acitretin. Dermatol Online J. 2011;15(17):3.

47. Monshi B, Richter L, Hashimoto T, et al. IgA pemphigus of subcorneal pustular dermatosis type. Successful therapy with combination of dapsone and acitretin. Hautarzt. 2012;63:482–6.
48. Darwich E, Munoz Santoz C, Mascaro JM Jr. Erosive pustular dermatosis of the scalp responding to acitretin. Arch Dermatol. 2011;147:252–3.
49. Carlesimo M, Narcisis A, Orsini D, et al. A case of lichen amyloidosis treated with acitretin. Clint Ter. 2011;162:e59–61.
50. Agrawal Y, Petkar KC, Sawant KK. Development, evaluation and clinical studies of acitretin loaded nanostructured lipid carriers for topical treatment of psoriasis. Int J Pharm. 2010;401:93–102.

Alitretinoin

32

Introduction

Alitretinoin, also referred to as 9-*cis*-retinoic acid, is an endogenous first-generation retinoid, routinely present in the skin and circulation. It is acquired following isomerization of tretinoin [1]. Though initially approved by the FDA for topical therapy in localized Kaposi sarcoma (KS), alitretinoin is now utilized both systemically and topically for treating many other dermatologic disorders. Of late, the systemic use of alitretinoin has elaborated propitious outcomes in recalcitrant hand eczema, owing to which it is licensed for this indication in many countries of the European union [2]. Besides, alitretinoin delineates a superior toxicity profile compared to other retinoids, making it a valuable option in the management of other retinoid responsive dermatoses as well.

Mechanism of Action

A distinctive uniqueness of alitretinoin rests on its potential to bind to all subclasses of retinoic acid receptors (RARs) and retinoid X receptors (RXRs). Upon receptor binding, a battery of responses ensue, which finally culminate in protein expression, essential for growth and regulation [3]. In general, the pharmacodynamic sketch of alitretinoin can be split into:

1. Anti-inflammatory and immunomodulatory effects
2. Anti-proliferative and apoptotic effects

A. K. Bubna, *Therapeutics in Dermatology - Essentials for Clinical Practice*, https://doi.org/10.1007/978-981-95-3791-4_32

Anti-inflammatory and Immunomodulatory Effects

By suppressing expression of chemokine receptors and terminating recruitment of inflammatory cells, alitretinoin exhibits its anti-inflammatory and immunomodulatory effects [4]. Besides, alitretinoin notably exhausts the tally of macrophages and activated dendritic cells, two major contributors of TNF-α, thereby considerably reducing inflammation [5]. Other inflammatory mediators diminished by alitretinoin include IL-4, IL-1β and IL-12p40 [6, 7]. Alitretinoin also inhibits production of nitric oxide (NO), secondary to stimulation by other cytokines and lipopolysaccharides, further bringing about immunomodulation by downregulating activity of leucocytes [8].

Anti-proliferative and Apoptotic Effects

RARs and RXRs are responsible for the anti-proliferative and apoptotic effects of alitretinoin, respectively. These facets of alitretinoin are of specific use in the treatment of Kaposi sarcoma (KS). Following binding of alitretinoin to RARs and RXRs in patients of KS, the expression of IL-6 receptors, as well as of viral encoded oncogenes occupying lesions of KS are downregulated [9, 10].

Pharmacokinetics

Following oral intake, the absorption of alitretinoin is variable, with absorption being augmented after intake of food. Besides, alitretinoin is strongly bound to plasma proteins, and its volume of distribution transcends the extracellular volume. The metabolism of alitretinoin occurs in the liver with the CYP3A4 isoenzyme to form 4-oxoalitretinoin. The $t_{1/2}$ of alitretinoin is 2–10 h, with excretion of the drug occurring through the kidneys. Alitretinoin and its 4-oxo metabolite do not accumulate like other systemic retinoids, and therefore after 1 month of stoppage of alitretinoin, pregnancy can be planned [11]. Interestingly, topical alitretinoin lacks extensive systemic exposure [7].

Clinical Uses

Chronic Hand Eczema

Hand eczemas are a group of dermatoses frequently confronted by all dermatologists. Lesions in chronic hand eczema (CHE) vary from erythema and vesiculation at one end of the spectrum to scaling and fissuring at the other. Symptoms include pruritus and pain [12]. The mechanism by means of which alitretinoin improves signs/symptoms in CHE remains obscure, but is propounded that by activating RXRs, alitretinoin stimulates Th2 immune functions, thereby alleviating the pathology observed in CHE [13, 14]. The use of alitretinoin in CHE have shown promising results. Bollag and Ott [14] conducted an exploratory open-labelled study in 1999, with 38 patients who had recalcitrant CHE. The morphologic patterns of CHE encountered in this study were hyperkeratotic palmar eczema, finger-tip eczema, pompholyx and discoid eczema. Patients were administered 20–40 mg of oral alitretinoin for a period of 1–5 months. At the end of the study, 89% of patients assessed by the treating physician showed very good clinical responses. Side effects encountered were transient headache, flushing, conjunctivitis and cheilitis.

In 2004, Ruzicka et al. [15] further substantiated the finding of Bollag and Ott in a randomized double-blind placebo-controlled trial with 348 patients. Only patients who were refractory or intolerant to topical glucocorticoids for at least 4 weeks were enrolled in the study. Morphologic patterns of CHE included were hyperkeratotic hand eczema, finger-tip eczema and pompholyx. Patients were administered 10 mg, 20 mg and 40 mg of alitretinoin once daily along with a placebo group for the purpose of comparison. Treatment was instituted for a period of 12 weeks. At the end of the study, the physician's global assessment (PGA) scores were 27%, 39%, 41% and 53% for responders in the placebo, 10 mg, 20 mg and 40 mg groups, respectively. A significant dose-dependent outcome was demonstrated by the Cochrane Armitage trend test ($p < 0.001$) and evaluation of the total lesion/symptom score (TLSS) showed a 25%, 59%, 52% and 70.5% decrease of lesions in the placebo, 10 mg, 20 mg and 40 mg doses, respectively. Besides, results obtained showed a $p < 0.001$, which was significant as per the Kruskal–Wallis test. The Jonckheere–Terpstra trend test further highlighted the importance of dose dependence in alleviation of symptoms and signs following alitretinoin administration. Adverse effects were encountered only with the 40 mg dosed patients, which included flushing, headache, anaemia, hyperlipidaemia and reduced levels of thyroxine.

In 2008, Ruzicka et al. [16] conducted the "Benefit of Alitretinoin in Chronic Hand dermatitis (BACH)" study. This was a larger randomized double-blind placebo-controlled study enrolling a total of 1032 patients. Three groups were allotted, first the placebo group and second and third groups that received 10 and 30 mg of alitretinoin, respectively, for a period of 24 weeks. Morphologic patterns of CHE in this study were hyperkeratotic hand eczema, pompholyx and finger-tip eczema. At the end of 24 weeks, the PGA yielded an efficacy score of 17% in the placebo group, 28% in the 10 mg group and 48% in the 30 mg group. A modified TLSS at 24 weeks was 39%, 56% and 75% in the placebo, 10 mg and 30 mg groups, respectively. The result of this study was at par with the one conducted in 2004.

Further, R. Aguayo Leiva et al. [17] delineated alitretinoin to be effective in CHE recalcitrant to traditional treatment.

Psoriasis

Oral alitretinoin has outlined favorable outcomes in the treatment of palmoplantar pustular psoriasis [18], owing to its immunomodulatory effects on keratinocytes [19], fibroblasts [20], mast cells [21], dendritic cells [22] and T cells [23]. By suppressing the expression of chemokine receptors, alitretinoin intercepts chemotaxis of inflammatory cells [4]. In this way, it brings about a rapid abatement of plaques and pustules encountered in palmoplantar psoriasis. Alitretinoin has also been combined with biologic agents such as adalimumab and etanercept [24] in the management of palmoplantar hyperkeratotic psoriasis with successful outcomes. Nevertheless, more controlled trials are needed to exemplify the efficacy of alitretinoin in the treatment of psoriasis.

Kaposi Sarcoma

Alitretinoin (0.1% gel) is approved by the FDA (since 1999) for localized cutaneous Kaposi sarcoma (KS). In KS, alitretinoin inhibits neo-angiogenesis as well as multiplication of KS cells, apart from regulating keratinocyte differentiation [25]. Further, alitretinoin decreases coherence between malignant keratinocytes and plummets the tendency for malignant degeneration [26–28]. Systemic use of alitretinoin for KS, however, demonstrates mediocre improvement, with an unpropitious toxicity profile, thereby restricting its use [25]. Alitretinoin gel is applied as a twice daily schedule to begin with, and the frequency of application is slowly increased to four applications per day depending on individual endurance [29, 30]. Covering lesions of KS with ample amount of the drug and allowing it to dry for 3–5 min (before covering that area with clothing) is the suggested protocol. Additionally, the area is to be kept free from any form of occlusive dressing. Besides, there should be no contact of the drug with the surrounding normal skin or mucosal surfaces. Response may be seen as early as 2 weeks. With continued application, further improvement is achieved. Alitretinoin can be continued as long as patients benefit from it. Other modalities of treatment like cryotherapy can also be synergized with topical alitretinoin.

Cutaneous Lichen Planus (CLP)

In CLP, alitretinoin is used owing to its anti-inflammatory and immunomodulatory effects. Besides, its role in regulating cellular proliferation, differentiation and apoptosis also significantly contribute towards its beneficial effects in CLP. Molin and Ruzicka [31] delineated systemic alitretinoin (30 mg/day), along with topical glucocorticoids and keratolytic agents to be profitable in the management of CLP, with regression of lesions following a duration of 5–6 months. Besides, no adverse events were encountered. However, more controlled trials are necessary to fully evaluate the role of alitretinoin in CLP.

Nail Lichen Planus (NLP)

Lichen planus of the nails is generally refractory to most treatments. Alsenaid et al. [32] delineated profitability of alitretinoin in two patients with end-stage destructive pterygium, with quality improvement following administration of alitretinoin (30 mg/day) for 8–9 months. Besides, improvement had become visible as early as 2–4 months post institution of treatment. The authors thereby concluded that early institution of alitretinoin in NLP may circumvent formation of pterygium, thereby abrogating the disfiguring effects on the nail apparatus caused by the disease.

Atopic Dermatitis

Grahovac et al. [33] outlined remarkable clinical clearance of lesions in atopic dermatitis (AD) with alitretinoin in a series of six patients observed over a time frame of 3 months. Alitretinoin (30 mg/day) along with emollients and topical immunomodulators was the regimen followed in this report. Furthermore, alitretinoin was well tolerated by all patients in this study. Nevertheless, more robust clinical trials are warranted to strengthen the above observation.

Lichen Simplex Chronicus

D'Erme et al. [34] elucidated the promising role of systemic alitretinoin in a case of recalcitrant lichen simplex chronicus (LSC), given at a dose of 30 mg/day for a period of 3 months. The rationale for employing alitretinoin in LSC was linked with its immunomodulatory and anti-inflammatory effects on various cytokines implicated in LSC. The authors delineated pronounced amelioration in pruritus and resolution of lesions with no relapse. Therefore, alitretinoin can be contemplated as a substitute for recalcitrant LSC. Nonetheless, more clinical trials need to be conducted to verify the above observation.

Cutaneous T Cell Lymphoma

Amongst the retinoids, bexarotene is currently accepted by the FDA in the treatment of cutaneous T cell lymphoma (CTCL), systemically as well as topically. Bexarotene is a rexinoid and acts by promoting apoptosis of malignant cells [35, 36]. Like bexarotene, alitretinoin demonstrates propinquity for RXRs and in this way outlines efficacy in these patients. Molin and Ruzicka [37] elaborated alitretinoin (30 mg/day) to be highly effective in treating CTCL in two patients over a time frame of 4–5 months. Alitretinoin's favourable attributes in CTCL can be due to its anti-proliferative, immune-modulating and pro-apoptotic properties. However, more clinical trials with alitretinoin in CTCL are required to establish its use for this indication.

Photoaging

Baumann et al. [38] propounded alitretinoin (0.1%) gel to be effective and safe, when prescribed for photo-damaged skin. On binding to RARs and RXRs, alitretinoin induces TGF-β, which further stimulates collagen synthesis and helps in the repair of photo-damaged skin [39, 40]. Apart from improving photo-damaged skin, benign skin lesions such as actinic keratosis and seborrheic keratosis also show significant regression.

Pyogenic Granuloma

Maloney et al. [41] described alitretinoin (0.1%) gel to be effective in treating pyogenic granuloma (PG). Based on the similar histologic patterns of PG and KS, 0.1% alitretinoin gel was employed in two adult patients with PG. Of the two patients, one documented complete clinical resolution after 7 days, and the other patient highlighted complete clearance of lesions within 21 days. Besides, in none of the two patients did the condition relapse, after a year of follow-up. Hence, 0.1% alitretinoin gel can be a valid pain-free treatment modality for PG, especially in the paediatric population. However, larger clinical trials are warranted to substantiate the above findings.

Pityriasis Rubra Pilaris

Pityriasis rubra pilaris (PRP) is a chronic and relapsing papulosquamous disorder. Alitretinoin (30 mg/day) along with topical emollients for a period of 16 weeks outlined excellent results in a patient presenting with recalcitrant disease [42]. Besides, side effects encountered were minimal. Based on its anti-inflammatory and immunomodulatory profile on keratinocytes and leukocytes, alitretinoin is able to achieve the desired results. Hence, oral alitretinoin may prove to be a worthwhile option in treating patients with refractory PRP.

Darier's Disease

Darier's disease (DD) is an autosomal dominant genodermatosis presenting as warty, dirty and greasy plaques distributed over the seborrheic areas of the body. Treatment of DD is usually unsatisfactory. Zamiri and Munro [43], Letule et al. [11], Anuset et al. [44] and Barnstedt [45] have demonstrated efficacy of oral alitretinoin in the treatment of DD. Given at a dose of 30 mg daily, improvement was documented as early as 2 weeks after institution of therapy. Alitretinoin's positive role in DD can be explained owing to its effect on cell proliferation, differentiation, keratinization and immunomodulation. However, further clinical trials become decisive in deciding a full-fledged role of alitretinoin in DD.

Keratitis–Ichthyois–Deafness Syndrome

The utility of alitretinoin in the treatment of keratitis–ichthyosis–deafness (KID) syndrome has been propounded by Werchau et al. [46] and Prasad and Bygum [47]. Alitretinoin possesses the ability to induce expression of connexin, and therefore it may be of value in KID syndrome [48, 49]. Werchau et al. described the positive contribution by alitretinoin in accelerating the resolution of cutaneous lesions in a case of KID syndrome. Treatment was started with alitretinoin (10 mg/day) for a fortnight, following which the dose was escalated to 30 mg/day for another 5 months. Following therapy completion, the authors observed sizeable improvement in the skin lesions following alitretinoin use. An added advantage seen was the favourable toxicity profile as well. Prasad and Bygum further outlined alitretinoin to be profitable in a patient with KID syndrome, who also presented with dissecting cellulitis of the scalp. Alitretinoin therefore appears to be a valuable therapeutic alternative in these patients.

Contraindications

Absolute

- Pregnancy/lactation
- Hypersensitivity to alitretinoin

Relative

- Patients less than 18 years of age
- Patients allergic to peanuts and soya as alitretinoin capsules contain soya oil and sorbitol
- Hepatic/renal insufficiency
- Uncontrolled hypercholesterolemia
- Uncontrolled hypertriglyceridemia
- Uncontrolled hypothyroidism
- Hypervitaminosis A
- Patients concomitantly on tetracyclines

Special Precautions While Using Alitretinoin

Caution needs to be exercised while administering alitretinoin in the following scenarios.

Women of Child-Bearing Age

Because alitretinoin is a teratogenic drug, the prescribing dermatologist must be extremely careful while using the drug in this category of patients. The usage of a reliable form of contraception is mandatory, which should be continued for a month even after cessation of therapy [30].

Sun Exposure

Owing to the photo-sensitive properties of alitretinoin gel, it is recommended to minimize ultraviolet light exposure to the treated sites, and usage of a sunblock of SPF 15 or more [30].

Dietary Vitamin A Intake

The dietary intake of vitamin A should not exceed the recommended dietary intake value, because of the risk of hypervitaminosis A.

Drug Interactions

N,*N*-Diethyl-*m*-toluamide (DEET), a constituent of insect repellents, should not be concurrently used with alitretinoin gel. Toxicology studies in animals delineated expanded DEET toxicity when it was a component of the gel formulation [29]. Systemically, alitretinoin hobnobs only with the CYP3A4 enzyme, with no reported interactions with other CYP enzymes such as CYP1A2, 2C9, 2C19 or 2D6. Because of the strong ability of alitretinoin to bind to plasma proteins, the potential of alitretinoin's interactions with substrates of the enzyme CYP3A4 is significantly low. The interaction of alitretinoin with cyclosporine A and ketoconazole does not delineate any modification in their pharmacokinetic properties. However, levels of simvastatin are substantially lowered with concomitant alitretinoin administration; thus dose adjustments are mandatory to secure requisite therapeutic effects from simvastatin. Conversely, the pharmacokinetic profile of alitretinoin is unaffected by cyclosporine A or simvastatin, but ketoconazole elaborates notable elevation in the plasma concentrations of alitretinoin when both drugs are simultaneously given [50]. Similarly, no pertinent interactions are linked with ethinylestradiol/norgestimate oral contraceptive pills and alitretinoin, with no effect on the pharmacokinetic profile for both drugs. These pills can therefore be safely employed for contraception while on alitretinoin [51]. Though there are no pharmacokinetic interactions of alitretinoin and tetracycline, benign intracranial hypertension is a likely complication when both drugs are administered together, and therefore needs avoidance [52]. Further, alitretinoin should not be taken with vitamin A and other retinoids owing to the risk of hypervitaminosis A [53]. Systemic alitretinoin may increase the hepatotoxicity of methotrexate when given together and so must be avoided.

Preliminary Investigations to Be Undertaken Prior to Starting Alitretinoin

- Serum pregnancy test (in women of child-bearing potential)
- Complete blood count with platelets
- Hepatic profile
- Fasting lipid profile
- Renal profile

Adverse Effects

The major side effects seen with oral alitretinoin include headache, dry skin, alopecia, exfoliative dermatitis and hyperlipidaemia. Other side effects include myalgia, facial flushing, dyspnoea, hypertriglyceridemia, hypercalcemia and a decrease in the levels of thyroid stimulating hormone [53]. Topical alitretinoin is associated with erythema and oedema at application sites and rarely complications such as vesiculation, burning, exfoliation and paraesthesia may develop [7]. Alitretinoin like other retinoids is a teratogenic drug. However, owing to its very short $t_{1/2}$, after stopping the drug for a period of 1 month, pregnancy can be contemplated upon, thus proving to be advantageous over other retinoids in this regard.

Availability

Alitretinoin is available as soft capsules under the brand name Toctino (Basilea Medical Ltd., Guildford, England). Strengths available are 10 and 30 mg. Along with the drug, the capsule contains soyabean oil and sorbitol. The 10 mg capsule is brown in colour, whereas the 30 mg capsule has maroon hue.

Conclusion

To conclude, alitretinoin is employed for multiple dermatologic indications. As it has a very short $t_{1/2}$, it proves advantageous in women who are in the child-bearing age group. Further, because of its better safety profile, compared to isotretinoin and acitretin, it may prove to be a better first-line drug for the above indications in the near future.

References

1. Ghasri P, Scheinfeld N. Update on the use of alitretinoin in treating chronic hand eczema. Clin Cosmet Invest Dermatol. 2010;3:59–65.
2. English J. Alitretinoin for the treatment of chronic eczema of the hand. Clin Med Insights Dermatol. 2011;4:7–16.
3. Sami N, Harper JC. Topical retinoids. In: Wolverton SE, editor. Comprehensive dermatologic drug therapy. 2nd ed. Saunders: Elsevier; 2007. p. 625–41.
4. Werner B, Bresch M, Brenner FM, Lima HC. Comparative study of histopathological and immunohistochemical findings in skin biopsies from patients with psoriasis before and after treatment with acitretin. J Cut Pathol. 2008;35:302–10.
5. Shklovskaya E, O'Sullivan BJ, Ng LG, Roediger B, Thomas R, Weninger W, et al. Langerhans cells are committed to immune tolerance induction. Proc Natl Acad Sci USA. 2011;108:18049–54.
6. Bissonette R, Diepgen TL, Elsner P, English J, Graham-Brown RA, Homey B, et al. Redefining treatment options in chronic hand eczema. J Eur Acad Dermatol Venereol. 2010;24(Suppl 3):1–20.
7. Cheng C, Michaels J, Scheinfeld N. Alitretinoin: a comprehensive review. Expert Opin Investig Drugs. 2008;17(3):437–43.
8. Molin S, Ruzicka T. Alitretinoin: a new treatment option for chronic refractory hand eczema. Hautarzt. 2008;59:703–9.
9. Duvic M, Friedman-Kien A, Looney D, Miles SA, Myskowski PL, Scadden DT, et al. Topical treatment of cutaneous lesions of acquired immune deficiency syndrome related Kaposi's sarcoma using alitretinoin gel. Arch Dermatol. 2000;136:1461–9.
10. Bodsworth N, Bloch M, Bower M, Donnell D, Yocum R, International Panretin Gel Study Group. Phase III vehicle controlled, multi-centered study of topical alitretinoin gel 0.1% in cutaneous AIDS related Kaposi's sarcoma. Am J Clin Dermatol. 2001;2:77–87.
11. Letule V, Herzinger T, Ruzicka T, Molin S. Treatment of Darier disease with oral alitretinoin. Clin Exp Dermatol. 2013;38:523–5.
12. Gralund H, Erkko P, Erikson E, Reitamo S. Comparison of cyclosporine and topical betamethasone-7,21-dipropionate in the treatment of severe chronic hand eczema. Acta Derm Venereol. 1996;76:371–6.
13. Stephenson CB, Rasooly R, Jiang X, Ceddia MA, Weaver CT, Chandraratna RA, et al. Vitamin a enhances in vitro Th2 development via retinoid X receptor pathway. J Immunol. 2002;168:4495–503.
14. Bollag W, Ott F. Successful treatment of chronic hand eczema with oral 9-cis retinoic acid. Dermatology. 1999;199:308–12.
15. Ruzicka T, Larsen FG, Galewicz D, Horvath A, Coenraads PJ, Pedersen KT, et al. Oral alitretinoin(9-cis retinoic acid) therapy for chronic hand dermatitis in patients refractory to standard therapy. Arch Dermatol. 2004;140:1453–9.
16. Ruzicka T, Lynde CW, Jemec GB, Diepgen T, Berth-Jones J, Coenraads PJ, et al. Efficacy and safety of oral alitretinoin (9-cis retinoic acid) in patients with severe hand eczema refractory to topical corticosteroids: results of a randomized double blind, placebo controlled multicentre trial. Br J Dermatol. 2008;158:808–17.
17. Aguaya-Leiva R, Urrutia S, Jaen-Olasolo P. Response to treatment with oral alitretinoin in patients with chronic hand eczema that is refractory to treatment with potent topical corticosteroids: experience in 15 patients. Actas Dermosifilogr. 2011;102:616–22.
18. Irla N, Navarini AA, Yawalkar N. Alitretinoin abrogates innate inflammation in palmoplantar pustular psoriasis. Br J Dermatol. 2012;167:1170–4.
19. Sorenson S, Solvsten H, Politi Y, Kragballe K. Effects of vitamin D3 on keratinocyte proliferation and differentiation in vitro: modulation by ligands for retinoic acid and retinoid X receptors. Skin Pharmacol. 1997;10:144–52.

20. Xiao R, Kanekura T, Yoshida N, Higashi Y, Yan KL, Fukushige T, et al. 9-cis retinoic acid exhibits anti fibrotic activity via induction of cyclooxygenase-2 expression and prostaglandin E2 production in scleroderma fibroblasts. Clin Exp Dermatol. 2008;33:484–90.
21. Ko J, Yun CY, Lee JS, KiM DH, Yuk JE, Kim IS. Differential regulation of CC chemokine receptors by 9-cis retinoic acid in human mast cell line, HMC-1. Life Sci. 2006;79:1293–300.
22. Zapata-Gonzalez F, Rueda F, Petriz J, Domingo P, Villarroya F, de Madariaga A, et al. 9-cis retinoic acid(9cRA), a retinoid X receptor (RXR) ligand, exerts immunosuppressive effects on dendritic cells by RXR-dependant activation: inhibition of peroxisome proliferator-activated receptor gamma blocks some of the 9cRA activities and precludes them to mature phenotype development. J Immunol. 2007;178:6130–9.
23. Dawson HD, Collins G, Pyle R, Key M, Weeraratna A, Deep-Dixit V, et al. Direct and indirect effects of retinoic acid on human Th2 cytokine and chemokine expression by human T lymphocytes. BMC Immunol. 2006;7:27.
24. Meyer V, Goerge T, Luger TA, Beissert S. Successful treatment of palmoplantar hyperkeratotic psoriasis with combination of etanercept and alitretinoin. J Clin Aesthet Dermatol. 2011;4(4):45–6.
25. Schwartz RA, Micali G, Nasca RM, Scuderi L. Kaposi sarcoma: a continuing conundrum. J Am Acad Dermatol. 2008;59:179–206.
26. Levine AM, Tulpule A. Clinical aspects and management of AIDS-related Kaposi's sarcoma. Eur J Cancer. 2001;37:1288–95.
27. Massod R, Nagpal S, Zheng T, Cai J, Tulpule A, Smith DL, et al. Kaposi sarcoma is a therapeutic agent for vit D(3) receptor agonist. Blood. 2000;96:3188–94.
28. Aboulafia DM, Norris D, Henry D, Grossman RJ, Thomas J, Bundow D, et al. 9 cis retinoic acid capsules in the treatment of AIDS related Kaposi sarcoma: results of a phase 2 multicentre clinical trial. Arch Dermatol. 2003;139:178–86.
29. Cheer SM, Foster RH. Alitretinoin. Am J Clin Dermatol. 2000;1(5):307–14.
30. Ligand pharmaceuticals. Panretin(alitretinoin) prescribing information; 2006.
31. Molin S, Ruzicka T. Oral alitretinoin in lichen planus: two case reports. Acta Derm Venereol. 2010;90:523–4.
32. Alsenaid A, Eder I, Ruzicka T, Braun-Falco M, Wolf R. Successful treatment of nail lichen planus with alitretinoin: report of 2 cases and review of the literature. Dermatology. 2014;229(4):293–6. [Epub ahead of print].
33. Grahovac M, Molin S, Prinz JC, Ruzicka T, Wollenberg A. Treatment of atopic eczema with oral alitretinoin. Br J Dermatol. 2010;162:217.
34. D'Emre AM, Milanesi N, Agnoletti AF, Maio V, Massi D. Efficacy of treatment with oral alitretinoin in patient suffering from lichen simplex chronicus and severe atopic dermatitis of the hands. Dermatol Ther. 2014;27:21–3.
35. Zhang C, Hazarika P, Ni X, Weidner DA, Duvic M. Induction of apoptosis by bexarotene in cutaneous T-cell lymphoma cells: relevance to mechanism of therapeutic action. Clin Cancer Res. 2002;8:1234–40.
36. Budgin JB, Richardson SK, Newton SB, Wysocka M, Zaki MH, Benoit B, et al. Biological effects of bexarotene in cutaneous T-cell lymphoma. Arch Dermatol. 2005;141:315–21.
37. Molin S, Ruzicka T. Possible benefit of oral alitretinoin in T-lymphoproliferative diseases: a report of two patients with palmoplantar hyperkeratotic rhagadiform skin changes and mycosis fungoides or Sezary syndrome. Br J Dermatol. 2009;169:1420–1.
38. Baumann L, Vujevich J, Halem M, Martin LK, Kerdel F, Lazarus M, et al. Open label pilot study of alitretinoin gel 0.1% in the treatment of photoaging. Cutis. 2005;76:69–73.
39. Glick AB, Flanders KC, Danielpour D, Yuspa SH, Sporn MB. Retinoic acid induces transforming growth factor-beta 2 in cultured keratinocytes and mouse epidermis. Cell Regul. 1989;1:87–97.
40. Kim HJ, Bogdan NJ, D'Agostaro LJ, Gold LI, Bryce GF. Effect of topical retinoic acids on the levels of collagen mRNA during the repair of UVB-induced dermal damage in the hairless mouse and the possible role of TGF-beta as a mediator. J Invest Dermatol. 1992;98:359–63.

41. Maloney DM, Schmidt JD, Duvic M. Alitretinoin gel to treat pyogenic granuloma. J Am Acad Dermatol. 2002;47:969–70.
42. Molin S, Ruzicka T. Treatment of refractory pityriasis rubra pilaris with oral alitretinoin: case report. Br J Dermatol. 2010;163:221–2.
43. Zamiri M, Munro CS. Successful treatment with oral alitretinoin in women of child bearing potential with Darier's disease. Br J Dermatol. 2013;169(3):709–10.
44. Anuset D, Goutorbe C, Bernard P, Reguiai. Efficacy of oral alitretinoin for the treatment of Darier disease: a case report. J Am Acad Dermatol. 2014;71:e46–8.
45. Barnstedt SE. Successful treatment of Darier disease with oral alitretinoin. Hautarzt. 2012;63:139–41.
46. Werchau S, Toberer F, Enk A, Helmbold P. Keratitis-ichthyosis-deafness syndrome: response to alitretinoin and review of literature. Arch Dermatol. 2011;147:993–5.
47. Prasad SC, Bygum A. Successful treatment with alitretinoin of dissecting cellulitis of the scalp in keratitis-ichthyosis-deafness syndrome. Acta Derm Venereol. 2013;93(4):473–4.
48. Bertram JS, Vine AL. Cancer prevention by retinoids and carotenoids: independent action on a common target. Biochem Biophys Acta. 2005;1740(2):170–8.
49. Liu YB, Xu B, Wang JW, Fang HQ, Li JT, Li HJ, et al. Effects of all-trans retinoic acid on expression of connexin genes and gap junction communication in hepatocellular carcinoma cell lines [in Chinese]. Zhonghua Yi Xue Za Zhi. 2005;85(20):1414–8.
50. Schmitt-Hoffmann AH, Roos B, Sauer J, Spickermann J, Maaares J, Schoetzau A, et al. Pharmacokinetic interactions between alitretinoin and ketoconazole or simvastatin or cyclosporine A. Clin Exp Dermatol. 2011;36(Suppl 2):24–8.
51. Schmitt-Hoffmann AH, Roos B, Sauer J, Schleimer M, Schoetzau A, Leese PT, et al. Influence of alitretinoin on the pharmacokinetics of the oral contraceptive ethinylestradiol/norgestimate. Clin Exp Dermatol. 2011;36(Suppl 2):4–11.
52. Garnock-Jones KP, Perry CM. Alitretinoin in severe chronic hand eczema. Drugs. 2009;69(12):1625–34.
53. King T, McKenna J, Alexandroff AB. Alitretinoin for the treatment of severe chronic hand eczema. Patient Prefer Adherence. 2014;8:1629–34.

33 Bexarotene

Introduction

Bexarotene (BXT) is a third-generation synthetic retinoid that is indicated for treating skin manifestations of advanced stage cutaneous T cell lymphoma (CTCL) in adults unresponsive to at least one systemic treatment.

Mechanism of Action

BXT binds selectively to retinoid X receptors (RXRs) α, β and γ. Once activated, these receptors function as transcription factors and modulate cellular differentiation and proliferation, apoptosis and insulin sensitization [1].

In vitro, BXT has also shown to block growth of tumour cell lines that are of haematopoietic and squamous cell origin. Further, in vivo studies have elucidated BXT to play a role in tumour regression, as well as preventing tumour induction in some animal models.

Pharmacokinetics

BXT exhibits linear pharmacokinetics up to a dose of 650 mg/m^2. The elimination $t_{1/2}$ of BXT ranges from 1 to 3 h. Greater than 99% of BXT is bound to plasma proteins. BXT undergoes hepatic metabolism by glucuronidation and oxidation, leading to the formation of metabolites, 6 and 7-OH-BXT and 6 and 7-oxo-BXT, respectively. BXT should be consumed after food as this enhances its bioavailability. The elimination of BXT is by the faecal route. Renal elimination is not a significant pathway for BXT.

A. K. Bubna, *Therapeutics in Dermatology - Essentials for Clinical Practice*,
https://doi.org/10.1007/978-981-95-3791-4_33

Clinical Use

The US FDA has approved BXT for the treatment of CTCL [2–4].

BXT produces dose-dependent apoptosis of CTCL cell lines, as well as peripheral blood cells in patients with Sezary syndrome. Besides, BXT downregulates chemokine receptor 4 and E-selectin expression that influence malignant T cell trafficking to the skin [5–7]. Besides, BXT is used both as monotherapy and combination therapy in CTCL.

BXT monotherapy is employed for early as well as late-stage CTCL, with higher response rates obtained in early stage disease [8, 9]. However, Quereux et al. documented similar responses for both early- and late-stage CTCL, along with safe administration of the drug for 5 years [10].

Therapies combined with BXT for CTCL include PUVA, IFNα, extracorporeal photopheresis, vorinostat, methotrexate, denileukin diftitox, gemcitabine and pralatrexate [11–17]. Of the combinations utilized, superior long-term responses have been accounted with pralatrexate and denileukin diftitox [16, 17]. Interestingly, triple therapy consisting of BXT, INFα and extracorporeal photopheresis is in widespread use for erythrodermic mycosis fungoides [12].

Although combined BXT and PUVA therapies outline swifter responses in comparison to PUVA monotherapy (5.8 months vs 9.7 months), no significant response rates are observed while comparing both groups ($p = 0.57$). However, in early-stage disease (IA–IIA), fewer PUVA sessions are required to obtain the therapeutic effect [11].

Further, reports have elucidated an overall response rate of only 26% with vorinostat in combination with BXT, which is not superior to results from trials testing both drugs individually. Besides, this combined regimen is plagued with high rates of adverse events, including severe ones [9, 13]. Similarly, BXT and gemcitabine combination does not delineate satisfactory overall responses [15].

Dosing Schedule

The dosing schedule is described in Table 33.1.

Table 33.1 Approach to initiating bexarotene therapy for cutaneous T cell lymphoma

Time	Bexarotene administration	Monitoring	Management of side effects
Prior to treatment		Baseline: Complete blood count Basic metabolic panel Hepatic panel Thyroid profile Fasting lipid profile Creatinine kinase Also to determine if patient is on any medication that inhibit or induce CYP3A4	Dietary and life style modifications to minimize risk of hyperlipidaemia If preexisting laboratory abnormalities, administer: levothyroxine to achieve normal T_4 levels a fibrate (e.g. fenofibrate) to achieve triglyceride levels <200 mg/dL and HDL level > 50 mg/dL a statin to achieve LDL levels <160 mg/dL
Day 7 (i.e. 7 days prior to starting BXT)			Start fenofibrate 145–200 mg/day, regardless of baseline lipid levels. Atorvastatin may be added if needed. However, gemfibrozil should be avoided. Reduce dose in patients with decreased creatinine clearance
Day 0	Start BXT 150 mg/m^2 daily		Start levothyroxine 0.05 mg/day
Days 7–28		Free T_4 and fasting lipid panel every 1–2 weeks Monitor free T_4 as an indicator of hypothyroidism as BXT lowers TSH levels (central hypothyroidism)	Adjust levothyroxine and fibrate doses and/or add statin as required to keep laboratory values in target ranges Niacin represents another option for patients with combined hyperlipidaemia as patients receiving fibrates and statins concomitantly may be at an increased risk of rhabdomyolysis
Day 28	Increase the dose to BXT 300 mg/m^2 daily (may increase dose as early as Day 14 or, if more time is required to normalize lipid and free T_4 levels, then after day 28)		
Day 29 onward	Adjust BXT dose as needed depending on disease response up to 650 mg/m^2/day	Free T_4 and fasting lipid panel every 1–2 weeks until target range and after subsequent dose changes, otherwise every 1–2 months Complete blood counts every 1–2 months	As above; a triglyceride level of <400 mg/dL may be a more realistic target for some patients

Contraindications

Absolute

- Pregnancy
- Lactation
- Hypersensitivity to the drug
- Women of child-bearing potential without effective birth control measures
- Children ≤18 years of age

Relative

- History of pancreatitis
- Uncontrolled hypercholesterolemia
- Uncontrolled hypertriglyceridemia
- Hypervitaminosis A
- Uncontrolled thyroid disease
- Hepatic insufficiency
- Ongoing systemic infections

Pregnancy prescribing status: Category 'X'.

Adverse Effects

Haematological

- Leukopenia
- Hypochromic anaemia
- Blood dyscrasia
- Purpura

Endocrine

- Hypothyroidism [18]

Metabolic

- Hyperlipidaemia
- Hypercholesterolemia
- Increased hepatic transaminases

Central Nervous System

- Dizziness
- Insomnia
- Hyperesthesia
- Vertigo

Ocular

- Dry eyes
- Blepharitis
- Conjunctivitis
- Amblyopia

Ear

- Deafness

Gastrointestinal

- Nausea
- Vomiting
- Diarrhoea
- Dry mouth
- Constipation
- Flatulence
- Pancreatitis

Cutaneous

- Exfoliative dermatitis
- Pruritus
- Alopecia
- Dry skin

Musculoskeletal

- Bone pain
- Arthralgia
- Myalgia

Renal

- Albuminuria

Drug Interactions

- *Vitamin A*: Patients on BXT should limit vitamin A supplementation to ≤15,000 IU/day to avoid potential additive toxic effects.
- *Insulin, sulfonylureas and thiazolidinediones*: BXT potentially enhances action of these agents, resulting in hypoglycaemia. No case of hypoglycaemia associated with BXT monotherapy have been reported though.
- *Oral contraceptives*: BXT can potentially induce metabolic enzymes and thereby theoretically reduce efficacy of oestrogen and progesterone containing oral contraceptives. Thus, if treatment with BXT is intended in a woman with child-bearing potential, a reliable non-hormonal form of contraception is also required because BXT belongs to a therapeutic class for which human foetal malformation risk is high.

Conclusion

BXT is a retinoid found to be of value in CTCL. Caution must be exercised while administering BXT owing to its side effect profile.

References

1. Budgin JB, Richardson SK, Newton SB, et al. Biologic effects of bexarotene in cutaneous T cell lymphoma. Arch Dermatol. 2005;141:315–21.
2. Duvic M, Martin AG, Kim Y, et al. Phase 2 and 3 clinical trials of oral bexarotene (Targetrin capsules) for the treatment of refractory or persistent early-stage cutaneous T cell lymphoma. Arch Dermatol. 2001;137:581–93.
3. Duvic M, Hymes K, Heald P, et al. Bexarotene is effective and safe for treatment of refractory advanced stage cutaneous T cell lymphoma: multinational phase II-III trial results. J Clin Oncol. 2001;19:2456–71.
4. Gniadecki R, Assaf C, Bagot M, et al. The optimal use of bexarotene in cutaneous T cell lymphoma. Br J Dermatol. 2007;157:433–40.
5. Zhang C, Hazarika P, Ni X, Weidner DA, Duvic M. Induction of apoptosis by bexarotene in cutaneous T-cell lymphoma cells: relevance to mechanism of therapeutic action. Clin Cancer Res. 2002;8:1234–40.
6. Budgin JB, Richardson SK, Newton SB, Wysocka M, Zaki MH, Benoit B, et al. Biological effects of bexarotene in cutaneous T-cell lymphoma. Arch Dermatol. 2005;141:315–21.
7. Richardson SK, Newton SB, Bach TL, Budgin JB, Benoit BM, Lin JH, et al. Bexarotene blunts malignant T-cell chemotaxis in Sezary syndrome: reduction of chemokine receptor 4-positive lymphocytes and decreased chemotaxis to thymus and activation-regulated chemokine. Am J Hematol. 2007;82:792–7.

8. Talpur R, Ward S, Apisarnthanarax N, Breuer-Mcham J, Duvic M. Optimizing bexarotene therapy for cutaneous T-cell lymphoma. J Am Acad Dermatol. 2002;47:672–84.
9. Väkevä L, Ranki A, Hahtola S. Ten-year experience of bexarotene therapy for cutaneous T-cell lymphoma in Finland. Acta Derm Venereol. 2012;92:258–63.
10. Quéreux G, Saint-Jean M, Peuvrel L, Brocard A, Knol AC, Dréno B. Bexarotene in cutaneous T-cell lymphoma: third retrospective study of long-term cohort and review of the literature. Expert Opin Pharmacother. 2013;14:1711–21.
11. Whittaker S, Ortiz P, Dummer R, Ranki A, Hasan B, Meulemans B, et al. Efficacy and safety of bexarotene combined with psoralen-ultraviolet A (PUVA) compared with PUVA treatment alone in stage IB-IIA mycosis fungoides: final results from the EORTC Cutaneous Lymphoma Task Force phase III randomized clinical trial (NCT00056056). Br J Dermatol. 2012;167:678–87.
12. Panchal MR, Scarisbrick JJ. The utility of bexarotene in mycosis fungoides and Sézary syndrome. Onco Targets Ther. 2015;8:367–73.
13. Dummer R, Beyer M, Hymes K, Epping MT, Bernards R, Steinhoff M, et al. Vorinostat combined with bexarotene for treatment of cutaneous T-cell lymphoma: in vitro and phase I clinical evidence supporting augmentation of retinoic acid receptor/retinoid X receptor activation by histone deacetylase inhibition. Leuk Lymphoma. 2012;53:1501–8.
14. Kannangara AP, Levitan D, Fleischer AB Jr. Evaluation of the efficacy of the combination of oral bexarotene and methotrexate for the treatment of early-stage treatment-refractory cutaneous T-cell lymphoma. J Dermatolog Treat. 2009;20:169–76.
15. Illidge T, Chan C, Counsell N, Morris S, Scarisbrick J, Gilson D, Popova B, Patrick P, Smith P, Whittaker S, Cowan R. Phase II study of gemcitabine and bexarotene (GEMBEX) in the treatment of cutaneous T-cell lymphoma. Br J Cancer. 2013;109:2566–73.
16. Foss F, Demierre MF, DiVenuti G. A phase-1 trial of bexarotene and denileukin diftitox in patients with relapsed or refractory cutaneous T-cell lymphoma. Blood. 2005;106:454–7.
17. Talpur R, Thompson A, Gangar P, Duvic M. Pralatrexate alone or in combination with bexarotene: long-term tolerability in relapsed/refractory mycosis fungoides. Clin Lymphoma Myeloma Leuk. 2014;14:297–304.
18. Sherman SI. Etiology, diagnosis and treatment recommendations of central hypothyroidism associated with bexarotene therapy for cutaneous T cell lymphoma. Clin Lymphoma. 2003;3:249–52.

Part VII

Biologic Immunomodulators

Tumour Necrosis Factor α Antagonists

34

Adalimumab: Introduction

Adalimumab was introduced in 2003 for the management of various dermatological and non-dermatological indications. It is a fully human IgG1 recombinant monoclonal antibody that only targets tumour necrosis factor alpha (TNFα), with no interaction with either TNF (p55 and p75) receptors.

Mechanism of Action

The mechanism of action of adalimumab is elucidated in Fig. 34.1 [1].

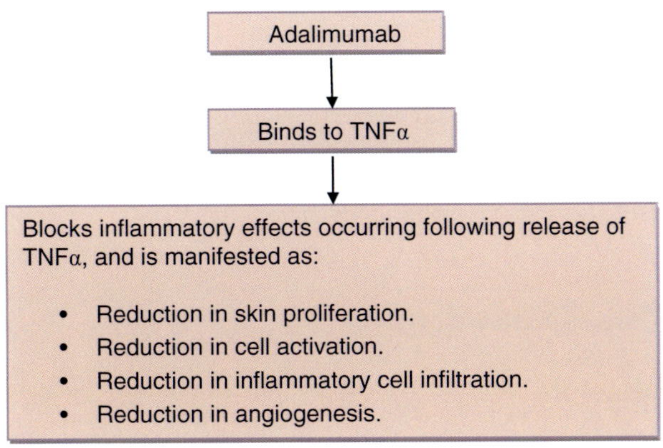

Fig. 34.1 Mechanism of action of adalimumab

A. K. Bubna, *Therapeutics in Dermatology - Essentials for Clinical Practice*, https://doi.org/10.1007/978-981-95-3791-4_34

Pharmacokinetics

Adalimumab is administered subcutaneously. Its bioavailability after a single subcutaneous injection is 64%. The $t_{1/2}$ of adalimumab is 14 days. Therapeutic effects of adalimumab are seen within 24 h to 7 days. By the end of a fortnight, maximum effects of the drug can be witnessed. The metabolism of adalimumab occurs by proteolysis. Fragments of the drug are excreted into bile and urine [2, 3].

Indications

FDA Approved

- Moderate to severe plaque type psoriasis.
- Psoriatic arthropathy.
- Hidradenitis suppurativa (HS).
- Rheumatoid arthritis.
- Juvenile idiopathic arthritis.
- Ankylosing spondylitis.
- Crohn's disease.
- Ulcerative colitis.

Off-Label

- Pyoderma gangrenosum (PG).
- Behcet's disease (BD).
- Wegener's granulomatosis (WG).
- Sarcoidosis.
- Pemphigus vulgaris (PV).
- Multicentric reticulohistiocytosis (MR).
- Alopecia areata (AA).
- Subcorneal pustular dermatosis (SCPD).

Contraindications

Absolute

- Known hypersensitivity to the drug.
- Concurrent administration of anakinra (IL-1 receptor antagonist).
- Active infections.
- Chronic/localized infections.
- Malignancies.

Relative

- Family history of demyelinating disease (including multiple sclerosis).

Pregnancy prescribing status: Category 'B'.

Clinical Uses

Psoriasis

Adalimumab is a valuable therapeutic agent for psoriasis unresponsive to conventional therapeutic modalities. Here, adalimumab is initiated as an 80 mg subcutaneous (SC) dose, followed by a second dose of 40 mg after 1 week. This 40 mg dose is then continued every other week for a total of 12–16 weeks. If no response is noticeable, then treatment may need reconsideration. In patients who respond to treatment, it is continued further as per the clinician's discretion. Besides, the safety profile of adalimumab is favourable with the most common side effects being upper respiratory tract infections, nasopharyngitis, headache and injection site reactions [4].

Hidradenitis Suppurativa

Literature has described association of hidradenitis suppurativa (HS) with Crohn's disease (with an increased activity of TNFα being common in both) [5].

Moul and Korman [6] were the first to describe successful treatment of Hurley stage III HS in a 67-year-old white man, where adalimumab 40 mg SC was administered once every other week. After 1 month of treatment, pain over his lesions had completely resolved, and drainage from his ears and axilla had considerably diminished. At 4 months of follow-up, improvement had become even more, with no drainage in the axilla, ears, retro-auricular region, and notable reduction in drainage from the patient's groins and perineum.

According to Blanco et al. [7], adalimumab should be used in HS only if the following criteria are fulfilled:

- HS recalcitrant to standard medical therapies,
- Lack of response to at least one systemic immunosuppressive/immunomodulatory drug,
- Multifocal active HS, and.
- At least 1 year of follow-up with insignificant response.

The recommended dose of adalimumab in HS patients (> 12 years of age, weighing > 60 kilograms) is 160mg subcutaneously on day 1, followed by 80mg on day

15. Thereafter, a maintenance dose of 40 mg is administered every week, or 80 mg every fortnightly. In patients whose weight range from 30 kilograms to less than 60 kilograms, adalimumab is dosed at 80 mg on day 1, followed by a maintenance schedule of 40 mg every other week, starting from day 8. Further, if clinical remission is noted, then the dose can be gradually tapered to 40 mg SC once every 3 weeks. Moreover, prior to starting adalimumab, specific antibiotics can be administered and continued for another 2 weeks after initiation of adalimumab therapy.

It was in May 2015 that the FDA approved adalimumab for the treatment of Hurley II and III stages of HS.

Pyoderma Gangrenosum

Heffernan et al. [8] demonstrated adalimumab to be an effective therapeutic agent in pyoderma gangrenosum (PG) unresponsive to aggressive topical therapies, and in those patients where systemic glucocorticoids or cyclosporine usage were risky, as in diabetes mellitus and hypertension. In their patient the dose of adalimumab administered was 80 mg SC per week for 2 weeks, followed by 40 mg/week for the next 6 months. By the end of 2 months, improvement had set in, and by 5.5 months, complete ulcer healing was documented.

Similarly, Hinterberger et al. [9] demonstrated the beneficial properties of adalimumab in PG. Their dosing schedule for adalimumab was 80 mg SC at week 0, 40 mg SC in week 1, followed by 40 mg every other week for 64 weeks. However, adalimumab was not completely stopped. A maintenance dose of 40 mg per month was continued.

Rationale behind the use of adalimumab in PG is the heightened levels of TNFα in these patients, owing to abnormal T cell responses.

Sweet's Syndrome

Agarwal et al. [10] demonstrated a dramatic, robust clinical response in case of subcutaneous sweet's syndrome (SS) in a middle-aged man unable to maintain with prednisolone (20 mg/day) and dapsone (200 mg/day). Adalimumab was given at a dose of 40 mg SC every week, with no relapses encountered at 6 months of follow-up.

Though adalimumab is proposed as a treatment option for SS, occurrence of paradoxical SS is a possibility. Keidel et al. [11] reported development of SS after adalimumab therapy for refractory relapsing polychondritis.

Behcet's Disease

Behcet's disease (BD) is a chronic systemic inflammatory disorder characterized by mucocutaneous, ocular, articular, vascular, gastrointestinal and central nervous system manifestations.

Adalimumab is successfully used in cases of BD refractory to both conventional treatment and infliximab therapy. Compared with infliximab, adalimumab offers several advantages such as the ability to self-administer at home, better patient compliance and an improved side effect profile. Adalimumab is administered at a dose of 40 mg SC every fortnightly in BD. Apart from improvement in cutaneous features, adalimumab demonstrates improvement in uveitis associated with BD [12–18].

With regard to severe aphthosis in BD, Perra et al. [19] documented complete response in 62.5% of their patients.

Similarly in intestinal BD, Tanida et al. [20] demonstrated adalimumab to be effective with marked improvement demonstrable after 52 weeks of treatment.

There is accumulating evidence that adalimumab is safe and effective for the treatment of serious manifestations of BD, with sparing effects of conventional immunosuppressive agents and glucocorticoids. However, long-term, large-scale studies are warranted to determine the efficacy and safety of adalimumab in BD.

Sarcoidosis

Adalimumab is reported to be successful in treating cutaneous sarcoidosis.

Heffernan and Smith [21] reported favourable responses in a 46-year-old black woman with sarcoidosis using adalimumab (40 mg SC per week), combined with pentoxifylline and hydroxychloroquine. Within 5 weeks of initiating adalimumab, improvement was observed.

Similarly, Philips et al. [22] reported excellent responses in a patient with ulcerative cutaneous sarcoidosis, after addition of adalimumab (40 mg SC per week), to the previous ongoing therapy consisting of prednisolone and hydroxychloroquine, within 9 weeks of combining adalimumab.

Pemphigus

Adalimumab (40 mg SC once in 2 weeks) was beneficial in a 41-year-old male with aggressive IgA pemphigus. In this patient, adalimumab was combined with mycophenolate mofetil (1 g/day). After the third dose of adalimumab, lesions cleared completely [23].

Multicentric Reticulohistiocytosis

Shanon et al. [24] described a 37-year-old female with multicentric reticulohistiocytosis (MR) along with erosive arthritis, improving significantly after addition of adalimumab (40 mg SC every other week) to her existing treatment that consisted of MMF, cyclosporine, prednisolone, simvastatin and tramadol.

Adverse Effects

Local Injection Site Reactions [25]

- Mild transient.
- Pruritus.
- Pain.
- Erythema.
- Urticarial plaques.

Hypersensitivity Reactions

- Anaphylaxis.
- Angioedema.

Cutaneous

- Skin infections.
- Allergic rash.
- Urticaria.
- Drug eruptions.
- Eczematous psoriasiform eruptions.
- Vasculitis.
- Ulcers.
- Actinic keratosis.
- Tumours.
- Treatment related plaque psoriasis and pustulosis [26].

Infections

- Incidence of serious infections is 1.7% like fungal pneumonia, septic arthritis and pyelonephritis [27, 28].
- Reactivation of hepatitis B may occur while on adalimumab treatment.
- Latent tuberculosis (TB) can progress to overt TB, or a new onset TB can occur.
- There can be dissemination of TB [29].
- Reactivation of TB usually occurs during the first 8 months of treatment.
- Opportunistic infections such as listeriosis [30], legionella pneumonia [31], aspergillosis, histoplasmosis, pneumocystosis, coccidioidomycosis, candidiasis and paracoccidiodomycois [32].

Malignancies

- Increased risk of developing both Hodgkin's and non-Hodgkin's lymphoma.
- Basal cell carcinoma.
- Squamous cell carcinoma.

Neurologic

- Increased incidence of new onset of or exacerbation of multiple sclerosis.
- Optic neuritis.
- Guillain-Barré syndrome.
- If neurological symptoms suggestive of demyelination develop, therapy should be withdrawn.

Hematologic

- Thrombocytopenia.
- Aplastic anaemia.
- Leukopenia.
- If any fever, bruising or bleeding is noticed, the need for immediate medical attention needs to be emphasized [33].

Cardiovascular

- Worsens the symptoms of congestive cardiac failure (CCF).
- Even cases of new CCF have been observed.

Hepatotoxicity

- There are conflicting reports of the possible role of adalimumab in causing hepatotoxicity.
- Increased risk of re-activation of hepatitis B and C [34].

Drug-Induced Lupus

- Autoantibodies to nuclear and double stranded DNA may develop in 3–12% of cases.
- However, development of overt systemic lupus erythematosus and lupus like syndrome is quite rare.

Drug Interactions

- *Anakinra*: Should not to be given together with adalimumab, owing to increased risk of serious infections and neutropenia.
- *Live attenuated vaccines*: To be similarly avoided.

Monitoring Guidelines

Baseline

- Clinical examination and history.
- Complete blood count (CBC).
- Erythrocyte sedimentation rate.
- C-reactive protein.
- Liver function tests (LFT).
- Urinalysis.
- Mantoux test.
- QuantiFERON TB gold test and T spot TB tests (these are interferon gamma release assays).
- Chest X-ray.
- HBsAg.
- Anti-hepatitis B core IgM antibody.
- Anti-hepatitis C antibody.
- ELISA (enzyme-linked immunosorbent assay).

Follow-Up

- Patient should be monitored once every 3–4 months with CBC and LFT.
- Also, patients must be monitored for the development of infections and consider appropriate diagnostic tests and institute treatment.

Special Populations

Geriatric

- Increased incidence of malignancy and infections.
- Needs to be very carefully planned in this population.

Paediatric

- Has been used only in juvenile idiopathic arthritis.
- There is an increased risk of developing hepatosplenic T cell lymphoma.
- Caution is therefore mandated in ages <4 years and weight < 15 kg.

Pregnancy

- Category 'B' drug.
- Should be used only after judging the risk–benefit ratio.
- To be used only in severe recalcitrant disease.
- Routine usage is not advisable as it crosses the placenta [35].

Lactation

- Can be used with caution.
- Case reports have demonstrated no adverse effects in infants [36].

Availability

Adalimumab is available in pre-filled syringes as a preservative free sterile solution containing 40 mg of the drug. The medicine should be kept in the refrigerator and warmed to room temperature 15 min before injection.

Conclusion

Adalimumab is a well-tolerated biological agent. It has demonstrated excellent efficacy in psoriasis and psoriatic arthritis. Judicious selection of patients appears to be an integral step while managing them with adalimumab in dermatologic clinics.

Infliximab: Introduction

Infliximab (IFX) is a chimeric IgG1 monoclonal antibody specific for TNFα only. Though originally used to manage Crohn's disease, IFX demonstrates benefit in a number of dermatological disorders.

Mechanism of Action

The mechanism of action of IFX is elaborated in Fig. 34.2 [37].

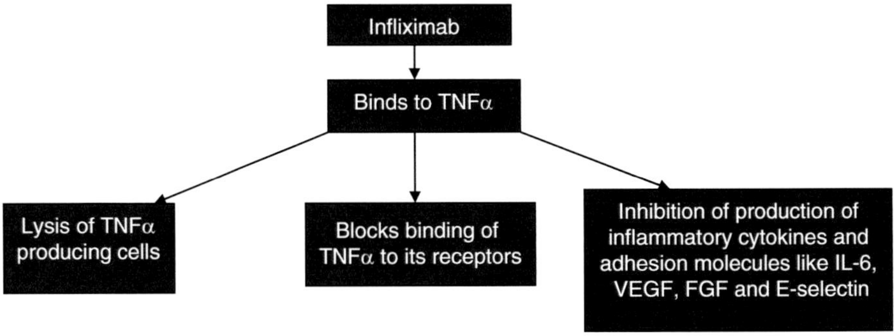

Fig. 34.2 Mechanism of action of infliximab

Pharmacokinetics

IFX is administered intravenously. Its $t_{1/2}$ ranges from 7 to 9 days. The metabolism of IFX occurs by proteolysis. Excretion occurs via the biliary and urinary route [37].

Indications

FDA Approved

- Psoriatic arthritis.
- Plaque type psoriasis.

Off-Label

Neutrophilic Dermatoses
- Pyoderma gangrenosum (PG).
- Behcet's disease (BD).

Vasculitis
- Wegener's granulomatosis (WG).
- Giant cell arteritis (GCA).

Granulomatous Dermatoses
- Sarcoidosis.
- Granuloma annulare (GA).
- Necrobiosis lipoidica.
- Granulomatous cheilitis.

Autoimmune Connective Tissue Disorders

- Dermatomyositis (DM).
- Relapsing polychondritis (RP).
- Polymyositis.

Others

- Graft versus host disease (GVHD).
- Hidradenitis suppurativa (HS).
- Multicentric reticulohistiocytosis.
- Pityriasis rubra pilaris (PRP).
- Reiter's disease.
- Subcorneal pustular dermatosis (SCPD).

Contraindications

Absolute

- Known hypersensitivity to the drug.
- Concurrent administration of anakinra (IL-1 receptor antagonist).
- Active infections.
- Chronic/localized infections, including tuberculosis.

Relative

- Family history of demyelinating disease (including multiple sclerosis).
- Congestive cardiac failure (with a dose of 5 mg/kg).

Pregnancy prescribing status: Category 'B'.

Clinical Uses

Psoriasis

IFX in psoriasis is used only when:

- The disease is severe with PASI score > 10,
- The disease is intolerant or unresponsive to standard treatment,
- The disease is unstable, severe and life-threatening such as generalized pustular psoriasis and erythrodermic psoriasis,
- A patient is suffering from psoriatic arthropathy unresponsive to conventional therapy, and.
- The disease requires repeated in-patient management for control.

In severe psoriasis and psoriatic arthropathy, IFX is administered at a dose of 5–10 mg/kg over a period of 2 h at 0, 2 and 6 weeks. It is then followed by repeat single infusions at 8–12-week intervals. Owing to its chimeric nature, neutralizing antibodies may form in some patients. Concomitant administration of methotrexate with IFX has shown to reduce the formation of these antibodies and prolong the efficacy of IFX [38, 39].

In a 3-year-old child with generalized pustular psoriasis, IFX (5 mg/kg dosing schedule) was effective in controlling the disease. However, after a year of treatment, IFX had to be stopped because of disease recurrence [40].

In a series of four patients, with recalcitrant erythrodermic psoriasis and psoriatic arthritis, which had been recalcitrant to other systemic therapies, a favourable response was documented following combined institution of IFX and methotrexate. The duration of treatment ranged from 9 months to 5 years [41].

Lisby et al. [42] successfully treated a patient of erythrodermic psoriasis with IFX (3 mg/kg) along with methotrexate. After a 14-week remission, relapse was observed in the form of guttate psoriasis and a session with IFX was repeated.

IFX is also effective in clearing lesions of dermatitis repens and psoriasis unguium [43, 44]. However, in a patient with palmoplantar pustulosis, IFX was associated with worsening of the condition [45].

Immunobullous Disorders

The expression of TNFα has been strongly documented in acantholytic cells associated with pemphigus [46]. Taking this feature into consideration, IFX may have a role in treating pemphigus.

Pardo et al. [47] demonstrated IFX to be effective in controlling lesions of pemphigus in a 62-year-old male. However, after 13 successful infusions of IFX (5 mg/kg, per infusion), there was a relapse of the condition, prompting cessation of IFX treatment.

Jacobi et al. [48] also demonstrated IFX to be effective in treating pemphigus. However, development of herpes zoster in their patient necessitated drug discontinuation.

Voigtlander et al. [49] and Bonifati et al. [50] demonstrated IFX to be effective in the treatment of subcorneal pustular dermatosis (SCPD) in individual case reports. However, more studies are required to test the efficacy of IFX in SCPD, whether responses associated with IFX are merely short term or sustained.

Connective Tissue Diseases

In systemic lupus erythematosus (SLE), TNFα is elevated at various stages in the course of the disease. The use of IFX in SLE is associated with decline in disease activity. However, levels of autoantibodies against double stranded DNA were found to be increased following IFX therapy [51].

In dermatomyositis (DM), the role of IFX is particularly noted for the myositis component of the disease [52, 53].

IFX also documents benefit in the treatment of Sjogren's syndrome (SjS). In an open-label study, 16 patients with active primary SjS were treated with IFX at a dose of 3 mg/kg. After 3 infusions at weeks 0, 2 and 6, clinical improvement was observed and persisted for 2 months during the follow-up period [54].

In addition, the above study was extended for 1 more year, enrolling 10 of 16 patients who experienced relapse of symptoms. After administering IFX [3 mg/kg (8 patients) and 5 mg/kg (2 patients)] once every 12 weeks, it is seen that repeated infusions of IFX can ameliorate symptoms of primary SjS for a long time period, without serious side effects [55].

Cutaneous Vasculitis

The efficacy of IFX has been observed in cases of childhood cutaneous polyarteritis nodosa [56], systemic manifestations of Takayasu's arteritis [57], Wegener's granulomatosis (WG) [58], Kawasaki's disease [59], Churg–Strauss syndrome [60] and giant cell arteritis (GCA) [61]. However, treatment failure of IFX along with other drugs has been reported in two patients with refractory vasculitis, secondary to hepatitis C-associated mixed cryoglobulinemia [62].

Further, the occurrence of cutaneous vasculitis with IFX has also been documented, so caution needs to be exercised while using IFX in this scenario [63].

Hidradenitis Suppurativa

Several case series with regard to treatment of hidradenitis suppurativa (HS) with IFX are documented.

Sullivan et al. [64] in a series of five patients reported IFX (5 mg/kg) to be effective in the treatment of HS. In some of the patients of this series, significant reduction in pain was documented, as early as 24 h after the first infusion of IFX. Further, all patients in this study rated IFX as the most effective therapy to date in their disease course.

However, Usmani et al. [65] in their case series did not associate IFX with efficacy in treating HS. Out of the four patients evaluated, two exhibited no improvement, and in the remaining two patients, severe adverse effects necessitated immediate withdrawal of IFX despite temporary response to the drug.

In another series of seven patients diagnosed with HS, moderate to marked improvement was noted in five patients after 6 weeks of initiation of therapy with IFX. However, effects obtained were transient [66].

Absolute avoidance of nicotine appears to be a prerequisite for treatment success of IFX in these patients. Overall, IFX does appear to be a valuable adjuvant to conventional therapeutic strategies for severe cases of HS, as well as an alternative to surgery in problematic cases. Further, in the sense of 'down-staging', IFX can help achieving an operable status in very severe cases of HS. However, controlled clinical studies are needed to determine the necessary duration of therapy more precisely.

Acne

IFX has been effectively used in a patient with acne conglobata and rheumatoid arthritis [67].

In four patients with SAPHO (synovitis, acne, pustulosis, hyperostosis, osteitis) syndrome, after three infusions of IFX (5 mg/kg), complete remission was observed, with patients being in remission for 1 full year [68].

Behcet's Disease

Interleukin (IL)-8, a chemotactic and activating factor for neutrophils, is elevated in patients with Behcet's disease (BD) and may serve as a parameter of disease activity [69].

TNFα is capable of increasing production and release of IL-8 in many target cells; therefore inhibiting TNFα appears a logical principle while treating patients of BD. Case reports of successful treatment of many patients with ocular, oral and genital involvement in BD exist with IFX, showing particularly good responses of lesions characterized by marked neutrophilic infiltrates [70, 71].

Sweet's Syndrome

Association of Sweet's syndrome (SS) with chronic inflammatory bowel disease is known. Case reports of patients with Crohn's disease and associated SS have shown very good effects of IFX on the symptoms of SS [72, 73].

No case reports currently exist in the treatment of SS, unassociated with Crohn's disease. Only limited recommendations on the use of TNFα inhibitors in the treatment of SS are available. It must be remembered that SS is often associated with infection, and treatment with IFX can aggravate them. Decreased immune response while on this drug can cause serious side effects, including sepsis as reported in a single case [72].

Pyoderma Gangrenosum

IFX is used for treating pyoderma gangrenosum (PG) associated with Crohn's disease, as well as those cases unassociated with it.

Brooklyn et al. [74], in a randomized, double-blind, placebo-controlled trial in 30 patients, clearly demonstrated IFX (5 mg/kg once) to be much superior when compared to placebo in treating PG. After 2 weeks of IFX infusion, in 46% of patients, improvement was noticeable in comparison to 6% of patients in the placebo group.

Combining IFX with low dose of methotrexate can help in prolonging treatment responses in PG. Also, this combination prevents formation of autoantibodies to IFX, thereby precluding reduction in efficacy, or the appearance of adverse infusion reactions related to IFX.

Pityriasis Rubra Pilaris

Manoharan et al. [75] reported IFX (5 mg/kg) to be of value in an adult patient with erythrodermic pityriasis rubra pilaris (PRP). Within 2 weeks of the first infusion, beneficial effects were noticed.

In another case report, moderate improvement in PRP with two infusions of IFX (5 mg/kg), combined with acitretin was documented [76].

Atopic Dermatitis

It is noted that patients with atopic dermatitis (AD) demonstrate elevated serum and tissue concentrations of TNFα, thereby allowing TNFα blockers to constitute an alternative option in treating severe cases of AD [77].

In an open, prospective, pilot study, nine adult patients with moderate to severe refractory AD received seven infusions of IFX at a dose of 5 mg/kg and were followed for 46 weeks. A significant improvement was noted in all patients, although it was not maintained for all 46 weeks in the vast majority [78].

Sarcoidosis

Satisfactory outcomes with IFX for sarcoidosis have been documented.

Doty et al. [79], in a retrospective review of 10 patients with various manifestations of sarcoidosis, including skin involvement in 6 cases, which were treated with IFX (5 mg/kg) in combination with prednisolone, noted the efficacy and safety of the drug. In five patients with cutaneous manifestations of sarcoidosis, clinical improvement of skin lesions was noted and in the remaining one patient, there was complete resolution of the rash. In 8 of 10 patients, treatment was well tolerated. In the remaining two, one developed hypertension, flushing and chest pain and the other developed angioimmunoblastic lymphoma, necessitating drug cessation.

Similar results were reported in another retrospective chart review of nine subjects with sarcoidosis who received IFX (3–5 mg/kg). The introduction of IFX allowed reduction in the dose of prednisolone/methotrexate and induced clinical improvement, including remission of skin lesions. Out of the nine subjects, one developed drug-induced lupus, thus emphasizing caution while using IFX [80].

Adverse Effects

Infusion Reactions

Infusion reactions have adverse effects that arise during an infusion and usually may continue up to 3 h after infusion. The side effects comprise headache, dyspnoea, flushing, nausea, taste perversions and injection site infiltrations.

These symptoms usually resolve if the infusion rate is reduced and adjunctive drugs such as anti-histamines and paracetamol are given. These drugs can also be given prior to the infusion as a precautionary measure. Serious cases may require epinephrine and systemic glucocorticoids [81].

Infections

Increased rate of the following infections has been encountered with IFX:

- Pneumonia.
- Cellulitis.
- Abscess.
- Sepsis.
- Reactivation of latent tuberculosis.
- Histoplasmosis.
- Pneumocystis infections.
- Reactivation of hepatitis B in patients who were HBsAg positive [82].

Increased Risk of Malignancies

- Lymphomas.
- Other lymphoproliferative disorders.

Neurologic Diseases

- Demyelinating diseases [83].

Anti-Drug Antibody Formation

These antibodies form due to the chimeric nature of IFX. An increase of these antibodies is associated with an increased clearance rate of IFX, increased incidence of infusion reactions and reduced efficacy of therapy.

The ways to combat this are:

- Concomitant immunomodulatory therapy with methotrexate,
- Pre-medication with oral steroids,
- Continuing with maintenance dose after induction,
- Increasing the dose of IFX per kilogram body weight, and.
- Shortening the dosing interval between doses [84].

Congestive Cardiac Failure

If the dose of IFX is increased from 5 to 10 mg/kg, the chances of increased mortality and morbidity has been demonstrated in patients with heart disease and therefore in these patients, caution needs to be exercised while administering IFX [85].

Hematologic

- Leukopenia.
- Neutropenia.
- Thrombocytopenia.
- Pancytopenia.

Availability

IFX is available as a lipophilized concentrate. Each vial contains 100 mg of IFX. It is re-constituted with 10 mL of sterile water. It is then dosed in 250 mL of 0.9% normal saline over 2 h. Clinical trials have shown efficacy with 3–5 mg/kg of IFX. It would therefore be reasonable to start IFX as 3 mg/kg/day. As IFX has a quick onset of action, this is of particular benefit in severe presentations of psoriasis.

Drug Interactions

- *Anakinra*: Not to be given together with IFX, as increased risk of serious infections and neutropenia.
- *Live attenuated vaccines*: To be similarly avoided.

Monitoring Guidelines

Baseline

- Clinical examination and history.
- Complete blood count (CBC).

- Erythrocyte sedimentation rate.
- C-reactive protein.
- Liver function tests (LFT).
- Urinalysis.
- Mantoux test.
- QuantiFERON TB gold test and T spot TB tests (these are interferon gamma release assays).
- Chest X-ray.
- HBsAg.
- Anti-hepatitis B core IgM antibody.
- Anti-hepatitis C antibody.
- ELISA (enzyme-linked immune solvent assay).

Follow-Up

- Patient should be monitored once every 3–4 months with CBC and LFT.
- Also, patients must be monitored for the development of infections and consider appropriate diagnostic tests and prompt institution of treatment, if any detected.

Conclusion

With the emergence of newer biologic agents, the use of IFX has somewhat reduced for psoriasis. Nevertheless, owing to its swift onset of action, it may be superior compared to other biologic agents to obtain the initial quick fix. However, the main disadvantage with IFX is the need for hospital admission, as it requires medical personnel to administer therapy. Another disadvantage with IFX is development of auto-antibodies. Despite these drawbacks, IFX is still utilized in many centres. The author personally considers IFX to be valuable in generalized pustular psoriasis to control the initial flare in those situations where cyclosporine is contraindicated.

Etanercept: Introduction

Etanercept (ETP) is a recombinant molecule comprising of the human TNFα p75 receptor and the F_c portion of human IgG1 molecule fused together. It is a fully human dimeric fusion protein that functions as a TNF inhibitor by binding to and inactivating TNFα, thereby preventing interaction with its cell surface receptors on target cells and blocking the pro-inflammatory responses [86].

Mechanism of Action

The mechanism of action of ETP is elaborated in Fig. 34.3 [87–90].

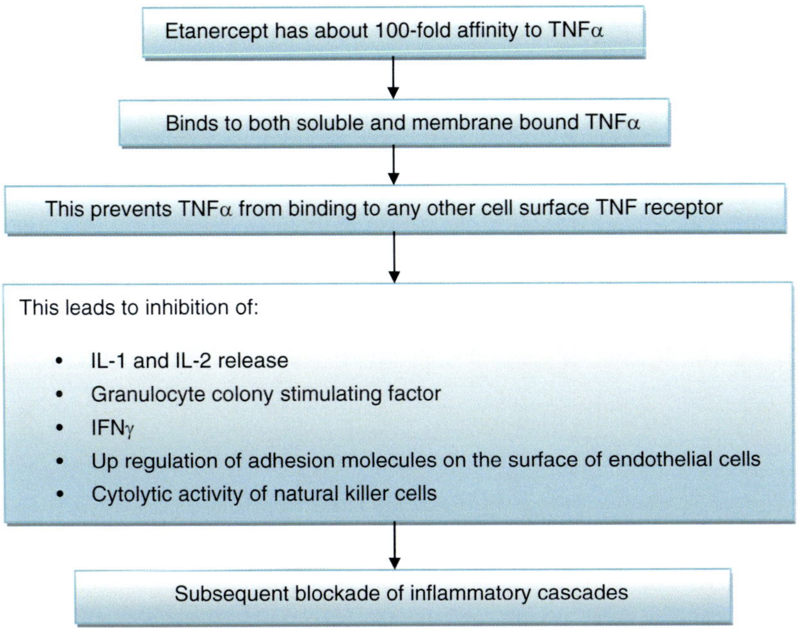

Fig. 34.3 Mechanism of action of etanercept

Pharmacokinetics

Given subcutaneously, ETP gets slowly absorbed, reaching peak levels within 2 days. The $t_{1/2}$ of ETP is 4.8 days, and its absolute bioavailability is 88%. The metabolism occurs via proteolysis. The elimination of the drug occurs via bile and urine [91–93].

Indications

FDA Approved

- Plaque type psoriasis.
- Psoriatic arthropathy.

Off-Label

Bullous Dermatoses

- Pemphigus vulgaris (PV).
- Cicatricial pemphigoid (CP).

Neutrophilic Dermatoses
- Behcet's disease (BD).
- Pyoderma gangrenosum (PG).
- Aphthous stomatitis.

Granulomatous Dermatosis
- Sarcoidosis.

Autoimmune Connective Tissue Disorders
- Dermatomyositis.
- Lupus erythematosus.
- Relapsing polychondritis (RP).

Others
- Hidradenitis suppurativa.
- Graft versus host disease.
- Multicentric reticulohistiocytosis.

Contraindications

Absolute

- Known hypersensitivity.
- Concurrent administration of anakinra (IL-1 receptor antagonist).
- Active infections.
- Chronic or localized infections including tuberculosis.
- Heart failure.

Relative

- Family history of demyelinating disease including multiple sclerosis.
- Malignancy within 5 years of the therapy being initiated.

Pregnancy prescribing status: Category 'B'.

Clinical Uses

Plaque, Pustular and Erythrodermic Psoriasis

Generally, ETP is used for those cases of psoriasis where the disease is resistant to conventional drugs, or when prolonged administration of conventional drugs has produced end organ toxicity. Further, in severe cases of psoriasis such as generalized pustular psoriasis and psoriatic erythroderma where cyclosporine is contraindicated, ETP can be utilized for the immediate quick fix.

Dosing usually begins with 50 mg of ETP given subcutaneously, twice weekly for 12 weeks. Sites for injection include the thighs, abdomen and upper arms. This needs to be rotated with at least 1 inch distance from the last site of injection. Generally, after 12 weeks, substantial clearance is obtained, following which ETP can be administered as 25 mg twice weekly subcutaneously. This can further be reduced to 25 mg once a week as per the clinical assessment, and then completely stopped. This usually takes around 6 months. Besides, no evidence of tachyphylaxis or formation of neutralizing antibodies have been reported with ETP [94–96].

For psoriatic arthropathy, ETP is given at a dose of 25 mg twice weekly. It is usually continued for a minimum of 12 weeks before any change in the dose is contemplated upon. ETP has been approved by the FDA for use in psoriatic arthropathy with methotrexate.

Pemphigus Vulgaris (PV)

PV is a bullous autoimmune disease characterized by autoantibodies against desmogleins 1 and 3, which are adhesion molecules in desmosomes of keratinocytes [97]. TNFα has been linked with the etiopathogenesis of PV, with evidence demonstrating that concentrations of this cytokine in the blister fluid is directly proportional to the clinical activity of the disease [98, 99].

Etanercept can be used alone or in combination with systemic steroids, azathioprine, methotrexate, dapsone and IVIG in PV [99]. The disease is usually successfully controlled within 1–1.5 months of treatment, with reduction in the number of bulla and fewer recurrences. Treatment, however, needs to be continued up to 4 months. Dose of etanercept employed is 50 mg twice weekly given subcutaneously (SC) [97].

Pityriasis Rubra Pilaris (PRP)

PRP is a papulosquamous disorder characterized by follicular hyperkeratosis and palmoplantar keratoderma, with a tendency for progression to erythroderma in some cases. Though etanercept is not a conventional line of management for PRP, in some recalcitrant cases it has been utilized.

Garcovich et al. [100] utilized etanercept 50 mg SC once weekly for PRP and reported 75% improvement for the same.

Similarly, Guedes et al. [101] reported good results in a 30-year-old patient with PRP who was administered etanercept 50 mg SC once a week.

The duration of treatment by both authors was 5 months.

Sarcoidosis

In sarcoidosis, reports utilizing etanercept have been mixed. Though there have been beneficial reports with etanercept for cutaneous sarcoidosis, results with pulmonary and ocular sarcoidosis have been disappointing.

Etanercept in sarcoidosis is usually administered at a dose of 25–50 mg SC/week. It is usually reserved as a second-line drug when treatment with steroids, hydroxychloroquine and methotrexate have failed [102, 103]. However, given the paucity of successful outcomes with etanercept in sarcoidosis, its usage should only be employed as a last resort.

SAPHO (Synovitis, Acne, Pustulosis, Hyperostosis and Osteitis) Syndrome

Etanercept given at 25 mg SC/week for 4 weeks has shown to be effective in SAPHO syndrome in a 27-year-old man who was unsuccessfully treated with antibiotics and isotretinoin. Etanercept heralded improvement in both cutaneous and arthritis components of the disease [104].

Acrodermatitis Continua of Hallopeau (ACH)

ACH is a localized form of pustular psoriasis characterized by formation of pustules on the distal phalanges of the hands and feet, onychodystrophy, paronychia and occasionally osteolysis of the adjacent phalanges.

Puig et al. [105] used etanercept 50 mg SC twice weekly, along with 10 mg of weekly oral methotrexate in ACH for 4 weeks. The response was favourable. However, on tapering both drugs, there was a relapse, with the intensity of paronychia and pain being more severe, incapacitating the patient's day-to-day activities. The treatment in this case was then switched to adalimumab, where the disease was controlled without any relapse.

Hidradenitis Suppurativa (HS)

HS is an inflammatory dermatosis characterized by deep, painful nodules and abscesses that progress to form fistulas, fibrotic plaques and retractile scars. Sites involved include axilla, perianal, submammary and/or inguinal regions.

Etanercept at 25–50 mg SC once or twice weekly for 24 weeks has shown to be effective in controlling the disease. However, once treatment is stopped, there is a high chance of relapse, and that should be borne in mind prior to initiating therapy with etanercept. Moreover, utilizing etanercept as a first-line therapy in HS is not justified [106].

Lupus Erythematosus (LE)

The use of etanercept in LE has been controversial. Some studies have reported that etanercept could even trigger LE, with some studies reporting it to be beneficial [107].

Norman et al. [108] described the case of a 42-year-old patient with subacute cutaneous LE unresponsive to antimalarials, methotrexate and prednisolone, who responded successfully after addition of etanercept 25 mg SC twice weekly to the above regimen.

However, Swale et al. [109] reported a case where etanercept administration resulted in systemic lupus erythematosus (SLE). Therefore, prior to administering etanercept for LE, the pros and cons need to be adequately weighed.

Dermatomyositis (DM)

DM is an autoimmune connective tissue disorder affecting the skin, along with inflammation of proximal striated muscles. Similar to LE, benefits of etanercept in DM is unclear.

In a randomized pilot trial of etanercept in DM wherein 50 mg weekly SC injections were administered to 11 patients, along with gradual taper of prednisolone 5 mg/day by week 24, a mixed response was witnessed. In five subjects, improvement in symptoms were noted, with worsening of symptoms in the remaining six [110].

Similarly, Lannone et al. [111], in their case series of five DM patients, receiving etanercept 25 mg SC twice weekly for 12 weeks, reported exacerbation of the disease in all patients, thereby warranting immediate cessation of etanercept therapy. These patients were later started on methotrexate and azathioprine, which improved disease manifestations in all patients.

Atopic Dermatitis (AD)

In AD, contrasting results have been witnessed following the use of etanercept. Rullan and Murase [112] treated two adults with AD using 50 mg SC etanercept twice weekly for 8–11 months. After this period, despite stopping etanercept therapy, these patients were in remission for almost 26–31 months. However, Buka et al. [113] demonstrated that etanercept was ineffective in their case series of two paediatric patients with AD.

Behcet's Disease (BD)

In a double-blind placebo-controlled study of 40 male patients with BD, it was seen that etanercept given 25 mg SC twice weekly for 4 weeks had an effective role in suppressing most mucocutaneous lesions. The drug had a clear effect on oral ulcers and nodular lesions, and the response was evident as early as the first week of therapy initiation. Almost half of the patients receiving etanercept were free of oral ulcers at the end of the study, compared to 5% of patients in the placebo group. However, etanercept did not affect skin pathergy reaction and skin responses to monosodium urate crystals, which were the primary end points in this study. As far as ocular symptoms were concerned, no mention of that were made in this study [114].

There have been other reports where etanercept has been shown to be effective in BD [115, 116].

Nonetheless, unfavourable responses with etanercept in BD have been reported. In these patients, administration of infliximab later helped in improvement of BD [117, 118].

Pyoderma Gangrenosum (PG)

PG is a neutrophilic dermatosis characterized by deep painful ulcers on the lower extremities with an autoimmune aetiology. Etanercept has been shown to be effective in refractory cases of PG.

McGowen et al. [119] reported etanercept to be a valuable drug while managing a 30-year-old patient with PG refractory to systemic glucocorticoids. Following addition of etanercept 100 mg/week SC, a good therapeutic response was achieved.

Similarly, Goldenburg and Jorizzo [120] demonstrated etanercept (25 mg SC twice weekly) along with prednisolone to be effective in a 30-year-old female patient with PG who also had autoimmune hepatitis.

In another case report of a 49-year-old patient with psoriatic arthritis and vegetative PG, improvement was noticed after 3 weeks of etanercept therapy [121].

Subcorneal Pustular Dermatosis (SCPD)

Berk et al. [122] reported etanercept (50 mg SC twice weekly) to be effective in two cases of SCPD. After 3 months of therapy, there was considerable reduction in the extent and severity of the disease.

Palmoplantar Pustulosis (PPP)

Bissionette et al. [123] reported etanercept (50 mg SC twice weekly for 3 months) to be effective in improving lesions of PPP.

Erythema Nodosum (EN)

EN is the most common panniculitis and represents the prototype of septal panniculitis. Boyd [124], in a 22-year-old female patient, with a 5-year history of EN with frequent relapses and failed treatments following conventional therapeutic modalities; demonstrated favourable response with etanercept (25 mg SC twice weekly). Within 5 months of treatment with etanercept, her EN resolved. Following this, the dose of etanercept was reduced to 25 mg/week, which she continued for 12 months without developing new lesions, thereby suggesting that etanercept can be a good alternative in resistant cases.

Availability

ETP 25 mg is available as a sterile preservative-free lipophilized powder that is reconstituted with 1 mL of supplied bacteriostatic water. The reconstituted solution has to be stored in the refrigerator and not frozen. It is stable for up to 14 days in the refrigerator.

ETP is also available as a 50 mg prefilled syringe. This too needs to be stored in the refrigerator and not frozen.

It should be allowed to return to room temperature for about 15 min prior to injection, to decrease injection site pain [125].

Drug Interaction

ETP should never be administered with anakinra, owing to increased risk of serious infections when used together [126].

Adverse Effects

Injection Site Reactions

- Erythematous, oedematous patch or plaque that may be asymptomatic, tender or pruritic. Treatment includes warm water compresses, topical steroids and oral antihistamines [125].

Precipitation of Tuberculosis

- This poses a major drawback for ETP use.

Malignancy Risk

- Lymphomas.

Reports of Exacerbating Quiescent Multiple Sclerosis and New Onset Demyelinating Disease Has Been Reported

- Symptoms include paraesthesia, confusion and optic neuritis.

Autoimmunity

- Antidrug antibodies are produced in a few patients on ETP, but these antibodies are not neutralizing unlike monoclonal antibodies, nor are they found to be associated with ineffective treatment. Positive anti-nuclear antibodies are reported, but in very few cases actually translate to drug-induced lupus. Further, these antibodies disappear when treatment is discontinued [125].

Drug Monitoring

Baseline

- Complete history and physical examination.
- Screen for underlying tuberculosis.
- Chest X-ray.
- Tuberculin test (not very useful in Indian setting).
- QuantiFERON gold assay (helps in detecting latent tuberculosis).
- Hemogram.
- Liver function tests.
- Renal function tests.
- Hepatitis B and C serology.
- Baseline ANA (anti-nuclear antibody).
- Urinalysis.
- HIV.

Follow-Up

- Once every 2–3 months to repeat a hemogram and liver function tests.

Comparison of TNFα Antagonists

The comparison of TNFα antagonists is elucidated in Table 34.1 [127].

Table 34.1 Comparison of TNFα antagonists

Feature	Etanercept	Infliximab	Adalimumab
Chemistry	Fusion protein of soluble TNF receptor p75 and fc fragment of human IgG	Chimeric human mouse anti-TNFα antagonist	Fully human IgG1 monoclonal antibody against TNFα
Mode of administration	Subcutaneous self- administration	Intravenous (I/V) injection, thereby needing the clinician to administer	Subcutaneous self-administration
Dosing	25–50 mg S/C twice weekly for 12 weeks, then 50 mg once weekly	5 mg/kg I/V at 0, 2, 6 weeks and then once every 8 weeks	80 mg S/C initially and then 40 mg S/C after 1 week, followed by 40 mg S/C every other week
Storage	Must be refrigerated at 2–8 °C and protected from sunlight	Must be refrigerated at 2–8 °C and protected from sunlight	Must be refrigerated at 2–8 °C and protected from sunlight
Onset of action	Slower onset	Early onset	Relatively early onset
Development of antibodies	Decreased chances compared to infliximab	Increases chances of developing autoantibodies	Less chances of developing autoantibodies

References

1. Smith CH, Anstey AV, Barker JN, et al. British association of dermatologists guidelines for biologic intervention for psoriasis 2009. Br J Dermatol. 2009;161:987–1019.
2. Traczewski P, Rudnicka L. Adalimumab in dermatology. Br J Clin Pharmacol. 2008;66:618–25.
3. Scheinfield N. Adalimumab (Humira): A brief review for dermatologists. J Dermatolog Treat. 2004;15:348–52.
4. Alawi EA, Mehlis SL, Gordon KB. Treating psoriasis with adalimumab. Ther Clin Risk Management. 2008;4:341–5.
5. Jacob S, Kerdel F. Biologics for hidradenitis suppurativa (Verneuil's disease in the era of biologics). In: Jemec GBE, Revuz J, Leydon JJ, editors. Hidradenitis suppurativa. Heidelberg: Springer; 2006. p. 145–9.
6. Moul DK, Korman NJ. Severe hidradenitis suppurativa treated with adalimumab. Arch Dermatol. 2006;142:1110–2.
7. Blanco R, Martinez-Taboada VM, Villa I, et al. Long-term successful adalimumab therapy in severe hidradenitis suppurativa. Arch Dermatol. 2009;145:580–4.
8. Heffernan MP, Anadkat MJ, Smith DI. Adalimumab for the treatment of pyoderma gangrenosum. Arch Dermatol. 2007;143:306–8.
9. Hinterberger L, Muller CSL, Vogt T, et al. Adalimumab: a treatment option for pyoderma gangrenosum after failure of systemic standard therapies. Dermatol Ther. 2012;2:6.
10. Agarwal A, Barrow W, Selim MA, et al. Refractory subcutaneous sweet's syndrome treated with adalimumab. JAMA Dermatol. 2016;152:842–4.
11. Keidel S, McColl A, Edmonds S. Sweet's syndrome after adalimumab therapy for refractory relapsing polychondritis. BMJ Case Rep. 2011;2011:bcr1020114935.
12. Van Laar JA, Missotten T, van Daele PL, et al. Adalimumab: a new modality for Behcet's disease? Ann Rheum Dis. 2007;66:565–6.

13. Bawazeer A, Raffa LH. Clinical experience with adalimumab in the treatment of ocular Behcet's disease. Ocul Immunol Inflamm. 2010;18:226–32.
14. Interlandi E, Lessese P, Olivieri I, et al. Adalimumab for treatment of severe Behcet's uveitis: a retrospective long term follow up study. Clin Exp Rheumatol. 2014;32:S58–62.
15. Leccese P, Latanza L, D'Angelo S, et al. Efficacy of switching to adalimumab in a patient with refractory uveitis of Behcet's disease to infliximab. Clin Exp Rheumatol. 2011;29:S93.
16. Mustaq B, Saeed T, Situnayake, et al. Adalimumab for sight threatening uveitis in Behcet's disease. Eye. 2007;21:824–5.
17. Takase K, Ohno S, Ideguchi H, et al. Successful switching to adalimumab in infliximab allergic patient with severe Behcet's disease related uveitis. Rheumatol Int. 2011;31:243–5.
18. Callejas-Rubio JL, Sachez-Cano D, Serrano JL, et al. Adalimumab therapy for refractory uveitis: a pilot study. J Ocul Pharmacol Ther. 2008;24:613–4.
19. Perra D, Alba MA, Callejas JL, et al. Adalimumab for the treatment of Behcet's disease: experience in 19 patients. Rheumatology. 2012;51:1825–31.
20. Tanida S, Inoue N, Kobayashi K, et al. Adalimumab for the treatment of Japanese patients with intestinal Behcet's disease. Clin Gastroenterol Hepatol. 2014:1–11.
21. Heffernan MP, Smith DJ. Adalimumab for treatment of cutaneous sarcoidosis. Arch Dermatol. 2006;142:17–9.
22. Philips MA, Lynch J, Azmi FH. Ulcerative cutaneous sarcoidosis responding to adalimumab. J Am Acad Dermatol. 2005;53:917.
23. Howell SM, Bessinger GT, Altman CE, et al. Rapid response of IgA pemphigus of the subcorneal pustular dermatosis subtype to treatment with adalimumab and mycofenolate mofetil. J Am Acad Dermatol. 2005;53:541–3.
24. Shannon SE, Schumacher HR, Self S, et al. Multicentric reticulohistiocytosis responding to tumor necrosis factor alpha inhibition in a renal transplant patient. J Rheumatol. 2005;32:565–7.
25. Salfeld J, Kupper H. Adalimumab. In: Boehncke WH, Radeke H, editors. Biologics in general medicine. Heidelberg: Springer; 2007. p. 14–31.
26. Aslanidis S, Pyrpasopoulou A, Douma S, et al. Tumor necrosis factor-α antagonist induced psoriasis: yet another paradox in medicine. Clin Rheumatol. 2008;27:377–80.
27. Weinberg JM. A review of safety of tumor necrosis factor inhibitors infliximab, etanercept, adalimumab. In: Weinberg JM, Burholtz R, editors. TNF-alpha inhibitors. Basel: Birkhauser Verlag; 2006. p. 115–27.
28. Scheinfeld N. Adalimumab: A review of side effects. Expert Opin Drug Saf. 2005;4:637–41.
29. Hernandez C, Cetner AS, Jordan JE, et al. Tuberculosis in the age of biologic therapy. J Am Acad Dermatol. 2008;59:363–80.
30. Slifman NR, Gershon SK, Lee JH, et al. Listeria monocytogenes infection as a complication of treatment with tumor necrosis factor neutralizing agents. Arthritis Rheum. 2003;48:319–24.
31. Tubach F, Ravaud P, Salmon CJH, et al. Emergence of legionella pneumophila pneumonia in patients receiving tumor necrosis factor antagonists. Clin Infect Dis. 2006;43:e95–100.
32. Bongartz T, Sutton AJ, Sweeting MJ, et al. Anti TNF antibody therapy in rheumatoid arthritis and the risk of serious infections and malignancies. Systematic review and meta analysis of rare harmful effects in randomized controlled trials. JAMA. 2006;295:2275–85.
33. Bessissow T, Renard M, Hoffman I, et al. Review article: non-malignant hematological complications of anti-tumor necrosis factor alpha therapy. Ailment Pharmacol Ther. 2012;36:312–23.
34. Brunasso AM, Puntoni M, Gulia A, et al. Safety of anti-tumor necrosis factor agents in patients with chronic hepatitis C infection: a systematic review. Rheumatology. 2011;50:1700–11.
35. Murase JE, Heller MM, Butler DC. Safety of dermatologic medications in pregnancy and lactation: part I. Pregnancy J Am Acad Dermatol. 2014;70:e1–e14.
36. Butler DC, Heller MM, Murase JE. Safety of dermatologic medications in pregnancy and lactation: part II. Lactation J Am Acad Dermatol. 2014;70:417–e1-e10.

37. Gottleib AB, Masud S, Ramamurthi R, et al. Pharmacodyanamic and pharmacokinetic response to anti tumor necrosis factor alpha monoclonal antibody (infliximab) treatment for moderate to severe psoriasis vulgaris. J Am Acad Dermatol. 2003;48:68–75.
38. Gottleib AB, Chaudhari U, Malcahy LD, et al. Infliximab monotherapy provides rapid and sustained benefit for plaque type psoriasis. J Am Acad Dermatol. 2003;48:829–35.
39. Gottleib AB, Evans r, Li S, et al. Infliximab induction therapy for patients with severe plaque type psoriasis: a randomized double blind placebo controlled trial. J Am Acad Dermatol. 2004;51:534–42.
40. Pereira TM, Vieira AP, Fernandes JC, et al. Anti-TNFα therapy in childhood pustular psoriasis. Dermatology. 2006;213:350–2.
41. Heikkila H, Ranki A, Cajanus S, et al. Infliximab combined with methotrexate as long term treatment for erythrodermic psoriasis. Arch Dermatol. 2005;141:1607–10.
42. Lisby S, Gniadecki R. Infliximab (remicade) for acute, severe, pustular and erythrodermic psoriasis. Acta Derm Venereol. 2004;84:247–8.
43. Mang R, Ruzika T, Stege H. Successful treatment of acrodermatitis continua of Hallopeau by the tumor necrosis factor alpha inhibitor infliximab (remicade). Br J Dermatol. 2004;150:379–80.
44. Bianchi L, Bergamin A, De Felice C, et al. Remission and time of resolution of nail psoriasis during infliximab therapy. J Am Acad Dermatol. 2005;52:736–7.
45. Michaelson G, Kajermo U, Michaelson A, et al. Infliximab can precipitate as well as worsen palmoplantar pustulosis: possible linkage to the expression of tumor necrosis factor alpha in the normal palmar eccrine sweat duct. Br J Dermatol. 2005;153:1243–4.
46. Lopez-Robles E, Avalos-Diaz E, Vega-Menaije E, et al. TNFα and IL-6 are mediators in the blistering process of pemphigus. Int J Dermatol. 2001;40:185–8.
47. Pardo J, Mercader P, Mahiques L, et al. Infliximab in the management of severe pemphigus vulgaris. Br J Dermatol. 2005;153:222–3.
48. Jacobi A, Schuler G, Hertl M. Rapid control of therapy refractory pemphigus vulgaris by treatment with tumor necrosis factor alpha inhibitor infliximab. Br J Dermatol. 2005;153:448–9.
49. Voigtlander C, Luftl M, Schuler G, et al. Infliximab (anti tumor necrosis factor alpha antibody): a novel, highly effective treatment of recalcitrant subcorneal pustular dermatosis (Sneddon Wilkinson disease). Arch Dermatol. 2001;137:1571–4.
50. Bonifati C, Trento E, Cordiali FP, et al. Early bot not lasting improvement of recalcitrant subcorneal pustular dermatosis (Sneddon Wilkinson disease) after infliximab therapy: relationship with variations in cytokine levels in suction blister fluids. Clin Exp Dermatol. 2005;30:662–5.
51. Aringer M, Steiner G, Graininger WB, et al. Effects of short term infliximab therapy on autoantibodies in systemic lupus erythematosus. Arthritis Rheum. 2007;56:274–9.
52. Selva-O'Callaghan A, Martinez-Costa X, Solans-Laque R, et al. Refractory adult dermatomyositis with pneumotosis cystoides intestinalis treated with infliximab. Rheumatology (Oxford). 2004;43:1196–7.
53. Dold S, Justiniano ME, Marquez J, et al. Treatment of early and refractory dermatomyositis with infliximab. A report of 2 cases. Clin Rheumatol. 2007;26:1186–8.
54. Steinfeld SD, Demols P, Salmon I, et al. Infliximab in patients with primary Sjogren's syndrome: A pilot study. Arthritis Rheum. 2001;44:2371–5.
55. Steinfeld SD, Demols P, Appelboom T. Infliximab in primary Sjogren's syndrome: one year follow up. Arthritis Rheum. 2002;46:3301–3.
56. Vega Gutierrez J, Rodriguez Prieto MA, Garcia Ruiz JM. Successful treatment of childhood cutaneous polyarteritis nodosa with infliximab. J Eur Acad Dermatol Venereol. 2007;21:570–1.
57. Della Rossa A, Tavoni A, Merlini G, et al. Two Takayasu arteritis patients successfully treated with infliximab: a potential disease modifying agent. Rheumatology (Oxford). 2005;44:1074–5.
58. Kleinert J, Lorenz M, Kostler W, et al. Refractory Wegner's granulomatosis responds to tumor necrosis factor blockade. Wien Klin Wochenschr. 2004;116:334–8.

59. Burns JC, Mason WH, Hauger SB, et al. Infliximab treatment for refractory Kawasaki's syndrome. J Pediatr. 2005;146:662–7.
60. Tiliakos AIV, Shaia S, Hostoffer R, et al. The use of infliximab in a patient with steroid dependant Churg-Strauss syndrome. J Clin Rheumatol. 2004;10:96–7.
61. Uthman I, Kanj N, Atweh S. Infliximab as monotherapy in giant cell arteritis. Clin Rheumatol. 2006;25:109–10.
62. Chandesris MO, Gayet S, Schleinitz N, et al. Infliximab in the treatment of refractory vasculitis secondary to hepatitis C associated mixed cryoglobulinemia. Rheumatology (Oxford). 2004;43:532–3.
63. McCain ME, Quinet RJ, Davis WE. Etanercept and infliximab associated with cutaneous vasculitis. Rheumatology (Oxford). 2002;41:116–7.
64. Sullivan TP, Welsh E, Kerdel FA, et al. Infliximab for hidradenitis suppurativa. Br J Dermatol. 2003;149:1046–9.
65. Usmani N, Clayton TH, Everett S, et al. Variable response of hidradenitis suppurativa to infliximab in four patients. Clin Exp Dermatol. 2007;32:204–5.
66. Fardet L, Dupuy A, Kerob D, et al. Infliximab in severe hidradenitis suppurativa: transient clinical efficacy in 7 consecutive patients. J Am Acad Dermatol. 2007;56:624–8.
67. Shirakawa M, Uramoto K, Harada FA. Treatment of acne conglobata with infliximab. J Am Acad Dermatol. 2006;55:344–6.
68. Massara A, Cavazzini PL, Trotta F. In SAPHO syndrome anti TNF alpha therapy may induce persistent amelioration of osteoarticular complaints, but may exacerbate cutaneous manifestations. Rheumatology (Oxford). 2006;45:730–3.
69. Zouboulis CC, Katsantonis J, Ketteler R, et al. Adamantiades-Behcet's disease: interleukin 8 is increase in serum of patients with active oral and neurological manifestations and is secreted by small vessel endothelial cells. Arch Dermatol Res. 2000;292:274–84.
70. Haugeberg G, Velken M, Johnson V. Successful treatment of genital ulcers with infliximab in Behcet's disease. Am Rheum Dis. 2004;63:744–5.
71. Goossens PH, Verburg RJ, Breedveld FC. Remission of Behcet's syndrome with tumor necrosis factor alpha blocking therapy. Ann Rheum Dis. 2001;60:637.
72. Matzkies FG, Manger B, Schmitt-Haendle M, et al. Severe septicemia in a patient with polychondritis and sweet's syndrome after initiation of treatment with infliximab. Ann Rheum Dis. 2003;62:81–2.
73. Foster EN, Nguyen KK, Sheikh RA, et al. Crohn's disease associated with sweet's syndrome and Sjogren's syndrome treated with infliximab. Clin Dev Immunol. 2005;12:145–9.
74. Brooklyn TN, Dunnill MG, Shetty A, et al. Infliximab for the treatment of pyoderma gangrenosum: a randomized double blind placebo controlled trial. Gut. 2006;55:505–9.
75. Manoharan S, White S, Gumpartthy K. Successful treatment of type II adult onset pityriasis rubra pilaris with infliximab. Australas J Dermatol. 2006;47:124–9.
76. Liao NC, Mutasim DF. Infliximab for the treatment of adult onset pityriasis rubra pilaris. Arch Dermatol. 2005;141:423–5.
77. Leung DY, Bieber T. Atopic dermatitis. Lancet. 2003;361:151–60.
78. Jacobi A, Antoni C, Manger B, et al. Infliximab in the treatment of moderate to severe atopic dermatitis. J Am Acad Dermatol. 2005;52(3 Pt 1):522–6.
79. Doty JD, Mazur JE, Judson MA. Treatment of sarcoidosis with infliximab. Chest. 2005;127:1064–71.
80. Sweiss NJ, Welsh MJ, Curran JJ, et al. Tumor necrosis factor inhibition as a novel treatment for refractory sarcoidosis. Arthritis Rheum. 2005;53:788–91.
81. Winterfield L, Menter A. Psoriasis and its treatment with infliximab—mediated tumor necrosis factor alpha blockade. Dermatol Clin. 2004;22:437–47.
82. Magro F, Pereira P, Carneiro F, et al. Reactive hepatitis in a patient with Crohn's disease successfully treated with infliximab: does tumor necrosis factor play a role in reactive hepatitis? Inflamm Bowel Dis. 2005;11:88–90.
83. Mohan N, Edwards ET, Cupps TR, et al. Demyelination occurring during anti-tumor necrosis alpha therapy for inflammatory arhtritides. Arthritis Rheum. 2001;44:2862–9.

84. Cheifetz A, Mayer L. Monoclonal antibodies, immunogenicity and associated infusion reactions. Mt Sinai J Med. 2005;72:250–6.
85. Khanna D, McMahon M, Furst DE. Anti tumor necrosis factor alpha and heart failure: what have we learned and where do we go from here? Arthriris Rheum. 2004;50:1040–50.
86. Smith CH, Anstey AV, Barker JN, et al. British association of dermatologists guidelines for use of biological interventions in psoriasis 2005. Br J Dermatol. 2005;153:486–97.
87. Mohler KM, Torrance DS, Smith CS, et al. Soluble tumor necrosis factor (TNF) receptors are effective therapeutic agents in lethal endotoxemia and function simultaneously as both TNF carriers and antagonists. J Immunol. 1993;151:1548–61.
88. Kauffman CL, Aria N, Toichi E, et al. A phase I study evaluating the safety, pharmacokinetics and clinical response of human IL-12 p40 antibody in subjects with plaque psoriasis. J Invest Dermatol. 2004;123:1037–44.
89. Vandenbroeck K, Alloza I, Gadina M, et al. Inhibiting cytokines of the interleukin-12 family: recent advances and novel challenges. J Pharm Pharmacol. 2004;56:145–60.
90. Banks RE, Patel PM, Selby PJ. Interleukin 12. A new clinical player in cytokine therapy. Br J Cancer. 1995;71:655–9.
91. Moreland LW, Schiff MH, Baugartner SW, et al. Etanercept therapy in rheumatoid arthritis. A randomized, controlled trial. Ann Intern Med. 1999;130:478–86.
92. Zhou H, Mayer PR, Wajdula J, et al. Unaltered etanercept pharmacokinetics with concurrent methotrexate in patients with rheumatoid arthritis. J Clin Pharmacol. 2004;44:1235–43.
93. Zhou H, Patat A, Parks V, et al. Absence of pharmacokinetic interaction between etanercept and warfarin. J Clin Pharmacol. 2004;44:543–50.
94. Elewski BE, Papp K, Zitnik R. Efficacy and safety of etanercept in patients with psoriasis. Results of a global phase III study. J Am Acad Dermatol. 2004;50:P159.
95. Leonardi CL, Elewski BE, Camisa C, et al. The efficacy and safety of etanercept in the re-treatment of psoriasis after relapse. J Am Acad Dermatol. 2004;50:P146.
96. Gottlieb AB, Gordon KB, Wang A, et al. Withdrawal from etanercept after successful clinical response in psoriasis patients. Disease characteristics and the durability of treatment response. J Am Acad Dermatol. 2004;50:146.
97. Fiorentio DF, Garcia M, Rehmus W, et al. A pilot study of etanercept treatment for pemphigus vulgaris. Arch Dermatol. 2011;147:117–8.
98. Lin MH, Hsu CK, Lee JY. Successful treatment of recalcitrant pemphigus vulgaris and pemphigus vegetans with etanercept and carbon dioxide laser. Arch Dermatol. 2005;141:680–2.
99. Tirado-Sanchez A, Bonifaz A, Monte de Oca-Sanchez G *et al.* Etanercept plus methotrexate: an effective combination therapy for recalcitrant pemphigus. J Res Med Sci 2015;20:317.
100. Garcovich S, DiGiampetruzzi AR, Antonelli G, et al. Treatment of refractory adult onset pityriasis rubra pilaris with TNFα antagonists: a case series. J Eur Acad Dermatol Venereol. 2010;24:881–4.
101. Guedes R, Leite L. Therapeutic hot line. Treatment of pityriasis rubra pilaris with etanercept. Dermatol Ther. 2011;24:285–6.
102. Guhl G, Diaz-Ley B, Fernandez-Herrera J. Off label use of biologic agents in the treatment of dermatosis; part 2: Etanercept, Efalizumab, Alefacept, rituximab, Daclizumab, Basiliximab, Omalizumab and Cetuximab. Actas Dermosifiliogr. 2008;99:5–33.
103. Tuchinda C, Wong HK. Etanercept for chronic progressive cutaneous sarcoidosis. J Drugs Dermatol. 2006;5:538–40.
104. Vilar-Alejo J, Dehesa L, De La Rosa-del RP, et al. SAPHO syndrome with unusual cutaneous manifestations treated successfully with etanercept. Acta Derm Venereol. 2010;90:531–2.
105. Puig L, Barco D, Vilarrosa E, et al. Treatment of acrodermatitis continua of Hallopeau with TNF blocking agents: case report and review. Dermatology. 2010;220:154–8.
106. Haslund P, Lee RA, Jemec G. Treatment of hidradenitis suppurativa with tumor necrosis factor alpha inhibitors. Acta Derm Venereol. 2009;89:595–600.
107. Tirado Sanchez A, De la Fuente-Garcia V, Ponce-Olivera RM. Off label uses of etanercept in dermatology. Rev Med Hosp Gen Mex. 2016;79:26–32.

108. Norman R, Greenberg RG, Jackson JM. Case repots of etanercept in inflammatory dermatoses. J Am Acad Dermatol. 2006;54(Suppl 2):S139–42.
109. Swale VJ, Perret CM, Denton CP, et al. Etanercept induced systemic lupus erythematosus. Clin Exp Dermatol. 2003;28:604–7.
110. Muscle study group. A randomized pilot trial of etanercept in dermatomyositis. Ann Neurol. 2011;70:427–36.
111. Lannone F, Scioscia C, Falappone PCF, et al. Use of etanercept in the treatment of dermatomyositis: a case series. The J of Rheumatology. 2006;33:1802–4.
112. Rullan P, Murase J. Two cases of chronic atopic dermatitis treated with soluble tumor necrosis factor receptor therapy. J Drugs Dermatol. 2009;8:873–6.
113. Buka RL, Resh B, Roberts B, et al. Etanercept is minimally effective in 2 children with atopic dermatitis. J Am Acad Dermatol. 2005;53:358–9.
114. Melikoglu M, Fresko I, Mat C, et al. Short term trial of etanercept in Behcet's disease: a double blind placebo controlled trial. J Rheumatol. 2005;32:98–105.
115. Sommer a, Altmeyer P, Kreuter A. A case of mucocutaneous Behcet's disease responding to etanercept. J Am Acad Dermatol. 2005;52:717–9.
116. Atzeni F, Sarzi-Puttini P, Capsoni F, et al. Successful treatment of resistant Behcet's disease with etanercept. Clin Exp Rheumatol. 2005;23:729.
117. Estrach C, Mpofu S, Moots RJ. Behcet's syndrome: response to infliximab after failure of etanercept. Rheumatology. 2002;41:1213–4.
118. Saurenman RK, Levin AV, Rose JB, et al. Tumor necrosis factor alpha inhibitors in the treatment of childhood uveitis. Rhematology. 2006;45:982–9.
119. McGowan JW, Johnson CA, Lynn A. Treatment of pyoderma gangrenosum with etanercept. J Drugs Dermatol. 2004;3:441–4.
120. Goldenburg G, Jorizzo JL. Use of etanercept in treatment of pyoderma gangrenosum in a patient with autoimmune hepatitis. J Dermatol Treat. 2005;16:347–9.
121. Carrera C, Mascaro JM Jr, Moreno-Romero JA, et al. Pyoderma vegetans associated with severe psoriatic arthritis: good response to etanercept. Dermatology. 2007;214:77–81.
122. Berk DR, Hurt MA, Mann C, et al. Sneddon Wilkinson's disease treated with etanercept: a report of two cases. Clin Exp Dermatol. 2008;34:347–51.
123. Bissonnette R, Poulin Y, Bolduc C, et al. Etanercept in the treatment of palmoplantar pustulosis. J Drugs Deramtol. 2008;7:940–6.
124. Boyd AS. Etanercept treatment of erythema nodosum. Skinmed. 2007;6:197–9.
125. Rajagopalan M, Vasani R. Etanercept: Indian perspective. Indian J Drugs Dermatol. 2014;1:50–2.
126. Burls A, Jobanputra P. The trials of anakinra. Lancet. 2004;364:827–8.
127. Rambhia KD, Khopkar US. Adalimumab. Indian J Drugs Dermatol. 2015;1:7–11.

Ustekinumab

35

Introduction

Ustekinumab is a human monoclonal antibody (mAb) generated from transgenic mice using techniques of genetic engineering. It targets and blocks the p40 subunit, which is shared by interleukin (IL)-12 and 23, thereby inhibiting ensuing signalling, differentiation and cytokine production, which is pivotal in inflammatory diseases. [1]

Pharmacokinetics

Following administration of a single subcutaneous (SC) dose of 45 mg/90 mg of ustekinumab, it attains a bioavailability of 78.3%, with a $t_{1/2}$ of 19.8/21.2 days [2].

The metabolism of ustekinumab occurs via catabolic pathways similar to endogenous IgG. There remains limited information on the main route of elimination of ustekinumab. It is considered that following degradation, ustekinumab is eliminated via the renal route [3].

Indications

FDA Approved

- Moderate to severe plaque psoriasis.
- Psoriatic arthropathy (PsA).

A. K. Bubna, *Therapeutics in Dermatology - Essentials for Clinical Practice*,
https://doi.org/10.1007/978-981-95-3791-4_35

Off-Label

- Hidradenitis suppurativa (HS).
- Lichen planus (LP).
- Pityriasis rubra pilaris (PRP).
- Behcet's disease (BD).
- Lupus erythematosus (LE).
- Alopecia areata (AA).
- Atopic dermatitis (AD).
- Pyoderma gangrenosum (PG).

Contraindications

Absolute

- Presence of active infections; more importantly latent or active tuberculosis, hepatitis B, C and HIV.
- Hypersensitivity to ustekinumab.

Relative

- PUVA sessions being received.
- Premalignant conditions.
- Demyelinating disease.
- Optic neuritis.
- Multiple sclerosis.
- Pregnancy/lactation.
- Congestive cardiac failure.
- Concurrent use of live vaccines.
- Marked elevated levels of hepatic transaminases.

Clinical Uses

Plaque Psoriasis

Psoriasis is a chronic inflammatory disorder with predominant cutaneous features, along with systemic involvement, affecting 1–3% of the global population, with plaque psoriasis accounting for 90% of the cases [4, 5]. According to the new psoriasis model, the interleukin (IL)-23/Th17 axis contributes significantly in the development of psoriasis [6]. The activation of Th17 by IL-23, and subsequent generation of pro-inflammatory cytokines such as IL-17, TNFα, IL-26 and IL-29 majorly promote recruitment of inflammatory cells, with eventual epidermal hyperplasia [7]. Ustekinumab blocks IL-23 and subsequently targets upstream cytokines; unlike downstream cytokines (viz TNFα and IL-17) targeted by other biologic agents, enabling ustekinumab to be dosed at lesser frequencies, when compared to other classes of biologic drugs [8]. Moreover, blockade of IL-23, also plummets levels of IL-17 and IL-22, furthering ustekinumab's anti-inflammatory effects [9].

The efficacy and safety of ustekinumab in plaque psoriasis has been illustrated through four large phase III randomized placebo-controlled trials (PHOENIX 1/2, PEARL and LOTUS) and one phase III randomized active comparator trial (ACCEPT) [10–14]. In both PHOENIX studies, Psoriasis Area Severity Index (PASI) 75 responses at week 12 was observed in 66.4–75.7% of ustekinumab-treated patients, which was strikingly greater than the placebo group (3–4%). Besides, with ongoing treatment, improvements were sustained and incidence of adverse effects did not reveal anything alarming [10, 11]. The PEARL and LOTUS studies correspondingly delineated statistically significant improvements of PASI 75 in the ustekinumab group when compared to placebo at week 12 ($p < 0.001$), which was maintained through week 36 [12, 13]. Further, in the ACCEPT trial, PASI 75 was observed in 67.5–73.8% of patients treated with ustekinumab and 56.8% of patients in the etanercept group, with comparable safety profiles in both groups [14]. Interestingly, consistent data regarding the efficacy and safety of ustekinumab has been noted through 5 years of follow-up, with dose escalation (90 mg every 8 weeks) resulting in greater reduction of psoriasis in those patients unresponsive to the lower dosing (45 mg) [15]. However, following cessation of ustekinumab therapy, exacerbation of psoriasis occurs in most patients. Unfortunately, currently there is no available data supporting the long-term use of ustekinumab, mandating further research in this field [16].

Though superior to etanercept in plaque psoriasis, PASI 90 values from randomized controlled trials (RCTs) have displayed ustekinumab's inferiority to secukinumab (57.6% vs 79%, respectively) and risankizumab (42% vs 75.3%, respectively) [17, 18]. Nevertheless, ustekinumab does have value in the management of plaque psoriasis and has been associated with rapid and clinically significant amelioration of moderate-to-severe plaque psoriasis, with apparent results as early as 2 weeks following treatment initiation, and maximum responses obtainable by 24 weeks of sustained therapy. Besides, it is the preferred biological in paediatric psoriasis, as well as adult patients with Crohn's disease. Furthermore, its widely spaced dosing schedule at week 0, 4 and then every 12 weeks, offers an added advantage over the older biological agents that require more frequent administration [10, 11, 15, 19].

Psoriatic Arthropathy

Psoriatic arthropathy (PsA) is a chronic inflammatory arthritis observed in around 20% of psoriasis patients, associated with diverse clinical features. Although there exist numerous therapeutic agents for PsA, discovering newer agents to treat PsA is readily embraced, owing to its refractoriness to various treatments [20].

Ustekinumab's efficacy in PsA has been substantiated by two phase III randomized placebo-controlled trials (PSUMMIT 1/2) and one randomized controlled active comparator trial (ECLIPSA) [21–23]. The PSUMMIT trials (at 24 weeks) delineated an American College of Rheumatology (ACR)-20 score in 42.4–49.5% of participants receiving ustekinumab, which was almost double when compared to the placebo group (20.2–22.8%) [21, 22], and in the ECLIPSA study (at 24 weeks), the primary end point (defined as the Spondylarthritis Research Consortium of Canada [SPARCC] index of 0) was demonstrated in 73.9% of subjects receiving ustekinumab and 41.7% of patients on TNFα blockers [23]. Besides, enthesitis also demonstrated a favourable response to ustekinumab, along with decline in radiologic disease progression [21–23]. This can be explained by the central role of the proinflammatory cytokine IL-23 in the development of enthesitis, with IL-23 blockade silencing the inflammatory effects of IL-23 sensitive cells in the entheses, and subsequent blockade of downstream inflammatory mediators such as IL-17, IL-22 and TNFα [24, 25]. However, synovitis in PsA does not show much response to ustekinumab, as synovitis in PsA is less sensitive to IL-12/23 inhibition [25].

Interestingly, systematic reviews and metanalysis have propounded the beneficial effects of combining ustekinumab with etanercept/adalimumab/golimumab/certolizumab in recalcitrant cases of PsA and psoriasis with dose adjustments (ustekinumab being administered as 90 mg/12 weekly in these special scenarios). This integrated approach can be of particular value in the management of patients presenting with both PsA and psoriasis unresponsive to biologic monotherapy. As various biologics act differently with regard to cutaneous psoriasis and PsA (owing to the different pathogenesis), this concoction could have a role to play. However, the risk of infections and cardiovascular disease cannot be undermined while initiating this approach. Although there have been reports without encountering any adverse effects, flares of herpes zoster, retro-tonsillar abscess, erysipelas and bacterial pneumonia have been confronted [26–28].

Pustular Psoriasis

Pustular psoriasis comprises a clinically heterogenous variant of psoriasis with both generalized and localized presentations. Generalized pustular psoriasis (GPP) usually has an acute or even a fulminating course, but subacute forms are also commonly encountered. Localized forms of pustular psoriasis are usually confined to the hands and feet and tends to have a chronic discourse.

Generalized Pustular Psoriasis

In GPP, there occurs a high risk of serious complications if appropriate treatment is not promptly instituted. Currently, there exist two case reports and one case series demonstrating successful management of GPP with ustekinumab [29–31].

Acrodermatitis Continua of Hollopeau

In acrodermatitis continua of Hollopeau (ACH), ustekinumab has proven to be highly advantageous, as represented in four case reports [32–35]. Apart from its conventional dosing, ustekinumab dose escalation (from 45 to 90 mg, even if body weight is <100 kg), in those cases of ACH where therapeutic responses are short-lived, can be attempted [32, 33]. Additionally, combining acitretin with ustekinumab in recalcitrant ACH is associated with a synergistic clinical outcome [34]. Generally, by 28 weeks of treatment with ustekinumab, acceptable lesional clearance is observed in ACH, with marked improvement in the Dermatology Life Quality Index (DLQI) [35].

Palmoplantar Pustulosis

Palmoplantar pustulosis (PPP) is a localized variant of pustular psoriasis characterized by sterile pustules along with erythematous-desquamative lesions involving the palms and soles. Responsiveness of PPP to ustekinumab has been mixed with profitable outcomes on one hand and poor to paradoxical responses on the other. Thc positive effects of ustekinumab in PPP has been linked to blockade of IL-23, which in turn prevents IL-17 secretion from Th17 cells, with consequent impediment of neutrophil influx and neutrophil-mediated inflammatory responses [36]. On the contrary, poor/paradoxical responses associated with ustekinumab have been attributed to stimulation of IFNα synthesis (following blockade of IL-23 and Th17 activity). Activation of T cells by IFNα goes on to produce TNFα and IL-17, which in turn sustain inflammatory cascades for the development of psoriatic plaques and pustules. Besides, serum in PPP patients demonstrate increased levels of IL-17 and IL-22-related cytokines, without significant elevation of IL-23 and IL-8 (thereby accounting as to why ustekinumab is not effective in every patient) [37, 38]. Currently, there exist only case reports and case series exemplifying the utility of ustekinumab in PPP [39–43], highlighting the need for RCTs to further strengthen these observations.

Palmoplantar Psoriasis(Non-pustular)

This type of psoriasis affects the skin of the palms and soles, featuring as hyperkeratotic plaques and causing significant functional disability. Often, response to this variant of psoriasis to treatment is delayed, accounted for by the presence of subclinical trauma and chronic pressure amounting to systematic koebnerization [44]. By antagonizing IL-23, ustekinumab indirectly blocks IL-22 and prevents occurrence of epidermal hyperplasia and acanthosis [45]. The utility of ustekinumab in non-pustular palmoplantar psoriasis has been elaborated in two case reports [44, 45].

Nail Psoriasis

Nail psoriasis (NP) commonly manifests in patients with plaque psoriasis and PsA, causing cosmetic disfigurement that profoundly distresses the patient. Treatment for NP can be quite challenging owing to the intricate nail anatomy compared to the usual skin. Besides, if NP is the sole manifestation of the disease, prior to starting any systemic therapy, both pros and cons need to be adequately weighed. A practical suggestion would be to initiate topical therapy, and if unresponsive, intramatriceal drug injections could be an avenue to contemplate upon, owing to the localized approach, with higher levels of safety and cost-effectiveness when compared to systemic therapy. Literature search revealed one open-label uncontrolled non-randomized study, one retrospective evaluation of NP from the PHOENIX trial and one case report depicting the beneficial role of ustekinumab in NP. [46–48] However, Iqarashi et al. [49] in their report failed to elucidate significant improvement in Nail Psoriasis Severity Index (NAPSI) with ustekinumab for NP in their report.

Hidradenitis Suppurativa

Hidradenitis suppurativa (HS) is a chronic, recurrent inflammatory skin disease arising from hair follicles, particularly affecting intertriginous zones, often associated with a systemic comorbidity [50]. The utility of ustekinumab in HS has been described in one phase II open label trial, one multicentre retrospective study and few case series [51–56]. The role of ustekinumab in HS is associated with inhibition of IL-23 and IL-12. It has been hypothesized that inflammation in HS is caused by abnormal Notch signalling. These signals induce differentiation of outer hair root sheath cells, which are destroyed easily and release keratins that trigger macrophage activation via Toll-like receptors. This consequently activates dendritic cells that release IL-23 to activate Th17 cells. Furthermore, IL-12 and IL-23 are also produced by $CD68^+$ and $CD32^+$ macrophages in lesions of HS. This subsequently deteriorates the balance between Th17 and regulatory T cells (Treg). By suppressing both IL-23 and IL-12, ustekinumab enables restoration of this imbalance [57, 58].

Despite the above postulation, Gkine and Bewley [59] displayed development of HS with ustekinumab in a 19-year-old Caucasian female treated for psoriasis. The reason for this remains unclear but has been suggested to be a probable paradox reaction to anti-IL-12/2. Physicians should therefore be aware of this potent complication, with ustekinumab in the event of which other treatment options of HS need consideration.

Pyoderma Gangrenosusm

Pyoderma gangrenosum (PG) is an ulcero-necrotic neutrophilic dermatoses characterized by painful ulcers commonly involving the lower extremities [60]. Currently, ustekinumab's efficacy in PG has only been highlighted in case reports.

Gonzalez et al. demonstrated ustekinumab to be effective in treating PG in a 29-year-old female with CD, who had failed to respond to adalimumab. Ustekinumab was initiated at a dose of 260 mg IV, following which the patient improved tremendously. Patient was then maintained on ustekinumab at 90 mg every 8 weekly. With this treatment, patient remained in remission [60].

A French report further established the profitability of ustekinumab in a 56-year-old lady with plaque psoriasis/PsA, wherein PG had been precipitated following adalimumab therapy. Following three doses of ustekinumab (45 mg SC, as per the standard protocol for plaque psoriasis), PG had completely healed along with clearance of psoriasis lesions [61].

Nunes and colleagues likewise outlined the utility of ustekinumab in treating PG in a patient with CD resistant to treatment with azathioprine, cyclosporine and infliximab. Complete healing of PG was witnessed after administration of the first dose of ustekinumab (520 mg IV). Patient was then maintained with ustekinumab 90 mg SC every 8 weeks [62].

Ustekinumab's role in PG was further highlighted in a report from North Carolina, wherein PG induced by secukinumab in a patient with psoriasis was successfully treated with ustekinumab (90 mg SC on weeks 0, 4 and then every 8 weeks). Significant improvement was noticed after two doses of ustekinumab, with almost complete re-epithelialization of the ulcer [63].

Another publication revealed ustekinumab in combination with Vacuum Assisted Closure (VAC) therapy to be highly effective in treating PG in a 62-year-old man who had been diagnosed with myelodysplastic syndrome (MDS). Ustekinumab (90 mg SC, standard psoriasis regimen) was commenced owing to failure of treatment with corticosteroids, thalidomide, infliximab, adalimumab and immunoglobins. Within 2 weeks of the first dose of ustekinumab, dramatic improvement was observed, following which VAC therapy was applied every 5 days to the ulcer. This treatment was continued for 8 weeks with complete healing occurring at 20 weeks. Ustekinumab was then continued every 8 weeks as maintenance for 18 months. This revealed surgical treatments to be advantageous along with biologic therapy, once the correct immunosuppressive environment was achieved, in treating PG. [64]

The role of ustekinumab in PG can be attributed to the heightened expression of IL-23 in tissue samples from PG lesions at both transcriptional and protein levels [65].

Atopic Dermatitis

Atopic dermatitis (AD) is a chronic inflammatory disorder of the skin characterized by intense pruritus and xerosis. The pathogenesis of AD is believed to be driven via a type 2 helper T-cell (Th2)-mediated immune response. However, during the chronic phase of the disease, there is a switch towards the Th1-mediated immune response wherein IL-12 comes into play and brings about this change [66–68]. Besides, based on Th1/Th2 cell responses, evidence suggests involvement of Th17 cells also in the immunopathology of AD. The exact mechanism of action of ustekinumab in AD is still not fully understood. Based on the above postulation, ustekinumab's role in AD occurs by the down-regulation of Th1 and Th17 inflammatory pathways once it binds to IL-12 and IL-23 [69, 70]. However, despite these conclusions, therapeutic effects of ustekinumab for AD has demonstrated disparity, ranging from complete responsiveness to no response at all, as demonstrated in RCTs, case series and case reports [71–75].

Interestingly, AD, following ustekinumab therapy, has also been observed. Ishuyi and coworkers reported emergence of AD in a 59-year man with psoriasis following ustekinumab treatment, with a SCORAD of 10 being reached after 172 weeks of ustekinumab therapy, and rapid improvement of AD after cessation of ustekinumab [76]. In another patient with concurrent psoriasis and AD, ustekinumab resulted in complete remission of psoriasis, but worsening of AD with SCORAD values increasing from 9 to 15, and improvement of AD with subsequent halting of ustekinumab treatment [77]. The underlying mechanism for this can be ascribed to IL-12 blockade as well as indirect IL-17 inhibition, resulting in an immunological imbalance, favouring an increased activity of the Th2 pathway. The resultant Th2 dominance in turn accounts for AD-like symptoms [77, 78]. This variation in clinical responses illustrates that ustekinumab may not be a very suitable agent in AD. Nonetheless, it can be tried as an unconventional drug in patients when treatment with approved biologic drugs have failed.

Alopecia Areata

Alopecia areata (AA) is an autoimmune disorder resulting in non-scarring alopecia with considerable impact on patient's quality of life. Although there exist a number of therapeutic agents for AA, which though effective, cannot be used for prolonged periods owing to safety concerns, and often cessation of treatment is heralded again by hair loss [79, 80]. Currently, ustekinumab's utility in AA has been outlined in case reports and case series alone. The role of ustekinumab in AA is contributed by its antagonistic action on IL-12, which enables development of naive T cells to Th1 cells [81].

Alesia and colleagues demonstrated hair regrowth in three paediatric patients following ustekinumab treatment. Two patients received a stat dose of 90 mg of ustekinumab and the third patient was given 90 mg of ustekinumab at months 0, 3 and 6. In all three patients, the SALT score improved by 71.43–100% [81]. Similarly, in another study, ustekinumab (90 mg SC) was found to be effective in AA, given at weeks 0, 4 and 16. Besides, in one patient with alopecia universalis improvement was substantial with regrowth of all body hair, eyebrows and all of the scalp at week 49 [82]. Again, ustekinumab's favourable effect in AA was iterated in a 39-year-old south Asian woman. Dosed at 90 mg (0, 4 and every 8 weeks) by 20 weeks, hair density had visibly increased [83].

Lupus Erythematosus

Lupus erythematosus (LE) is associated with dysregulation of the IL-17/IL-23 axis along with a reduction in the total number of T-regulatory FoxP3+ cells. Increased levels of IL-23 produced predominantly by dendritic cells and macrophages promote expansion of Th17 cells, which in turn elaborates IL-17 production; a cytokine significantly elevated in skin of patients with SLE and DLE. IL-17 further stimulates production of autoantibodies and inflammatory cytokines (TNFα, IL-1β, IL-6, IL-8, IL-22, etc.) and chemokines (CCL2, CCL7, CCL29, CXCL1 and CXCL5). There is thus an imbalance between pro- and anti-inflammatory cytokines with a deranged homeostasis. Ustekinumab in LE ameliorates this deranged homeostasis by preventing differentiation of T cells to Th17 via IL-12/23 inhibition [84–87].

Though there are a number of case reports where ustekinumab has been beneficial in LE, RCTs are currently lacking in this context [88–93]. However, despite the propitious effect of ustekinumab in LE, it has also reported to induce SCLE [94]. The cause of this reaction occurs secondary to diversion of T cell differentiation to the alternative pathway of T helper cell IL-22 production, via IL-6, leading to excess TNFα production and stimulation of inflammatory responses [95].

Bechet's Disease

The role of ustekinumab in Bechet's disease (BD) occurs via its antagonist activity against IL-23 and the associated Th17 pathway that plays a major role in BD [96]. Ustekinumab has demonstrated efficacy in two patients, with multi-refractory BD (unresponsive to colchicine, cyclosporine, methotrexate, azathioprine, anakinra and anti-TNFα agents) [97, 98]. In order to strengthen these findings, RCTs are warranted.

Pityriasis Rubra Pilaris

The exact mechanism of ustekinumab action in pityriasis rubra pilaris (PRP) is unclear. By its IL-12 and IL-23 blocking properties, and subsequent suppression of cytokine release/immune activation, ustekinumab has been used in patients with unremitting PRP. However, information of the effects ustekinumab on PRP does not meet the requirements of evidence-based medicine [99]. Currently, there exists only case reports describing the appositeness of ustekinumab in PRP [99–104].

Miscellaneous

In an anecdotal report, ustekinumab (45 mg SC in the standard psoriasis dosage) was associated with dramatic clinical improvement of recalcitrant oral lichen planus (LP) within 12 weeks in a 72-year-old female unresponsive to systemic/topical steroids, ciclosporin, acitretin and azathioprine [105]. It has been suggested that IL-23 is markedly elevated in LP lesions, which is suppressed by the antagonizing effects of ustekinumab on IL-23 and Th17/Tc17 cells [106].

Similarly, isolated reports have highlighted the utility of ustekinumab in Synovitis Acne Pustulosis Hyperostosis Osteitis (SAPHO) syndrome, bullous pemphigoid (BP), lichen planus pemphigoid and anti-laminin γ1 pemphigoid [107–110]. Interestingly, the occurrence of BP has been associated following ustekinumab therapy, suggesting other cytokine pathways responsible for the development of iatrogenic pemphigoid [111–113].

Adverse Effects

Cutaneous

- Pruritus [114].
- Exfoliative dermatitis [114]
- Bullous pemphigoid [111–113]
- Lupus erythematosus tumidus [115]
- Jessner–Kanof's lymphocytic infiltrate [115]
- Injection site erythema [114]

Extracutaneous

Common [116]

- Nasopharyngitis.
- Headache.
- Arthralgia.
- Fatigue.
- Bronchitis/upper respiratory tract infection.
- Sinusitis.
- Back pain.
- Abdominal pain and fever (in higher dosing schedules).

Serious [117]

- Severe infections or exacerbation/reactivation of existing infection (bacterial, viral, fungal, mycobacterial).
- Major adverse cardiovascular events (MACEs).
- Hypersensitivity reactions/anaphylaxis.
- Reversible posterior leukoencephalopathy syndrome.
- Cryptogenic organizing pneumonia.
- Interstitial or eosinophilic pneumonia.
- Non-melanoma skin cancer.

Drug Monitoring [118]

Baseline

- Routine blood tests: complete blood counts (CBC), liver function test (LFT), renal function test (RFT), C-reactive protein (CRP), erythrocyte sedimentation rate (ESR), serum electrolytes.
- Varicella antibody status should be clarified, and vaccination considered in appropriate patients.
- Screening for tuberculosis: chest X-ray and interferon-gamma release assay.
- Hepatitis B, C and HIV tests.
- Pregnancy test needs to be done in females where pregnancy is a possibility.

Ongoing [119–121]

- Routine blood tests including, CBC, urea, electrolytes, LFTs, CRP, ESR need to be done every 4–6 months.
- Retesting for Hepatitis and HIV needs consideration if clinically indicated.
- Patients must be monitored clinically for development of severe infections (including TB), jaundice, malignancy, non-infectious pneumonia, posterior reversible encephalopathy syndrome or serious skin conditions such as exfoliative dermatitis. Patients should be encouraged to report any concerning symptoms.
- Clinical monitoring for efficacy should be carried out using disease-specific measuring systems for psoriasis, psoriatic arthritis and inflammatory bowel disease.
- There are experimental data to suggest that monitoring serum drug levels may be beneficial during ustekinumab treatment, but this is not the current standard for care.

Administration [122–124]

Ustekinumab is available for injection in prefilled syringes and vials. The drug is administered by either subcutaneous injection or intravenous infusion. The dosage and administration recommendations depend on the particular indication for treatment and patient's weight.

Dosage Forms and Strengths

Subcutaneous Injection*:*

- Injection 45 mg/0.5 mL or 90 mg/mL solution in a prefilled syringe.
- Injection 45 mg/0.5 mL solution in a single dose vial.

Intravenous Infusion

- Injection: 130 mg/26 mL (5 mg/mL) in a single dose vial.

Dosage and Administration

- ***Psoriasis and psoriatic arthropathy adult SC recommended dosage:***
  - Less than or equal to 100 kg: 45 mg given at week 0, 4 and then every 12 weeks.
  - Greater than 100 kg: 90 mg given at weeks 0, 4 and then every 12 weeks.
- ***Psoriasis paediatric SC recommended dosage:***
  - Weight < 60 kg: 0.75 mg/kg.
  - Weight 60–100 kg: 45 mg.
  - Weight > 100 kg: 90 mg.
- In inflammatory bowel disease, an initial intravenous weight-based infusion is given followed by a SC maintenance schedule.
  - Initial infusion dosage:
    - Weight < 55 kg: 260 mg (2 vials).
    - Weight 55–85 kg: 390 mg (3 vials).
    - Weight 85 kg: 520 mg (4 vials).
  - SC maintenance dose:
    - 90 mg every 8 weeks after the initial IV infusion.

Renal dosing (including haemodialysis and peritoneal dialysis) and hepatic dosing are undefined.

Use in Specific Populations

Pregnancy

Although there are several cases of pregnant patients treated safely with ustekinumab—mostly in gastroenterological indications—the German S3 guideline and also the SmPC (summary of product characteristic) do not currently recommended using this medication for psoriasis during gestation [125].

Lactation

Only few reports exist on the use of ustekinumab during lactation. The substance was found in breast milk in four out of six breastfeeding patients with chronic inflammatory bowel disease (IBD). The highest concentration (0.72–1.57 mg/mL) was measured during a period of 12–72 h after drug administration. The breastfed infants did not demonstrate any negative effects with it. Despite this, owing to limited evidence, ustekinumab is not currently recommended in lactating mothers [125].

Paediatric

Ustekinumab can be used in paediatric patients with psoriasis. Besides, it is a safe and effective treatment option for paediatric and adolescent Crohn's disease and Crohn's-like IBD [126].

Drug Interactions [3]

Concomitant Therapies

Methotrexate, cyclosporine, azathioprine and CS used along with ustekinumab did not appear to influence the overall safety and efficacy of the drug.

CYP450 Substrates

Ustekinumab can normalize the formation of CYP450 enzymes; therefore, patients receiving concomitant CYP450 substrates, particularly those with a narrow therapeutic index monitoring for therapeutic effects (e.g. warfarin) or drug concentration (e.g. ciclosporin), should be considered and the individual dose of the drug should be adjusted as needed.

Allergen Immunotherapy

Ustekinumab may reduce the protective effect of allergen immunotherapy, and thus increase the risk of an allergic reaction to a dose of allergen immunotherapy. Caution therefore is required in patients receiving or those who have received allergen immunotherapy, particularly for anaphylaxis.

Conclusion

Ustekinumab is a good biological drug for the treatment of psoriasis and PsA. Besides, it is the biologic of choice for paediatric patients with psoriasis owing to its weight-based dosing schedule. Moreover, currently, ustekinumab has found to be effective in a number of off-label dermatological indications. Furthermore, it is tolerated well by patients with minimal side effects. Nevertheless, there are reports of serious adverse effects following ustekinumab usage. All these points need to be carefully evaluated prior to prescribing ustekinumab.

References

1. Cingoz O. Ustekinumab. MAbs. 2009;1:216–21.
2. Adedokun OJ, Xu Z, Gasink C, Jacobstein D, Szapary P, Johanns J, et al. Pharmacokinetics and exposure response relationships of Ustekinumab in patients with Crohn's disease. Gastroenterology. 2018;154:1660–71.
3. FDA approved drug products: Stelara (Ustekinumab) injection for subcutaneous and intravenous use: https://www.accessdata.fda.gov/drugsatfda_docs/label/2016/761044lbl.pdf
4. Rendon A, Schäkel K. Psoriasis pathogenesis and treatment. Int J Mol Sci. 2019;20:1475.
5. Armstrong AW, Read C. Pathophysiology, clinical presentation, and treatment of psoriasis: a review. JAMA Dermatol. 2020;323:1945–60.
6. Piskin G, Sylva-Steenland RM, Bos JD, Teunissen MB. In vitro and in situ expression of IL-23 by keratinocytes in healthy skin and psoriasis lesions: enhanced expression in psoriatic skin. J Immunol. 2006;176:1908–15.
7. Hawkes JE, Yan BY, Chan TC, Krueger JG. Discovery of the IL-23/IL-17 signaling pathway and the treatment of psoriasis. J Immunol. 2018;201:1605–13.
8. Girolomoni G, Strohal R, Puig L, Bachelez H, Barker J, Boehncke WH, et al. The role of IL-23 and the IL-23/T_H 17 immune axis in the pathogenesis and treatment of psoriasis. J Eur Acad Dermatol Venereol. 2017;31:1616–26.
9. Guo W, Luo C, Wang C, Zhu Y, Wang X, Gao X, et al. Protection against Th17 cells differentiation by an interleukin-23 receptor cytokine-binding homology region. PLoS One. 2012;7:e45625.
10. Leonardi CL, Kimball AB, Papp KA, Yeilding N, Guzzo C, Wang Y, PHOENIX 1 Study Investigators, et al. Efficacy and safety of ustekinumab, a human interleukin-12/23 monoclonal antibody, in patients with psoriasis: 76-week results from a randomised, double-blind, placebo-controlled trial (PHOENIX 1). Lancet. 2008;371:1665–74.
11. Papp KA, Langley RG, Lebwohl M, Krueger GG, Szapary P, Yeilding N, PHOENIX 2 Study Investigators, et al. Efficacy and safety of ustekinumab, a human interleukin-12/23 monoclonal antibody, in patients with psoriasis: 52-week results from a randomised, double-blind, placebo-controlled trial (PHOENIX 2). Lancet. 2008;371:1675–84.
12. Tsai TF, Ho JC, Song M, Szapary P, Guzzo C, Shen YK, et al. Efficacy and safety of ustekinumab for the treatment of moderate-to-severe psoriasis: a phase III, randomized, placebo-controlled trial in Taiwanese and Korean patients (PEARL). J Dermatol Sci. 2011;63:154–63.
13. Zhu X, Zheng M, Song M, Shen YK, Chan D, Szapary PO, Wang B. Efficacy and safety of ustekinumab in Chinese patients with moderate to severe plaque-type psoriasis: results from a phase 3 clinical trial (LOTUS). J Drugs Dermatol. 2013;12:166–74.
14. Griffiths CE, Strober BE, van de Kerkhof P, Ho V, Fidelus-Gort R, Yeilding N, ACCEPT Study Group, et al. Comparison of ustekinumab and etanercept for moderate-to-severe psoriasis. N Engl J Med. 2010;362:118–28.
15. Kimball AB, Papp KA, Wasfi Y, Chan D, Bissonnette R, Sofen H, PHOENIX 1 Investigators, et al. Long-term efficacy of ustekinumab in patients with moderate-to-severe psoriasis treated for up to 5 years in the PHOENIX 1 study. J Eur Acad Dermatol Venereol. 2013;27:1535–45.
16. Chiu HY, Hui RC, Tsai TF, Chen YC, Liao NF, Chen PH, Lai PJ, Wang TS, Huang YH. Predictors of time to relapse following ustekinumab withdrawal in patients with psoriasis who had responded to therapy: an 8-year multicenter study. J Am Acad Dermatol. 2023;88:71–8.
17. Thaçi D, Blauvelt A, Reich K, Tsai TF, Vanaclocha F, Kingo K, et al. Secukinumab is superior to ustekinumab in clearing skin of subjects with moderate to severe plaque psoriasis: CLEAR, a randomized controlled trial. J Am Acad Dermatol. 2015;73:400–9.
18. Gordon KB, Strober B, Lebwohl M, Augustin M, Blauvelt A, Poulin Y, et al. Efficacy and safety of risankizumab in moderate-to-severe plaque psoriasis (UltIMMa-1 and UltIMMa-2):

results from two double-blind, randomised, placebo-controlled and ustekinumab-controlled phase 3 trials. Lancet. 2018;392:650–61.
19. Krueger GG, Langley RG, Leonardi C, Yeilding N, Guzzo C, Wang Y, CNTO 1275 Psoriasis Study Group, et al. A human interleukin-12/23 monoclonal antibody for the treatment of psoriasis. N Engl J Med. 2007;356:580–92.
20. Karmacharya P, Chakradhar R, Ogdie A. The epidemiology of psoriatic arthritis: a literature review. Best Pract Res Clin Rheumatol. 2021;359:419–29.
21. McInnes IB, Kavanaugh A, Gottlieb AB, Puig L, Rahman P, Ritchlin C, PSUMMIT 1 Study Group, et al. Efficacy and safety of ustekinumab in patients with active psoriatic arthritis: 1 year results of the phase 3, multicentre, double-blind, placebo-controlled PSUMMIT 1 trial. Lancet. 2013;382:780–9.
22. Ritchlin C, Rahman P, Kavanaugh A, McInnes IB, Puig L, Li S, PSUMMIT 2 Study Group, et al. Efficacy and safety of the anti-IL-12/23 p40 monoclonal antibody, ustekinumab, in patients with active psoriatic arthritis despite conventional non-biological and biological anti-tumour necrosis factor therapy: 6-month and 1-year results of the phase 3, multicentre, double-blind, placebo-controlled, randomised PSUMMIT 2 trial. Ann Rheum Dis. 2014;73:990–9.
23. Araujo EG, Englbrecht M, Hoepken S, Finzel S, Kampylafka E, Kleyer A, et al. Effects of ustekinumab versus tumor necrosis factor inhibition on enthesitis: results from the enthesial clearance in psoriatic arthritis (ECLIPSA) study. Semin Arthritis Rheum. 2019;48:632–7.
24. Reinhardt A, Yevsa T, Worbs T, Lienenklaus S, Sandrock I, Oberdörfer L, et al. Interleukin-23-dependent γ/δ T cells produce Interleukin-17 and accumulate in the Enthesis, aortic valve, and ciliary body in mice. Arthritis Rheumatol. 2016;68:2476–86.
25. Sherlock JP, Joyce-Shaikh B, Turner SP, Chao CC, Sathe M, Grein J, et al. IL-23 induces spondyloarthropathy by acting on ROR-γt+ CD3+CD4-CD8- entheseal resident T cells. Nat Med. 2012;18:1069–76.
26. Huynh D, Kavanaugh A. Psoriatic arthritis: current therapy and future approaches. Rheumatology (Oxford). 2015;54:20–8.
27. Gniadecki R, Bang B, Sand C. Combination of antitumour necrosis factor-α and anti-interleukin-12/23 antibodies in refractory psoriasis and psoriatic arthritis: a long-term case-series observational study. Br J Dermatol. 2016;174:1145–6.
28. Nast A, Jacobs A, Rosumeck S, Werner RN. Efficacy and safety of systemic Long-term treatments for moderate-to-severe psoriasis: a systematic review and meta-analysis. J Invest Dermatol. 2015;135:2641–8.
29. Daudén E, Santiago-et-Sánchez-Mateos D, Sotomayor-López E, García-Díez A. Ustekinumab: effective in a patient with severe recalcitrant generalized pustular psoriasis. Br J Dermatol. 2010;163:1346–7.
30. Storan ER, O'Gorman SM, Markham T. Generalized pustular psoriasis treated with ustekinumab. Clin Exp Dermatol. 2016;41:689–90.
31. Arakawa A, Ruzicka T, Prinz JC. Therapeutic efficacy of interleukin 12/interleukin 23 blockade in generalized pustular psoriasis regardless of IL36RN mutation status. JAMA Dermatol. 2016;152:825–8.
32. Cymerman RM, Cohen DE. Treatment of Acrodermatitis continua of Hallopeau with Ustekinumab as monotherapy. JAMA Dermatol. 2016;152:346–8.
33. Adas A, Dadban A, Arnault JP, Chaby G, Lok C. Acrodermatitis continua of Hallopeau response to optimized biological therapy. Dermatol Online J. 2019;25:16.
34. Saunier J, Debarbieux S, Jullien D, Garnier L, Dalle S, Thomas L. Acrodermatitis continua of Hallopeau treated successfully with ustekinumab and acitretin after failure of tumour necrosis factor blockade and anakinra. Dermatology. 2015;230:97–100.
35. Shi L, Zeng L, Huang X, Wang B, Zhang Y, Zhang G. Acrodermatitis continua of Hallopeau successfully treated with Ustekinumab: a case report and literature review. Clin Cosmet Investig Dermatol. 2023;16:951–7.
36. Yilmaz SB, Cicek N, Coskun M, Yegin O, Alpsoy E. Serum and tissue levels of IL-17 in different clinical subtypes of psoriasis. Arch Dermatol Res. 2012;304:465–9.

37. Elliott M, Benson J, Blank M, Brodmerkel C, Baker D, Sharples KR, et al. Ustekinumab: lessons learned from targeting interleukin-12/23p40 in immune-mediated diseases. Ann N Y Acad Sci. 2009;1182:97–110.
38. Murakami M, Hagforsen E, Morhenn V, Ishida-Yamamoto A, Iizuka H. Patients with palmoplantar pustulosis have increased IL-17 and IL-22 levels both in the lesion and serum. Exp Dermatol. 2011;20:845–7.
39. Pinto-Almeida T, Torres T, Sanches M, Selores M. Treatment of palmoplantar pustulosis with ustekinumab--the importance of interfering with the IL23/Th17 pathway. Eur J Dermatol. 2013;23:916–7.
40. Bertelsen T, Kragballe K, Johansen C, Iversen L. Efficacy of ustekinumab in palmoplantar pustulosis and palmoplantar pustular psoriasis. Int J Dermatol. 2014;53:e464–6.
41. Gerdes S, Franke J, Domm S, Mrowietz U. Ustekinumab in the treatment of palmoplantar pustulosis. Br J Dermatol. 2010;163:1116–8.
42. Morales-Múnera C, Vilarrasa E, Puig L. Efficacy of ustekinumab in refractory palmoplantar pustular psoriasis. Br J Dermatol. 2013;168:820–4.
43. Buder V, Herberger K, Jacobi A, Augustin M, Radtke MA. Ustekinumab in the treatment of palmoplantar pustular psoriasis – a case series of nine patients. J Dtsch Dermatol Ges. 2016;14:1108–13.
44. Bulai Livideanu C, Lahfa M, Mazereeuw-Hautier J, Paul C. Efficacy of ustekinumab in palmoplantar psoriasis. Dermatology. 2010;221:321–3.
45. Nuño-González A, Gómez de la Fuente E, Vicente-Martín FJ, López-Estebaranz JL. Psoriasis hiperqueratósica palmoplantar con excelente respuesta a ustekinumab [Good response of hyperkeratotic palmoplantar psoriasis to ustekinumab]. Actas Dermosifiliogr. 2012;103:169–70.
46. Patsatsi A, Kyriakou A, Sotiriadis D. Ustekinumab in nail psoriasis: an open-label, uncontrolled, nonrandomized study. J Dermatolog Treat. 2013;24:96–100.
47. Rich P, Bourcier M, Sofen H, Fakharzadeh S, Wasfi Y, Wang Y, PHOENIX 1 Investigators, et al. Ustekinumab improves nail disease in patients with moderate-to-severe psoriasis: results from PHOENIX 1. Br J Dermatol. 2014;170:398–407.
48. Rallis E, Kintzoglou S, Verros C. Ustekinumab for rapid treatment of nail psoriasis. Arch Dermatol. 2010;146:1315–6.
49. Igarashi A, Kato T, Kato M, Song M, Nakagawa H, Japanese Ustekinumab Study Group. Efficacy and safety of ustekinumab in Japanese patients with moderate-to-severe plaque-type psoriasis: long-term results from a phase 2/3 clinical trial. J Dermatol. 2012;39:242–52.
50. Sabat R, Jemec GBE, Matusiak Ł, Kimball AB, Prens E, Wolk K. Hidradenitis suppurativa. Nat Rev Dis Primers. 2020;6:18.
51. Takeda K, Kikuchi K, Kanazawa Y, Yamasaki K, Aiba S. Ustekinumab treatment for hidradenitis suppurativa. J Dermatol. 2019;46:1215–8.
52. Blok JL, Li K, Brodmerkel C, Horvátovich P, Jonkman MF, Horváth B. Ustekinumab in hidradenitis suppurativa: clinical results and a search for potential biomarkers in serum. Br J Dermatol. 2016;174:839–46.
53. Romaní J, Vilarrasa E, Martorell A, Fuertes I, Ciudad C, Molina-Leyva A. Ustekinumab with intravenous infusion: results in hidradenitis Suppurativa. Dermatology. 2020;236:21–4.
54. Sánchez-Martínez EM, García-Ruiz R, Moneva-Léniz LM, Mateu-Puchades A. Effectiveness and safety of ustekinumab in patients with hidradenitis suppurativa using intravenous induction. Dermatol Ther. 2020;33:e14054.
55. Gulliver WP, Jemec GB, Baker KA. Experience with ustekinumab for the treatment of moderate to severe hidradenitis suppurativa. J Eur Acad Dermatol Venereol. 2012;26:911–4.
56. Scholl L, Hessam S, Garcovich S, Bechara FG. High-dosage ustekinumab for the treatment of severe hidradenitis suppurativa. Eur J Dermatol. 2019;29:659–61.
57. Ali N, Zirak B, Rodriguez RS, Pauli ML, Truong HA, Lai K, et al. Regulatory T cells in skin facilitate epithelial stem cell differentiation. Cell. 2017;169:1119–1129.e11.
58. Schlapbach C, Hänni T, Yawalkar N, Hunger RE. Expression of the IL-23/Th17 pathway in lesions of hidradenitis suppurativa. J Am Acad Dermatol. 2011 Oct;65(4):790–8.

59. Gkini MA, Bewley AP. Development of hidradenitis suppurativa in a patient treated with ustekinumab for her psoriasis: a potential paradoxical reaction? Dermatol Ther. 2018;31:e12742.
60. López González J, Lázaro Sáez M, Moreno Moraleda I, Hernández MÁ. Pyoderma gangrenosum solved by ustekinumab therapy. Gastroenterol Hepatol. 2021;44:299–300.
61. Benzaquen M, Monnier J, Beaussault Y, Rouby F, Berbis P. Pyoderma gangrenosum arising during treatment of psoriasis with adalimumab: effectiveness of ustekinumab. Australas J Dermatol. 2017;58:e270–1.
62. Nunes G, Patita M, Fernandes V. Refractory pyoderma Gangrenosum in a patient with Crohn's disease: complete response to Ustekinumab. J Crohns Colitis. 2019;13:812–3.
63. Petty AJ, Whitley MJ, Balaban A, Ellington K, Marano AL. Pyoderma gangrenosum induced by secukinumab in a patient with psoriasis successfully treated with ustekinumab. JAAD Case Rep. 2020;6:731–3.
64. Nieto D, Sendagorta E, Rueda JM, Herranz P. Successful treatment with ustekinumab and vacuum-assisted closure therapy in recalcitrant myelodysplastic syndrome-associated pyoderma gangrenosum: case report and literature review. Clin Exp Dermatol. 2019;44:116–9.
65. Guenova E, Teske A, Fehrenbacher B, Hoerber S, Adamczyk A, Schaller M, et al. Interleukin 23 expression in pyoderma gangrenosum and targeted therapy with ustekinumab. Arch Dermatol. 2011;147:1203–5.
66. Leung DY, Boguniewicz M, Howell MD, Nomura I, Hamid QA. New insights into atopic dermatitis. J Clin Invest. 2004;113:651–7.
67. Nomura T, Kabashima K, Miyachi Y. The panoply of αβT cells in the skin. J Dermatol Sci. 2014;76:3–9.
68. Nakajima S, Kitoh A, Egawa G, Natsuaki Y, Nakamizo S, Moniaga CS, et al. IL-17A as an inducer for Th2 immune responses in murine atopic dermatitis models. J Invest Dermatol. 2014;134:2122–30.
69. Weaver CT, Hatton RD, Mangan PR, Harrington LE. IL-17 family cytokines and the expanding diversity of effector T cell lineages. Annu Rev Immunol. 2007;25:821–52.
70. Koga C, Kabashima K, Shiraishi N, Kobayashi M, Tokura Y. Possible pathogenic role of Th17 cells for atopic dermatitis. J Invest Dermatol. 2008;128:2625–30.
71. Khattri S, Brunner PM, Garcet S, Finney R, Cohen SR, Oliva M, et al. Efficacy and safety of ustekinumab treatment in adults with moderate-to-severe atopic dermatitis. Exp Dermatol. 2017;26:28–35.
72. Saeki H, Kabashima K, Tokura Y, Murata Y, Shiraishi A, Tamamura R, et al. Efficacy and safety of ustekinumab in Japanese patients with severe atopic dermatitis: a randomized, double-blind, placebo-controlled, phase II study. Br J Dermatol. 2017;177:419–27.
73. Nic Dhonncha E, Clowry J, Dunphy M, Buckley C, Field S, Paul L. Treatment of severe atopic dermatitis with ustekinumab: a case series of 10 patients. Br J Dermatol. 2017;177:1752–3.
74. Shroff A, Guttman-Yassky E. Successful use of ustekinumab therapy in refractory severe atopic dermatitis. JAAD Case Rep. 2014;1:25–6.
75. Samorano LP, Hanifin JM, Simpson EL, Leshem YA. Inadequate response to ustekinumab in atopic dermatitis - a report of two patients. J Eur Acad Dermatol Venereol. 2016;30:522–3.
76. Ishiuji Y, Umezawa Y, Asahina A, Fukuta H, Aizawa N, Yanaba K, et al. Exacerbation of atopic dermatitis symptoms by ustekinumab in psoriatic patients with elevated serum immunoglobulin E levels: report of two cases. J Dermatol. 2018;45:732–4.
77. Guttman-Yassky E, Krueger JG. Atopic dermatitis and psoriasis: two different immune diseases or one spectrum? Curr Opin Immunol. 2017;48:68–73.
78. Weiss D, Schaschinger M, Ristl R, Gruber R, Kopp T, Stingl G, et al. Ustekinumab treatment in severe atopic dermatitis: Down-regulation of T-helper 2/22 expression. J Am Acad Dermatol. 2017;76:91–97.e3.
79. Park KY, Jang WS, Son IP, Choi SY, Lee MY, Kim BJ, et al. Combination therapy with cyclosporine and psoralen plus ultraviolet a in the patients with severe alopecia areata: a retrospective study with a self-controlled design. Ann Dermatol. 2013;25:12–6.

80. Açıkgöz G, Calışkan E, Tunca M, Yeniay Y, Akar A. The effect of oral cyclosporine in the treatment of severe alopecia areata. Cutan Ocul Toxicol. 2014;33:247–52.
81. Aleisa A, Lim Y, Gordon S, Her MJ, Zancanaro P, Abudu M, et al. Response to ustekinumab in three pediatric patients with alopecia areata. Pediatr Dermatol. 2019;36:e44–5.
82. Guttman-Yassky E, Ungar B, Noda S, Suprun M, Shroff A, Dutt R, et al. Extensive alopecia areata is reversed by IL-12/IL-23p40 cytokine antagonism. J Allergy Clin Immunol. 2016;137:301–4.
83. Elkady A, Bonomo L, Amir Y, Vekaria AS, Guttman-Yassky E. Effective use of ustekinumab in a patient with concomitant psoriasis, vitiligo, and alopecia areata. JAAD Case Rep. 2017;3:477–9.
84. Tanasescu C, Balanescu E, Balanescu P, Olteanu R, Badea C, Grancea C, et al. IL-17 in cutaneous lupus erythematosus. Eur Intern Med. 2010;21:202–7.
85. Mok MY, Wu HJ, Lo Y, Lau CS. The relation of interleukin 17 (IL-17) and IL-23 to Th1/Th2 cytokines and disease activity in systemic lupus erythematosus. J Rheumatol. 2010;37:2046–52.
86. Maczynska I, Millo B, Ratajczak-Stefańska V, Maleszka R, Szych Z, Kurpisz M, et al. Proinflammatory cytokine (IL-1beta, IL-6, IL-12, IL-18 and TNF-alpha) levels in sera of patients with subacute cutaneous lupus erythematosus (SCLE). Immunol Lett. 2006;102:79–82.
87. Solomon GJ, Magro CM. Foxp3 expression in cutaneous T-cell lymphocytic infiltrates. J Cutan Pathol. 2008;35:1032–9.
88. De Souza A, Ali-Shaw T, Strober BE, Franks AG Jr. Successful treatment of subacute lupus erythematosus with ustekinumab. Arch Dermatol. 2011;147:896–8.
89. Winchester D, Duffin KC, Hansen C. Response to ustekinumab in a patient with both severe psoriasis and hypertrophic cutaneous lupus. Lupus. 2012;21:1007–10.
90. Dahl C, Johansen C, Kragballe K, Olesen AB. Ustekinumab in the treatment of refractory chronic cutaneous lupus erythematosus: a case report. Acta Derm Venereol. 2013;93:368–9.
91. Chyuan IT, Tsai TH, Chang TH, Wu CS. Ustekinumab treatment in a patient with psoriasis and systemic lupus erythematosus. Lupus. 2015;24:650–1.
92. Varada S, Gottlieb AB, Merola JF, Saraiya AR, Tintle SJ. Treatment of coexistent psoriasis and lupus erythematosus. J Am Acad Dermatol. 2015;72:253–60.
93. Romero-Maté A, García-Donoso C, Hernández-Núñez A, Martínez-Morán C, Moreno-Torres A, Borbujo-Martínez J. Successful treatment of recalcitrant discoid lupus erythematosus with ustekinumab. Dermatol Online J. 2017;23:13030.
94. Tierney E, Kirthi S, Ramsay B, Ahmad K. Ustekinumab-induced subacute cutaneous lupus. JAAD Case Rep. 2019;5:271–3.
95. Lowe GC, Henderson CL, Grau RH, Hansen CB, Sontheimer RD. A systematic review of drug-induced subacute cutaneous lupus erythematosus. Br J Dermatol. 2011;164:465–72.
96. Mirouse A, Barete S, Desbois AC, Comarmond C, Sene D, Domont F, et al. Long term outcome of ustekinumab therapy for Behcet's disease. Arthritis Rheumatol. 2019;71:1727–32.
97. Baerveldt EM, Kappen JH, Thio HB, van Laar JA, van Hagen PM, Prens EP. Successful long-term triple disease control by ustekinumab in a patient with Behcet's disease, psoriasis and hidradenitis suppurativa. Ann Rheum Dis. 2013;72:626–7.
98. Lopalco G, Fabiani C, Venerito V, Lapadula G, Iannone F, Cantarini L. Ustekinumab efficacy and safety in mucocutaneous multi-refractory Behçet's disease. Clin Exp Rheumatol. 2017;35(Suppl 108):130–1.
99. Di Stefani A, Galluzzo M, Talamonti M, Chiricozzi A, Costanzo A, Chimenti S. Long-term ustekinumab treatment for refractory type I pityriasis rubra pilaris. J Dermatol Case Rep. 2013;7:5–9.
100. Wohlrab J, Kreft B. Treatment of pityriasis rubra pilaris with ustekinumab. Br J Dermatol. 2010;163:655–6.
101. Eytan O, Qiaoli L, Nousbeck J, van Steensel MA, Burger B, Hohl D, et al. Increased epidermal expression and absence of mutations in CARD14 in a series of patients with sporadic pityriasis rubra pilaris. Br J Dermatol. 2014;170:1196–8.

102. Chowdhary M, Davila U, Cohen DJ. Ustekinumab as an alternative treatment option for chronic pityriasis rubra pilaris. Case Rep Dermatol. 2015;7:46–50.
103. Feldmeyer L, Mylonas A, Demaria O, Mennella A, Yawalkar N, Laffitte E, et al. Interleukin 23-helper T cell 17 Axis as a treatment target for Pityriasis Rubra pilaris. JAMA Dermatol. 2017;153:304–8.
104. Aragón-Miguel R, Prieto-Barrios M, Calleja-Algarra A, Velasco-Tamariz V, Andres-Lencina JJ, Ortiz-Romero P, et al. Refractory pityriasis rubra pilaris with good response after treatment with ustekinumab. J Dtsch Dermatol Ges. 2018;16:1022–5.
105. Solimani F, Pollmann R, Schmidt T, Schmidt A, Zheng X, Savai R, et al. Therapeutic targeting of Th17/Tc17 cells leads to clinical improvement of lichen planus. Front Immunol. 2019;10:1808.
106. Lu R, Zeng X, Han Q, Lin M, Long L, Dan H, et al. Overexpression and selectively regulatory roles of IL-23/IL-17 axis in the lesions of oral lichen planus. Mediat Inflamm. 2014;2014:701094.
107. Wendling D, Aubin F, Verhoeven F, Prati C. IL-23/Th17 targeted therapies in SAPHO syndrome. A case series. Joint Bone Spine. 2017;84:733–5.
108. Loget F, Plée P, Antonicelli F, Bernard P, Loget J, Plée J. A successful treatment with ustekinumab in a case of relapsing bullous pemphigoid associated with psoriasis. J Eur Acad Dermatol Venereol. 2017;31:e228–30.
109. Knisley RR, Petropolis AA, Mackey VT. Lichen planus pemphigoides treated with ustekinumab. Cutis. 2017;100:415–8.
110. Majima Y, Yagi H, Tateishi C, Groth S, Schmidt E, Zillikens D, Koga H, Hashimoto T, Tokura Y. A successful treatment with ustekinumab in a case of antilaminin-γ1 pemphigoid associated with psoriasis. Br J Dermatol. 2013;168:1367–9.
111. Le Guern A, Alkeraye S, Vermersch-Langlin A, Coupe P, Vonarx M. Bullous pemphigoid during ustekinumab therapy. JAAD Case Rep. 2015 Oct;1:359–60.
112. Nakayama C, Fujita Y, Watanabe M, Shimizu H. Development of bullous pemphigoid during treatment of psoriatic onycho-pachydermo periostitis with ustekinumab. J Dermatol. 2015;42:996–8.
113. Onsun N, Sallahoglu K, Dizman D, Su Ö, Tosuner Z. Bullous pemphigoid during ustekinumab therapy in a psoriatic patient. Eur J Dermatol. 2017;27:81–2.
114. Colquhoun M, Kemp AK. Ustekinumab. In: StatPearls [Internet]. Treasure Island (FL): StatPearls Publishing; 2023. Available at https://www.ncbi.nlm.nih.gov/books/NBK570645/.
115. Guarneri C, Lentini M, Polimeni G, Giuffrida R, Cannavò SP. Ustekinumab-induced drug eruption resembling lymphocytic infiltration (of Jessner-Kanof) and lupus erythematosus tumidus. Br J Clin Pharmacol. 2016;81:792–4.
116. Lebwohl M, Leonardi C, Griffiths CE, Prinz JC, Szapary PO, Yeilding N, et al. Long-term safety experience of ustekinumab in patients with moderate-to-severe psoriasis (part I of II): results from analyses of general safety parameters from pooled phase 2 and 3 clinical trials. J Am Acad Dermatol. 2012;66:731–41.
117. Gordon KB, Papp KA, Langley RG, Ho V, Kimball AB, Guzzo C, et al. Long-term safety experience of ustekinumab in patients with moderate to severe psoriasis (part II of II): results from analyses of infections and malignancy from pooled phase II and III clinical trials. J Am Acad Dermatol. 2012;66:742–51.
118. Smith CH, Yiu ZZN, Bale T, Burden AD, Coates LC, Edwards W, British Association of Dermatologists' Clinical Standards Unit, et al. British Association of Dermatologists guidelines for biologic therapy for psoriasis 2020: a rapid update. Br J Dermatol. 2020;183:628–37.
119. Holroyd CR, Seth R, Bukhari M, Malaviya A, Holmes C, Curtis E, et al. The British Society for Rheumatology biologic DMARD safety guidelines in inflammatory arthritis-executive summary. Rheumatology (Oxford). 2019;58:220–6.
120. Lamb CA, Kennedy NA, Raine T, Hendy PA, Smith PJ, Limdi JK, et al. British Society of Gastroenterology consensus guidelines on the management of inflammatory bowel disease in adults. Gut. 2019;68(Suppl 3):s1–s106.

121. Tsakok T, Wilson N, Dand N, Loeff FC, Bloem K, Baudry D, British Association of Dermatologists biologic and Immunomodulators register (BADBIR) study group and the psoriasis stratification to optimise relevant therapy (PSORT) consortium, et al. Association of Serum Ustekinumab Levels with clinical response in psoriasis. JAMA Dermatol. 2019;155:1235–43.
122. Landells I, Marano C, Hsu MC, Li S, Zhu Y, Eichenfield LF, et al. Ustekinumab in adolescent patients age 12 to 17 years with moderate-to-severe plaque psoriasis: results of the randomized phase 3 CADMUS study. J Am Acad Dermatol. 2015 Oct;73(4):594–603.
123. Sands BE, Sandborn WJ, Panaccione R, O'Brien CD, Zhang H, Johanns J, UNIFI Study Group, et al. Ustekinumab as induction and maintenance therapy for ulcerative colitis. N Engl J Med. 2019;381:1201–14.
124. Feagan BG, Sandborn WJ, Gasink C, Jacobstein D, Lang Y, Friedman JR, UNITI–IM-UNITI Study Group, et al. Ustekinumab as induction and maintenance therapy for Crohn's disease. N Engl J Med. 2016;375:1946–60.
125. Balakirski G, Gerdes S, Beissert S, Ochsendorf F, von Kiedrowski R, Wilsmann-Theis D. Therapy of psoriasis during pregnancy and breast-feeding. J Dtsch Dermatol Ges. 2022;20:653–83.
126. Takeuchi I, Arai K, Kyodo R, Sato T, Tokita K, Hirano Y, et al. Ustekinumab for children and adolescents with inflammatory bowel disease at a tertiary children's hospital in Japan. J Gastroenterol Hepatol. 2021;36:125–30.

IL-17 Antagonists

36

Secukinumab: Introduction

Secukinumab is an interleukin-17A antagonist, and the first in this class to be employed for the treatment of psoriasis.

Mechanism of Action

Secukinumab is a fully human immunoglobin IgG_1 monoclonal antibody that selectively binds to IL-17A and inhibits its interaction with the IL-17 receptor family [1]. Because of this blockade, inflammatory cascades generated by IL-17 cannot proceed further, thereby halting disease progression. Further details of secukinumab's mechanism of action in relation to the respective disease are outlined in appropriate sections.

Pharmacokinetics

Following a single subcutaneous (SC) dose of 150 mg or 300 mg, C_{max} for secukinumab is achieved after 6–7 days of administration. Steady state concentrations of the drug are obtained by 24 weeks, following the weekly dosing regimen suggested for psoriasis. The concentration of secukinumab in lesional and non-lesional skin of patients with plaque psoriasis varies from 27% to 40% at one and two weeks after a single SC dose of 300 mg. The $t_{1/2}$ of secukinumab is 27 days [2].

Metabolism of secukinumab occurs via catabolic pathways, wherein secukinumab gets degraded into small peptides and amino acids. Main route of secukinumab elimination is via intracellular catabolism and therefore renal impairment is not likely to influence the overall pharmacokinetic profile of secukinumab [3].

A. K. Bubna, *Therapeutics in Dermatology - Essentials for Clinical Practice*,
https://doi.org/10.1007/978-981-95-3791-4_36

Indications

FDA Approved

- Moderate to severe plaque psoriasis (including paediatric psoriasis in patients ≥6 years of age) [4].
- Psoriatic arthropathy (PsA) (including active juvenile psoriatic arthritis in children aged 2 years or older) [4].
- Ankylosing spondylitis [5].
- Hidradenitis suppurativa (HS) [6].

Off Label [7–9]

- Pyoderma gangrenosum (PG).
- Atopic dermatitis (AD).
- Lichen planus (LP).
- Pityriasis rubra pilaris (PRP).
- Behcet's disease (BD).
- Allergic contact dermatitis (ACD).

Contraindications

Absolute [10]

- Presence of active infections; more importantly latent or active tuberculosis, hepatitis B, C and HIV.
- Hypersensitivity to secukinumab.

Relative [11]

- PUVA sessions being received.
- Premalignant conditions.
- Demyelinating disease.
- Optic neuritis.
- Multiple sclerosis.
- Pregnancy/lactation.
- Congestive cardiac failure.
- Inflammatory bowel disease.
- Concurrent use of live vaccines.
- Marked elevated levels of hepatic transaminases.

Clinical Uses

Plaque Psoriasis

The role of secukinumab in psoriasis is linked to its antagonist effect against IL-17, which is elevated in both serum and skin of patients affected with psoriasis [12, 13]. Further, greater levels of IL-17 is associated with increased severity of psoriasis [14].

Interleukin-17 plays an important role contributing to the aberrant activity of keratinocytes, and activation of immune cells, along with raised levels of other inflammatory cytokines (that include IL-6, IL-1β and TNFα), ultimately resulting in abnormal epidermal differentiation and proliferation [15–17].

Secukinumab acts by its inhibitory effect on inflammation secondary to IL-17A blockade. In moderate to severe plaque psoriasis, secukinumab serves as a valuable therapeutic agent. Besides, secukinumab has a rapid onset of action, with therapeutic responses evident as early as 4 weeks following treatment initiation; and effects being sustained and long lasting [18–21].

Four large scale studies have substantiated the efficacy of secukinumab (300 mg/150 mg at week 0, 1, 2, 3, 4 and then monthly) in moderate-to-severe plaque psoriasis; with the 300 mg dosing being more effective, and demonstrating greater percentage of patients with Psoriasis Area Severity Index (PASI)-75 (6.4–10%), PASI-90 (12.3–20%) and PASI-100 (9.7–34.6%) in comparison to the 150 mg regimen [18–20].

Besides, secukinumab is superior to etanercept and ustekinumab in the management of psoriasis, with statistically significant outcomes [18, 21].

Currently, the approved dosing regimen of secukinumab is 300 mg SC at weeks 0, 1, 2, 3 and 4, followed by monthly maintenance dosing, starting at week 8 [1].

However, some patients respond only partially to this dosing; or display disease relapse in between maintenance injections. In such scenarios, increasing the frequency of maintenance dosing every 2–3 weeks has shown to provide clinical benefit, without any increase in the incidence of adverse effects. Therefore, in patients not responding adequately to the currently approved secukinumab regimen, dose optimization can be a valuable option, before considering drug discontinuation [22].

Palmoplantar Psoriasis

Palmoplantar psoriasis (PPP) describes plaque psoriasis present over the palms and soles. This variant of psoriasis is quite difficult to treat, often resulting in higher levels of impairment in health-related quality of life (HR-QoL), with psychological, physical and occupational repercussions [23].

Secukinumab serves as a safe and valuable treatment option in those cases of PPP, where conventional therapy is ineffective. Both 300 mg and 150 mg regimens have been used in PPP, with better therapeutic responses obtained utilizing the former dosing [24, 25].

In a double-blind randomized control trial (RCT), following 16 weeks of therapy, 19.2% more patients receiving 300 mg of secukinumab had achieved the primary end point (Primary end point was Palmoplantar Investigator's Global Assessment wherein '0' corresponded to clear palms/soles and 1 represented almost clear palms/soles; at 16 weeks), in comparison to those receiving 150 mg [24]. However, at 2.5 years, the difference in the mean palmoplantar Psoriasis Area Severity Index (ppPASI) amelioration between both dosing schedules was 6.8%, with both groups delineating improved clinical responses to secukinumab [25].

In another report, ppPASI 75 and 100 at week 16 (with secukinumab 300 mg), was seen in 38% and 23.8% patients respectively [26].

Secukinumab thus brings a sustained and continuous improvement in PPP, with acceptable long term clinical outcomes, and a positive impact on HR-QoL.

Nail Psoriasis

Nail involvement is common in psoriasis patients and is associated with significant pain, impaired finger mobility/function; along with loss of manual dexterity (in severe cases) [27].

Often nail psoriasis is associated with PsA, further causing impairment in HR-QoL. A number of topical and systemic therapies have been employed in nail psoriasis (NP). Owing to the distinctive anatomy of the nail unit, sufficient concentrations of active topical drugs may not be achieved in the involved nail, making topical treatment frequently ineffective [28].

In NP, secukinumab has been used systematically, as well as by intramatriceal injections [29, 30].

Systemic secukinumab has shown to provide long term sustainability of treatment effect in NP, with mean NAPSI improvements of 73.7% (300 mg dosing) and 63.6% (150 mg dosing) after 2.5 years of treatment, and can be considered a valuable alternative to treat NP unresponsive to conventional anti-psoriatic therapy [29].

Intramatriceal injections with low dose secukinumab (7.5 mg–30 mg/ml) has been found to be quick, effective, safe as well as economic, in the management of NP, with 42.9–80% improvement following 3 months of therapy [30].

It is suggested that durability of secukinumab in NP is connected with its ability in antagonising release of IL-17A from innate immune cells, which other biologics generally fail to target [29].

Psoriatic Arthropathy

PsA is a chronic inflammatory arthritis found in around 20% of patients with psoriasis [20].

Clinical manifestations of PsA are diverse evolving over time from a monoarticular pattern to polyarticular involvement. Currently, with considerable progress in understanding disease pathogenesis; a number of new therapies have been outlined for PsA. Secukinumab is among the newer agents developed for the management of PsA.

Levels of IL-17, as well as its receptor IL-17RA, are elevated in the synovial tissue. This pathologic increase proceeds to an abnormal upregulation of matrix metalloproteinases and cytokines like IL-6 and IL-8 that significantly contribute to joint/bone changes in PsA. Targeting IL-17 and its receptor IL-17RA, and preventing this inflammatory cascade from occurring, is the role played by secukinumab in PsA [31, 32].

The efficacy and safety of secukinumab has been assessed in 2 large studies in adults with active PsA, with gratifying results.

In both studies, patients had PsA for at least 5 years and were unable to continue methotrexate or systemic corticosteroids. In all patients a minimum of 3 swollen/tender joints were present despite treatment with non-steroidal anti-inflammatory drugs (NSAIDs), corticosteroids or disease modifying antirheumatic drugs (DMRDs). The common primary end point in these studies was achievement of American College of Rheumatology 20 (ACR-20) response at week 24 following initiation of treatment with secukinumab.

Study 1: This study consisted of 4 groups. Group 1 received 300 mg of secukinumab, group 2 got 150 mg, group 3 obtained 75 mg and group 4 received placebo. The dosing given was as per the schedule employed in plaque psoriasis. At 24 weeks, ACR-20 was witnessed in 54% of the 300 mg group, 51% of the 150 mg group, 29% of the 75 mg group and 15% of the placebo group. Responses were maintained until week 52 in the groups receiving 300 mg and 150 mg of secukinumab. Besides, the drug was tolerated well with no serious adverse reactions [33].

Study 2: Here subjects received intravenous (IV) secukinumab (10 mg/kg at weeks 0, 2 and 4 followed by SC administration of either 150 mg/75 mg once in 4 weeks). Unlike other studies dose dependent improvement was not observed here. Overall, 50% of participants receiving 150 mg, achieved ACR-20 at 24 weeks and 50.5% receiving 75 mg of secukinumab attained ACR-20 at 24 weeks. Moreover, these results were sustained at week 52. Importantly, this study did not utilise the 300 mg dose, unlike other studies [34].

In both studies, patients tolerated the drug well, with no significant adverse events. Secukinumab can therefore be considered highly efficacious and safe in patients with PsA.

Pustular Psoriasis

Pustular psoriasis (PP) is one of the subtypes of psoriasis very difficult to treat. Often therapy for PP is a prolonged one, warranting selection of a drug that is effective, yet at the same time associated with low levels of toxicity.

Traditional agents employed in pustular psoriasis, particularly in the generalised variant; include acitretin, cyclosporine and methotrexate, which though effective are limited by their slower onset of action and serious side effects [35].

Though currently not approved by the FDA for pustular psoriasis, secukinumab's efficacy in GPP has been clearly documented. Besides in Japan, it is approved for coverage of health insurance in pustular psoriasis [36].

Various reports have highlighted the efficacy of secukinumab in pustular psoriasis, with improvements evident as early as 3 days of receiving the first dose, and excellent control of lesions by 12 weeks [37–43].

Hidradenitis Suppurativa

HS is a chronic, inflammatory, recurrent, debilitating, follicular disease that usually presents after puberty and is characterized by painful, deep seated inflamed lesions in the apocrine gland bearing areas of the body, most commonly the axillary, inguinal and anogenital regions. It is observed that patients with HS have high serum levels of IL-17A, which in turn facilitates recruitment of neutrophils and provides a positive feedback in maintaining the population of proinflammatory Th17 cells [44, 45].

IL-17 induces the release of several chemokines; majorly CXCL1, CXCL8 and CCL20. It further acts on the nod-like receptor protein 3 (NLRP 3) inflammasome and stimulates production of TGFβ, IL-1β, IL-6 and TNFα from macrophages, which are pivotal for Th17 differentiation and proliferation [46, 47].

- TGFβ sets into motion RAR-related orphan receptor gamma-γt (a transcription factor), necessary for generation of Th17 cells [48].
- IL-1β and IL-6 independently downregulate Foxp3 (a transcription factor), consequently resulting in decreased levels of regulatory T cells (Tregs) [49].
- TNFα promotes rapid induction of IL-1β, IL-6, IL-8 and IL-2, as well as adhesion molecules in monocytes and macrophages, perpetuating a relentlessly progressive cycle in the pathogenesis of HS [50].

By antagonizing IL-17A, secukinumab prevents the generation of these inflammatory cascades, and thus helps in the treatment of HS.

Recently, secukinumab was approved for the management of HS [6], the dosing being slightly different than that used in psoriasis. Response to secukinumab (300 mg given every 2 weekly, and 4 weekly) were assessed in clinical trials. At 16 weeks; HS clinical response (HiSCR) was seen in 45% of patients receiving the drug every 2 weeks, and in 42% patients receiving secukinumab every 4 weeks in one clinical trial; and in 42% of patients (biweekly secukinumab) and 45% of patients (monthly secukinumab) in another clinical trial, concluding no significant difference in improvement with the biweekly dosing schedule. Besides, secukinumab was well tolerated with no issues related to safety [51].

In previous reports though, the label dosing regimen of psoriasis was found effective and safe in treating HS [52–57].

However, Prussik and colleagues [53], despite witnessing meaningful improvement in HS with the approved dosing regimen of psoriasis, felt the need for dose escalation, owing to higher levels of IL-17A in HS, when compared to psoriasis.

Interestingly, Marasca and coworkers [58], reported precipitation of HS in a 47-year-old male receiving secukinumab for psoriasis. Currently, the mechanism for this paradoxical reaction needs elucidation.

Pyoderma Gangrenosum

PG is a rare neutrophilic dermatosis characterised by painful, inflammatory papules, pustules or vesiculopustules that progressively expand and finally ulcerate. Although generally associated with an underlying malignancy or an inflammatory condition, 50% of PG patients demonstrate an idiopathic aetiology [59].

Secukinumab has a role in PG, owing to the given effect of IL-17 on neutrophil migration [60].

IL-17 and its receptors are increasingly expressed in the lesional skin of PG. IL-17 promotes release of chemokines that facilitate neutrophilic migration, and triggers secretion of IL-6, GM-CSF and IL-8, all of which significantly contribute in the pathogenesis of PG. Moreover, Th17 counts are notably elevated in PG, with reduction in levels of Tregs. By blocking IL-17, secukinumab antagonizes the subsequent chain of inflammatory events and in this way helps in PG. [61–63]

McPhie and Kirchhof [64] demonstrated secukinumab (300 mg, standard dosing regimen) to be highly effective in bringing about significant improvement of PG in a 50 year old woman who had failed previous treatments with systemic corticosteroids and methotrexate. Following 4 weeks of initiation of therapy with secukinumab, patient's pain had ameliorated by 70–80%, and after 3 months there was no pain with complete healing of skin ulceration.

Garcia et al. [65], also reported the effectiveness of secukinumab in the treatment of PG, along with prednisolone (30 mg/day). Here, secukinumab (300 mg) was initially dosed as per the psoriasis induction and maintenance protocol, but after 16 weeks of treatment, secukinumab was administered fortnightly. Lesions highlighted a partial positive response with secukinumab, unlike previous failed attempts with cyclosporine, adalimumab, ustekinumab, etanercept and methotrexate. However, complete clinical recovery was not documented.

A study from Germany, on the other hand stated secukinumab to be ineffective in a patient with PG. [66]

Moreover, there have been reports elucidating secukinumab precipitating PG.

A Japanese publication outlined the development of PG in a 47 year of woman with PsA who was started on secukinumab following development of palmoplantar pustulosis 4 months after treatment with adalimumab. Secukinumab did result in improvement of psoriatic lesions, but lead to the development of PG following 4 months of therapy with the drug [67].

This finding was reiterated in 2 individual reports, wherein PG was induced by secukinumab in both patients having moderate-to-severe plaque psoriasis [68, 69].

It is suggested that inhibition of IL-17A can paradoxically increase IL-23 production, which in turn facilitates development of PG. [60]

It thus becomes essential to keep this therapeutic paradox of secukinumab in mind, prior to its prescription for this indication.

Atopic Dermatitis

Atopic dermatitis (AD) is a highly heterogenous disease having diverse subtypes and displaying varied immune activation. This makes room for additional therapeutic strategies while managing patients with AD [70].

Of late, increased Th17 skewing in paediatric and Asian AD patients has been ascertained and it has been observed that Th17 related markers show an obvious correlation with AD severity [70, 71].

A 22-year-old Asian man with AD demonstrated significant improvement following treatment with secukinumab (300 mg, as per the induction and maintenance dosing schedule for psoriasis), following failed topical and systemic therapies, including cyclosporine. After 16 weeks of therapy, SCORAD reduced from 84.5 to 28.2 with impressive improvement in erythema and pruritus. Besides, Th1 markers (IFNα and CXCL10) had also significantly decreased; and expression of filaggrin/loricrin (epidermal differentiation markers) were restored to normal levels post treatment with secukinumab [9].

However, Ungar and colleagues [72] in their analysis were unable to obtain any benefit with secukinumab for AD. They suggested that although in some populations IL-17 targeting may have some benefit, owing to the increased microbial burden; as a whole IL-17 is certainly not a valid therapeutic target in majority patients with AD, as this disorder integrates numerous cytokines in its pathogenesis.

More studies are therefore mandated to vehemently emphasize the utility of secukinumab for AD.

Lichen Planus

Lichen planus (LP) is a common, chronic relapsing inflammatory disease involving the skin and mucous membranes, with a refractory course [73].

Solimani et al. [74], delineated the propitious role of secukinumab in 3 patients with LP, with resolution of lesions within 12–48 weeks of treatment.

The role of secukinumab in LP can be linked to the pathogenic role of Th17/Tc17 and T cell derived IL-17A that induces and perhaps also perpetuates the inflammatory response in LP. The notion that Th17/Tc17 cells are responsible for the generation of IL-17 is bolstered by the presence of $CD4^+$/$IL17^+$ and $CD8^+$/$IL\text{-}17^+$ cells lined along the dermal-epidermal junction in close proximity to apoptotic epidermal keratinocytes (a distinctive finding in LP) [75].

The favourable profile of secukinumab in LP was further highlighted by Rezzag-Mahcena et al. [76], in a 66-year-old male with genital LP who was unresponsive to topical corticosteroids/calcineurin inhibitors, hydroxychloroquine, acitretin (up to 40 mg/day) and methotrexate (6 months of 25 mg SC/week). Following 12 weeks of secukinumab (300 mg, conventional dosing for psoriasis), complete resolution was witnessed at 9 months of follow up.

However, despite these encouraging reports of secukinumab in LP, anomalous occurrence of LP (including oral, genital and hypertrophic variants) has been documented following its administration in psoriasis patients [77–79].

It is postulated that following IL-17 neutralization with secukinumab, there is upregulation of dendritic cells and an increase in type 1 interferon, that in turn leads to the development of LP [77].

Further, oral candidiasis secondary to immune suppression can trigger the development of oral LP, in patients receiving secukinumab [77, 79].

Nevertheless, LP seen in these settings is usually not severe enough to demand cessation of secukinumab.

Pityriasis Rubra Pilaris

PRP is a rare papulosquamous disease with an unknown cause. There are a number of drugs in the therapeutic armamentarium of PRP, with newer drugs continually being added to the existing list.

Secukinumab (300 mg, according to the psoriasis dosing schedule) has been reported to be effective in the management of PRP refractory to conventional treatment, with resolution of pruritus and erythema within 4–8 weeks of treatment; and palmoplantar keratoderma by 24 weeks [80, 81].

However, in other reports, a mixed response to secukinumab was observed, with significant improvement in 2 patients, not very satisfactory results in 1, and paradoxical worsening of PRP in another [82, 83].

The role of secukinumab in PRP is associated with upregulation of helper T cell 17 cytokines, including IL-17A, IL-17F and IL-22 in lesional skin of PRP patients (which it antagonizes) [84]. These cytokines are thought to drive keratinocyte proliferation and vascular dysfunction, observed in PRP [85].

As there exists a report of paradoxical PRP exacerbation with secukinumab, this needs to be kept in mind, prior to its prescription in PRP.

Overall, though, secukinumab has been well tolerated in patients with PRP.

Behçet's Disease

BD is a systemic vasculitis that presents with a heterogenous clinical picture. Mucosal lesions of the oral cavity and genitalia are the most recognizable features in BD and negatively impact patients' quality of life [86].

Di Scala et al. [87], evaluated the efficacy and safety of secukinumab in 5 patients with BD, with complete resolution of articular and mucocutaneous lesions following 3–9 months of therapy.

Fagni and colleagues [88] further propounded the favourable profile of secukinumab in the treatment of refractory BD, in 15 patients. Previous therapy given to these patients included corticosteroids, colchicine, methotrexate, azathioprine and hydroxychloroquine. Dosing of secukinumab was either 150 mg/month (9 patients) or 300 mg/month (6 patients). Out of the 9 patients receiving 150 mg/month of secukinumab, 4 were switched to the 300 mg/month dosing at 3 months and 3 patients were switched to the 300 mg/month dosing at 6 months, owing to inadequate therapeutic responses with the lower dosing of secukinumab. Following 3 months of treatment, 66.7% of patients had achieved complete/partial response with respect to control of mucosal/articular manifestations that sharply increased from 86.7% at 6 months to 100% at 24 months.

However, in 9 patients relapse of the disease was seen, 5 of whom, were not available for follow up. In one patient, increasing the dose from 150 mg to 300 mg was sufficient to obtain clinical response. In 2 patients, spontaneous remission was attained within the subsequent follow up and in the other patient complete response was obtained with introduction of methotrexate to the treatment regimen.

Moreover, most patients tolerated treatment well, except for candida infection occurring in 2 patients, gingivitis in one patient and vertigo/mild mood disorders in another patient. However, there were no serious side effects reported.

The unique attributes of mucosal and articular phenotypes of BD, along with an increased prevalence of peripheral spondylarthritis like features such as enthesopathy and inconstant axial involvement strongly hint the justification of using anti IL-17 drugs for BD [89].

Allergic Contact Dermatitis

Although used in an open label phase II trial for ACD, secukinumab did not demonstrate notable improvements. Out of 4 patients treated with secukinumab (300 mg at weeks 0,1,2,3,4 and 8), one patient demonstrated minor improvements in the physician's global assessment (PGA) score from 3 to 2; and the DLQI reducing from 16 to 3. However, in the remaining 3 patients, lesions had either worsened or remained the same [90].

Further studies with a larger sample size are thus needed to determine the utility of secukinumab for this indication.

Alopecia Areata

In a randomised trial of 7 AA patients getting secukinumab (300 mg as per the dosing schedule of plaque psoriasis), none of the patients experienced the primary outcome of 50% reduction in SALT score. Out of the 7, only one demonstrated partial hair regrowth, one had worsening of hair loss and status of the remaining two was *sine quo* [91].

Again, more research in this regard is mandatory prior to using secukinumab in AA.

Adverse Effects [92, 93]

Most Common

- Nasopharyngitis.
- Upper respiratory tract infections.
- Diarrhoea.

Others

Cutaneous

- Urticaria.
- Pruritus.
- Pyoderma.
- Mucocutaneous candidiasis.
- Injection site reactions.
- Non-melanoma skin cancer.
- Melanoma.

Extra Cutaneous

- Hypertension.
- Arthralgia/back pain.
- Bladder cancer.
- Thyroid cancer.

Despite these adverse effects, overall safety profile of secukinumab leaves it highly recommendable. According to product labelling, in clinical trials, doses of 30 mg/kg IV have been administered without toxicity. However, all patients should be monitored for any signs/symptoms of toxicity and adverse reactions in the event of an overdose. There exists no antidote for secukinumab currently, with management being purely supportive.

Drug Monitoring [94]

Baseline

- Complete blood count/hemogram.
- Erythrocyte sedimentation rate.

- C-reactive protein.
- Liver function test.
- Renal function test.
- Serum electrolytes.
- Anti-nuclear antibody.
- Anti-dsDNA antibody.
- Screening for hepatitis and human immunodeficiency virus.
- Chest X-ray.
- Tuberculin skin testing or QuantiFERON gold test.
- Pregnancy test in females of child bearing age.
- Serology for varicella zoster and measles (if clinically indicated).
- Urinalysis.

Ongoing Monitoring

- Evaluation of response to treatment is measurable by respective assessment scores; i.e. PASI, DLQI at 3 months initially and subsequently every 6 months.
- A complete blood count and hemogram needs to be repeated at 3 months and then every 6 months.
- Liver and renal function tests, electrolytes and urinalysis need similar evaluation.

Use in Specific Populations

Pregnancy

There aren't sufficient well controlled trials yet for the use of secukinumab in pregnancy. However, pre-clinical embryo-foetal development studies observed no adverse outcomes after SC administration of secukinumab, during organ development at 30 times maximum recommended human dose. The exposure of secukinumab though, was relatively short in these studies. Therefore, secukinumab must be used in pregnancy only if the potential benefit justifies potential risk to the foetus [95].

Nursing Mothers

As secukinumab has a high molecular weight, its concentration in maternal milk is likely to be very low. Secukinumab is also partially destroyed in the infant's gastrointestinal tract. However, significant research is still needed in this regard. Clinicians should thus be cautious still, while prescribing secukinumab during breast feeding [96].

Paediatric Use

Secukinumab has been approved by the FDA for the management of paediatric psoriasis in patients ≥6 years of age, and active juvenile psoriatic arthritis in children aged 2 years or older [4].

Geriatric Use

Although no response differences were seen between older/younger patients who received secukinumab, the number of patients aged ≥65 years was not sufficient to demonstrate potential differences [97].

Drug Interactions [97]

Live Vaccines

Prior to starting secukinumab therapy, all appropriate immunizations according to the current immunization guidelines needs to be administered to all patients. However, live vaccines are contraindicated in patients receiving secukinumab.

Non-live Vaccines

These can be given along with secukinumab. The clinical effectiveness of meningococcal and influenza vaccines has not been assessed with secukinumab.

Cytochrome (CY) P_{450} Substrates

As the formation of CYP450 enzymes can be altered by increased levels of certain cytokines (e.g., IL-1, IL-6, IL-10, TNFα, IFN) during chronic inflammation, secukinumab can potentially alter the concentrations of CYP substrate drugs with a narrow therapeutic index.

Warning and Precautions [97]

Infections

Serious infections have occurred with secukinumab. Caution should be exercised when the use of secukinumab is contemplated upon in patients with chronic infection or history of recurrent infection. If a serious infection arises, then secukinumab needs immediate discontinuation, till resolution of the infection.

Tuberculosis

Secukinumab should never be used in patients with active tuberculosis (TB) infection. In patients with a history of latent/active TB for whom an adequate treatment course is not confirmatory, anti-TB therapy may need to be given prior to starting treatment with secukinumab.

Inflammatory Bowel Disease

Caution needs to be exercised while prescribing secukinumab in patients with Crohn's disease (CD), as exacerbation of CD (serious in some cases) has been observed.

Availability and Administration

Secukinumab comes as readymade prefilled syringes available in all standard pharmacies, or a sensory ready pen that requires storage at a temperature of 2–8 °C [98].

Prior to administration, the pen or prefilled syringe must be kept aside for 20–30 minutes until room temperature is reached.

Next, product reconstitution is done with 10 ml of sterile distilled water, followed by gentle stirring to dissolve the powder and kept aside for 10mins. Lastly, the solution is inspected to be free of any residual particulate matter or any discoloration following which it needs to be promptly administered.

Secukinumab is given SC at sites such as the upper arm, thigh and abdomen. Previously injected or tender, bruised, inflamed and indurated areas are avoided.

Conclusion

Secukinumab has proven to be a valuable drug in the management of psoriasis and HS. Apart from its efficacy for these indications, the use of secukinumab in PG, BD, LP and PRP has further expanded its dermatologic horizon. Nevertheless, in some of these off-label indications, the phenomenon of therapeutic paradox has been encountered with secukinumab, making it imperative for the dermatologist to evaluate all aspects in relation to the drug as well as the recipient, prior to its prescription.

Ixekizumab: Introduction

Ixekizumab is a fully humanized monoclonal IgG4 antibody, that selectively binds to interleukin (IL)-17A and inhibits IL-17A—IL-17 receptor interaction. This blockade subsequently prevents generation of IL-17 dependent inflammatory cascades, thereby halting disease progression [99, 100].

Pharmacokinetics

Following subcutaneous (SC) administration, peak plasma concentrations of ixekizumab are achieved within 4–7 days; with a volume of distribution of approximately 6 litres, clearance of 0.0147 L/h, and $t_{1/2}$ of around 12 days [101]. Being a humanized IgG4 monoclonal antibody, ixekizumab gets degraded into small peptides/amino acids via catabolic pathways; similar to endogenous IgG. Bioavailability of ixekizumab depends upon the site of SC injection (ranging from 61–80%), with availability being highest when injected into the thigh. Main route of elimination for ixekizumab is yet to be characterized [102].

Indications [103–108]

FDA approved

- Moderate-to-severe plaque psoriasis in adults and children ≥6 years of age.
- Genital Psoriasis.
- Active Psoriatic arthritis.
- Active ankylosing spondylitis.
- Active non-radiographic axial spondylarthritis with objective signs of inflammation.

Off Label

- Hidradenitis suppurativa.
- Pyoderma gangrenosum.
- Lichen planopilaris.
- Pityriasis rubra pilaris.
- Bullous pemphigoid.

Contraindications [103–108]

Absolute

- Presence of active infections, more importantly latent or active tuberculosis, hepatitis B, C and HIV.
- Hypersensitivity to ixekizumab.
- Active inflammatory bowel disease.

Relative

- Recent suicidality.
- Presence of zoster antibody.
- Underlying malignancy.

Clinical Uses

Plaque Psoriasis

Psoriasis is a chronic inflammatory disorder affecting 1–3% of the global population, with plaque psoriasis accounting for 90% of the cases [109, 110]. Heightened expression (almost six-fold) of IL-17A advances immune dysregulation in psoriasis [111]. IL-17A contributes to activation and recruitment of neutrophils to the psoriatic epidermis [112], promotes inhibition of neutrophil apoptosis [113], enhances angiogenesis [114], assists release of inflammatory cytokines and chemokines like TNFα, IL-1, IL-6 and CCL20 [115], and reduces expression of filaggrin (that results in impaired skin barrier function) [116]. By neutralizing IL-17, ixekizumab antagonizes the above responses and heralds clinical and histologic improvement in psoriasis, as early as 2 weeks of therapy [117]. Additionally, ixekizumab is associated with significant subsidence of pain and pruritus in psoriasis (by 4 weeks of treatment), that dramatically improves the quality of life (QoL) of patients [118]. Owing to rapid skin clearance delivered by ixekizumab, discontinuation rates associated with it are quite low [119].

Clinical trials have demonstrated ixekizumab to be superior to etanercept, ustekinumab, adalimumab, guselkumab, brodalumab and secukinumab, in plaque psoriasis [118, 120–124]. Though having similar pharmacodynamic and bioavailability properties as secukinumab, ixekizumab has about 50–100 times greater affinity for IL-17, and therefore delineates superior therapeutic outcomes (both short-term and long-term) when compared to secukinumab. Because of this, ixekizumab is also preferred in obese patients, who require higher secukinumab dosage [125].

On juxtaposing ixekizumab with IL-23 antagonists, it is seen that the onset of action is faster with ixekizumab, with a greater percentage of patients delineating a

PASI ≤3 at week 16 for ixekizumab (73%), followed by guselkumab (65%), risankizumab (63%) and tildrakizumab (43%). However, by week 52 this description changes slightly, with a higher number of patients experiencing PASI ≤3 with risankizumab (95%), followed by ixekizumab (88%), guselkumab (87%) and tildrakizumab (74%), thus making risankizumab a better option for long term therapy. This facet is linked to the longer drug survival for risankizumab with respect to ixekizumab. Nevertheless, though inferior to risankizumab, drug survival for ixekizumab is superior to guselkumab and tildrakizumab, making it safe and effective for long term therapy (even up to 5 years). [126–132]

Besides, ixekizumab is effective in those patients with moderate-to-severe psoriasis who have failed to respond to TNFα inhibitors, ustekinumab and secukinumab [133, 134]. Interestingly, the effectiveness of ixekizumab in biologic-experienced patients versus biologic-naïve patients has demonstrated contrasting results, with some reports outlining no significant impact on the average PASI improvement in both groups, whereas others delineating superior PASI 90 and PASI 100 response rates in biologic-naïve patients [135–137]. This observation can be ascribed to the different populations involved in these studies, suggesting that responder enriched populations can benefit from long term treatment with ixekizumab in the same measure regardless of previous biologic exposure, unlike the overall population in real-world settings wherein the likelihood of experiencing greater benefit with ixekizumab is more for biologic-naïve patients [137]. However, it is noted that with an increase in the number of prior biologic therapies, there is a tendency for reduction in the response with ixekizumab [138, 139], with notable disparity in the persistence rates of ixekizumab in biologic-naïve and biologic-experienced patients at 12 months (69.4% vs 57.4%), 24 months (60.8% vs 43.7%) and 36 months (51.9% vs 36.2%) [140], thereby making contemplation essential prior to the introduction of ixekizumab in such scenarios. Also, as biologics are expensive compared to traditional systemic management, a complete cost-effective perspective needs evaluation before considering a biologic shift, as there occur a subset of patients who tend to lose responsiveness with biologics. [141, 142]

The recommended dose of ixekizumab is 160 mg SC at week 0 followed by 80 mg SC every 2 weeks for 12 weeks, and 80 mg SC every 4 weeks thereafter [102]. However, as frequent dosing is expensive and burdensome, a modified dosing has been suggested, wherein after the 160 mg induction dose, 80 mg of ixekizumab is administered at week 2, 4 and 8, and every 8 weeks thereafter. This modified regimen has shown to be effective, along with considerable reduction in the cost by around 41.2%, and a saving of 6818 USD per patient, in the first year of treatment [143].

Moreover, ixekizumab is a viable and effective treatment option for moderate-to-severe psoriasis in children ≥6 years, both as a first line agent, as well as following treatment failure with other common therapeutic options [131, 144]. Additionally, ixekizumab is effective in treating psoriasis involving difficult areas like palms, soles, scalp and genitalia, with rapid relief of lesions along with good safety and manageability [144]. PASI 90 and 100 responses with ixekizumab are evident within 12 weeks of starting therapy [120, 121, 123, 128, 145, 146].

Genital Psoriasis

Genital Psoriasis (GP) is commonly encountered in patients with inverse psoriasis and less frequently in those with plaque psoriasis. Occasionally GP maybe the only presentation encountered. In men, glans penis is the commonly affected site, whereas vulvar involvement is primarily observed in women. Because of involvement of genitals, problems associated with sexual function potentially impair the QoL of these patients [147].

Current treatment guidelines support systemic therapies for GP when other treatment options fail, even in patients with lower Body Surface Area (BSA) involvement [148]. A major advantage of ixekizumab in GP is its rapidity of action, associated with significant improvement of the static Physician Global Assessment-Genitalia (sPGA-G) scores as early as week 1, and clinically meaningful improvements in genital itch and Health related (HR)-QoL, along with notable reduction in the negative impact of GP with regard to frequency of sexual activity, by 12 weeks of treatment [149]. Besides, results produced with ixekizumab in GP are consistent and sustained with ongoing therapy [150].

Nail Psoriasis

Nail Psoriasis (NP) is one of the most difficult-to-treat variants of psoriasis. In 5–10% of cases, it has an isolated manifestation, lacking any form of cutaneous involvement [151]. Besides, nail involvement often portents PsA, making it essential for clinicians to begin early treatment in all cases of NP, so that long term outcomes can be improved [152].

Ixekizumab exhibits higher rates of nail clearance in psoriasis when compared to etanercept, ustekinumab, adalimumab and guselkumab [153]. Additionally, simultaneous complete resolution of NP and plaque psoriasis is observed to be numerically greater with ixekizumab at all-time points when compared to the above biologic drugs, except for PASI 100 at week 24 versus guselkumab where both ixekizumab and guselkumab achieved similar levels of complete skin clearance [153, 154]. Generally by 8 weeks statistically significant improvement in the Nail Psoriasis Severity Index score is observed with ixekizumab, with complete clearance occurring as early as 16 and 20 weeks in patients with moderate NP and significant NP respectively [155]. Furthermore, ixekizumab maintains sustained levels of improvement through 5 years, along with acceptable levels of safety [156].

Palmoplantar Psoriasis

Palmoplantar psoriasis (PPP) describes plaque psoriasis present over the palms and soles. This variant of psoriasis is quite difficult to treat, often resulting in higher levels of impairment in the HR-QoL, with psychological, physical and occupational repercussions [23].

In a post-hoc analysis, it was seen that ixekizumab enabled quick improvement of PPP that was sustained up to 5 years in adult patients and 2 years in paediatric patients. Within 4 weeks, palmoplantar(pp)PASI 100 was observed in 38.9%–52.9% of adult patients in various reports, that had increased to 83.5%–96% in 1 year; with sustained improvements ranging from 90.2%–96.6% at 5 years. Likewise in paediatric patients, ppPASI 100 at week 4 was observed in 21.4% of patients, that had increased to 90% at week 108 [157].

Ixekizumab's rapid and sustained effects make it a valuable agent for PPP.

Generalized Pustular Psoriasis

Generalized pustular psoriasis (GPP) is a distinctive variant of psoriasis that is very difficult to treat. As therapy for GPP is often protracted, selection of an effective drug with a favourable toxicity profile becomes mandatory. Traditional agents utilised in GPP include acitretin, cyclosporine and methotrexate, which though effective are limited by their slower onset of action and side effects [158].

Though currently not approved by the US-FDA for this indication, ixekizumab's efficacy in GPP has been documented in various reports [158–162].

Erythrodermic Psoriasis

Erythrodermic psoriasis (EP) is a severe variant of psoriasis presenting as generalized erythema and desquamation involving ≥90% of the BSA [163]. Often EP is associated with systemic symptoms, which can become life threatening if immediate/appropriate treatment is not instituted [164]. Growing body of evidence supports the safety/efficacy of biologics in rapidly achieving near total clearance of EP, particularly with IL-17 antagonists, of which ixekizumab is capable of achieving almost complete clearance of lesions within 8–12 weeks of treatment [165–167]. Theoretically the role of IL-17 and its interaction with other cytokines in severe cases of psoriasis is well established, and this forms the basis for the use of ixekizumab in EP [168]. Besides, ixekizumab has been found to be safe and effective in treating EP in patients with HIV and thyroid cancer, as well as drug induced EP [169–171].

Currently, there are no RCTs comparing ixekizumab with placebo for EP, with literature search revealing 4 prospective open-label single-arm studies describing the utility of ixekizumab in EP. [162, 172–174] Three of them evaluated ixekizumab treatment in the same cohort of 8 EP patients at different time points of treatment [162, 172, 173]. At week 12, PASI75 was achieved in all patients(which was maintained at week 52), and PASI90 was obtained in 62.5% of the participants(which increased to 75% at week 52) [162, 172]. Between week 52 and week 192, owing to adverse effects(elevated hepatic transaminases and positive mycobacterium tuberculosis test), 2 patients discontinued treatment, and at week 192, one of the 6 patients delineated a Global Improvement Score of resolved, while in the remaining

5 patients an improved score was documented. Even so, all patients tolerated the drug well [173]. In a different study, 5 EP patients were given ixekizumab every 2 weekly and reported PASI75 and PASI90 in 50% and 25% of patients, respectively at week 12; and PASI75 and PASI90 in 75% and 25% of patients respectively, at week 20, with good safety and tolerability. [174]

A recent real-life cohort study that compared secukinumab with ixekizumab in EP, could not confirm the efficacy of ixekizumab, as only 1 patient out of 3 completed three months of treatment, without attaining PASI90 at week 48 [175]. However, in a case series of 9 patients with EP who failed secukinumab, ixekizumab was successful in achieving PASI50 in 7 patients at week 12, of which 4 patients achieved PASI75 and one PASI90 [176]. Superior response of ixekizumab with respect to secukinumab is attributed to the structural difference between the two, and a higher affinity and stability of ixekizumab toward IL-17A [177]. Other publications elucidating the beneficial properties of ixekizumab in EP are confined to case reports/series [167, 178, 179]. Interestingly, withdrawal of ixekizumab in patients with plaque psoriasis has been associated with precipitation of EP [180].

Psoriatic Arthropathy

Psoriatic arthropathy (PsA) is a chronic, immune mediated inflammatory arthritis with a progressive course, associated with joint damage, dactylitis, enthesitis and axial involvement [181]. Increased levels of IL-17A producing cells are present in the peripheral blood, synovial tissue/fluid and cutaneous plaques in patients with PsA [182]. IL-17A triggers activation and trafficking of immune cells and induces release of proinflammatory cytokines and chemokines, that attract neutrophils and monocytes, and stimulates production of matrix metalloproteases and receptor activator of nuclear factor kappa-β ligand, that majorly contribute to cartilage and bone destruction [183]. Based on these findings, specific inhibition of IL-17A represents an emerging targeted approach in the management of PsA [184].

Therapeutic responses with ixekizumab in PsA is observed as early as 1 week following treatment initiation. Besides, apart from symptomatic improvement, ixekizumab is associated with significant improvement in enthesitis, and dactylitis along with notable reduction in radiologic progression of joint damage [185, 186]. Additionally, the safety profile of ixekizumab in PsA is acceptable with mild-to-moderate transient injection site reactions being the commonest adverse event encountered [185, 186].

Hidradenitis Suppurativa

Hidradenitis suppurativa (HS) is a chronic, autoinflammatory cutaneous disorder affecting hair follicles in apocrine gland rich areas of the body. Severe manifestations of HS considerably impair QoL of patients [187]. Although the exact pathogenesis of HS in unknown, IL-17 pathway is considered to play an important role in this immunopathological process [188].

In HS, IL-17 is over expressed, not only in lesional and perilesional tissue, but also in unaffected skin, expounding the occurrence of subclinical inflammatory processes even prior to the development of active disease [189]. Moreover, elevated levels of IL-17 induce proteins like LL37/cathelicidin, S100A7, S100A8 and S100A9 that promote cytokine/chemokine expression and keratinocyte proliferation, thereby perpetuating a progressive feed forward loop, eventuating in potential tissue damage [190, 191]. IL-17 further acts on nod-like receptor protein-3 (NLRP-3) inflammasome and stimulates production of TGFβ, IL-1β, IL-6 and TNFα from macrophages, crucial for Th17 differentiation and proliferation [192].

Transforming growth factor (TGF)β sets into motion RAR-related orphan receptor gamma-γt (a transcription factor), necessary for generation of Th17 cells [193]; IL-1β and IL-6 independently downregulate Foxp3 (another transcription factor), consequently resulting in reduced levels of regulatory T cells [49]; and TNFα rapidly promotes induction of IL-1β, IL-6, IL-8, IL-2 and adhesion molecules in monocytes and macrophages, generating a relentlessly progressive pathogenic cycle for HS [194].

Ixekizumab, by binding to IL-17A, inhibits a major portion of the inflammatory cascade in HS [195]. However, as ixekizumab does not target IL-17F transcripts in lesional tissue, receptor signalling related with IL-17F continues. Nevertheless, synergism of IL-17F associated with IL-17A in the inflammatory process is stopped, allowing considerable reduction in the inflammatory cycle [190].

Currently, the efficacy of ixekizumab in HS is confined to case reports/series [196–199].

Pyoderma Gangrenosum

Pyoderma gangrenosum (PG) is a rare debilitating disease presenting as rapidly evolving painful, irregular ulcers with a violaceous and erythematous edge [200].

Kao and colleagues [201], described targeted therapy with ixekizumab (label dosing) to be effective in PG in their series of 4 patients. Within a period of 12–47 weeks, significant clearance of lesions was observed, with no adverse events being reported.

Diseased skin in PG is characterized by an increased expression of IL-17, that facilitates neutrophilic migration, triggers secretion of IL-6, IL-8 and GM-CSF, and reduces levels of regulatory T cells. By antagonizing IL-17, ixekizumab reverses this disturbed homeostasis, and normalizes the cytokine milieu, thereby accelerating PG resolution [61, 62, 202, 203]. However, development of PG in patients receiving ixekizumab for psoriasis has been reported [204]. This occurs due to paradoxical upregulation of IL-23, following IL-17A inhibition (secondary to disruption of the IL-23/IL-17A axis) [204]. It therefore becomes mandatory for clinicians to keep this therapeutic paradox in mind prior to prescribing ixekizumab for PG.

Lichen Planopilaris

Lichen planopilaris (LPP) is a lymphocytic primary cicatricial alopecia whose treatment is challenging and responses with conventional therapeutic agents remain disappointing [205]. In an anecdotal report, highly satisfactory responses to ixekizumab (label dosing) were witnessed in a 30-year-old woman with linear LPP. At week 12 of ixekizumab therapy, her lichen planopilaris activity index had reduced to 0 from 6 (initial visit score). Additionally, the response obtained was maintained at week 20, with complete hair re-growth and improved appearance of the linear forehead depression [206]. Currently, the mechanism of ixekizumab in LPP still needs elucidation.

Pityriasis Rubra Pilaris

Pityriasis rubra pilaris (PRP) is a rare papulo-squamous disorder characterized by keratotic follicular papules, palmoplantar keratoderma and erythematous patches [207]. Upregulation of Th17 cytokines IL-17A, IL-17F and IL-22 have been found in skin samples of PRP patients; and reduction in levels of expression of these cytokines parallel clinical and histologic improvement of the disease [84]. Based on this observation, IL-17 inhibitors may have a role in the treatment of PRP. Several reports have demonstrated ixekizumab to be effective in the management of PRP [207–211].

Bullous Pemphigoid

Of late, an association between psoriasis and bullous pemphigoid (BP) has been propounded with a 1.5 times greater likelihood of developing BP in patients with psoriasis [212]. Neutrophil elastase, identified along the basement membrane zone (BMZ) of psoriatic plaques can compromise the BMZ integrity, thereby exposing sequestered antigens and evoking a secondary autoimmune disease [213, 214]. Furthermore, a shared pathogenic role of pro-inflammatory cytokines (like IL-1, IL-17 and IL-23), and neutrophil activity responsible for the degradation of mature proteins has been hypothesized in both psoriasis and BP [212].

In addition, IL-17/IL-23 upregulate expression of proteases and facilitate cleavage of the extracellular domain of BP180, with eventual blister formation [215, 216]. Moreover, the relevance of IL-17A in the pathogenesis of BP has been exemplified by its ability to upregulate cytokine and related genes in the skin of BP patients, and activate neutrophils to release neutrophil elastase. Even so, in animal models IL-17A has been associated with BP [217].

Based on these findings, the utility of IL-17A blockers as a therapeutic agent in BP has been suggested. At present there exist only 2 case reports that have demonstrated the utility of ixekizumab in BP. In both patients (63-year-old man and 37-year-old woman), there was co-existent psoriasis, and both were on systemic steroids and methotrexate, with aggravation of psoriatic plaques and formation of new blisters as steroids were tapered. For this, ixekizumab was added to the regimen, and at week 20, psoriatic lesions were almost relieved, and no new blisters resurfaced. Besides, both patients tolerated the treatment well with no adverse effects. [218, 219] Although, the effects of ixekizumab in BP appear promising allowing a practical method to effectively taper glucocorticoids and methotrexate, further exploration in this avenue becomes essential to validate the above findings.

Adverse Effects [220, 221, 223]

Most Common Reactions

- Nasopharyngitis.
- Upper respiratory tract infection.
- Sinusitis.
- Pharyngitis.
- Injection site reactions.

Others

Cutaneous

- Folliculitis.
- Candidiasis (Oral).
- Dermatophytosis.
- Pruritus.
- Vitiligo.
- Urticaria and angioedema.

Extracutaneous

- Fatigue.
- Nausea.
- Cough.
- Oropharyngeal pain.
- Urinary tract infection.
- Hypertension.

Serious Adverse Effects Leading to Drug Discontinuation

- Neutropenia.
- Sciatica.
- Staphylococcal infection.
- Generalized rash.
- Kaposi's varicelliform eruption.

Drug Monitoring

Baseline

- Complete blood count/hemogram.
- Erythrocyte sedimentation rate.
- C-reactive protein.
- Liver function test.
- Renal function test.
- Serum electrolytes.
- Anti-nuclear antibody.
- Anti-dsDNA antibody.
- Screening for hepatitis and human immunodeficiency virus.
- Chest X-ray.
- Tuberculin skin testing or QuantiFERON gold test.
- Pregnancy test in females of child bearing age.
- Serology for varicella zoster and measles (if clinically indicated).
- Urinalysis.

Ongoing

- Evaluation of response to treatment is measurable by respective assessment scores; i.e. PASI, DLQI at 3 months initially and subsequently every 6 months.
- A complete blood count and hemogram needs to be repeated at 3 months and then every 6 months.
- Liver and renal function tests, electrolytes and urinalysis need similar evaluation.

Use in Specific Populations

Pregnancy

Available data from published literature and pharmacovigilance databases for usage of ixekizumab in pregnancy is currently insufficient to evaluate for drug associated risk of birth defects, miscarriage or other adverse maternal/foetal outcomes. As human IgG is capable of crossing the placental barrier, ixekizumab may be transmitted from the mother to the foetus, but various studies have confirmed an overall favourable safety profile of ixekizumab. Moreover, the risk of spontaneous abortion following ixekizumab exposure is constant with that observed in the general population for this age demographic [222]. However, contraception in susceptible women is advised during and for 10 weeks post therapy. The US-FDA has not assigned any pregnancy category to this molecule yet [223].

Lactation

As ixekizumab is a large protein molecule (molecular weight: 146,000 Da), amount in breast milk is likely to be very low. Besides, it is also likely to get partially destroyed in the infant's gastrointestinal tract, making its absorption very minimal. Though considered acceptable by some professional guidelines in breast feeding, caution needs to be exercised especially while nursing a newborn or preterm infant. Waiting for at least 2 weeks post-partum to resume therapy may minimize transfer to the infant [224]. This is suggested owing to wider gaps in the breast alveolar cells during the first few days of lactation leading to more ready passage of immunoglobulins via the breast milk. With passage of time these gaps narrow down, making immunoglobulin transfer minimal [223].

Paediatric Use

Ixekizumab is approved by the US-FDA in the management of paediatric psoriasis in patients ≥6 years of age (in March 2021). Safety and effectiveness of ixekizumab in other paediatric indications and paediatric subjects <6 years of age is not established yet [131].

Geriatric Use

A retrospective observational study delineated optimal efficacy and safety of ixekizumab in elderly psoriasis patients throughout a 1-year treatment period, confirming the results showcased in the drug product information, and reporting responses in elderly patients to be higher when compared to younger individuals [223].

Availability and Administration

Ixekizumab injection is a stable, preservative free, odourless and clear to slightly yellow solution, available in a single-dose prefilled autoinjector or prefilled syringe to deliver 80 mg of ixekizumab. It needs to be removed from the refrigerator (non-freezer compartment) 30 minutes prior to administration. Ixekizumab needs to be protected from light, and should be injected only if the solution is clear/slightly yellow and free from particles. The prefilled syringe/autoinjector should not be shaken. Subcutaneous injections of ixekizumab are administered over the thighs, upper arms or abdomen and these sites are rotated with each dose to prevent skin damage. Additionally, bruised/diseased/damaged skin needs to be avoided [226].

Drug Interactions

Live Vaccines

These need to be avoided in patients receiving ixekizumab [102].

Cytochrome P_{450} Substrates

As formation of CYP450 enzymes can be altered by increased levels of certain cytokines (eg IL-1, IL-10, TNFα, IFN) during chronic inflammation, ixekizumab can potentially alter the concentration of CYP substrate drugs with a narrow therapeutic index [102]. It is theorized that ixekizumab can neutralize the effects, and lower blood plasma concentrations of drugs metabolized by CYP450 enzymes and therefore in such cases drug monitoring becomes mandatory [227].

Warnings and Precautions

Tuberculosis

Patients need to be evaluated for tuberculosis (TB) prior to initiating treatment with ixekizumab. If active TB infection is identified, ixekizumab cannot be given. In patients with a past history of latent or active TB in whom an adequate treatment course cannot be conformed, anti-TB treatment needs consideration. All patients on ixekizumab need to be monitored for signs and symptoms of active TB during and after treatment [226].

Hypersensitivity Reactions

Serious hypersensitivity reactions have occurred with ixekizumab, including anaphylaxis. In such cases, ixekizumab needs to be discontinued immediately, with administration of appropriate rescue therapy [226].

Inflammatory Bowel Disease

Ixekizumab has been associated with an increased risk of precipitating and exacerbating IBD. During treatment with ixekizumab, these aspects need to be adequately monitored and if detected, treatment with ixekizumab needs to be stopped, followed by appropriate medical management for the same. [226]

Conclusion

Ixekizumab has proven to be a valuable drug in the management of psoriasis. Apart from its efficacy in psoriasis, use of ixekizumab in HS, PG, LPP, PRP and BP have further expanded its dermatologic horizon. Nevertheless, in some of these off-label indications, the phenomenon of therapeutic paradox has been encountered with ixekizumab, making it imperative for dermatologists to evaluate all aspects in relation to the drug as well as the recipient, prior to its prescription.

Brodalumab: Introduction

Brodalumab is a fully human monoclonal antibody that targets the interleukin-17 receptor A (IL-17RA), effectively blocking the activity of multiple pro-inflammatory IL-17 cytokines [228]. It is this unique mechanism of action that distinguishes brodalumab from other IL-17 inhibitors, contributing to its superior efficacy in various forms of psoriasis. The US Food and Drug Administration (FDA) in 2017 approved brodalumab for the treatment of moderate-to-severe plaque psoriasis in adults who were recalcitrant to other systemic therapies [229].

Pharmacokinetics

After subcutaneous (SC) injection, brodalumab is absorbed with a bioavailability of approximately 55%. It undergoes slow absorption, reaching peak serum concentrations by 3 days. Brodalumab exhibits non-linear pharmacokinetics, with a $t_{1/2}$ of 10.9 days. Clearance of brodalumab involves degradation into small peptides and amino acids via catabolic pathways similar to endogenous IgG, and hepatic impairment is not expected to influence its elimination [229].

Indications

FDA Approved

- Moderate to severe plaque psoriasis.

Off Label

- Psoriatic arthropathy (PsA).
- Hidradenitis suppurativa (HS).
- Pyoderma gangrenosum (PG).
- Pityriasis rubra pilaris (PRP).

Clinical Uses

Plaque Psoriasis

Psoriasis is a chronic inflammatory disorder with predominant cutaneous features, along with systemic involvement, affecting 1–3% of the global population with plaque psoriasis accounting for 90% of the cases [110]. Pathogenesis of psoriasis involves a complex series of immunologic events. Following a/an genetic/environmental trigger in susceptible individuals, dendritic cells are activated and release IL-23/IL-12, which in turn activates Th17, Th1 and Th22 cells to produce IL-17, IL-22, TNFα and numerous other cytokines [230–232]. Emerging data state IL-17 to play a crucial role in orchestrating inflammation in psoriasis [233, 234]. The IL-17 cytokine family consists of 6 cytokines (IL-17A to 17F) and five receptors (IL-17RA to IL-17RE) [235]. These receptors are expressed on keratinocytes, dendritic cells and a variety of immune cells, mediating responses to IL-17 cytokines [235]. Aberrant differentiation and proliferation of keratinocytes, and production of proinflammatory cytokines occur following stimulation by IL-17 ligands, resulting in neutrophil recruitment and further perpetuation of inflammation [236, 237]. Besides, IL-17A downregulates filaggrin expression and disrupts the normal skin barrier function [238]. Moreover, neutrophils, mast cells and Tc17 cells present in psoriatic plaques produce IL-17A, furthering the progression of an uninterrupted inflammatory cycle [239]. IL-17C, the most abundant cytokine in psoriatic plaques, upregulates levels of IL-17A, IL-17F and TNFα, all of which synergistically bring about downstream gene activation, and establish a pro-inflammatory milieu [16, 239]. Additionally, excessive expression of IL-17E (IL-25) in psoriatic skin facilitates enhanced inflammation via recruitment of immune cells (including monocytes and neutrophils), that predominantly contribute to plaque formation and proliferation in psoriasis [240].

Brodalumab selectively binds to the A subunit of the IL-17R and blocks the activity of pro-inflammatory cytokines IL-17A, IL-17F, IL-17A/F heterodimer, IL-17C and IL-17E(IL-25), promoting anti-inflammatory effects and ameliorating clinical symptoms associated with psoriasis [241, 242]. Furthermore, brodalumab regularizes abnormal expression of keratinocyte expressed genes like KRT6A, IL1F6, chemokine CXCL6 and antimicrobial peptide gene S100A7A [243]; and revamps mRNA levels of IL-17 modulated keratinocyte derived factors like cathelicidin, KRT16, CCL18 and CCL20 [244]. Besides, cytokines not directly regulated by IL-17R (like IL-22 and IL-23) also plummet following brodalumab treatment, with levels of IL-17A, IL-17C and IL-17F confirming those of healthy individuals, eventuating in disease remission and manifesting clinically as resolved lesions [244].

Brodalumab has the most rapid onset of action, obtaining 50% improvement of the baseline Psoriasis Area and Severity Index (PASI) by 1.8–2.6 weeks, when compared to ixekizumab (1.9–2.3 weeks), secukinumab (3–4.3 weeks), adalimumab (~3.5 weeks), infliximab (~3.7 weeks), guselkumab (~3.8 weeks), ustekinumab (~5.1 weeks), tildrakizumab (5.6–5.7 weeks) and etanercept (6.5–10.9 weeks), making it a good choice for treating unstable and severe forms of psoriasis that require immediate responses [245–247]. Following brodalumab treatment, a rapid and dramatic reduction of pruritus (by 2 weeks) is witnessed, resulting in better sleep, and alleviation of depressive symptoms, manifesting overall in an improved quality of life (QoL) [248–250].

IL-17A has emerged as a potential mediator of itch symptoms in psoriasis by modulating pruritogenic neuronal signalling at the level of the dorsal root ganglion and spinal cord neurons. Brodalumab's role in alleviating pruritus can be accounted by its ability to selectively block signalling via IL-17RA, resulting in reduction of inflammation in lesional skin, as well as pruritogenic effects in the spinal cord, and in this way facilitates skin clearance, along with amelioration of pruritus. [249, 251] However, it needs to be stated that other molecular mediators of itch like nerve growth factor, substance P and calcitonin-gene related peptide are also involved in psoriasis, against which brodalumab is ineffective [249]. Additionally, brodalumab affects anxiety and depression in a more direct way, and not just indirectly by improving itch and lesional clearance of psoriasis; the exact mechanism for which still needs elucidation [252].

Within 12 weeks of brodalumab therapy, lesional skin resembles non-lesional skin at both cellular and molecular levels [253]. Furthermore, the effectiveness of brodalumab increases with ongoing therapy, and is maintained even at 5 years of treatment [254–257]. This long-term effect is linked to the drug survival (DS) of brodalumab, and currently DS is considered a useful measure in evaluating the long term treatment success of biologics (encompassing factors like drug efficacy, safety and patient adherence) in real world settings [258]. DS rates for brodalumab range from 85–89.9% at 1 year, and 77.3–80% at 2 years [259]. Interestingly in a real-life setting, a notable brodalumab survival of 85.64% at 3 years was demonstrated [254]. However, in the analysis by Elgaard et al. [260], low brodalumab survival of 65.7% and 57.2% after 1 and 2 years respectively, was reported. These low values were attributed to the very high percentage of bio-experienced patients (>90%) and the low number of patients followed up for the whole period in this study. In a retrospective evaluation, DS for brodalumab was highest at week 16 and 28 (80% vs 90%), followed by ixekizumab (73% vs 83%), guselkumab (65% vs 82%), risankizumab (63% vs 86%), secukinumab (60% vs 72%) and tildrakizumab (43% vs 68%). However, at week 52, this description changed slightly with maximum DS being for risankizumab (95%), followed by ixekizumab (88%), guselkumab (87%), brodalumab (82%), secukinumab (80%) and tildrakizumab (74%) [261]. Another study comparing the DS over a 2-year period specifically for IL-17 inhibitors, reported highest DS for brodalumab (80%), followed by ixekizumab (79%) and secukinumab (75%). The higher DS of brodalumab though, was not statistically significant [262].

In this aspect, risankizumab and guselkumab certainly illustrate superiority for long-term therapy with regard to brodalumab. Nevertheless, the high sustainability of brodalumab for long term therapy cannot be undermined [254–257]. Considering the diverse range of systemic therapies available, DS therefore plays a crucial role in guiding the clinician for selecting the most suitable option in treating patients with psoriasis [263, 264].

Based on PASI responses, systemic meta-analysis reveal brodalumab to be superior to apremilast, TNFα blockers and ustekinumab in the management of psoriasis [265, 266]. On the other hand, although brodalumab, ixekizumab and secukinumab delineate almost similar PASI75 and 90 responses at 12 weeks, greater PASI100 rates are obtained with brodalumab during the same timepoints, along with better overall maintenance at 1 year [267]. The ability of brodalumab to block the effects of all cytokines that interact with the IL-17RA is likely to contribute to the higher efficacy observed with brodalumab in comparison to secukinumab/ixekizumab, whose effects are limited to IL-17A antagonism [268]. Besides, brodalumab is effective in patients who have failed prior treatment with ixekizumab/secukinumab, outlining PASI75, 90 and 100 response rates of 76%, 50% and 32% respectively, within 4-months of therapy [269]. Interestingly, patients responding to brodalumab in this scenario elucidate lower baseline levels of TNFα and IL-6 [270].

Of importance, patients receiving brodalumab without prior exposure to IL-17A inhibitors show five-fold higher PASI 90 and 100 responses at week 36, as well as PASI75 and 90 responses at week 48, when compared to those with previous exposure to these drugs [271]. Indeed, a reduced efficacy is recognised to occur also for other biologics, when switching between the same class [271, 272]. However, switching to brodalumab following an eczematous reaction secondary to secukinumab/ixekizumab is associated with significant improvement of eczema, followed by remission of both eczema and psoriasis without any reduction in its efficacy [271]. By blocking IL-17RA, apart from antagonizing IL-17A, brodalumab also prevents over expression of the IL-17C isoform that is responsible for triggering an autocrine stimulation loop on keratinocytes (possibly involved in the eczematous reaction) driven by Th17 and Th2, thereby making brodalumab a valuable switch over drug in patients developing eczema following secukinumab/ixekizumab therapy [273].

Of note, switching from ustekinumab to brodalumab has been effective in attaining PASI 75, 90 and 100 responses as early as week 12, with gradual improvement at week 52, in those demonstrating inadequate responses to ustekinumab [274]. Besides, in patients who have failed previous biologic therapies (mainly TNFα blockers), brodalumab is 3 times more effective than ustekinumab as per PASI 100 values [275]. Also, brodalumab switching is effective in patients non-responsive to IL-23 inhibitors [269]. Nonetheless, despite the positive findings of brodalumab in patients with failed prior biologic therapy, there occur a subset of patients who tend to lose responsiveness to biologics; and as biologic therapy is expensive compared to traditional systemic management, a complete cost effective perspective warrants attention prior to considering a biologic switch [142, 276].

Following secondary failure with brodalumab, re-administration of brodalumab after a short wash out period has shown retrieval of its initial efficacy in psoriatic patients [255, 277]. The mechanism of secondary failure to brodalumab remains unclear and may possibly occur due to altered immunogenicity, closely connected to a complex cytokine imbalance, and activation of secondary pathways in disease induction and/or exacerbation [277]. Besides, antidrug antibodies against brodalumab appear to be a rare phenomenon and this maybe another reason as to why the efficacy of brodalumab is not compromised [278]. Interestingly, both quantifiable and sub-quantifiable levels of brodalumab enable PASI75 responses by 3 months. This can be accounted for by target mediated drug disposition for brodalumab, resulting in highly variable drug clearance rates at low drug concentrations. However, in patients with suboptimal levels of brodalumab, chances of relapses are greater [279, 280].

Furthermore, brodalumab exhibits versatility, as its efficacy extends across a wide spectrum of patients burdened with a range of comorbid diseases and established risk factors for poor psoriasis outcome [254]. In this regard, obese patients benefit with brodalumab. Surprisingly, results regarding the efficacy of brodalumab in obese and overweight patients have been mixed with some studies stating no significant statistical association between PASI responses and body weight or Body Mass Index (BMI), and others demonstrating significantly higher PASI 100 responses in non-obese individuals [142, 254, 281]. Bioavailability rather than BMI, therefore serves as a more important criteria to assess the response of brodalumab, with quantifiable levels of brodalumab in the circulation being necessary for its efficacy [279].

Nevertheless, the role of BMI cannot be negated because quantifiable levels of brodalumab tend to be higher in non-obese individuals. Also, patients with quantifiable levels of brodalumab delineate maintenance of IL-6 levels, but in patients where levels of brodalumab are not quantifiable, IL-6 levels increase after 12 weeks of treatment and is often considered the cytokine preceding production of IL-17 [282]. Even so, IL-6 production may increase as a result of a feedback loop in which IL-6 production is sustained, which in turn is maintained in this state by Th17 cells [283]. Thus, when this loop is not broken effectively in patients with sub-quantifiable levels of brodalumab, Th17 feedback stimulation of IL-6 production accounts for raised IL-6 levels, that promotes inflammation by augmenting IL-17 production. Besides, excess adipose tissue represents a fundamental reservoir of inflammatory cytokines and adipokines with repercussions in skin inflammation [284]. In such situations, the clinical judgement of the dermatologist becomes paramount whether or not to initiate treatment with brodalumab.

Label dosing of brodalumab is 210 mg at weeks 0, 1 and 2, and then every 2 weekly [285]. Interestingly, off-label dosing with brodalumab has been attempted by gradually prolonging the interval of administration (depending on the response) by 1 week (group A) or dosing at regular intervals of 4, 6 or 8 weeks (group B). It was observed that in group A, 25% of patients achieved complete skin clearance and in group B, 33.3% of patients obtained skin clearance with the application of the modified dosing schedule [286]. Although conventional dosing is more effective, based on clinical judgement, the treating dermatologist can attempt dose modification for the purpose of reducing financial burden on patients, and at the same time maintaining the therapeutic response [286].

Scalp Psoriasis

Scalp psoriasis (SP) is estimated to occur in ~80% of psoriatic patients [287]. It is characterized by erythematous plaques and silvery white scales, or diffuse involvement of the scalp. Lesions extend up to the hairline and may be associated with bleeding, pruritus and altered skin integrity [288]. Besides, SP portents a poor QoL owing to its clear visibility, leading to substantial negative psychosocial impairment [288]. In addition, topical therapy for SP is challenging owing to the presence of hair, that can alter correct treatment application and penetration. Also, patients may not be compliant to long term topical therapy because of the greasy texture of most topical agents, including the ordeal of daily application. Despite these barriers arising from topical therapies, systemic therapy in SP is typically reserved for severe cases [289]. Currently, there are no RCTs evaluating the efficacy of brodalumab for SP; available data being confined to post hoc analysis and sub-analysis of prior phase 3 and phase 2 trials [290, 291].

Post-hoc analysis of the AMAGINE-1 study, demonstrated improvement rates from baseline in the mean Psoriasis Scalp Severity Index (PSSI) within 2 weeks in patients receiving brodalumab (label dosing) versus placebo (67.6% vs 6.7%, $p = 0.001$). Besides, treatment responses with brodalumab were maintained at week 12 (PSSI75 and PSSI100 improvement was seen in 92.8% and 63.4% patients respectively, receiving brodalumab, and in 9.5% and 3.2% of patients respectively, who were on placebo) [290]. The effectiveness of brodalumab was further confirmed in a sub-analysis of a phase 2, RCT from Japan, wherein the mean PSSI improvement rate of 94.5% after 12 weeks of therapy with brodalumab (label dosing) from baseline, versus 12.6% of placebo-treated patients ($p < 0.001$) was reported [291].

Further, in an analysis of 25 patients by Cacciapuoti et al. [292] the mean baseline PSSI value of 20.33 reduced to 15.70 (at week 4), 4.29 (at week 24) and 2.46 (at week 52) following brodalumab treatment [292]. Besides in all reports, adverse events were mild, not requiring treatment discontinuation. Brodalumab's unique mechanism of action of IL-17RA blockade prompts faster onset of responses when compared to other biologicals, making it a valuable option for SP, enabling quicker remission and an overall improvement in patient QoL [292].

Nail Psoriasis

Nail psoriasis (NP) affects approximately 50–80% of patients with plaque psoriasis. Although, finger nails are more frequently involved than toenails, >50% of patients with NP have both sites affected [288]. Also, the intricate nail anatomy, prevents effective penetration of topical agents accounting for treatment failure [155]. Furthermore, NP is an important marker for the development of PsA, making it essential to promptly treat NP [293]. Besides, NP dramatically affects patients QoL with increased emotional and psychologic burden [288].

Systemic therapy is often considered inappropriate by dermatologists if cutaneous manifestations of psoriasis are minimal, especially when the number of psoriatic nails affected are low [294]. Nevertheless, systemic therapy with biologics have demonstrated efficacy in treating NP, although the effects are delayed and less pronounced when compared to the effects in cutaneous psoriasis. Recent trials have suggested that the maximum effects with biologics in NP may not be reached for up to 1 year or even beyond [29, 290, 295]. Amongst biologic drugs, based on a recent network metanalysis (NMA) evaluating results over 24–26 weeks, it was observed that ixekizumab had the highest response rates, with the Surface Under the Cumulative Ranking (SUCRA) curve value of 96.9%, followed by brodalumab (78.7%), adalimumab (61.7%), guselkumab (58%), ustekinumab (37.5%), infliximab (17.2%) and placebo (0%) [295].

In a post-hoc analysis of phase 3 studies that evaluated patients with moderate-to-severe NP who received either brodalumab (label dosing) or ustekinumab (label dosing) through week 52, it was observed that brodalumab was associated with significantly greater rates of complete clearance of NP (NAil Psoriasis Severity Index [NAPSI] 0) at weeks 12, 36 and 52 (7.9%, 54.2% and 63.8% respectively) versus ustekinumab (2.2%, 33.7% and 39.1% respectively; $p < 0.05$). Additionally, patients receiving brodalumab had significantly reduced rates of NAPSI from weeks 12 to 36 (5.3 to 1.7) compared to ustekinumab (6.7 to 2.9; $p < 0.05$) [290].

Improvement of NP was also reported in a sub-analysis of a phase 2, randomized placebo-controlled trial which after 12 weeks of evaluation, demonstrated brodalumab (label dosing) to be superior to placebo (mean ± SD of NAPSI improvement: 47.6 ± 35.2 versus 9.6 ± 86.2 respectively) [291].

In an open-label, single centre, unblinded study in patients with severe NP, brodalumab (label dosing) outlined statistically significant improvements in NAPSI for fingers and toes at weeks 12 and 24, with respect to baseline values ($p < 0.01$). Besides, improvement was witnessed in the HR-QoL, with mean DLQI values plummeting from 22.8 at baseline to 3.7 at week 24 ($p < 0.001$) [296].

Despite the favourable profile of brodalumab in NP in the above publications, more RCTs are warranted to further strengthen its profile in treating NP.

Genital Psoriasis

Genital psoriasis (GP) is commonly encountered in patients with inverse psoriasis and less frequently in those with plaque psoriasis. Occasionally, GP maybe the only presentation encountered. In men, glans penis is the commonly affected site, whereas vulvar involvement is primarily observed in women. Because of involvement of genitals, problems associated with sexual function potentially impair the QoL of these patients [147].

To date, only ixekizumab has been formally investigated for its efficacy and safety in GP, with promising results [297, 298]. In a 48-week retrospective study of 69 patients with GP, brodalumab (label dosing) enabled achievement of static-Physician Global Assessment of genitalia (s-PGA-G) 0/1 in 83% of patients at week

16 and 100% of patients at week 24 and 48 [299]. Apart from this report, currently no data outlining the efficacy of brodalumab in GP exists, making it essential to conduct RCTs to confirm the above findings.

Palmoplantar Psoriasis

Palmoplantar psoriasis (PPP) describes plaque psoriasis present over the palms and soles. This variant of psoriasis is quite difficult to treat often resulting in higher levels of impairment in the HR-QoL, with psychological, physical and occupational repercussions [23].

In a retrospective study assessing the efficacy of brodalumab (label dosing) for PPP in 54 patients; the mean palmoplantar (PP) PASI reduced from 3.5 at baseline to 0.4 at week 16 and 0.2, both at week 24 and 48 [299].

Politou et al. [300], evaluated the efficacy of brodalumab in 4 patients with PPP who had failed to respond to secukinumab. At week 16, all of them achieved complete skin clearance with brodalumab.

Erythrodermic Psoriasis

Erythrodermic psoriasis (EP) is a rare and severe variant of psoriasis presenting as generalised redness and desquamation, involving >90% of the Body Surface Area, and affecting 1–2.25% of psoriatic patients [165]. Despite, the complex interplay between Th1, Th2 and Th17 inflammatory pathways in EP pathophysiology, recent findings elucidate IL-17 responses to be the pivotal signal contributing to evolution of clinical events in EP [301]. Although not currently approved by the FDA for EP, brodalumab has been effective in the treatment of EP as demonstrated in one open-label trial, with other reports confined to individual cases and case series [302–305].

Pustular Psoriasis

Pustular psoriasis consists of a clinically heterogenous group of disorders characterized by varying clinical phenotypes. Both generalized and localized variants have been identified, that are often recalcitrant to nearly all forms of therapy. Excessive IL-17 signalling is thought to play an important role on the pathogenesis of psoriasis [306], and increased Th17 cells as well as levels of IL-17 have been reported in patients with pustular psoriasis, making IL-17 antagonists a valuable option for its management [307, 308].

Generalized Pustular Psoriasis

Generalized pustular psoriasis (GPP) is a distinctive variant of psoriasis that is often difficult to treat. As therapy for GPP is often protracted, selection of an effective drug with a favourable toxicity profile becomes mandatory. Gene expression profiling of skin biopsies from GPP have demonstrated higher expression of IL-36α, IL-36γ and IL-1β, when compared to IFNγ and IL-17A [309]. Owing to this feature, currently spesolimab (an anti-IL-36 drug) has been approved for the management of GPP. Nonetheless, increased levels of IL-17 as well as IL-17 producing cells in both blood and skin have been identified in patients with GPP [310, 311]. In an open label multicentre long-term phase 3 study, brodalumab significantly improved symptoms of GPP patients throughout 52 weeks and demonstrated favourable safety profiles without any new warning signals. Of the 12 patients evaluated, PASI 75, 90 and 100 responses at 12 weeks were obtained in 58.3%, 33.3% and 25% of patients respectively; and at week 52, PASI 75, 90 and 100 responses were seen in 83.3%, 83.3% and 58.3% of patients respectively. Besides, of the 12 patients, 6 had received prior biologic treatment (adalimumab, infliximab and ustekinumab), with 5 of the patients showing Clinical Global Impression of improvement as 'improved' or 'remission', and was linked to the different mechanism of action of brodalumab, with regard to the above-mentioned biologics [305].

Despite the favourable profile of brodalumab in the above report, the need for RCTs become essential to further confirm the above observation.

Acrodermatitis Continua of Hallopeau

Acrodermatitis continua of Hallopeau (ACH) is a rare variant of localized PP, presenting as recurrent eruptions of sterile pustules affecting only the distal phalanges of the hands and feet, sometimes precipitating onychodystrophy and angioedema [312]. Although many drugs have been used to treat ACH, success rates have been highly variable as a result of which, no concrete treatment guidelines exist for ACH [313]. Currently the utility of brodalumab in ACH is limited to 3 case reports [314–316].

Studies have demonstrated heightened expression of IL-17A and IL-17F in lesions of ACH [317]. This may explain the reason for the success of brodalumab in patients failing to respond to ixekizumab and secukinumab, because of its broader spectrum of action in targeting all IL-17 ligands.

Palmoplantar Pustular Psoriasis

Palmoplantar pustular psoriasis (PPPP) is a variant of pustular psoriasis characterized by the presence of sterile pustules on the palms and soles, in addition to indurated scaly psoriatic plaques on the palms/soles as a localized form, or as part of skin lesions distributed elsewhere on the body [318]. Despite the relatively small area of involvement, PPPP profoundly effects patient QoL due to the greater incidence of disease-related pain and functional limitation. Currently, no standardized therapy exists for PPPP, and although the efficacy of biologic drugs for plaque psoriasis has been widely demonstrated, limited data exist for the utility of biologics specifically for PPPP that has been refractory to many treatments. Recent studies have elaborated IL-17A, IL-17C and IL-17F positivity in lesions of PPPP [308, 319]. These findings support brodalumab's use in the treatment of PPPP. Currently the utility of brodalumab in PPPP is confined to case reports and series, with conflicting outcomes, including paradoxical eruption of palmoplantar pustulation [320–323]. It is speculated that blockade of IL-17A may precipitate increased production of inflammatory cytokines upstream of IL-17A, or there is an upregulation of the Th1 pathway with enhanced production of IL-12 and TNFα that potentially mediate this paradoxical reaction.[339]

Psoriatic Arthropathy

PsA is a chronic, immune mediated inflammatory arthritis with a progressive course, associated with joint damage, dactylitis, enthesitis and axial involvement.[340] Increased levels of IL-17 producing cells are present in the peripheral blood, synovial tissue/fluid and cutaneous plaques in patients with PsA [182]. Among the IL-17 ligands, IL-17A is the most important, followed by IL-17F and IL-17E (IL-25). IL-17F is the closest member to IL-17A, outlining 50% sequence identity with IL-17A. Although IL-17F is less active than IL-17A, it certainly appears to be important biologically due to the associated synergism with IL-17A and TNFα, allowing attainment of pro-inflammatory gene signature levels almost synonymous to IL-17A [324, 325]. Both IL-17A and IL-17F trigger activation and trafficking of immune cells and induces release of proinflammatory cytokines and chemokines, that attract neutrophils and monocytes, stimulating release of matrix metalloproteases and receptor activator of κβ-ligand, that majorly contribute to cartilage and bone destruction [183].

Interestingly, whereas both IL-17A and IL-17F are pro-inflammatory, IL-17E (IL-25) can downregulate such an effect (as an endogenous control of the inflammatory response) [326]. Theoretically, blockade of the IL-17RA, would not only block IL-17A and IL-17F, but also inhibit IL-17E binding, thus possibly reducing its anti-inflammatory effects [327]. However, increase in levels of IL-17E occur as a compensatory mechanism to decrease inflammation following escalation of IL-17A/F levels, and when the IL-17RA is blocked, the requirement for this compensation may not be essential [327]. In this way brodalumab is capable of producing clinically meaningful improvements in arthritis, enthesitis and dactylitis in patients with PsA. Clinical improvements in PsA are evident within 4 weeks of therapy initiation with brodalumab [328, 329].

Hidradenitis Suppurativa

HS is a chronic autoinflammatory follicular disorder, classically involving those body parts rich in apocrine glands, and clinically manifesting as nodules, abscesses and draining sinuses. Apart from significant physical disability, HS also has a profound impact on the emotional aspect of life [187].

Recently, the IL-17 pathway has been identified as a major player in HS pathogenesis [331]. In HS, IL-17 is expressed, not only in lesional and perilesional tissue, but also in unaffected skin; expounding the occurrence of subclinical inflammatory processes even prior to the development of active disease [189]. Moreover, elevated levels of IL-17 induce proteins like IL37/cathelicidin, S100A7, S100A8 and S100A9 that promote cytokine/chemokine expression and keratinocyte proliferation, thereby perpetuating a progressive feed forward loop, eventuating in potential tissue damage [191, 332]. IL-17 further acts on nod-like receptor protein-3(NCRP-3) inflammasome and stimulates production of TGFβ, IL-1β, IL-6 and TNFα from macrophages, crucial for Th17 differentiation and proliferation [47].

Transforming growth factor (TGF)-β sets into motion RAR-related orphan receptor gamma-γt (a transcription factor), necessary for generation of Th17 cells [330]; IL-1β and IL-6 independently downregulate Foxp3 (another transcription factor), consequently resulting in reduced levels of regulatory T cells [49]; and TNFα rapidly promotes induction of IL-1β, IL-6, IL-8, IL-2 and adhesion molecules in monocytes and macrophages, generating a relentless progressive pathogenic cycle for HS [50].

Even so, in HS patients, elevated levels of IL-17 A/C/F transcripts and $CD4^+$ IL-17 T cells have been identified in lesional tissue, with increased IL-17A serum levels of these patients [331]. IL-17A and IL-17F, work synergistically in promoting inflammation in HS. They act on IL-17C and promote production of other inflammatory cytokines, including IL-17A and IL-17F, thereby establishing a well-coordinated inflammatory cascade that is continuous and self-perpetuating [332]. Brodalumab by its unique mechanism of blocking IL-17RA, antagonizes IL-17A, IL-17C and IL-17F, thereby inhibiting all 3 cytokines and breaking the inflammatory feedback loop which eventuates in amelioration of inflammation, manifesting clinically as resolution of lesions. Besides, it proves superior to ixekizumab and secukinumab owing to its ability to supress other cytokines not targeted by them. [331, 333] Propitious effects of brodalumab in HS have been demonstrated in open label studies, as well as case series/reports. [333–339]

Pyoderma Gangrenosum

PG is a burdensome, painful neutrophilic dermatosis characterized by rapidly evolving painful, irregular ulcers with a violaceous and erythematous edge [340]. It can present in isolation or in association with other immunological conditions like inflammatory bowel disease [340].

Currently, the efficacy of brodalumab has been outlined in two publications [341, 342]. Diseased skin in PG is characterized by an increased expression of multiple IL-17 isoforms (IL-17A, IL-17C and IL-17F), that facilitate neutrophilic migration, trigger secretion of IL-6, IL-8 and GM-CSF; and plummet levels of regulatory T cells. Additionally, these isoforms upregulate CXCL1, and CXCL8 (IL-8) that again mediate neutrophil chemotaxis and potentially perpetuate the inflammatory cascade [61, 343].

Brodalumab, by blocking multiple IL-17 isoforms contributes in rapid resolution of PG. Besides, the high recapture rate of brodalumab allows it to be effective even following temporary suspension [342, 344]. However, development of PG in patients receiving brodalumab for psoriasis has been reported following biologic switching from adalimumab, secukinumab and ustekinumab [345–347]. This occurs secondary to compensatory upregulation of IL-23 following IL-17RA inhibition that disrupts the IL-23/IL-17 axis [346, 347]. Additionally, there is also disruption in the TNFα dependent apoptotic pathway, furthering cytokine disequilibrium, eventually precipitating PG. [345] Interestingly, patients with heterozygous polymorphisms within the promoter region of IL-6 genes have been associated with an increased susceptibility for the development of PG. This occurs due to exaggerated IL-6 production in these patients that skew the patients' immune responses towards a Th17 phenotype and this genetically determined milieu, when coupled with brodalumab mediated inhibition of IL-17 associated physiological regulatory functions, results in exaggeration of the preexisting Th17 response, that possibly precipitates PG. [346] The clinician should therefore be aware of this therapeutic paradox prior to prescribing brodalumab for PG.

Pityriasis Rubra Pilaris

PRP is a rare inflammatory dermatosis characterized by keratotic follicular papules coalescing into scaly orange-red plaques. Although easy to diagnose, treatment is often challenging, as a result of which newer agents to treat PRP are being explored constantly. Of late, upregulated expression of Th17 cytokines (IL-17A, IL-17F and IL-22) as well as TNF, IL-6, IL-12, IL-23 and IL-1β have been demonstrated in PRP [84]. Based on these findings, the utility of brodalumab in PRP has been propounded. Currently though, the efficacy of brodalumab in PRP is confined to case reports [348–351], with the need for RCTs to strengthen this observation. One major advantage of brodalumab in PRP is its rapidity of action in both lesional clearance, and alleviation of pruritus.

Adverse Effects

Common

Common adverse events encountered with brodalumab include arthralgia, headache, fatigue, diarrhoea, myalgia, nausea, oropharyngeal pain, neutropenia and influenza [352].

Cutaneous

Injection Site Reactions

Brodalumab has been associated with a very low prevalence (0.5–1.4%) of injection site reactions [353].

Subacute Cutaneous Lupus Erythematosus

Development of subacute cutaneous lupus erythematosus (SCLE) has been described in an isolated report on brodalumab for plaque psoriasis, with complete resolution of symptoms following cessation of brodalumab. Induction of SCLE with brodalumab is attributed to a paradoxical reaction in genetically predisposed individuals wherein a complex manipulation of immune mediated inflammatory reaction occurs, that in turn precipitates SCLE [354]. Nonetheless, more reports become essential to further link this association.

Acquired Ichthyosis

In an anecdotal report, development of acquired ichthyosis (AI) in a psoriatic patient on brodalumab therapy has been described. The mechanism postulated for this occurrence was an imbalance of the cytokine profile following IL-17RA blockade that altered the normal functioning of enzymes involved in the cornification process [355]. Nevertheless, further studies are mandated to clearly define the cause of AI following brodalumab therapy.

Miscellaneous

These include palmoplantar pustulosis, alopecia areata and PG. [323, 356]

Infections

In phase I, II and III studies, no case of TB reactivation following brodalumab therapy was reported. Even so, in an extension study at 108 weeks, there was a similar conclusion [357]. Although no serious fungal infections have been reported with brodalumab, onychomycosis has been described in a patient receiving brodalumab, that led to the patient discontinuing treatment with brodalumab [358].

Malignancies

Malignancy rates from a long-term clinical trial and 1-, 2- and 3-year US pharmacovigilance studies in patients receiving brodalumab were 0.9, 1.0, 0.8 and 1.1 events/100 patient years respectively [358].

In the above analysis, 37 malignancies were described in 32 patients. Dermatologic malignancies included squamous cell carcinoma, basal cell carcinoma and malignant melanoma. Other malignancies reported were hepatic, lung, gall bladder, renal, prostate, ovarian, endometrial, plasma cell myeloma and other unspecified neoplasms. However, none of the reported malignancies were deemed related to brodalumab. Of the 32 patients, 10 continued treatment with brodalumab and 18 discontinued. In the remaining 4 patients, treatment status was unknown [358].

Black Box warning
A rare, but worrisome adverse effect associated with brodalumab in psoriasis patients is the occurrence of suicidal ideation and behaviour. The US-FDA has therefore issued a black box warning regarding the association of brodalumab with suicidality. This causation though, has been disputed in literature, with the suggestion that untreated or insufficiently treated disease could majorly contribute for the same [359, 360].

Drug Monitoring

Baseline

- Complete blood count/hemogram.
- Erythrocyte sedimentation rate.
- C-reactive protein.
- Liver function test.
- Renal function test.
- Serum electrolytes.
- Anti-nuclear antibody.
- Anti-dsDNA antibody.
- Screening for hepatitis and human immunodeficiency virus.
- Chest X-ray.
- Tuberculin skin testing or QuantiFERON gold test.
- Pregnancy test in females of child bearing age.
- Serology for varicella zoster and measles (if clinically indicated).
- Urinalysis.

Ongoing

- Evaluation of response to treatment is measurable by respective assessment scores; i.e. PASI, DLQI at 3 months initially and subsequently every 6 months.
- A complete blood count and hemogram needs to be repeated at 3 months and then every 6 months.
- Liver and renal function tests, electrolytes and urinalysis need similar evaluation.

Use in Special Populations

Pregnancy/lactation

Although no contraindication exists for the usage of brodalumab in pregnancy/lactation, monoclonal antibodies are known to actively be transported through the placenta, especially in the third trimester, and gets excreted in modest amounts in breast milk. Risk and benefits to the mother require assessment before initiation or discontinuation of brodalumab [361].

Crohn's Disease

In patients with Crohn's disease, brodalumab is contraindicated. If a patient develops Crohn's disease while taking brodalumab, it needs to be discontinued, otherwise Crohn's disease can progress disproportionately with ongoing brodalumab therapy [362].

Infections

In patients having a non-resolving infection, brodalumab needs to be discontinued [363]. Screening for tuberculosis (TB) is essential prior to initiation of brodalumab therapy. If acute tubercular infection is detected, brodalumab should not be given. In patients with latent TB or history of active/latent TB with unconfirmed treatment, anti-tubercular treatment needs to be started before administering brodalumab because of the risk of activation of latent TB [364].

Paediatric

Efficacy and safety data of brodalumab in the paediatric population with moderate to severe psoriasis in not yet characterized. However, based on the adult population data regarding brodalumab, it could become an excellent therapeutic option for paediatric psoriasis in the future, given the rapid therapeutic onset and high skin clearance rates associated with it [144].

Geriatric

Brodalumab is seen to be an effective and safe therapeutic option for treating psoriasis in patients ≥65 years. Besides, adverse events do not seem to differ from those reported in younger patients, despite the greater frequency of comorbidities in the elderly population [365].

Availability and Administration

Brodalumab injection is available as a single-dose prefilled syringe containing 210 mg of the drug, which can only be used one time. It needs to be removed from the refrigerator 30 minutes prior to administration. The prefilled syringe should not be shaken. Subcutaneous injections of brodalumab are administered over the thighs, upper arms or abdomen and these sites are rotated with each dose to prevent skin damage. Additionally, bruised/diseased/damaged skin needs to be avoided [229].

Future Direction

Currently in highly recalcitrant cases of psoriasis, the need for combining conventional anti-psoriatic agents with brodalumab is an avenue for future exploration. Besides, evaluating various dosing schedules for brodalumab is another arena open for further study. This facet can enable dose titration with brodalumab in specific cases with the aim of reducing side effects, as well as alleviating the financial burden associated with brodalumab therapy.

Conclusion

Brodalumab has emerged as a highly effective treatment option for various forms of psoriasis and other inflammatory skin conditions. Its unique mechanism of action, targeting the IL-17RA and blocking multiple IL-17 cytokines has shown rapid and sustained efficacy, not only in moderate-to-severe plaque psoriasis but also in difficult to treat psoriasis variants, and few other dermatoses, thereby highlighting its versatility. While common adverse effects are generally mild, occurrence of rare serious adverse events necessitates ongoing monitoring and research. Overall, brodalumab represents a significant advancement in the management of IL-17-mediated inflammatory dermatoses, offering hope to patients who have not responded to other biologic therapies. Further studies are warranted to fully understand its long-term safety and efficacy across diverse patient populations.

References

1. Novartis Pharmaceuticals. Costenyx[package insert]. East Hanover, NJ; Revised June 2018. Available at https://www.novartis.com/us-en/sites/novartis_us/files/cosentyx.pdf.
2. Bruin G, Hockey HP, La Stella P, Sigurgeirsson B, Fu R, Patekar M, et al. Comparison of pharmacokinetics, safety and tolerability of secukinumab administered subcutaneously using different delivery systems in healthy volunteers and in psoriasis patients. Br J Clin Pharmacol. 2020;86:338–51.
3. Roman M, Madkan VK, Chiu MW. Profile of secukinumab in the treatment of psoriasis: current perspectives. Ther Clin Risk Manag. 2015;11:1767–77.

4. Narbutt J, Niedźwiedź M, Lesiak A, Ceryn J, Skibińska M. Secukinumab for the treatment of psoriasis in pediatrics: patient selection and acceptability. Patient Prefer Adherence. 2023;17:421–31.
5. Aboobacker S, Kurn H, Al Aboud AM. Secukinumab. [Updated 2023 Jun 20]. In: StatPearls [Internet]. Treasure Island (FL): StatPearls Publishing; 2023 Jan-. Available from: https://www.ncbi.nlm.nih.gov/books/NBK537091/
6. Novartis. FDA approves Novartis Cosentyx® as the first new biologic treatment option for hidradenitis suppurativa patients in nearly a decade. Press release. Published online October 31, 2023. Accessed October 31, 2023. https://www.novartis.com/us-en/news/media-releases/fda-approves-novartis-cosentyx-first-new-biologic-treatment-option-hidradenitis-suppurativa-patients-nearly-decade.
7. Wu KK, Dao H Jr. Off-label dermatologic uses of IL-17 inhibitors. J Dermatolog Treat. 2022;33:41–7.
8. Mital R, Gray A, Minta A, Almhana F, Amin S, Hydol-Smith J, Mallela T, Kaffenberger BH. Novel and off-label biologic use in the Management of Hidradenitis Suppurativa, pyoderma Gangrenosum, lichen planus, and seborrheic dermatitis: a narrative review. Dermatol Ther (Heidelb). 2023;13:77–94.
9. Noda S, Hashim P, Khattri S, Shroff A, Guttman-Yassky E. 224 successful use of secukinumab in an asian patient with severe refractory atopic dermatitis. J Invest Dermatol. 2016;136:S40.
10. Smith CH, Jabbar-Lopez ZK, Yiu ZZ, Bale T, Burden AD, Coates LC, et al. British Association of Dermatologists guidelines for biologic therapy for psoriasis 2017. Br J Dermatol. 2017;177:628–36.
11. Blair HA. Secukinumab: a review in moderate to severe pediatric plaque psoriasis. Paediatr Drugs. 2021;23:601–8.
12. Kagami S, Rizzo HL, Lee JJ, Koguchi Y, Blauvelt A. Circulating Th17, Th22, and Th1 cells are increased in psoriasis. J Invest Dermatol. 2010 May;130(5):1373–83.
13. Zaba LC, Cardinale I, Gilleaudeau P, Sullivan-Whalen M, Suárez-Fariñas M, Fuentes-Duculan J, et al. Amelioration of epidermal hyperplasia by TNF inhibition is associated with reduced Th17 responses. J Exp Med. 2007;204:3183–94.
14. Zhang L, Yang XQ, Cheng J, Hui RS, Gao TW. Increased Th17 cells are accompanied by FoxP3(+) Treg cell accumulation and correlated with psoriasis disease severity. Clin Immunol. 2010;135:108–17.
15. Malakouti M, Brown GE, Wang E, Koo J, Levin EC. The role of IL-17 in psoriasis. J Dermatolog Treat. 2015;26:41–4.
16. Lowes MA, Russell CB, Martin DA, Towne JE, Krueger JG. The IL-23/T17 pathogenic axis in psoriasis is amplified by keratinocyte responses. Trends Immunol. 2013;34:174–81.
17. Harper EG, Guo C, Rizzo H, Lillis JV, Kurtz SE, Skorcheva I, et al. Th17 cytokines stimulate CCL20 expression in keratinocytes in vitro and in vivo: implications for psoriasis pathogenesis. J Invest Dermatol. 2009;129:2175–83.
18. Langley RG, Elewski BE, Lebwohl M, Reich K, Griffiths CE, Papp K, ERASURE Study Group; FIXTURE Study Group, et al. Secukinumab in plaque psoriasis—results of two phase 3 trials. N Engl J Med. 2014;371:326–38.
19. Blauvelt A, Prinz JC, Gottlieb AB, Kingo K, Sofen H, Ruer-Mulard M, ; FEATURE Study Group, et al. Secukinumab administration by pre-filled syringe: efficacy, safety and usability results from a randomized controlled trial in psoriasis (FEATURE). Br J Dermatol 2015; 172:484–493.
20. Paul C, Lacour JP, Tedremets L, Kreutzer K, Jazayeri S, Adams S, ; JUNCTURE Study Group, et al. Efficacy, safety and usability of secukinumab administration by autoinjector/pen in psoriasis: a randomized, controlled trial (JUNCTURE). J Eur Acad Dermatol Venereol 2015; 29:1082–1090.
21. Bagel J, Blauvelt A, Nia J, Hashim P, Patekar M, de Vera A, et al. Secukinumab maintains superiority over ustekinumab in clearing skin and improving quality of life in patients with moderate to severe plaque psoriasis: 52-week results from a double-blind phase 3b trial (CLARITY). J Eur Acad Dermatol Venereol. 2021;35:135–42.

22. Phung M, Georgakopoulos JR, Ighani A, Giroux L, Yeung J. Secukinumab dose optimization in adult psoriasis patients: a retrospective, multicenter case series. JAAD Case Rep. 2018;4:310–3.
23. Pettey AA, Balkrishnan R, Rapp SR, Fleischer AB, Feldman SR. Patients with palmoplantar psoriasis have more physical disability and discomfort than patients with other forms of psoriasis: implications for clinical practice. J Am Acad Dermatol. 2003;49:271–5.
24. Gottlieb AB, Kubanov A, van Doorn M, Sullivan J, Papp KA, You R, et al. Sustained efficacy of secukinumab in patients with moderate-to-severe palmoplantar psoriasis: 2·5-year results from GESTURE, a randomized, double-blind, placebo-controlled trial. Br J Dermatol. 2020;182:889–99.
25. Gottlieb A, Sullivan J, van Doorn M, Kubanov A, You R, Parneix A, et al. Secukinumab shows significant efficacy in palmoplantar psoriasis: results from GESTURE, a randomized controlled trial. J Am Acad Dermatol. 2017;76:70–80.
26. Galluzzo M, Talamonti M, Atzori L, Bardazzi F, Campanati A, Di Cesare A, et al. Secukinumab for the treatment of palmoplantar psoriasis: a 2-year, multicenter, real-life observational study. Expert Opin Biol Ther. 2022;22:547–54.
27. Lawry M. Biological therapy and nail psoriasis. Dermatol Ther. 2007;20:60–7.
28. De Berker D. Management of nail psoriasis. Clin Exp Dermatol. 2000;25:357–62.
29. Reich K, Sullivan J, Arenberger P, Jazayeri S, Mrowietz U, Augustin M, et al. Secukinumab shows high and sustained efficacy in nail psoriasis: 2.5-year results from the randomized placebo-controlled TRANSFIGURE study. Br J Dermatol. 2021;184:425–36.
30. He F, Long F, Tu J, Yin Z. Intramatricial low-dose secukinumab injection for nail psoriasis. Indian J Dermatol Venereol Leprol. 2021;87:116–9.
31. Karmacharya P, Chakradhar R, Ogdie A. The epidemiology of psoriatic arthritis: a literature review. Best Pract Res Clin Rheumatol. 2021;35:101692.
32. Raychaudhuri SP, Raychaudhuri SK, Genovese MC. IL-17 receptor and its functional significance in psoriatic arthritis. Mol Cell Biochem. 2012;359:419–29.
33. McInnes IB, Mease PJ, Kirkham B, Kavanaugh A, Ritchlin CT, Rahman P, et al. FUTURE 2 study group. Secukinumab, a human anti-interleukin-17A monoclonal antibody, in patients with psoriatic arthritis (FUTURE 2): a randomised, double-blind, placebo-controlled, phase 3 trial. Lancet. 2015;386:1137–46.
34. Mease PJ, McInnes IB, Kirkham B, Kavanaugh A, Rahman P, van der Heijde D, et al. FUTURE 1 study group. Secukinumab inhibition of interleukin-17A in patients with psoriatic arthritis. N Engl J Med. 2015;373:1329–39.
35. Crowley JJ, Pariser DM, Yamauchi PS. A brief guide to pustular psoriasis for primary care providers. Postgrad Med. 2021;133:330–44.
36. Fujita H, Terui T, Hayama K, Akiyama M, Ikeda S, Mabuchi T, et al. Japanese dermatological association guidelines development Committee for the Guidelines for the management and treatment of generalized pustular psoriasis. Japanese guidelines for the management and treatment of generalized pustular psoriasis: the new pathogenesis and treatment of GPP. J Dermatol. 2018;45:1235–70.
37. Li J, Gao X, Ma L, Fang Y. Secukinumab for the treatment of generalized pustular psoriasis: a case report. Medicine (Baltimore). 2023;102:e33693.
38. Yeung J, Valbuena V. Successful use of secukinumab in pustular psoriasis. JAAD Case Rep. 2016;2:470–2.
39. Madanagobalane S. Secukinumab in generalized pustular psoriasis. Indian Dermatol Online J. 2018;9:464–6.
40. Xue G, Lili M, Yimiao F, Miao W, Xiaohong Y, Dongmei W. Case report: successful treatment of acute generalized pustular psoriasis of puerperium with secukinumab. Front Med. 2022;9:1072039.
41. Mrowietz U, Bachelez H, Burden AD, Rissler M, Sieder C, Orsenigo R, et al. Secukinumab for moderate-to-severe palmoplantar pustular psoriasis: results of the 2PRECISE study. J Am Acad Dermatol. 2019;80:1344–52.

42. Ho PH, Tsai TF. Successful treatment of refractory juvenile generalized pustular psoriasis with secukinumab monotherapy: a case report and review of published work. J Dermatol. 2018;45:1353–6.
43. Imafuku S, Honma M, Okubo Y, Komine M, Ohtsuki M, Morita A, et al. Efficacy and safety of secukinumab in patients with generalized pustular psoriasis: a 52-week analysis from phase III open-label multicenter Japanese study. J Dermatol. 2016;43:1011–7.
44. Melnik BC, John SM, Chen W, Plewig G. T helper 17 cell/regulatory T-cell imbalance in hidradenitis suppurativa/acne inversa: the link to hair follicle dissection, obesity, smoking and autoimmune comorbidities. Br J Dermatol. 2018;179:260–72.
45. Matusiak Ł, Szczęch J, Bieniek A, Nowicka-Suszko D, Szepietowski JC. Increased interleukin (IL)-17 serum levels in patients with hidradenitis suppurativa: implications for treatment with anti-IL-17 agents. J Am Acad Dermatol. 2017;76:670–5.
46. Goldburg SR, Strober BE, Payette MJ. Hidradenitis suppurativa: epidemiology, clinical presentation, and pathogenesis. J Am Acad Dermatol. 2020;82:1045–58.
47. Korn T, Bettelli E, Oukka M, Kuchroo VK. IL-17 and Th17 cells. Annu Rev Immunol. 2009;27:485–517.
48. Quesniaux V, Ryffel B, Di Padova. Central role of Th17 cells in adaptive immune responses. In: Quesniaux V, Ryffel B, Di Padova F, editors. IL-17, IL-22 and their producing cells. Role in inflammation and autoimmunity. 2nd ed. Berlin/Heidelberg, Germany: Springer; 2013. p. 71–89.
49. Ikeda S, Saijo S, Murayama MA, Shimizu K, Akitsu A, Iwakura Y. Excess IL-1 signaling enhances the development of Th17 cells by downregulating TGF-β-induced Foxp3 expression. J Immunol. 2014;192:1449–58.
50. Moran B, Sweeney CM, Hughes R, Malara A, Kirthi S, Tobin AM, et al. Hidradenitis Suppurativa Is Characterized by Dysregulation of the Th17:Treg Cell Axis, Which Is Corrected by Anti-TNF Therapy. J Invest Dermatol. 2017;137:2389–95.
51. Kimball AB, Jemec GBE, Alavi A, Reguiai Z, Gottlieb AB, Bechara FG, et al. Secukinumab in moderate-to-severe hidradenitis suppurativa (SUNSHINE and SUNRISE): week 16 and week 52 results of two identical, multicentre, randomised, placebo-controlled, double-blind phase 3 trials. Lancet. 2023;401(10378):747–61.
52. Casseres RG, Prussick L, Zancanaro P, Rothstein B, Joshipura D, Saraiya A, et al. Secukinumab in the treatment of moderate to severe hidradenitis suppurativa: results of an open-label trial. J Am Acad Dermatol. 2020;82:1524–6.
53. Prussick L, Rothstein B, Joshipura D, Saraiya A, Turkowski Y, Abdat R, et al. Open-label, investigator-initiated, single-site exploratory trial evaluating secukinumab, an anti-interleukin-17A monoclonal antibody, for patients with moderate-to-severe hidradenitis suppurativa. Br J Dermatol. 2019;181:609–11.
54. Villegas-Romero I, Collantes-Rodríguez C, Valenzuela-Ubiña S, Jiménez-Gallo D. Moderate to severe hidradenitis Suppurativa successfully treated with secukinumab. Actas Dermosifiliogr. 2020;111:696–8.
55. Schuch A, Fischer T, Boehner A, Biedermann T, Volz T. Successful treatment of severe recalcitrant hidradenitis Suppurativa with the interleukin-17A antibody Secukinumab. Acta Derm Venereol. 2018;98:151–2.
56. Thorlacius L, Theut Riis P, Jemec GBE. Severe hidradenitis suppurativa responding to treatment with secukinumab: a case report. Br J Dermatol. 2018;179:182–5.
57. Jørgensen AR, Yao Y, Thomsen SF. Therapeutic response to Secukinumab in a 36-year-old woman with hidradenitis Suppurativa. Case Rep Dermatol Med. 2018;2018:8685136.
58. Marasca C, Megna M, Balato A, Balato N, Napolitano M, Fabbrocini G. Secukinumab and hidradenitis suppurativa: friends or foes? JAAD Case Rep. 2019;5:184–7.
59. Pereira N, Brites MM, Gonçalo M, Tellechea O, Figueiredo A. Pyoderma gangrenosum--a review of 24 cases observed over 10 years. Int J Dermatol. 2013;52:938–45.
60. Alavi A, French LE, Davis MD, Brassard A, Kirsner RS. Pyoderma Gangrenosum: an update on pathophysiology, diagnosis and treatment. Am J Clin Dermatol. 2017;18:355–72.

61. Ortega-Loayza AG, Friedman MA, Reese AM, Liu Y, Greiling TM, Cassidy PB, et al. Molecular and cellular characterization of pyoderma Gangrenosum: implications for the use of gene expression. J Invest Dermatol. 2022;142:1217–1220.e14.
62. Wang EA, Steel A, Luxardi G, Mitra A, Patel F, Cheng MY, et al. Classic ulcerative pyoderma Gangrenosum is a T cell-mediated disease targeting follicular adnexal structures: a hypothesis based on molecular and Clinicopathologic studies. Front Immunol. 2018;8:1980.
63. Caproni M, Antiga E, Volpi W, Verdelli A, Venegoni L, Quaglino P, et al. The Treg/Th17 cell ratio is reduced in the skin lesions of patients with pyoderma gangrenosum. Br J Dermatol. 2015;173:275–8.
64. McPhie ML, Kirchhof MG. Pyoderma gangrenosum treated with secukinumab: a case report. JCMS Case Rep. 2020;8:1–3.
65. García M, Madrid González M, Prada Lobato JM. Secukinumab for pyoderma gangrenosum: a case report. Med Clin (Barc). 2019;152:246.
66. Herberger K, Dissemond J, Brüggestrat S, Sorbe C, Augustin M. Biologics and immunoglobulins in the treatment of pyoderma gangrenosum - analysis of 52 patients. J Dtsch Dermatol Ges. 2019;17:32–41.
67. Jin K, Matsuzaki Y, Akasaka E, Nakano H, Sawamura D. Pyoderma gangrenosum triggered by switching from adalimumab to secukinumab. J Dermatol. 2019;46:e108–9.
68. Wollina U, Schönlebe J, Fürll C. Pyoderma gangrenosum induced by secukinumab-a late paradoxical drug reaction. Dermatol Ther. 2020;33:e13161.
69. Petty AJ, Whitley MJ, Balaban A, Ellington K, Marano AL. Pyoderma gangrenosum induced by secukinumab in a patient with psoriasis successfully treated with ustekinumab. JAAD Case Rep. 2020;6:731–3.
70. Noda S, Suárez-Fariñas M, Ungar B, Kim SJ, de Guzman Strong C, Xu H, et al. The Asian atopic dermatitis phenotype combines features of atopic dermatitis and psoriasis with increased TH17 polarization. J Allergy Clin Immunol. 2015;136:1254–64.
71. Czarnowicki T, He H, Krueger JG, Guttman-Yassky E. Atopic dermatitis endotypes and implications for targeted therapeutics. J Allergy Clin Immunol. 2019;143:1–11.
72. Ungar B, Pavel AB, Li R, Kimmel G, Nia J, Hashim P, et al. Phase 2 randomized, double-blind study of IL-17 targeting with secukinumab in atopic dermatitis. J Allergy Clin Immunol. 2021;147:394–7.
73. Wagner G, Rose C, Sachse MM. Clinical variants of lichen planus. J Dtsch Dermatol Ges. 2013;11:309–19.
74. Solimani F, Pollmann R, Schmidt T, Schmidt A, Zheng X, Savai R, et al. Therapeutic targeting of Th17/Tc17 cells leads to clinical improvement of lichen planus. Front Immunol. 2019;10:1808.
75. Schmidt T, Solimani F, Pollmann R, Stein R, Schmidt A, Stulberg I, et al. T_H1/T_H17 cell recognition of desmoglein 3 and bullous pemphigoid antigen 180 in patients with lichen planus. J Allergy Clin Immunol. 2018;142:669–72.
76. Rezzag-Mahcene C, Cardot-Leccia N, Lacour JP, Montaudié H, Passeron T. Successful treatment of recalcitrant genital lichen planus with secukinumab. J Eur Acad Dermatol Venereol. 2021;35:e321–3.
77. Doolan BJ, Anderton H, Christie M, Dolianitis C. Cutaneous lichen planus induced by Secukinumab. J Clin Exp Dermatol Res. 2017;9:1.
78. Daye M, Temiz SA, Gümüş S, Kılınç F. Secukinumab-induced Oral lichen planus: a report of case and review of literature. İstanbul Med J. 2021;22:235–7.
79. Komori T, Honda T, Endo Y, Kaku Y, Otsuka A, Kabashima K. Oral lichen planus associated with candidiasis during secukinumab treatment. J Dermatol. 2017;44:e60–1.
80. Gauci ML, Jachiet M, Gottlieb J, Madeleine-Chambrin I, Rybojad M, Bagot M, et al. Successful treatment of type II pityriasis rubra pilaris with secukinumab. JAAD Case Rep. 2016;2:462–4.
81. Schuster D, Pfister-Wartha A, Bruckner-Tuderman L, Schempp CM. Successful treatment of refractory Pityriasis Rubra pilaris with Secukinumab. JAMA Dermatol. 2016;152:1278–80.

82. Bonomo L, Levitt JO. Secukinumab emerges as a rapidly effective therapy for pityriasis rubra pilaris. Cutis. 2018;101:367–9.
83. Wain T, Choy B, Satchell AC, Woods JA, Frew JW. Secukinumab in pityriasis rubra pilaris: a case series demonstrating variable response and the need for minimal clinical datasets. JAAD Case Rep. 2018;4:500–5.
84. Feldmeyer L, Mylonas A, Demaria O, Mennella A, Yawalkar N, Laffitte E, et al. Interleukin 23-helper T cell 17 Axis as a treatment target for Pityriasis Rubra pilaris. JAMA Dermatol. 2017;153:304–8.
85. Boudreaux BW, Pincelli TP, Bhullar PR, Patel MH, Brumfiel CM, Li X, et al. Secukinumab for the treatment of adult onset pityriasis rubra pilaris: a single arm clinical trial with transcriptomic analysis. Br J Dermatol. 2022;187:650–8.
86. Fabiani C, Vitale A, Orlando I, Sota J, Capozzoli M, Franceschini R, et al. Quality of life impairment in Behçet's disease and relationship with disease activity: a prospective study. Intern Emerg Med. 2017;12:947–55.
87. Di Scala G, Bettiol A, Cojan RD, Finocchi M, Silvestri E, Emmi G. Efficacy of the anti-IL 17 secukinumab in refractory Behçet's syndrome: a preliminary study. J Autoimmun. 2019;97:108–13.
88. Fagni F, Bettiol A, Talarico R, Lopalco G, Silvestri E, Urban ML, et al. Long-term effectiveness and safety of secukinumab for treatment of refractory mucosal and articular Behçet's phenotype: a multicentre study. Ann Rheum Dis. 2020;79:1098–104.
89. Hatemi G, Fresko I, Tascilar K, Yazici H. Increased enthesopathy among Behçet's syndrome patients with acne and arthritis: an ultrasonography study. Arthritis Rheum. 2008;58:1539–45.
90. Todberg T, Zachariae C, Krustrup D, Skov L. The effect of treatment with anti-interleukin-17 in patients with allergic contact dermatitis. Contact Derm. 2018;78:431–2.
91. Guttman-Yassky E, Nia JK, Hashim PW, Mansouri Y, Alia E, Taliercio M, et al. Efficacy and safety of secukinumab treatment in adults with extensive alopecia areata. Arch Dermatol Res. 2018;310:607–14.
92. Ordenes-Cavieres G, Andino-Navarrete R. Secukinumab for plaque psoriasis. Medwave. 2018;18:e7364.
93. Bodemer C, Kaszuba A, Kingo K, Tsianakas A, Morita A, Rivas E, et al. Secukinumab demonstrates high efficacy and a favourable safety profile in paediatric patients with severe chronic plaque psoriasis: 52-week results from a phase 3 double-blind randomized, controlled trial. J Eur Acad Dermatol Venereol. 2021;35:938–47.
94. Smith BJ, Nuccio BC, Graves KY, McMillan VM. Preparing patients for biologic medications for dermatologic and rheumatic diseases. JAAPA. 2018;31:23–8.
95. Warren RB, Reich K, Langley RG, Strober B, Gladman D, Deodhar A, et al. Secukinumab in pregnancy: outcomes in psoriasis, psoriatic arthritis and ankylosing spondylitis from the global safety database. Br J Dermatol. 2018;179:1205–7.
96. Drugs and lactation database (LactMed®) [internet]. National Institute of child health and human development: Bethesda (MD); 2023. Secukinumab.
97. Cada DJ, Baker DE, Panther SG, Ingram K. Secukinumab. Hosp Pharm. 2015;50:714–27.
98. Garnock-Jones KP. Secukinumab: a review in moderate to severe plaque psoriasis. Am J Clin Dermatol. 2015;16:323–30.
99. Dong J, Goldenberg G. New biologics in psoriasis: an update on IL-23 and IL-17 inhibitors. Cutis. 2017;99:123–7.
100. Preuss CV, Quick J. Ixekizumab[updated 2023 July 4]. In: StatPearls[Internet]. Treasure Island(FL): StatPearls Publishing; 2023. Available from: https://www.ncbi.nlm.nih.gov/books/NBK431088/.
101. Jackson K, Chua L, Velez de Mendizabal N, Pitou C, Rodriguez Capriles C, Paller AS, Lansang P, Seyger MM, Papp K, IXORA-PEDS Study Group. Population pharmacokinetic and exposure–efficacy analysis of ixekizumab in paediatric patients with moderate-to-severe plaque psoriasis (IXORA-PEDS). Br J Clin Pharmacol. 2022;88:1074–86.
102. Taltz®. Summary of product characteristics. Accessed March 01, 2022. https://www.ema.europa.eu/en/documents/product-information/taltz-epar-product-information-en.pdf.

103. Blegvad C, Skov L, Zachariae C. Ixekizumab for the treatment of psoriasis: an update on new data since first approval. Expert Rev Clin Immunol. 2019;15:111–21.
104. Brownstone ND, Hong J, Mosca M, Hadeler E, Liao W, Bhutani T, Koo J. Biologic treatments of psoriasis: an update for the clinician. Biologics Targets Ther. 2021;15:39–51.
105. Pavelka K. Targeted and biological drugs in the treatment of inflammatory rheumatic diseases. Vnitr Leka. 2021;67:195–200.
106. Atzeni F, Carriero A, Boccassini L, D'Angelo S. Anti-IL-17 agents in the treatment of axial spondyloarthritis. Immunotargets Ther. 2021;10:141–53.
107. Cather JC, Young CT, Young MS, Cather JC. Ixekizumab for the treatment of pediatric patients with moderate to severe plaque psoriasis. Expert Opin Biol Ther. 2021;21:983–90.
108. Kearns DG, Uppal S, Chat VS, Wu JJ. Comparison of guidelines for the use of Interleukin-17 inhibitors for psoriasis in the United States, Britain, and Europe: a critical appraisal and comprehensive review. J Clin Aesthet Dermatol. 2021;14:55–9.
109. Rendon A, Schäkel K. Psoriasis pathogenesis and treatment. Int J Mol Sci. 2019;20:1475.
110. Armstrong AW, Read C. Pathophysiology, clinical presentation, and treatment of psoriasis: a review. JAMA. 2020;323:1945–60.
111. Diotallevi F, Campanati A, Radi G, Molinelli E, Offidani A. Ixekizumab for treatment of moderate to severe plaque psoriasis: real world clinical experience. G Ital Dermatol Venereol. 2020;155:739–43.
112. Laan M, Cui ZH, Hoshino H, Lötvall J, Sjöstrand M, Gruenert DC, et al. Neutrophil recruitment by human IL-17 via C-X-C chemokine release in the airways. J Immunol. 1999;162:2347–52.
113. Lynde CW, Poulin Y, Vender R, Bourcier M, Khalil S. Interleukin 17A: toward a new understanding of psoriasis pathogenesis. J Am Acad Dermatol. 2014;71:141–50.
114. Numasaki M, Fukushi J, Ono M, Narula SK, Zavodny PJ, Kudo T, et al. Interleukin-17 promotes angiogenesis and tumor growth. Blood. 2003;101:2620–7.
115. Krueger JG, Fretzin S, Suárez-Fariñas M, Haslett PA, Phipps KM, Cameron GS, et al. IL-17A is essential for cell activation and inflammatory gene circuits in subjects with psoriasis. J Allergy Clin Immunol. 2012;130:145–54.e9.
116. Gutowska-Owsiak D, Schaupp AL, Salimi M, Selvakumar TA, McPherson T, Taylor S, Ogg GS. IL-17 downregulates filaggrin and affects keratinocyte expression of genes associated with cellular adhesion. Exp Dermatol. 2012;21:104–10.
117. Kreuger J, Fretzin S, Farinas M, et al. Interleukin-17A is an essential cytokine to sustain pathogenic cell activation and inflammatory gene circuits in psoriasis vulgaris. Br J Dermatol. 2011;165:e6.
118. Blauvelt A, Papp K, Gottlieb A, Jarell A, Reich K, Maari C, et al. A head-to-head comparison of ixekizumab vs. guselkumab in patients with moderate-to-severe plaque psoriasis: 12-week efficacy, safety and speed of response from a randomized, double-blinded trial. Br J Dermatol. 2020;182:1348–58.
119. Craig S, Warren RB. Ixekizumab for the treatment of psoriasis: up-to-date. Expert Opin Biol Ther. 2020;20:549–57.
120. Griffiths CE, Reich K, Lebwohl M, van de Kerkhof P, Paul C, Menter A, et al. Comparison of ixekizumab with etanercept or placebo in moderate-to-severe psoriasis (UNCOVER-2 and UNCOVER-3): results from two phase 3 randomised trials. Lancet. 2015;386:541–51.
121. Reich K, Pinter A, Lacour JP, Ferrandiz C, Micali G, French LE, et al. Comparison of ixekizumab with ustekinumab in moderate-to-severe psoriasis: 24-week results from IXORA-S, a phase III study. Br J Dermatol. 2017;177:1014–23.
122. Blauvelt A, Shi N. Comparison of real-world treatment patterns among patients with psoriasis treated with ixekizumab or adalimumab. Patients Prefer Adherence. 2020;14:517–27.
123. Megna M, Potestio L, Camela E, Fabbrocini G, Ruggiero A. Ixekizumab and brodalumab indirect comparison in the treatment of moderate to severe psoriasis: results from an Italian single-center retrospective study in a real-life setting. Dermatol Ther. 2022;35:e15667.

124. Warren RB, Brnabic A, Saure D, Langley RG, See K, Wu JJ, et al. Matching-adjusted indirect comparison of efficacy in patients with moderate-to-severe plaque psoriasis treated with ixekizumab vs. secukinumab. Br J Dermatol. 2018;178:1064–71.
125. Paul C. Ixekizumab or secukinumab in psoriasis: what difference does it make? Br J Dermatol. 2018;178:1003–5.
126. Mastorino L, Dapavo P, Susca S, Cariti C, Siliquini N, Verrone A, Stroppiana E, et al. Drug survival and clinical effectiveness of secukinumab, ixekizumab, brodalumab, guselkumab, risankizumab, tildrakizumab for psoriasis treatment. J Dtsch Dermatol Ges. 2024;22:34–42.
127. Leonardi C, Reich K, Foley P, Torii H, Gerdes S, Guenther L, et al. Efficacy and safety of Ixekizumab through 5 years in moderate-to-severe psoriasis: Long-term results from the UNCOVER-1 and UNCOVER-2 Phase-3 randomized controlled trials. Dermatol Ther (Heidelb). 2020;10:431–47.
128. Blauvelt A, Lebwohl MG, Mabuchi T, Leung A, Garrelts A, Crane H, et al. Long-term efficacy and safety of ixekizumab: a 5-year analysis of the UNCOVER-3 randomized controlled trial. J Am Acad Dermatol. 2021;85:360–8.
129. Lebwohl MG, Gordon KB, Gallo G, Zhang L, Paul C. Ixekizumab sustains high level of efficacy and favourable safety profile over 4 years in patients with moderate psoriasis: results from UNCOVER-3 study. J Eur Acad Dermatol Venereol. 2020;34:301–9.
130. Leonardi C, Maari C, Philipp S, Goldblum O, Zhang L, Burkhardt N, et al. Maintenance of skin clearance with ixekizumab treatment of psoriasis: three-year results from the UNCOVER-3 study. J Am Acad Dermatol. 2018;79:824–830.e2.
131. Paller AS, Seyger MMB, Magariños GA, Pinter A, Cather JC, Rodriguez-Capriles C, et al. Long-term efficacy and safety of up to 108 weeks of Ixekizumab in pediatric patients with moderate to severe plaque psoriasis: the IXORA-PEDS randomized clinical trial. JAMA Dermatol. 2022;158:533–41.
132. Mastorino L, Dapavo P, Burzi L, Rosset F, Giunipero di Corteranzo I, Leo F, et al. Drug survival, effectiveness and safety of ixekizumab for moderate-to-severe psoriasis up to 5 years. J Eur Acad Dermatol Venereol. 2024;38:568–75.
133. Sherman S, Cohen ES, Amitay-Laish I, Hodak E, Pavlovsky L. IL-17A inhibitor switching–efficacy of ixekizumab following secukinumab failure. a single-center experience. Acta Derm Venereol. 2019;99:769–73.
134. Herrera-Acosta E, Garriga-Martina GG, Suárez-Pérez JA, Martínez-García EA, Herrera-Ceballos E. Comparative study of the efficacy and safety of secukinumab vs ixekizumab in moderate-to-severe psoriasis after 1 year of treatment: real-world practice. Dermatol Ther. 2020;33:e13313.
135. Chiricozzi A, Megna M, Giunta A, Carrera CG, Dapavo P, Balato A, et al. Ixekizumab is effective in the long-term management in moderate-to-severe plaque psoriasis: results from an Italian retrospective cohort study (the LOTIXE study). J Dermatolog Treat. 2023;34:2246606.
136. Malagoli P, Dapavo P, Pavia G, Amoruso F, Argenziano G, Bardazzi F, et al. Real life long-term efficacy and safety of ixekizumab in moderate-to-severe psoriasis: a 192 weeks multicentric retrospective study-IL PSO (Italian landscape psoriasis). Dermatol Ther. 2022;35:e15608.
137. Lynde C, Riedl E, Maul JT, Torres T, Pinter A, Fabbrocini G, et al. Comparative effectiveness of biologics across subgroups of patients with moderate-to-severe plaque psoriasis: results at week 12 from the PSoHO study in a real-world setting. Adv Ther. 2023;40:869–86.
138. Torres T, Puig L, Vender R, Lynde C, Piaserico S, Carrascosa JM, et al. Drug survival of IL-12/23, IL-17 and IL-23 inhibitors for psoriasis treatment: a retrospective multi-country, multicentric cohort study. Am J Clin Dermatol. 2021;22:567–79.
139. Wade R, Sharif-Hurst S, Dias S. Patient characteristics as effect modifiers for psoriasis biologic treatment response: an assessment using network meta-analysis subgroups. Syst Rev. 2020;9:132.
140. Wang C, Torisu-Itakura H, Hanada T, Matsuo T, Cai Z, Osaga S, et al. Treatment persistence of interleukin-17 inhibitor class drugs among patients with psoriasis in Japan: a retrospective database study. J Dermatolog Treat. 2023;34:2229465.

141. Hendrix N, Ollendorf DA, Chapman RH, Loos A, Liu S, Kumar V, et al. Cost-effectiveness of targeted pharmacotherapy for moderate to severe plaque psoriasis. J Manag Care Spec Pharm. 2018;24:1210–7.
142. Megna M, Balato A, Napolitano M, Gallo L, Caso F, Costa L, et al. Psoriatic disease treatment nowadays: unmet needs among the "jungle of biologic drugs and small molecules". Clin Rheumatol. 2018;37:1739–41.
143. Ye LR, Yan BX, Chen XY, Chen SQ, Chen JQ, Man XY, Chinese Psoriasis Real World Evidence Research Group (CPRWERG). Extended dosing intervals of ixekizumab for psoriasis: a single-center, uncontrolled, prospective study. J Am Acad Dermatol. 2022;86:1348–50.
144. Ruggiero A, Portarapillo A, Megna M, Patruno C, Napolitano M. Management strategies for pediatric moderate-to-severe plaque psoriasis: spotlight on biologics. Pediatric Health Med Ther. 2023;14:435–51.
145. Leonardi C, Matheson R, Zachariae C, Cameron G, Li L, Edson-Heredia E, et al. Anti-interleukin-17 monoclonal antibody ixekizumab in chronic plaque psoriasis. N Engl J Med. 2012;366:1190–9.
146. Gordon KB, Blauvelt A, Papp KA, Langley RG, Luger T, Ohtsuki M, et al. Phase 3 trials of Ixekizumab in moderate-to-severe plaque psoriasis. N Engl J Med. 2016;375:345–56.
147. Meeuwis KA, de Hullu JA, Massuger LF, van de Kerkhof PC, van Rossum MM. Genital psoriasis: a systematic literature review on this hidden skin disease. Acta Derm Venereol. 2011;91:5–11.
148. American Academy of Dermatology Work Group, Menter A, Korman NJ, Elmets CA, Feldman SR, Gelfand JM, et al. Guidelines of care for the management of psoriasis and psoriatic arthritis: section 6. Guidelines of care for the treatment of psoriasis and psoriatic arthritis: case-based presentations and evidence-based conclusions. J Am Acad Dermatol. 2011;65:137–74.
149. Ryan C, Menter A, Guenther L, Blauvelt A, Bissonnette R, Meeuwis K, et al. Efficacy and safety of ixekizumab in a randomized, double-blinded, placebo-controlled phase IIIb study of patients with moderate-to-severe genital psoriasis. Br J Dermatol. 2018;179:844–52.
150. Calianno G, Esposito M, Fidanza R, Palmieri M, Fargnoli MC. Ixekizumab improves disease severity, clinical symptoms and quality of life in patients with genital psoriasis: a 24-week real-life experience. Dermatol Ther. 2021;34:e14993.
151. Langley RG, Daudén E. Treatment and management of psoriasis with nail involvement: a focus on biologic therapy. Dermatology. 2010;221(Suppl 1):29–42.
152. Girolomoni G, Griffiths CE, Krueger J, Nestle FO, Nicolas JF, Prinz JC, et al. Early intervention in psoriasis and immune-mediated inflammatory diseases: a hypothesis paper. J Dermatolog Treat. 2015;26:103–12.
153. Elewski BE, Blauvelt A, Gallo G, Wolf E, McKean-Matthews M, Burge R, et al. Simultaneous nail and skin clearance in Ixekizumab head-to-head trials for moderate-to-severe psoriasis and psoriatic arthritis. Dermatol Ther (Heidelb). 2022;12:911–20.
154. Blauvelt A, Leonardi C, Elewski B, Crowley JJ, Guenther LC, Gooderham M, et al. A head-to-head comparison of ixekizumab vs. guselkumab in patients with moderate-to-severe plaque psoriasis: 24-week efficacy and safety results from a randomized, double-blinded trial. Br J Dermatol. 2021;184:1047–58.
155. Wasel N, Thaçi D, French LE, Conrad C, Dutronc Y, Gallo G, et al. Ixekizumab and Ustekinumab efficacy in nail psoriasis in patients with moderate-to-severe psoriasis: 52-week results from a phase 3, head-to-head study (IXORA-S). Dermatol Ther (Heidelb). 2020;10:663–70.
156. Egeberg A, Kristensen LE, Vender R, Zaheri S, El Baou C, Gallo G, et al. Sustained resolution of nail psoriasis through 5 years with Ixekizumab: a post-hoc analysis from UNCOVER-3. Acta Derm Venereol. 2022;102:adv00787.
157. Menter MA, Armstrong A, Kircik L, Gniadecki R, Garrelts A, See K, McKean-Matthews M, Bagel J. 41824 palmoplantar psoriasis complete clearance is achieved rapidly and sustained with ixekizumab treatment in adult and pediatric patients with moderate-to-severe plaque psoriasis. J Am Acad Dermatol. 2023;89:AB203.

158. Serrano L, Carlberg V, Holland K. Rapid efficacy of Ixekizumab for pediatric acute generalized pustular psoriasis. Skin. 2021;5:667–71.
159. Megna M, Abategiovanni L, Annunziata A, Torta G, Peduto T, Fabbrocini G, Lauro W. Generalized pustular psoriasis rapidly and successfully treated with ixekizumab in a Caucasian patient. Dermatol Ther. 2022;35:e15382.
160. Burlando M, Salvi I, Paravisi A, Cozzani E, Parodi A. Severe generalized pustular psoriasis successfully treated with Ixekizumab: a case report. Case Rep Dermatol. 2022;14:326–9.
161. Gargiulo L, Pavia G, Ibba L, Fiorillo G, Bressan A. Generalized pustular psoriasis and plaque psoriasis successfully treated with Ixekizumab. Clin Exp Dermatol Ther. 2022;7:183.
162. Saeki H, Nakagawa H, Nakajo K, Ishii T, Morisaki Y, Aoki T, et al. Efficacy and safety of ixekizumab treatment for Japanese patients with moderate to severe plaque psoriasis, erythrodermic psoriasis and generalized pustular psoriasis: results from a 52-week, open-label, phase 3 study (UNCOVER-J). J Dermatol. 2017;44:355–62.
163. Shao S, Wang G, Maverakis E, Gudjonsson JE. Targeted treatment for Erythrodermic psoriasis: rationale and recent advances. Drugs. 2020;80:525–34.
164. Lo Y, Tsai TF. Updates on the treatment of Erythrodermic psoriasis. Psoriasis (Auckl). 2021;11:59–73.
165. Reynolds KA, Pithadia DJ, Lee EB, Liao W, Wu JJ. A systematic review of treatment strategies for erythrodermic psoriasis. J Dermatolog Treat. 2021;32:49–55.
166. Moy AP, Murali M, Kroshinsky D, Duncan LM, Nazarian RM. Immunologic overlap of helper T-cell subtypes 17 and 22 in Erythrodermic psoriasis and atopic dermatitis. JAMA Dermatol. 2015;151:753–60.
167. Bernardini N, Skroza N, Tolino E, Mambrin A, Anzalone A, Balduzzi V, et al. IL-17 and its role in inflammatory, autoimmune, and oncological skin diseases: state of art. Int J Dermatol. 2020;59:406–11.
168. Bernardini N, Skroza N, Proietti I, Mambrin A, Marchesiello A, Tolino E, et al. Erythrodermic psoriasis successfully treated with anti IL-17: a case series. Acta Dermatovenerol Croat. 2021;29:191–5.
169. Pangilinan MCG, Sermswan P, Asawanonda P. Use of anti-IL-17 monoclonal antibodies in HIV patients with Erythrodermic psoriasis. Case Rep Dermatol. 2020;12:132–7.
170. Vinaixa Aranzazu A, Morillas-Lahuerta V, Blanco De Tord M, Carrascosa Carrillo JM. Ixekizumab for the treatment of erythrodermic psoriasis triggered by durvalumab-tremelimumab in a cancer patient. Eur J Dermatol. 2021;31:564–5.
171. Pinto-Pulido EL, Polo-Rodríguez I, González-Cañete M, García-Verdú E, Piteiro-Bermejo AB, Medina-Montalvo S. Ixekizumab treatment for drug-induced erythrodermic psoriasis. Dermatol Ther 2022; 35: e15863.
172. Saeki H, Nakagawa H, Ishii T, Morisaki Y, Aoki T, Berclaz PY, et al. Efficacy and safety of open-label ixekizumab treatment in Japanese patients with moderate-to-severe plaque psoriasis, erythrodermic psoriasis and generalized pustular psoriasis. J Eur Acad Dermatol Venereol. 2015;29:1148–55.
173. Okubo Y, Mabuchi T, Iwatsuki K, Elmaraghy H, Torisu-Itakura H, Morisaki Y, et al. Long-term efficacy and safety of ixekizumab in Japanese patients with erythrodermic or generalized pustular psoriasis: subgroup analyses of an open-label, phase 3 study (UNCOVER-J). J Eur Acad Dermatol Venereol. 2019;33:325–32.
174. Morita A, Okubo Y, Morisaki Y, Torisu-Itakura H, Umezawa Y. Ixekizumab 80 mg every 2 weeks treatment beyond week 12 for Japanese patients with generalized pustular psoriasis and Erythrodermic psoriasis. Dermatol Ther (Heidelb). 2022;12:481–94.
175. Avallone G, Cariti C, Dapavo P, Ortoncelli M, Conforto L, Mastorino L, et al. Real-life comparison between secukinumab and ixekizumab in the treatment of pustular and erythrodermic psoriasis. J Eur Acad Dermatol Venereol. 2022;36:e574–6.
176. Lo Y, Tsai TF. Clinical experience of ixekizumab in the treatment of patients with history of chronic erythrodermic psoriasis who failed secukinumab: a case series. Br J Dermatol. 2019;181:1106–7.

177. Liu L, Lu J, Allan BW, Tang Y, Tetreault J, Chow CK, et al. Generation and characterization of ixekizumab, a humanized monoclonal antibody that neutralizes interleukin-17A. J Inflamm Res. 2016;9:39–50.
178. Megna M, Gallo L, Balato N, Balato A. A case of erythrodermic psoriasis successfully treated with ixekizumab. Dermatol Ther. 2019;32:e12825.
179. Trovato E, Orsini C, Russo F, Cortonesi G, Rubegni P. Ixekizumab as treatment of erythrodermic psoriasis. Dermatol Ther. 2021;34:e14868.
180. Potter KA, Motaparthi K, Schoch JJ. Erythrodermic psoriasis after discontinuation of ixekizumab. JAAD Case Rep. 2017;4:22–3.
181. De Vlam K, Gottlieb AB, Mease PJ. Current concepts in psoriatic arthritis: pathogenesis and management. Acta Derm Venereol. 2014;94:627–34.
182. Jandus C, Bioley G, Rivals JP, Dudler J, Speiser D, Romero P. Increased numbers of circulating polyfunctional Th17 memory cells in patients with seronegative spondylarthritides. Arthritis Rheum. 2008;58:2307–17.
183. Raychaudhuri SP. Role of IL-17 in psoriasis and psoriatic arthritis. Clin Rev Allergy Immunol. 2013;44:183–93.
184. Menon B, Gullick NJ, Walter GJ, Rajasekhar M, Garrood T, Evans HG, et al. Interleukin-17+ CD8+ T cells are enriched in the joints of patients with psoriatic arthritis and correlate with disease activity and joint damage progression. Arthritis Rheumatol. 2014;66:1272–81.
185. Mease PJ, van der Heijde D, Ritchlin CT, Okada M, Cuchacovich RS, Shuler C, et al. Ixekizumab, an interleukin-17A specific monoclonal antibody, for the treatment of biologic-naive patients with active psoriatic arthritis: results from the 24-week randomised, double-blind, placebo-controlled and active (adalimumab)-controlled period of the phase III trial SPIRIT-P1. Ann Rheum Dis. 2017;76:79–87.
186. Mease PJ, Smolen JS, Behrens F, Nash P, Leage SL, Li L, et al. A head-to-head comparison of the efficacy and safety of ixekizumab and adalimumab in biological-naïve patients with active psoriatic arthritis: 24-week results of a randomised, open-label, blinded-assessor trial. Ann Rheum Dis. 2020;79:123–31.
187. Nguyen TV, Damiani G, Orenstein LA, Hamzavi I, Jemec GB. Hidradenitis suppurativa: an update on epidemiology, phenotypes, diagnosis, pathogenesis, comorbidities and quality of life. J Eur Acad Dermatol Venereol. 2021;35:50–61.
188. Rosales Santillan M, Morss PC, Porter ML, Kimball AB. Biologic therapies for the treatment of hidradenitis suppurativa. Expert Opin Biol Ther. 2020;20:621–33.
189. Del Duca E, Morelli P, Bennardo L, Di Raimondo C, Nisticò SP. Cytokine pathways and investigational target therapies in hidradenitis suppurativa. Int J Mol Sci. 2020;21:8436.
190. Fletcher JM, Moran B, Petrasca A, Smith CM. IL-17 in inflammatory skin diseases psoriasis and hidradenitis suppurativa. Clin Exp Immunol. 2020;201:121–34.
191. Lima AL, Karl I, Giner T, Poppe H, Schmidt M, Presser D, et al. Keratinocytes and neutrophils are important sources of proinflammatory molecules in hidradenitis suppurativa. Br J Dermatol. 2016;174:514–21.
192. Korn T, Betteli E, Oukka M, Kuchroo VK. IL-17 and Th17 cells. Annu Rev Immunol. 2009;27:485–517.
193. Di Padova F, Ryffel B, Quesniaux V. Central role of Th17 cells in adaptive immune responses. In: Quesniaux V, Ryffel B, Padova F, editors. IL-17, IL-22 and their producing cells: role in inflammation and autoimmunity. 2nd ed. Basel: Springer Basel; 2013. p. 71–89.
194. Moran B, Sweeney CM, Hughes R, Malara A, Kirthi S, Tobin AM, et al. Hidradenitis suppurativa is characterized by dysregulation of the Th17: Treg cell axis, which is corrected by anti-TNF therapy. J Invest Dermatol. 2017;137:2389–95.
195. Hotz C, Boniotto M, Guguin A, Surenaud M, Jean-Louis F, Tisserand P, Ortonne N, Hersant B, Bosc R, Poli F, Bonnabau H. Intrinsic defect in keratinocyte function leads to inflammation in hidradenitis suppurativa. J Invest Dermatol. 2016;136:1768–80.
196. Megna M, Ruggiero A, Di Guida A, Patrì A, Fabbrocini G, Marasca C. Ixekizumab: an efficacious treatment for both psoriasis and hidradenitis suppurativa. Dermatol Ther. 2020;33:e13756.

197. Reardon K, Levin J, Levin C. Severe hidradenitis suppurativa with herpes simplex virus 1 superinfection and clinical responsiveness to ixekizumab. JAAD Case Rep. 2021;9:7–8.
198. Esme P, Botsali A, Akoglu G, Caliskan E. An anti-interleukin-17A monoclonal antibody, ixekizumab, in the treatment of resistant hidradenitis suppurativa: a case series. Skin Appendage Disord. 2022;8:342–5.
199. Gul MI, Singam V, Hanson C, Neill BC, Aires DJ, Rajpara AN. Remission of refractory PASH syndrome using ixekizumab and doxycycline. J Drugs Dermatol. 2020;19:1123.
200. Maronese CA, Pimentel MA, Li MM, Genovese G, Ortega-Loayza AG, Marzano AV. Pyoderma gangrenosum: an updated literature review on established and emerging pharmacological treatments. Am J Clin Dermatol. 2022;23:615–34.
201. Kao AS, King AD, Bardhi R, Daveluy S. Targeted therapy with ixekizumab in pyoderma gangrenosum: a case series and a literature overview. JAAD Case Rep. 2023;37:49–53.
202. Alavi A, French LE, Davis MD, Brassard A, Kirsner RS. Pyoderma gangrenosum: an update on pathophysiology, diagnosis and treatment. Am J Clin Dermatol. 2017;18:355–72.
203. Antiga E, Volpi W, Verdelli A, Venegoni L, Quaglino P, Fabbri P, et al. The Treg/Th17 cell ratio is reduced in the skin lesions of patients with pyoderma gangrenosum. Br J Dermatol. 2015;173:275–8.
204. Pollack IR, Wolner ZJ, Hammett J, Swerlick RA. Pyoderma gangrenosum in a patient on ixekizumab. JAAD Case Rep. 2021;16:152–4.
205. Sperling LC, Nguyen JV. Commentary: treatment of lichen planopilaris: some progress, but a long way to go. J Am Acad Dermatol. 2010;62:398–401.
206. Ahmed H, Petkar M, Steinhoff M. Successful treatment of rare linear lichen planopilaris with Ixekizumab. J Dermatol Treat. 2023;34:2201364.
207. Chastagner M, Hoelt P, Kanitakis J, Jullien D, Villani AP. Successful treatment of TNFα inhibitor-resistant pityriasis rubra pilaris with ixekizumab and acitretin. Eur J Dermatol. 2019;29:218–20.
208. Liu YT, Wang SS. Ixekizumab successfully treated severe pityriasis rubra pilaris after COVID-19 vaccination. Skin Health Dis. 2022;3:e139.
209. Hanfstingl K, Pekar-Lukacs A, Motz R, Guenova E, Hoetzenecker W. Successful treatment of Pityriasis Rubra pilaris with Ixekizumab. Case Rep Dermatol. 2018;10:97–100.
210. Heibel MD, Heibel HD. Successful treatment of type I pityriasis rubra pilaris with ixekizumab. JAAD Case Rep. 2018;4:774–6.
211. Haynes D, Strunck JL, Topham CA, Ortega-Loayza AG, Kent G, Cassidy PB, et al. Evaluation of ixekizumab treatment for patients with pityriasis rubra pilaris: a single-arm trial. JAMA Dermatol. 2020;156:668–75.
212. Kridin K, Ludwig RJ, Schonmann Y, Damiani G, Cohen AD. The bidirectional association between bullous pemphigoid and psoriasis: a population-based cohort study. Front Med. 2020;7:511.
213. Glinski W, Jarzabek-Chorzelska M, Kuligowski M, Pierozynska-Dubowska M, Glinska-Ferenz M, Jabłonska S. Basement membrane zone as a target for human neutrophil elastase in psoriasis. Arch Dermatol Res. 1990;282:506–11.
214. Chan LS, Vanderlugt CJ, Hashimoto T, Nishikawa T, Zone JJ, Black MM, et al. Epitope spreading: lessons from autoimmune skin diseases. J Invest Dermatol. 1998;110:103–9.
215. Le Jan S, Plée J, Vallerand D, Dupont A, Delanez E, Durlach A, et al. Innate immune cell-produced IL-17 sustains inflammation in bullous pemphigoid. J Invest Dermatol. 2014;134:2908–17.
216. Plée J, Le Jan S, Giustiniani J, Barbe C, Joly P, Bedane C, et al. Integrating longitudinal serum IL-17 and IL-23 follow-up, along with autoantibodies variation, contributes to predict bullous pemphigoid outcome. Sci Rep. 2015;5:18001.
217. Chakievska L, Holtsche MM, Künstner A, Goletz S, Petersen BS, Thaci D, et al. IL-17A is functionally relevant and a potential therapeutic target in bullous pemphigoid. J Autoimmun. 2019;96:104–12.
218. Xiao Y, Gu Y, Xia D, Zhou X, Li W. Ixekizumab successfully treated refractory psoriasis concurrent bullous pemphigoid. J Dermatol. 2023;50:e76–8.

219. Lu L, Yu Y, Zhang J, Fan X, Qi Y, Lin B. Incidental amelioration of bullous pemphigoid during ixekizumab treatment for psoriasis. J Dermatol. 2022;49:e13–5.
220. Strober B, Leonardi C, Papp KA, Mrowietz U, Ohtsuki M, Bissonnette R, et al. Short-and long-term safety outcomes with ixekizumab from 7 clinical trials in psoriasis: etanercept comparisons and integrated data. J Am Acad Dermatol. 2017;76:432–40.
221. Guenther JS, Ahronowitz I, Worswick S. Kaposi's Varicelliform eruption after treatment with Ixekizumab in a patient with Pityriasis Rubra pilaris. Cureus. 2023;15:e38395.
222. Egeberg A, Iversen L, Kimball AB, Kelly S, Grace E, Patel H, et al. Pregnancy outcomes in patients with psoriasis, psoriatic arthritis, or axial spondyloarthritis receiving ixekizumab. J Dermatol Treat. 2022;33:2503–9.
223. Prabhu SS, Suvarna P. Biological agents in pregnancy and lactation–a rational approach. J Skin Sex Transm Dis. 2019;1:54–60.
224. Drugs and lactation database (LactMed®) [internet]. Bethesda (MD): National Institute of Child Health and Human Development; 2006. Ixekizumab. [Updated 2023 Nov 15]. Available from: https://www.ncbi.nlm.nih.gov/books/NBK500805/
225. Megna M, Cinelli E, Balato A, Gallo L, Fabbrocini G. Efficacy and safety of ixekizumab in a group of 16 elderly patients with psoriasis over a 1-year period. Journal of the Eur Acad Dermatol Venereol. 2020;34:e152–3.
226. US Food and Drug Administration. TALTZ (ixekizumab) injection, for subcutaneous use. Highlights of prescribing information. 2016. https://www.pharma.us.novartis.com/sites/www.pharma.us.novartis.com/files/cosentyx.pdf. Accessed 7 Jan 2020.
227. Armanious M, Vender R. A review of drug-drug interactions for biologic drugs used in the treatment of psoriasis. J Cutan Med Surg. 2021;25:38–44.
228. Armstrong A, Fried R, Koo J, Gottlieb A, Jackson A. Mechanism of action of brodalumab may correlate with efficacy in patients with inflammatory skin diseases. J Drugs Dermatol. 2023;22:994–1000.
229. Valeant Pharmaceuticals North America LLC. SILIQ (brodalumab) injection, for subcutaneous use: prescribing information. Bridgewater (NJ): Valeant Pharmaceuticals North America LLC; 2017. Available from: https://www.accessdata.fda.gov/drugsatfda_docs/label/2017/761032lbl.pdf
230. Baliwag J, Barnes DH, Johnston A. Cytokines in psoriasis. Cytokine. 2015;73:342–50.
231. Kim J, Krueger JG. The immunopathogenesis of psoriasis. Dermatol Clin. 2015;33:13–23.
232. Nestle FO, Kaplan DH, Barker J. Psoriasis. N Engl J Med. 2009;361:496–509.
233. Miossec P, Korn T, Kuchroo VK. Interleukin-17 and type 17 helper T cells. N Engl J Med. 2009;361:888–98.
234. Pène J, Chevalier S, Preisser L, Vénéreau E, Guilleux MH, Ghannam S, et al. Chronically inflamed human tissues are infiltrated by highly differentiated Th17 lymphocytes. J Immunol. 2008;180:7423–30.
235. Gaffen SL. Structure and signalling in the IL-17 receptor family. Nat Rev Immunol. 2009;9:556–67. Erratum in: Nat Rev Immunol. 2009;9:747.
236. Kirkham BW, Kavanaugh A, Reich K. Interleukin-17A: a unique pathway in immune-mediated diseases: psoriasis, psoriatic arthritis and rheumatoid arthritis. Immunology. 2014;141:133–42.
237. Gooderham M, Posso-De Los Rios CJ, Rubio-Gomez GA, Papp K. Interleukin-17 (IL-17) inhibitors in the treatment of plaque psoriasis: a review. Skin Therapy Lett. 2015;20:1–5.
238. Silfvast-Kaiser A, Paek SY, Menter A. Anti-IL17 therapies for psoriasis. Expert Opin Biol Ther. 2019;19:45–54.
239. Girolomoni G, Mrowietz U, Paul C. Psoriasis: rationale for targeting interleukin-17. Br J Dermatol. 2012;167:717–24.
240. Senra L, Mylonas A, Kavanagh RD, Fallon PG, Conrad C, Borowczyk-Michalowska J, et al. IL-17E (IL-25) enhances innate immune responses during skin inflammation. J Invest Dermatol. 2019;139:1732–1742.e17.
241. Green L, Weinberg JM, Menter A, Soung J, Lain E, Jacobson A. Clinical and molecular effects of Interleukin-17 pathway blockade in psoriasis. J Drugs Dermatol. 2020;19:138–43.

242. Pinter A, Bonnekoh B, Hadshiew IM, Zimmer S. Brodalumab for the treatment of moderate-to-severe psoriasis: case series and literature review. Clin Cosmet Investig Dermatol. 2019;12:509–17.
243. Russell CB, Rand H, Bigler J, Kerkof K, Timour M, Bautista E, et al. Gene expression profiles normalized in psoriatic skin by treatment with brodalumab, a human anti-IL-17 receptor monoclonal antibody. J Immunol. 2014;192:3828–36.
244. Papp KA, Reid C, Foley P, Sinclair R, Salinger DH, Williams G, et al. Anti-IL-17 receptor antibody AMG 827 leads to rapid clinical response in subjects with moderate to severe psoriasis: results from a phase I, randomized, placebo-controlled trial. J Invest Dermatol. 2012;132:2466–9.
245. Egeberg A, Andersen YM, Halling-Overgaard AS, Alignahi F, Thyssen JP, Burge R, et al. Systematic review on rapidity of onset of action for interleukin-17 and interleukin-23 inhibitors for psoriasis. J Eur Acad Dermatol Venereol. 2020;34:39–46.
246. Papp KA, Lebwohl MG. Onset of action of biologics in patients with moderate-to-severe psoriasis. J Drugs Dermatol. 2018;17:247–50.
247. Blauvelt A, Papp KA, Lebwohl MG, Green LJ, Hsu S, Bhatt V, et al. Rapid onset of action in patients with moderate-to-severe psoriasis treated with brodalumab: a pooled analysis of data from two phase 3 randomized clinical trials (AMAGINE-2 and AMAGINE-3). J Am Acad Dermatol. 2017;77:372–4.
248. Dawn A, Yosipovitch G. Treating itch in psoriasis. Dermatol Nurs. 2006;18:227–33.
249. Stull C, Grossman S, Yosipovitch G. Current and emerging therapies for itch Management in Psoriasis. Am J Clin Dermatol. 2016;17:617–24.
250. Remröd C, Sjöström K, Svensson Å. Pruritus in psoriasis: a study of personality traits, depression and anxiety. Acta Derm Venereol. 2015;95:439–43.
251. Moynes DM, Vanner SJ, Lomax AE. Participation of interleukin 17A in neuroimmune interactions. Brain Behav Immun. 2014;41:1–9.
252. Andersch-Björkman Y, Micu E, Seifert O, Lonne-Rahm SB, Gillstedt M, Osmancevic A. Effects of brodalumab on psoriasis and depressive symptoms in patients with insufficient response to TNF-α inhibitors. J Dermatol. 2023;50:1401–14.
253. Tomalin LE, Russell CB, Garcet S, Ewald DA, Klekotka P, Nirula A, et al. Short-term transcriptional response to IL-17 receptor-a antagonism in the treatment of psoriasis. J Allergy Clin Immunol. 2020;145:922–32.
254. Gargiulo L, Ibba L, Malagoli P, Amoruso F, Argenziano G, Balato A, et al. Brodalumab for the treatment of plaque psoriasis in a real-life setting: a 3 years multicenter retrospective study-IL PSO (Italian landscape psoriasis). Front Med (Lausanne). 2023;10:1196966.
255. Papp K, Menter A, Leonardi C, Soung J, Weiss S, Pillai R, et al. Long-term efficacy and safety of brodalumab in psoriasis through 120 weeks and after withdrawal and retreatment: subgroup analysis of a randomized phase III trial (AMAGINE-1). Br J Dermatol. 2020;183:1037–48.
256. Lebwohl MG, Blauvelt A, Menter A, Papp KA, Guenthner S, Pillai R, et al. Efficacy, safety, and patient-reported outcomes in patients with moderate-to-severe plaque psoriasis treated with Brodalumab for 5 years in a Long-term, open-label, phase II study. Am J Clin Dermatol. 2019;20:863–71.
257. Reich K, Iversen L, Puig L, Lambert J, Mrowietz U, Kaplan Saday K, et al. Long-term efficacy and safety of brodalumab in moderate-to-severe plaque psoriasis: a post hoc pooled analysis of AMAGINE-2 and -3. J Eur Acad Dermatol Venereol. 2022;36:1275–83.
258. Costanzo A, Malara G, Pelucchi C, Fatiga F, Barbera G, Franchi A, et al. Effectiveness end points in real-world studies on biological therapies in psoriasis: systematic review with focus on drug survival. Dermatology. 2018;234:1–12.
259. Caldarola G, Galluzzo M, Bernardini N, Botti E, De Luca E, De Simone C, et al. Long-term effectiveness of Brodalumab for the treatment of moderate-to-severe psoriasis: a real-life multicenter study of up to 3 years in a real-life Italian cohort. Dermatol Pract Concept. 2024;14:e2024152.

260. Elgaard CDB, Iversen L, Hjuler KF. Single-Centre real-world study on drug survival and effectiveness of Brodalumab for treatment of psoriasis and psoriatic arthritis. Drugs R D. 2023;23:155–63.
261. Mastorino L, Dapavo P, Susca S, Cariti C, Siliquini N, Verrone A, et al. Drug survival and clinical effectiveness of secukinumab, ixekizumab, brodalumab, guselkumab, risankizumab, tildrakizumab for psoriasis treatment. J Dtsch Dermatol Ges. 2024;22:34–42.
262. Kojanova M, Hugo J, Velackova B, Cetkovska P, Fialova J, Dolezal T, BIOREP Study Group, et al. Efficacy, safety, and drug survival of patients with psoriasis treated with IL-17 inhibitors - brodalumab, ixekizumab, and secukinumab: real-world data from The Czech Republic BIOREP registry. J Dermatolog Treat. 2022;33:2827–37.
263. Schaeffer L, Ben-Anaya N, Sorbe C, Rustenbach SJ, Mrowietz U, Augustin M. Real-world outcomes and drug survival of brodalumab: results from the German psoriasis registry PsoBest. J Dermatolog Treat. 2024;35:2340107.
264. No DJ, Inkeles MS, Amin M, Wu JJ. Drug survival of biologic treatments in psoriasis: a systematic review. J Dermatolog Treat. 2018;29:460–6.
265. Sawyer L, Fotheringham I, Wright E, Yasmeen N, Gibbons C, Holmen MA. The comparative efficacy of brodalumab in patients with moderate-to-severe psoriasis: a systematic literature review and network meta-analysis. J Dermatolog Treat. 2018;29:557–68.
266. Lebwohl M, Strober B, Menter A, Gordon K, Weglowska J, Puig L, et al. Phase 3 studies comparing brodalumab with ustekinumab in psoriasis. N Engl J Med. 2015;373:1318–28.
267. Farahnik B, Beroukhim K, Nakamura M, Abrouk M, Zhu TH, Singh R, et al. Anti-IL-17 agents for psoriasis: a review of phase III data. J Drugs Dermatol. 2016;15:311–6.
268. Garber K. Anti-IL-17 mAbs herald new options in psoriasis. Nat Biotechnol. 2012;30:475–7.
269. Menter A, Armstrong A, Van Voorhees A, Liu C, Jacobson A. Brodalumab to the rescue: efficacy and safety of Brodalumab in patients with psoriasis and prior exposure or inadequate response to biologics. Dermatol Ther (Heidelb). 2020;10:615–21.
270. Loft N, Bregnhøj A, Fage S, Nielsen CH, Enevold C, Zachariae C, et al. Effectiveness of brodalumab after previous treatment failure of interleukin-17A inhibitors in patients with psoriasis. Dermatol Ther. 2021;34:e15106.
271. Galluzzo M, Caldarola G, De Simone C, Bernardini N, Moretta G, Pallotta S, et al. Use of brodalumab for the treatment of chronic plaque psoriasis: a one-year real-life study in the Lazio region, Italy. Expert Opin Biol Ther. 2021;21:1299–310.
272. Costa L, Perricone C, Chimenti MS, Del Puente A, Caso P, Peluso R, et al. Switching between biological treatments in psoriatic arthritis: a review of the evidence. Drugs R D. 2017;17:509–22.
273. Caldarola G, Pirro F, Di Stefani A, Talamonti M, Galluzzo M, D'Adamio S, et al. Clinical and histopathological characterization of eczematous eruptions occurring in course of anti-IL-17 treatment: a case series and review of the literature. Expert Opin Biol Ther. 2020;20:665–72.
274. Langley RG, Armstrong AW, Lebwohl MG, Blauvelt A, Hsu S, Tyring S, et al. Efficacy and safety of brodalumab in patients with psoriasis who had inadequate responses to ustekinumab: subgroup analysis of two randomized phase III trials. Br J Dermatol. 2019;180:306–14.
275. Papp KA, Gordon KB, Langley RG, Lebwohl MG, Gottlieb AB, Rastogi S, et al. Impact of previous biologic use on the efficacy and safety of brodalumab and ustekinumab in patients with moderate-to-severe plaque psoriasis: integrated analysis of the randomized controlled trials AMAGINE-2 and AMAGINE-3. Br J Dermatol. 2018;179:320–8.
276. Hendrix N, Ollendorf DA, Chapman RH, Loos A, Liu S, Kumar V, et al. Cost-effectiveness of targeted pharmacotherapy for moderate to severe plaque psoriasis. J Manag Care Spec Pharm. 2018;24(1):210–1217.
277. Tampouratzi E, Sfaelos K, Talaiporou K, Douvali T, Katsantonis J. Brodalumab seems to recover its therapeutic efficacy after a relatively short "washout" period with anti-TNF agents: a successful pattern for double-switch therapy. Acta Dermatovenerol Croat. 2023;31:48–50.
278. Thomas LW, Lee EB, Wu JJ. Systematic review of anti-drug antibodies of IL-17 inhibitors for psoriasis. J Dermatolog Treat. 2019;30:110–6.

279. Enevold C, Loft N, Bregnhøj A, Zachariae C, Iversen L, Skov L, et al. Circulating Brodalumab levels and therapy outcomes in patients with psoriasis treated with Brodalumab: a case series. JAMA Dermatol. 2022;158:762–9.
280. Timmermann S, Hall A. Population pharmacokinetics of brodalumab in patients with moderate to severe plaque psoriasis. Basic Clin Pharmacol Toxicol. 2019;125:16–25.
281. Mastorino L, Cariti C, Susca S, Boskovic S, Aquino C, Ortoncelli M, et al. Brodalumab efficacy in bio-naïve psoriasis patients: real-life experience of 202 subjects up to 48 weeks. J Dermatolog Treat. 2022;33:3211–3.
282. Neuner P, Urbanski A, Trautinger F, Möller A, Kirnbauer R, Kapp A, et al. Increased IL-6 production by monocytes and keratinocytes in patients with psoriasis. J Invest Dermatol. 1991;97:27–33.
283. Camporeale A, Poli V. IL-6, IL-17 and STAT3: a holy trinity in auto-immunity? Front Biosci (Landmark Ed). 2012;17:2306–26.
284. Chiricozzi A, Raimondo A, Lembo S, Fausti F, Dini V, Costanzo A, et al. Crosstalk between skin inflammation and adipose tissue-derived products: pathogenic evidence linking psoriasis to increased adiposity. Expert Rev Clin Immunol. 2016;12:1299–308.
285. Blair HA. Brodalumab: a review in moderate to severe plaque psoriasis. Drugs. 2018;78:495–504.
286. Sermsaksasithorn P, Wongtada C, Chaaim V, Chongpison Y, Asawanonda P. On and off-label uses of interleukin-17 inhibitors for patients with plaque-type psoriasis in Thailand: a real-world study. J Dermatolog Treat. 2022;33:2963–74.
287. Blakely K, Gooderham M. Management of scalp psoriasis: current perspectives. Psoriasis (Auckl). 2016;6:33–40.
288. Aldredge LM, Higham RC. Manifestations and management of difficult-to-treat psoriasis. J Dermatol Nurses Assoc. 2018;10:189–97.
289. Sarma N. Evidence and suggested therapeutic approach in psoriasis of difficult-to-treat areas: palmoplantar psoriasis, nail psoriasis, scalp psoriasis, and intertriginous psoriasis. Indian J Dermatol. 2017;62:113–22.
290. Elewski B, Rich P, Lain E, Soung J, Lewitt GM, Jacobson A. Efficacy of brodalumab in the treatment of scalp and nail psoriasis: results from three phase 3 trials. J Dermatolog Treat. 2022;33:261–5.
291. Nakagawa H, Niiro H, Ootaki K, Japanese Brodalumab Study Group. Brodalumab, a human anti-interleukin-17-receptor antibody in the treatment of Japanese patients with moderate-to-severe plaque psoriasis: efficacy and safety results from a phase II randomized controlled study. J Dermatol Sci. 2016;81:44–52.
292. Cacciapuoti S, Potestio L, Guerrasio G, Fabbrocini G, Scalvenzi M, Ruggiero A, et al. Effectiveness of Brodalumab in patients with moderate-to-severe plaque psoriasis located in difficult-to-treat areas. Clin Cosmet Investig Dermatol. 2023;16:2637–44.
293. Sobolewski P, Walecka I, Dopytalska K. Nail involvement in psoriatic arthritis. Reumatologia. 2017;55:131–5.
294. Rigopoulos D, Stathopoulou A, Gregoriou S. Small molecules and biologics in the treatment of nail psoriasis. Skin Appendage Disord. 2020;6:134–41.
295. Reich K, Conrad C, Kristensen LE, Smith SD, Puig L, Rich P, et al. Network meta-analysis comparing the efficacy of biologic treatments for achieving complete resolution of nail psoriasis. J Dermatolog Treat. 2022;33:1652–60.
296. Gregoriou S, Tsiogka A, Tsimpidakis A, Nicolaidou E, Kontochristopoulos G, Rigopoulos D. Treatment of nail psoriasis with brodalumab: an open-label unblinded study. J Eur Acad Dermatol Venereol. 2021;35:e299–301.
297. Guenther L, Potts Bleakman A, Weisman J, Poulin Y, Spelman L, Burge R, et al. Ixekizumab results in persistent clinical improvement in moderate-to-severe genital psoriasis during a 52 week, randomized, placebo-controlled, phase 3 clinical trial. Acta Derm Venereol. 2020;100:adv00006.

298. Merola JF, Ghislain PD, Dauendorffer JN, Potts Bleakman A, Brnabic AJM, Burge R, et al. Ixekizumab improves secondary lesional signs, pain and sexual health in patients with moderate-to-severe genital psoriasis. J Eur Acad Dermatol Venereol. 2020;34:1257–62.
299. Mastorino L, Celoria V, Macagno N, Cariti C, Susca S, Siliquini N, et al. Effectiveness of Brodalumab on scalp, palmoplantar, and genital psoriasis: a descriptive pilot study. Dermatol Ther. 2023;2023:1793535.
300. Politou M, Pompou M, Afroditi KI, Giannoukos A, Nikolaos F. 18501 twenty patients with moderate to severe psoriasis succesfully treated with brodalumab after a failed treatment with secukinumab. J Am Acad Dermatol. 2020;83:AB214.
301. Xing X, Liang Y, Sarkar MK, Wolterink L, Swindell WR, Voorhees JJ, et al. IL-17 responses are the dominant inflammatory signal linking inverse, Erythrodermic, and chronic plaque psoriasis. J Invest Dermatol. 2016;136:2498–501.
302. Bernardini N, Skroza N, Tolino E, Mambrin A, Balduzzi V, Marchesiello A, et al. Recurrent erythrodermic psoriasis and polycythemia successfully treated with brodalumab. Dermatol Ther. 2020;33:e14338.
303. Megna M, Fabbrocini G, Ferrillo M, Cinelli E. Erythrodermic psoriasis successfully and rapidly treated with brodalumab: report of two cases. Dermatol Ther. 2020;33:e14351.
304. Mota F, Mendes-Bastos P. Erythrodermic psoriasis successfully treated with Brodalumab: a case series. Actas Dermosifiliogr. 2023;114:547–9.
305. Yamasaki K, Nakagawa H, Kubo Y, Ootaki K, Japanese Brodalumab Study Group. Efficacy and safety of brodalumab in patients with generalized pustular psoriasis and psoriatic erythroderma: results from a 52-week, open-label study. Br J Dermatol. 2017;176:741–51.
306. Lowes MA, Kikuchi T, Fuentes-Duculan J, Cardinale I, Zaba LC, Haider AS, et al. Psoriasis vulgaris lesions contain discrete populations of Th1 and Th17 T cells. J Invest Dermatol. 2008;128:1207–11.
307. Yilmaz SB, Cicek N, Coskun M, Yegin O, Alpsoy E. Serum and tissue levels of IL-17 in different clinical subtypes of psoriasis. Arch Dermatol Res. 2012;304:465–9.
308. Bissonnette R, Nigen S, Langley RG, Lynde CW, Tan J, Fuentes-Duculan J, et al. Increased expression of IL-17A and limited involvement of IL-23 in patients with palmo-plantar (PP) pustular psoriasis or PP pustulosis; results from a randomised controlled trial. J Eur Acad Dermatol Venereol. 2014;28:1298–305.
309. Cai Y, Xue F, Quan C, Qu M, Liu N, Zhang Y, et al. A critical role of the IL-1β-IL-1R signaling pathway in skin inflammation and psoriasis pathogenesis. J Invest Dermatol. 2019;139:146–56.
310. Teraki Y, Tanaka S, Hitomi K, Izaki S. A case of generalized psoriasiform and pustular eruption induced by infliximab: evidence for skin-homing Th17 in the pathogenesis. Br J Dermatol. 2010;163:1347–51.
311. Yasukawa S, Dainichi T, Kokuba H, Moroi Y, Urabe K, Hashimoto T, et al. Bullous pemphigoid followed by pustular psoriasis showing Th1, Th2, Treg and Th17 immunological changes. Eur J Dermatol. 2009;19:69–71.
312. Smirnova LM, Vertieva EY, Olisova OY, Anpilogova EM. Outcomes of various types of therapy in patients with treatment-resistant acrodermatitis continua of Hallopeau. Biologics. 2019;13:83–7.
313. Galluzzo M, D'Adamio S, Teoli M, Bianchi L, Talamonti M. Biologic therapy for acrodermatitis continua of Hallopeau: successful treatment with secukinumab and review of the literature. Dermatol Ther. 2019;32:e12899.
314. Bardazzi F, Di Altobrando A, Lacava R. Brodalumab in the treatment of recalcitrant acrodermatitis continua of Hallopeau. Dermatol Ther. 2020;33:e14301.
315. Milani-Nejad N, Kaffenberger J. Treatment of recalcitrant Acrodermatitis continua of Hallopeau with Brodalumab. J Drugs Dermatol. 2019;18:1047.
316. Passante M, Dastoli S, Nisticò SP, Bennardo L, Patruno C. Effectiveness of brodalumab in acrodermatitis continua of Hallopeau: a case report. Dermatol Ther. 2020;33:e13170.

317. Navarini AA, Burden AD, Capon F, Mrowietz U, Puig L, Köks S, ERASPEN Network, et al. European consensus statement on phenotypes of pustular psoriasis. J Eur Acad Dermatol Venereol. 2017;31:1792–9.
318. Griffiths CE, Christophers E, Barker JN, Chalmers RJ, Chimenti S, Krueger GG, et al. A classification of psoriasis vulgaris according to phenotype. Br J Dermatol. 2007;156:258–62.
319. Murakami M, Hagforsen E, Morhenn V, Ishida-Yamamoto A, Iizuka H. Patients with palmoplantar pustulosis have increased IL-17 and IL-22 levels both in the lesion and serum. Exp Dermatol. 2011;20:845–7.
320. Nakao M, Asano Y, Kamata M, Yoshizaki A, Sato S. Successful treatment of palmoplantar pustular psoriasis with brodalumab. Eur J Dermatol. 2018;28:538–9.
321. Takahashi H, Sato K, Takagi A, Iizuka H. Brodalumab-induced palmar pustular eruption and joint swelling accompanied by muscle pains in two cases of psoriasis. J Dermatol. 2018;45:e325–6.
322. Pinter A, Wilsmann-Theis D, Peitsch WK, Mössner R. Interleukin-17 receptor a blockade with brodalumab in palmoplantar pustular psoriasis: report on four cases. J Dermatol. 2019;46:426–30.
323. Mössner R, Pinter A. Paradoxical palmoplantar pustulosis induced by secukinumab and brodalumab: a report of three cases. Eur J Dermatol. 2020;30:177–8.
324. Zrioual S, Ecochard R, Tournadre A, Lenief V, Cazalis MA, Miossec P. Genome-wide comparison between IL-17A- and IL-17F-induced effects in human rheumatoid arthritis synoviocytes. J Immunol. 2009;182:3112–20.
325. Hot A, Miossec P. Effects of interleukin (IL)-17A and IL-17F in human rheumatoid arthritis synoviocytes. Ann Rheum Dis. 2011;70:727–32.
326. Kleinschek MA, Owyang AM, Joyce-Shaikh B, Langrish CL, Chen Y, Gorman DM, et al. IL-25 regulates Th17 function in autoimmune inflammation. J Exp Med. 2007;204:161–70.
327. Miossec P. Update on interleukin-17: a role in the pathogenesis of inflammatory arthritis and implication for clinical practice. RMD Open. 2017;3:e000284.
328. Mease PJ, Genovese MC, Greenwald MW, Ritchlin CT, Beaulieu AD, Deodhar A, et al. Brodalumab, an anti-IL17RA monoclonal antibody, in psoriatic arthritis. N Engl J Med. 2014;370:2295–306.
329. Mease PJ, Helliwell PS, Hjuler KF, Raymond K, McInnes I. Brodalumab in psoriatic arthritis: results from the randomised phase III AMVISION-1 and AMVISION-2 trials. Ann Rheum Dis. 2021;80:185–93.
330. Quesniaux V, Ryffel B, Di Padova F. Central role of Th17 cells in adaptive immune responses. In: Quesniaux V, Ryffel B, Di Padova F, editors. IL-17, IL-22 and their producing cells: role in inflammation and autoimmunity. 2nd ed. Heidelberg/New York/Dordrecht/London: Springer; 2013. p. 71–89.
331. Kashetsky N, Mufti A, Alabdulrazzaq S, Lytvyn Y, Sachdeva M, Rahat A, et al. Treatment outcomes of IL-17 inhibitors in hidradenitis Suppurativa: a systematic review. J Cutan Med Surg. 2022;26:79–86.
332. Ramirez-Carrozzi V, Sambandam A, Luis E, Lin Z, Jeet S, Lesch J, et al. IL-17C regulates the innate immune function of epithelial cells in an autocrine manner. Nat Immunol. 2011;12:1159–66.
333. Frew JW, Navrazhina K, Grand D, Sullivan-Whalen M, Gilleaudeau P, Garcet S, et al. The effect of subcutaneous brodalumab on clinical disease activity in hidradenitis suppurativa: an open-label cohort study. J Am Acad Dermatol. 2020;83:1341–8.
334. Yoshida Y, Oyama N, Iino S, Shimizu C, Hasegawa M. Long-standing refractory hidradenitis suppurativa responded to a brodalumab monotherapy in a patient with psoriasis: a possible involvement of Th17 across the spectrum of both diseases. J Dermatol. 2021;48:916–20.
335. Tampouratzi E, Kanni T, Katsantonis J, Douvali T. Case report: treating a co-existence of hidradenitis suppurativa and psoriasis with different therapeutic approaches. F1000Res. 2019;8:2002.

336. Arenbergerova M, Arenberger P, Marques E, Gkalpakiotis S. Successful treatment of recalcitrant gluteal hidradenitis suppurativa with brodalumab after anti-TNF failure. Int J Dermatol. 2020;59:733–5.
337. Vagnozzi E, Bruni M, Esposito M, Fargnoli MC. Brodalumab for severe hidradenitis suppurativa: a case of clinico-radiologic improvement and literature review. J Dermatolog Treat. 2023;34:2270091.
338. Kearney N, Hughes R, Kirby B. Treatment of hidradenitis suppurativa with brodalumab in biologic treatment failures: experiences from a specialty clinic. Clin Exp Dermatol. 2023;48:790–2.
339. Frew JW, Navrazhina K, Sullivan-Whalen M, Gilleaudeau P, Garcet S, Krueger JG. Weekly administration of brodalumab in hidradenitis suppurativa: an open-label cohort study. Br J Dermatol. 2021;184:350–2.
340. Maronese CA, Pimentel MA, Li MM, Genovese G, Ortega-Loayza AG, Marzano AV. Pyoderma Gangrenosum: an updated literature review on established and emerging pharmacological treatments. Am J Clin Dermatol. 2022;23:615–34.
341. Huang CM, Tsai TF. Use of brodalumab for the treatment of pyoderma gangrenosum: a case report. Dermatol Sin. 2021;39:57–8.
342. Tee MW, Avarbock AB, Ungar J, Frew JW. Rapid resolution of pyoderma gangrenosum with brodalumab therapy. JAAD Case Rep. 2020;6:1167–9.
343. Ahn C, Negus D, Huang W. Pyoderma gangrenosum: a review of pathogenesis and treatment. Expert Rev Clin Immunol. 2018;14:225–33.
344. Lebwohl M, Cather J, Armstrong A, Van Voorhees A, Jacobson A. Recapture rate of Brodalumab in patients with a lapse in treatment. J Drugs Dermatol. 2020;19:384–7.
345. Salvia G, Bevilacqua M, Manzo Margiotta F, Michelucci A, Granieri G, Fidanzi C, et al. Switch from adalimumab to brodalumab as a possible trigger factor for the onset of pyoderma gangrenosum. Australas J Dermatol. 2024;65:e111–3.
346. Aromolo IF, Maronese CA, Moltrasio C, Boggio F, Violetti SA, Avallone G, et al. Genetic findings in a patient with paradoxical pyoderma gangrenosum induced by brodalumab. Clin Exp Dermatol. 2023;48:293–5.
347. Sadik CD, Thieme M, Zillikens D, Terheyden P. First emergence of pyoderma gangraenosum, palmoplantar pustulosis and sacroiliitis in a psoriasis patient associated with switching from secukinumab to brodalumab. J Eur Acad Dermatol Venereol. 2019;33:e406–7.
348. Amat-Samaranch V, Cubiró X, Tubau C, Garcia-Melendo C, Puig L. Response of pityriasis rubra pilaris to brodalumab after primary failure to ustekinumab. Int J Dermatol. 2021;60:e112–4.
349. De Felice C, Graceffa D, Morrone A, Bonifati C. Familial pityriasis rubra pilaris successfully treated with brodalumab. Int J Dermatol. 2020;59:885–7.
350. Khan U, Shihab N, Phelps RG, Lebwohl M. Successful treatment of Pityriasis Rubra pilaris with Brodalumab. SKIN J Cut Med. 2020;4:139–42.
351. De Rosa A, Gambardella A, Licata G, Alfano R, Argenziano G. Successful treatment of Pityriasis rubra pilaris with brodalumab. Australas J Dermatol. 2020;61:e249–51.
352. Lebwohl M, Koo J, Leonardi C, Armstrong A, Rawnsley N, Goehring E, Jacobson A. Brodalumab: 4-year US pharmacovigilance report. J Drugs Dermatol. 2023;22:419–22.
353. Thomaidou E, Ramot Y. Injection site reactions with the use of biological agents. Dermatol Ther. 2019;32:e12817.
354. Ang E, Hadjieconomou S, Kalavala M. Brodalumab-induced subacute cutaneous lupus erythematosus. Clin Exp Dermatol. 2021;46:926–7.
355. Mantovani L, Schenetti C, Montinari E, Pacetti L, Schettini N, Borghi A, et al. A possible case of brodalumab-induced ichthyosis. J Dtsch Dermatol Ges. 2023;21:288–90.
356. Murphy MJ, Cohen JM, Vesely MD, Damsky W. Paradoxical eruptions to targeted therapies in dermatology: a systematic review and analysis. J Am Acad Dermatol. 2022;86:1080–91.
357. Yamaguchi Y, Takatsu N, Ootaki K, Nakagawa H. Long-term safety of brodalumab in Japanese patients with plaque psoriasis: an open-label extension study. J Dermatol. 2020;47:569–77.

358. Lebwohl M, Leonardi C, Armstrong A, Rawnsley N, Alexander B, Goehring E Jr, Kerdel F, Jacobson A. Three-year U.S. pharmacovigilance report of brodalumab. Dermatol Ther. 2021;34:e15105. Erratum in: Dermatol Ther. 2022;35:e15664.
359. Lebwohl MG, Papp KA, Marangell LB, Koo J, Blauvelt A, Gooderham M, et al. Psychiatric adverse events during treatment with brodalumab: analysis of psoriasis clinical trials. J Am Acad Dermatol. 2018;78:81–89.e5.
360. Machado MO, Stergiopoulos V, Maes M, Kurdyak PA, Lin PY, Wang LJ, et al. Depression and anxiety in adults with hidradenitis Suppurativa: a systematic review and meta-analysis. JAMA Dermatol. 2019;155:939–45.
361. Golbari NM, Basehore BM, Zito PM. Brodalumab. [Updated 2023 Aug 8]. In: StatPearls [Internet]. Treasure Island (FL): StatPearls Publishing; 2024 Jan-. Available from: https://www.ncbi.nlm.nih.gov/books/NBK470324/
362. Monks G, Rivera-Oyola R, Lebwohl M. The psoriasis decision tree. J Clin Aesthet Dermatol. 2021;14:14–22.
363. He C, Xue C, Zhu G, Kang P. Efficacy and safety of interleukin-17 inhibitors in the treatment of chronic rheumatic diseases: a combined and updated meta-analysis. J Clin Pharm Ther. 2021;46:895–906.
364. Kaushik SB, Lebwohl MG. Psoriasis: which therapy in which patient: focus on special populations and chronic infection. J Am Acad Dernatol. 2019;80:43–53.
365. Phan C, Beneton N, Delaunay J, Reguiai Z, Boulard C, Fougerousse AC, The Groupe d'Etudes Multicentriques (GEM) RESOPSO, et al. Effectiveness and safety of anti-interleukin-17 therapies in elderly patients with psoriasis. Acta Derm Venereol. 2020;100:adv00316.

IL-23 Antagonists

37

Guselkumab: Introduction

Guselkumab is a humanized monoclonal IgG1 lambda IL-23p19 antibody, and the first in this group to get approval by the US FDA for the treatment of moderate-to-severe chronic plaque psoriasis in adults, who are candidates for systemic therapy/phototherapy [1].

Pharmacokinetics

Following a single 100 mg subcutaneous (SC) injection, guselkumab reaches a C_{max} of 5–12 mcg/ml in approximately 5–6 days. The absolute bioavailability of guselkumab is around 49%, with a mean volume of distribution ranging from 7 to 10 litres, and $t_{1/2}$ of 14.6 days. Metabolism occurs via catabolic pathways into small peptides and amino acids. Elimination occurs via both renal and faecal routes [2, 3].

Mechanism of Action

Guselkumab binds to the p19 subunit of the IL-23 receptor and antagonizes its effects. IL-23 has a key role in a number of diseases, stimulating many inflammatory processes that include:

- Differentiation of naïve T-helper (Th) cells to Th17 cells, responsible for IL-17 production [4].
- Inhibition of differentiation of regulatory T (Treg) cells, thus blocking generation of the anti-inflammatory cytokine IL-10 [5].

A. K. Bubna, *Therapeutics in Dermatology - Essentials for Clinical Practice*, https://doi.org/10.1007/978-981-95-3791-4_37

- Activation of Th17 and Th1 cells with subsequent release of IL-22 and TNFα [6].
- Promotion of differentiation of CD8+ T cells to cytotoxic T cells (Tc17) that along with mast cells and neutrophils further increase IL-17 production when stimulated by IL-23 [7, 8].

Once IL-23 release is blocked, these inflammatory cascades come to a halt, and in this way, guselkumab brings about its therapeutic effects.

Indications

FDA Approved

- Moderate-to-severe chronic plaque psoriasis.
- Psoriatic arthropathy.

Off-Label

- Hidradenitis suppurativa.
- Pyoderma gangrenosum.
- Pityriasis rubra pilaris.
- Lichen planus.
- Stewart-Treves angiosarcoma.

Contraindications

Absolute

- Presence of active infections; more importantly latent or active tuberculosis, hepatitis B and C and HIV.
- Hypersensitivity to guselkumab.

Relative

- PUVA sessions being received.
- Premalignant conditions.
- Demyelinating disease.
- Optic neuritis.
- Multiple sclerosis.
- Pregnancy/lactation.
- Congestive cardiac failure.
- Concurrent use of live vaccines.
- Marked elevated levels of hepatic transaminases.

Clinical Uses

Plaque Psoriasis

IL-23 is a pro-inflammatory cytokine, closely implicated in the pathogenesis of psoriasis. Produced by plasmacytoid dendritic cells, IL-23 triggers a cascade of events bringing about differentiation of naïve T lymphocytes to Th17 lymphocytes that produces IL-17, a potent inflammatory cytokine that stimulates keratinocyte proliferation and induces release of IFNα, IFNβ and cathelicidin that further mediate IL-23 release, ultimately setting up a relentlessly progressive inflammatory cycle [9, 10]. Guselkumab acts against the IL-23p19 subunit of IL-23 receptor and thus prevents IL-23 binding and subsequent progression of inflammation (Fig. 37.1) [11].

Guselkumab is administered subcutaneously with a lower frequency of administration (100 mg at weeks 0 and 4 and then 8 weekly), compared to other biologics, with therapeutic responses persisting over time even after drug discontinuation, thereby demonstrating a long-term efficacy [12].

The reason for this long-term effect of guselkumab is attributed to inhibition of the IL-23p19 subunit that has broader impact on inflammatory cytokines involved in psoriasis. Tissue-resident memory T cells are responsible for the persistence and recurrence of psoriasis, which in turn is sustained in their pathogenic state by localized IL-23 produced by various subtypes of antigen presenting cells. Blocking this pathway therefore enables a durable response and a low incidence of disease recurrence [13, 14].

Additionally, guselkumab has a lower risk of reactivation of tuberculosis and viral hepatitis and is not associated with de novo onset or worsening of

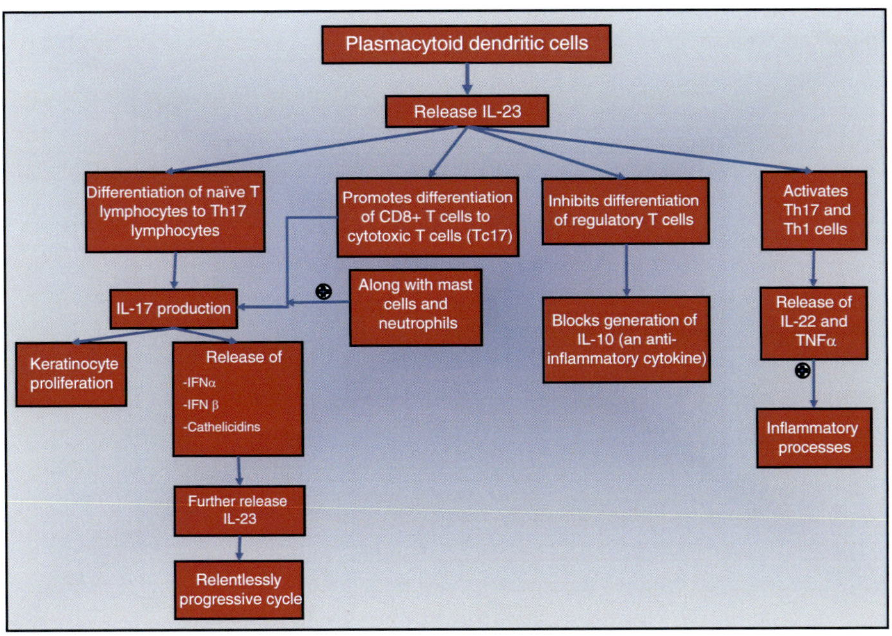

Fig. 37.1 Mechanism of action of guselkumab in psoriasis

inflammatory bowel disease (IBD) in treated patients, making it a safe and effective biologic in these patients [15].

Furthermore, guselkumab demonstrates superiority to adalimumab, ustekinumab and secukinumab, with more consistent responses, in the management of chronic plaque psoriasis [16–18].

Besides, significant benefit with guselkumab is observed in those patients where ustekinumab is ineffective, making guselkumab an ideal switch over drug in such scenarios [17].

In comparison with tildrakizumab, however, no advantage has been observed with guselkumab. Both drugs were equally potent and safe in treating psoriasis patients [19].

Various studies have outlined the efficacy of guselkumab in chronic plaque psoriasis [16–18, 20, 21].

Guttate Psoriasis

Guttate psoriasis (GP) is an uncommon variant of psoriasis, classically associated with an underlying streptococcal infection. However, GP has also been observed de novo with no recent infection [22].

Complete resolution of GP was first described by Hall et al. [22], after a single dose of guselkumab.

Another report illustrated complete remission of sunburn-induced guttate psoriasis following six doses of guselkumab, with cure maintained on drug cessation. The onset of GP in this case was connected to the activation of IL-23/IL-17 by various cytokines and keratinocytes, following sunburn in a genetically predisposed individual [23, 24].

Nail Psoriasis

Nail psoriasis (NP) presents with heterogenous clinical patterns. As the nail unit is closely linked to the extensor tendon fibres and periosteum of the distal phalanx, psoriasis of the nails is often associated with PsA [25].

Owing to the distinctive anatomy of the nail unit, it becomes mandatory for practitioners to have a detailed understanding regarding the therapeutic aspects in relation to NP, in order to obtain better clinical outcomes and an improved quality of life (QoL) [26, 27].

Though often associated with plaque psoriasis, in 5–10% of patients, NP can present as an isolated finding [28].

Guselkumab is effective in NP, with a longer remission period following withdrawal, when compared to cutaneous psoriasis. Besides, it is seen that less severe nail disease (lower baseline Nail Psoriasis Severity Index [NAPSI]) and lower PASI scores at week 16 following treatment are associated with greater probability of near or complete NP clearance (NAPSI 0/1) at weeks 24 and 48, thereby attributing a direct association between skin and nail responsiveness to guselkumab [29].

Additionally, cigarette smoking is associated with a negative impact on treatment response with guselkumab in NP, possibly due to local angiopathic factors, koebnerization and systemic effects of cigarette smoke [30].

Interestingly, no statistically significant association has been observed with guselkumab in relation to Body Mass Index (BMI) and the probability of obtaining NAPSI 0/1. This caries significance because obesity is a common comorbidity in psoriasis patients, and in cutaneous psoriasis, guselkumab has demonstrated PASI 90 to be more likely in patients with BMI < 25 kg/m^2 than in those having a BMI > 30 kg/m^2 [31–33].

Further, NAPSI 0/1 responses at weeks 24 and 48 with guselkumab are not impacted in patients who have previously received TNFα antagonist biologic agents, making it an ideal drug for NP even in bio-experienced individuals [21, 34].

A study from Tokyo delineated a significant reduction in the NAPSI score by 1.2 and 1.5 for patients receiving 50 mg and 100 mg of guselkumab (standard schedule), respectively, compared to a mere 0.2 for the placebo group at week 16. At week 52, the mNAPSI score had further reduced by 2.8 and 2.7 in the 50 mg and 100 mg guselkumab groups respectively [21].

A prospective, non-interventional, multicentre study assessed the utility of guselkumab (100 mg, label dosing) over a 52-week period for moderate-to-severe plaque psoriasis, with NAPSI scoring being included as one of the secondary end points. Among the 303 study subjects, 297 had a NAPSI ≥ 1 at week 0. The mNAPSI decreased from 4.2 at baseline to 1.2 at week 52, and the mean number of affected nails reduced from 6.8 at baseline to 3.3 at week 28 and 2.3 at week 52 [35].

Foley et al. [34] compared the response of guselkumab with adalimumab and placebo from the VOYAGE 1 and 2 trials for psoriasis in specific body regions, including the nails. Of the 1829 randomized patients, 1049 (57.4%) had fingernail psoriasis at baseline among which 928 (50.7%) patients had a fingernail-Physician Global Assessment (f-PGA) score ≥ 2. At week 16, 46.7% of patients receiving guselkumab achieved a f-PGA score of 0 or 1, when compared to 15.2% of patients who received placebo. The f-PGA score of 0 or 1, however, were comparable in guselkumab (60%) and adalimumab (64.3%) treated patients at week 24.

Jo et al. [36] evaluated the efficacy of guselkumab in the Asian population for different variants of psoriasis, including NP, using data from VOYAGE 1 and 2 trials. Guselkumab elaborated greater improvement than placebo in the target NAPSI at week 16 in the Asian subpopulation (mean improvement 35.4% vs 10.8%; $p = 0.021$). However, number of Asian patients obtaining the target NAPSI score of 0 with guselkumab was almost similar to that for placebo (9.1% vs 12%; $p = 0.617$). On comparing guselkumab and adalimumab at week 24, f-PGA scores of 0 or 1 were achieved in 63.6% and 54.8% of patients, respectively, and f-PGA score 0 was seen in 22.7% patients and 16.1% patients, respectively. The improvements in target NAPSI were maintained at week 24 and were comparable to those for adalimumab (mean improvement 39.9% vs 35.9%), with similar proportions of patients in the guselkumab (20%) and adalimumab (21.1%) groups achieving a 100% improvement in the target NAPSI.

Another study demonstrated ixekizumab to be more effective in NP than guselkumab [37].

Currently, with this preliminary data of newer biologic drugs for NP, establishing the drug of choice would not be very practical. More data and dedicated head on comparative trials of these drugs in NP become imperative to establish an evidence-based treatment algorithm for the same.

Palmoplantar Psoriasis (Non-pustular)

Palmoplantar psoriasis (PPP) is a variant of psoriasis characterized by hyperkeratotic and fissured plaques evolving the palms and soles and often recalcitrant to treatment [38].

At present, no gold standard therapy is recognized for PPP, despite the availability of broad and effective biologic treatment options for moderate-to-severe plaque psoriasis.

Moreover, clinical trials for PPP have been challenging because many patients do not meet typical inclusion criteria needed for these trials, owing to the low body surface area (BSA) involvement, often <10% [39].

In a multicentre placebo-controlled trial evaluating the efficacy of guselkumab for PPP, though the primary end point of ppPASI 75 response at 16 weeks (guselkumab 35.9%, placebo 28.2%, $p = 0.533$) was not met, more pronounced numerical improvements favouring guselkumab were seen for more stringent efficacy end points such as ppIGA 0/1 response at week 16 (guselkumab 34.6%, placebo 15.4%) and ppPASI90 response at week 16 (guselkumab 24.4%, placebo 15.4%). Regarding the quality of life, greater proportion of subjects in the guselkumab group reported a DLQI 0/1 score at week 16 compared with the placebo group (19.2% vs 7.7%), respectively. Besides, significant reduction of serum IL-17A, IL-17F and IL-22 was observed at week 16 from baseline in the guselkumab group, but not in those patients receiving placebo [40].

Currently, apart from the above trial, no other publication exists on assessing guselkumab for non-pustular PPP.

More studies are therefore warranted to better understand the impact of guselkumab treatment for this variant of psoriasis.

Palmoplantar Pustulosis

Palmoplantar pustulosis presents as multiple, sterile pustules/vesiculopustules, crusting and erythema involving the palms and soles and is considered a localized variant of pustular psoriasis [41].

The clinical efficacy of SC injections of guselkumab (200 mg at weeks 0 and 4) was assessed for moderate-to-severe palmoplantar pustulosis that had been unresponsive to topical steroids, vitamin D3 analogues, etretinate and phototherapy, in a randomized double-blind placebo-controlled clinical trial. At week 16, there was significant reduction in the mean (SD) Palmoplantar Pustulosis Severity Index (PPSI) total scores from baseline in the guselkumab group (−3.3[2.43]) versus placebo group (−1.8[2.09]). This reduction was maintained at week 24 in the guselkumab group (−3.9[2.47]) versus placebo group (−2.5[2.78]). Regarding biomarkers, notable reduction from baseline in circulating IL-17A levels was observed at weeks 4 and 16 for guselkumab-treated patients, while no remarkable change was noted in the placebo group [42].

In a phase 3 RCT, patients were assigned to receive guselkumab (100 mg) (n = 54), guselkumab (200 mg) (n = 52) or placebo (n = 53) for palmoplantar pustulosis. A significantly higher proportion of patients in the guselkumab (100 mg) group achieved a ppPASI 50 response (57.4%) at week 16, when compared to the guselkumab (200 mg) (36.5%) and placebo (34%) groups. However, the proportions of patients achieving a ppPASI 50 response increased over time, and at week 52, 83.3% of patients in the guselkumab (100 mg) group and 84.6% of patients in the guselkumab (200 mg) group demonstrated this change. Besides, there was remarkable improvement in the DLQI and PGA scores (of cleared and almost cleared) in both guselkumab groups when compared to the placebo group [43].

In another study, guselkumab demonstrated efficacy on palmoplantar pustulosis through week 60 with sustenance of efficacy until week 84, along with considerable improvement in HR-QoL. At week 60, ppPASI 50 was 79.6%, 84.6%, 80% and 80.8% in the guselkumab (100 mg), guselkumab (200 mg), placebo to guselkumab (100 mg) and placebo to guselkumab (200 mg) groups, respectively, which had increased to 88.9%, 95.3%, 85.7% and 87.5%, respectively, at week 84 [44].

The propitious effects of guselkumab in palmoplantar pustulosis is connected to significant reduction of levels of cytokines like IL-17A, IL-17F and IL-22 that are considerably elevated here and correlate with ppPASI disease scores. Guselkumab therapy results in 1.8- to three-fold reduction of these cytokines by week 72, with greater levels of reduction in IL-22 that is crucial in bringing about an overall better ppPASI improvement [45].

Psoriatic Arthropathy

Psoriatic arthropathy (PsA) is a heterogenous inflammatory disorder associated with peripheral joint inflammation, enthesitis, dactylitis, axial disease along with cutaneous and nail involvement along with significant physical and psychologic repercussions.

The IL-23/Th17 axis has shown to be critical in the pathogenesis of PsA (including enthesitis and dactylitis) [46].

A recent report has demonstrated the capability of resident myeloid cells, in producing IL-23 within the enthesis of normal human subjects [47], that in turn permits downstream IL-17A expression and induces IL-22 and TNF release, thereby eliciting articular symptoms and subsequent joint damage. Further, IL-17A has shown to have an equal role in bone remodelling by stimulating osteoclastogenesis and facilitating expression of the receptor activator of nuclear factor κβ ligand (an osteoclast differentiation factor) in osteoclast supporting cells, furthering joint destruction [48].

As IL-23 is involved in the regulation of numerous cytokines in the pathogenesis of PsA, targeting IL-23 individually results in the inhibition of all other cytokines.

Guselkumab, by blocking the IL-23 receptor, prevents generation of inflammatory cascades in PsA. Besides, as it selectively binds to the p19 subunit, it spares IL-12, a cytokine associated with protection from autoimmune inflammation and T-cell exhaustion, giving it an added advantage [49–51].

Various studies have highlighted the utility of guselkumab in the treatment of PsA [52–55].

Hidradenitis Suppurativa

Hidradenitis suppurativa (HS) is a chronic inflammatory condition of hair follicles and can severely affect patients physically and psychologically. The pathogenesis of HS occurs secondary to immune dysregulation, with increased levels of pro-inflammatory cytokines in lesional skin [56]. IL-23 is involved in the differentiation of Th17 cells and thus plays a major role in HS, as both IL-23 and Th17 are elevated in lesional skin of HS, and serum levels of IL-17A produced by Th17 correlate with severity of inflammation in HS [57, 58]. This upregulation supports the rationale for guselkumab in the treatment of HS.

However, in many HS patients, guselkumab has not been effective, suggesting other cells (that are IL-23 independent) to be involved in the pathophysiology of HS [59].

Alternatively, despite the cellular effects of guselkumab on psoriatic lesional tissue, its uptake in lesions/fistulas of HS is generally less efficient that may account for its reduced efficacy in HS [13].

Although positive outcomes of guselkumab have been demonstrated in case reports/series, phase 2 studies have not confirmed this positive trend, suggesting guselkumab to be effective in only a subgroup of HS patients [60–65].

Interestingly, guselkumab has shown to be advantageous in the management of paradoxical HS, as well as HS in patients with paradoxical psoriasiform reactions, following treatment with adalimumab [66–68].

Additionally, guselkumab has been effective in treating HS patients with other comorbidities like Crohn's disease [69–71].

Pyoderma Gangrenosum

Pyoderma gangrenosum (PG) is a rare ulcerative neutrophilic dermatosis, often resistant to various forms of treatment. IL-23, a cytokine implicated in neutrophilic diseases, has shown promise as a potential target in the management of PG. [72]

Additionally, IL-23 plays an essential role in advancing and bolstering Th17 cells, resulting in IL-17 production, that further boosts neutrophilic recruitment, thus setting up a relentlessly progressive inflammatory cycle [73].

Baier and Barak [74] were the first to demonstrate the profitability of guselkumab (100 mg, monthly dosing) in a 60-year-old woman having ulcerative PG that was rapidly progressive with evident tendons, ligaments and muscles on inspection. Prior treatment with adalimumab and infliximab was ineffective, with relapse occurring following an initial favourable response to ustekinumab (linked to the development of neutralizing antibodies). Within 3 months of guselkumab treatment, tremendous improvement of the lesion was evident with 95% reepithelialization.

The use of a modified dose regimen for PG (guselkumab (SC) 200 mg [week 0], 100 mg [week 4], 100 mg [week 10] and 100 mg [week 16]) was described to achieve complete healing of PG in a 49-year-old lady who had been recalcitrant to intralesional steroids, dapsone, systemic prednisolone, Epifix biologic dressings, cyclosporine and adalimumab [75].

In another report, guselkumab (100 mg, SC, label dosing) was highly effective in the management of ulcerative PG in a 78-year-old woman [76].

Pityriasis Rubra Pilaris

Pityriasis rubra pilaris (PRP) is a rare idiopathic papulosquamous disorder characterized by perifollicular keratotic papules that essentially coalesce to form orange-red scaly plaques and palmoplantar keratoderma [77].

The IL-23/Th17 axis is closely involved in the pathogenesis of PRP [78].

By blocking IL-23 release, guselkumab converts Th17 cells to regulatory T cells (Tregs) and eventually modifies the immune disbalance. [79]

Currently, there exist only case reports delineating the utility of guselkumab in PRP [80–82].

Lichen Planus

Lichen planus (LP) is a common, chronic relapsing inflammatory disorder of the skin and mucous membranes which often poses a major therapeutic challenge due to its refractory course.

IL-23 has been expounded as one of the key drivers of pro-inflammatory pathogenic Th17 cells that are increasingly identified in lesions of both mucocutaneous and oral LP [83]. By impelling B lymphocyte-induced maturation protein 1 (BLIMP 1), Th17 cells prompt the pathogenesis in LP, which if not controlled takes on a progressive course [84]. Guselkumab's role in LP is linked to its inhibitory role against IL-23 release with subsequent antagonism of the entire inflammatory cascade [85].

Solimani et al. [86] reported guselkumab (100 mg SC, label dosing) to be highly effective in a 72-year-old female with recalcitrant erosive LP of the tongue for 5 years that had been unresponsive to systemic/topical corticosteroids. Progressive amelioration of lesions was observed following initiation of guselkumab therapy with complete resolution by week 30.

Stewart-Treves Angiosarcoma

Stewart-Treves angiosarcoma (STA) is a rare cutaneous angiosarcoma that has a high rate of metastasis [87].

Immunohistochemical research has propounded IL-23 to have a significant role in tumour angiogenesis via stimulating the Th17 pathway and eventual IL-17 production [88]. Additionally, IL-23 inhibits apoptosis and recruits neutrophils and macrophages to the tumour site, promoting production of other cytokines, including vascular endothelial growth factor that further supports tumour progression [89, 90].

Esbeen and colleagues [91] reported pronounced clinical improvement of STA of the left forearm in an 87-year-old woman following guselkumab (100 mg SC, monthly for 3 months) treatment. After 3 months of therapy, substantial reduction in tumour size and forearm lymphoedema were observed. Also, satellite nodules that were attached to the lesion showed considerable regression. Apart from fatigue and headache, lasting for few days following injection, no other side effects were encountered.

Adverse Effects [92]

Common

Infections

- URTI.
- Gastroenteritis.
- Dermatophytes.
- Herpes simplex.

These are usually mild, not requiring treatment interruption

- Injection site reactions.
- Arthralgia.
- Bronchitis.
- Diarrhoea.
- Gastroenteritis.

Rare

Occurrence of bullous pemphigoid and vitiligo secondary to guselkumab has been described in two individual case reports [93, 94].

The occurrence of these cutaneous adverse effects may be due to the alteration of cytokine pathways resulting in cytokine imbalances responsible for the immunopathogenic mechanism encountered here [95, 96].

Drug Monitoring

Baseline

- Routine blood tests: complete blood counts (CBC), liver function test (LFT), renal function test (RFT), CRP, ESR, serum electrolytes.
- Varicella antibody status should be clarified, and vaccination considered in appropriate patients.
- Screening for tuberculosis: chest X-ray and interferon-gamma release assay.
- Hepatitis B and C and HIV tests.
- Pregnancy test needs to be done in females where pregnancy is a possibility.

Ongoing

- Routine blood tests including CBC, urea, electrolytes, LFTs, CRP and ESR need to be done every 4–6 months.
- Retesting for hepatitis and HIV needs consideration if clinically indicated.
- Patients must be monitored clinically for development of severe infections (including TB), jaundice, malignancy, noninfectious pneumonia, posterior reversible encephalopathy syndrome or serious skin conditions like exfoliative dermatitis. Patients should be encouraged to report any concerning symptoms.
- Clinical monitoring for efficacy should be carried out using disease-specific measuring systems for psoriasis, psoriatic arthritis and inflammatory bowel disease.
- There are experimental data to suggest that monitoring serum drug levels may be beneficial during ustekinumab treatment, but this is not the current standard for care.

Availability, Administration and Dosing

Guselkumab injection is available as single-dose (100 mg/ml) prefilled syringes and as single-dose (100 mg/ml) one-press patient-controlled injectors.

It is dosed as 100 mg SC at weeks 0 and 4 and every 8 weekly.

It appears as a clear and colourless to light yellow solution that may contain small translucent particles. It needs to be stored at 2° to 8 °C, protected from light until use and should not be shaken. It needs to be kept out of the refrigerator 30 min prior to injection.

Injection sites include front of thighs, lower abdomen (except for a 2-inch area around the umbilicus) or back of the arms (if administered by another person) and must not be erythematous, indurated, scaly or affected by psoriasis [92].

Use in Specific Populations

Pregnancy

Based on available data, it is not known if taking guselkumab increases the chance of birth defects. Because guselkumab is an antibody, transfer of the medication to the foetus might be low in early pregnancy, when organogenesis takes place.

Further, currently, it is not known if guselkumab can result in any other pregnancy complications or behavioural and learning issues [97].

Lactation

At present, no information is available on the clinical use of guselkumab during lactation. As guselkumab has a large molecular weight of around 144,000 Da, likelihood of its secretion in breast milk is very low [98].

Besides, guselkumab gets destroyed in the infant's gastrointestinal tract making its absorption unlikely [99].

However, guselkumab still needs to be used with caution in this scenario, especially while nursing neonates. Waiting for at least 2 weeks postpartum to resume treatment may minimize transfer to the infant [100].

Paediatric

To date, there are no clinical trials delineating the efficacy/safety of guselkumab in the paediatric population. Scientific evidence for the same is represented in few case reports wherein patients who were unresponsive to conventional anti-psoriasis treatment and at least one biologic drug achieved almost complete clinical remission with guselkumab without encountering any side effects [101, 102]. Despite insufficient data, guselkumab can be a valuable add-on in the therapeutic armamentarium of paediatric psoriasis.

Geriatric

Currently, data on guselkumab therapy for elderly patients in real-world clinical practice is scant. Nonetheless, available phase III trials have demonstrated it to be effective and safe in elderly patients with no difference from younger patients [103].

Drug Interactions

Vaccines

Currently, no specific data are available regarding guselkumab interaction with simultaneous administration of live vaccines. However, live vaccines are contraindicated when systemic immunosuppressive/immunomodulant therapies are administered [104].

In high-risk situations though, wherein potential risk of infection is considered to outweigh the risk related to administration of live vaccines, vaccination can be considered following an infectious disease consultation. Live vaccines can be given 2–4 weeks prior to initiating therapy or after temporarily halting treatment for 1–3 months, so then an adequate immune response is obtained [104].

On the other hand, non-live vaccines can be given concomitantly while administering guselkumab [104].

Cytochrome P450 Substrates

Upon initiation of guselkumab in patients receiving concomitant cytochrome P 450 (CYP450) substrates, particularly those with a narrow therapeutic index needs careful monitoring with consideration of dose adjustment if required [105].

Conclusion

Guselkumab is a newer agent for the management of psoriasis and PsA. It is also useful in the treatment of HS, PG, PRP and LP. Recently, its utility in STA and its propensity to reduce tumour size can have a promising role in the field of oncology.

Risankizumab: Introduction

Risankizumab is a humanized IgG1 monoclonal antibody that selectively binds to the p19 subunit of interleukin (IL)-23 and restricts its interaction with the IL-23 receptor, thereby arresting downstream IL-23-dependent cell signalling and pro-inflammatory effects [106]. Currently, risankizumab has been approved by the US Food and Drug Administration (FDA) for the treatment of patients with moderate-to-severe chronic plaque psoriasis, who are candidates for systemic therapy/phototherapy, and active psoriatic arthritis (PsA) [107]. Additionally in Japan, risankizumab has been approved for generalized pustular psoriasis (GPP) and erythrodermic psoriasis (EP) [108].

Pharmacokinetics

Risankizumab delineates pharmacokinetic features in tune with typical monoclonal antibodies, with no obvious target-mediated disposition following intravenous (IV) or subcutaneous administration [108]. For dermatologic indications, it is administered subcutaneously (SC) and obtains peak plasma concentrations after 3–14 days of dosing. Bioavailability of risankizumab is 89% and its $t_{1/2}$ is approximately 28 days. Being an IgG monoclonal antibody, risankizumab gets degraded via catabolic pathways into small peptides and amino acids similar to endogenous IgE and is not expected to undergo metabolism by hepatic enzymes or renal elimination [108].

Indications

FDA Approved

- Moderate-to-severe chronic plaque psoriasis.
- Active psoriatic arthropathy.

Off-Label

- Hidradenitis suppurativa (HS).
- Pyoderma gangrenosum (PG).
- Pityriasis rubra pilaris (PRP).
- Alopecia areata (AA).

Clinical Uses

Plaque Psoriasis

Psoriasis is a chronic inflammatory disorder with predominant cutaneous features, along with systemic involvement, affecting 1–3% of the global population, with plaque psoriasis accounting for 90% of the cases [109].

IL-23 is a pro-inflammatory cytokine closely implicated in the pathogenesis of psoriasis. Produced by plasmacytoid dendritic cells, IL-23 drives IL-17 expression, facilitating neutrophilic chemotaxis and uncontrolled proliferation of keratinocytes [110]. Apart from IL-17, other cytokines produced following IL-23 stimulation include IL-6 and TNFα that further sustain the inflammatory cycle [9]. Risankizumab attaches to the p19 subunit of IL-23 receptor, thereby preventing IL-23 binding and subsequent progression of inflammation [11]. Blockade of IL-23 additionally restores regulatory T-cell function, impedes functioning of pathogenic Th17 cells and downregulates tissue resident memory T cells [111].

Risankizumab is dosed at 150 mg (two 75 mg injections) SC at weeks 0 and 4 and then every 12 weekly thereafter. Beneficial effects of risankizumab are evident within 4 weeks of treatment initiation, which is sustained and continuous as treatment progresses [112]. Moreover, the efficacy of risankizumab is maintained between dosages, with no fluctuation in its effectiveness, making the 12 weekly dose interval apt [113]. Additionally, risankizumab enables considerable reduction in itching, burning and redness in psoriasis and helps improve the quality of life (QoL) (as pruritus is frequently reported as the most burdensome symptom in psoriasis) [113, 114].

Clinical trials have demonstrated risankizumab to be superior to adalimumab, ustekinumab, secukinumab and tildrakizumab in plaque psoriasis [113, 115–117], whereas guselkumab delineates synonymous results with regard to clinical outcomes, adverse event frequencies and discontinuation rates when compared to risankizumab [118, 119]. Besides, faster clinical responses are observed with risankizumab when juxtaposed with guselkumab and tildrakizumab, owing to its stronger affinity and higher selective inhibition of the IL-23/17 axis [120]. A close proximity in the onset of action of risankizumab and IL-17 inhibitors is witnessed, with risankizumab scoring above them by having the ability to maintain long-term responses and exhibiting better safety profiles [121]. This facet is attributed to the longer drug survival (DS) associated with risankizumab, unlike the shorter DS that characterize IL-17 blockers, thereby making risankizumab a suitable option for prolonged and effective therapy in psoriasis [122]. Interestingly, DS has been considered a valuable tool to evaluate the therapeutic success of drugs in real-life studies [122].

Furthermore, risankizumab is effective in patients with prior failure to ustekinumab, secukinumab, TNFα blockers, ixekizumab and guselkumab, with no compromise in its efficacy even in patients unresponsive to more than one biologic drug [112, 120, 123, 124]. Despite risankizumab delineating faster responses in bio-naïve patients in reaching PASI90, PASI75 and PASI<3 from week 16 to 40 when compared to bio-experienced patients, these differences eventually fade with almost similar outcomes in both patient groups by week 52, thereby confirming the overall efficacy of risankizumab in both settings [125]. However, in reports by Borroni et al. [126], and Mastorino et al. [127], risankizumab's efficacy delineated reduction in patients who had failed two or more biologics, thereby making contemplation essential prior to the introduction of risankizumab in such scenarios. Also, as biologics are expensive compared to traditional systemic management, a complete cost-effective perspective needs evaluation before considering a biologic shift (as there are a subset of patients who tend to lose responsiveness to biologics) [128, 129].

Therapeutic outcomes in patients with high Body Mass Index (BMI) are mixed concerning risankizumab, with some reports highlighting no significant difference in obtaining PASI90 and 100 responses in overweight and obese patients, and others reporting better clinical outcomes in patients with BMI < 25 [120, 126, 127, 130–133]. In obese individuals who obtained similar clinical outcomes as nonobese patients following risankizumab therapy, it is suggested that despite blood levels of the drug being 30% lower in obese patients, levels reached are within the therapeutic range, occupying an area close to the maximum response in the response curve. Even so, varying conclusions regarding this parameter needs to be kept in mind [126, 127, 133].

Smoking has shown to considerably affect treatment responses with risankizumab, significantly reducing the occurrence of PASI100 responses when compared to nonsmokers [127].

Additionally, risankizumab is effective in ameliorating psoriatic lesions in difficult to treat areas like the scalp, palms/soles and nails, with best responses being observed in the scalp, followed by the palms/soles and then the nails [123, 134].

To date, there are no clinical trials demonstrating the efficacy and safety of risankizumab in the paediatric population. Nevertheless, owing to its high compliance, efficacy and acceptable safety profile, risankizumab can represent a very useful drug for childhood psoriasis [135].

Even in real-life settings, risankizumab has delineated utility [126, 136].

Genital Psoriasis

Genital psoriasis (GP) is commonly encountered in patients with inverse psoriasis and less frequently in those with plaque psoriasis. Occasionally, GP may be the only presentation encountered. In men, glans penis is commonly affected, whereas vulvar involvement is primarily observed in women. Because of genital involvement, problems associated with sexual function potentially impair the QoL in these patients [137]. Current treatment guidelines support systemic therapies for GP when other treatment options fail, even in patients with lower body surface area (BSA) involvement [138].

To date, only ixekizumab has been formally investigated for its efficacy and safety in GP, with promising results [139, 140]. In a head-to-head real-life study comparison with ixekizumab, risankizumab was found to be equally effective in achieving almost clear or clear genital skin both at weeks 16 and 24. Seventy percent and 95% of the risankizumab cohorts achieved sPGA-G 1/0 at weeks 16 and 24, respectively, with 68.8% and 93.8% of ixekizumab subjects achieving sPGA-G 1/0 at weeks 16 and 24, respectively [141].

Erythrodermic Psoriasis

EP is a rare, life-threatening subtype of psoriasis involving 75–90% of the BSA [142]. Recent guidelines advocate the usage of infliximab and ustekinumab as first-line drugs for EP [143, 144].

However, these studies were conducted prior to the approval of risankizumab for moderate-to-severe plaque psoriasis. As Th17 cells are the second predominant cells following Th2 cells in EP, risankizumab can be considered a valid choice for treating EP [145]. Besides, in Japan, risankizumab has received global approval for EP in adults [146]. Improvement is visible after the first injection of risankizumab in EP, and complete resolution of lesions occurs after the third dose. Additionally; pruritus, myalgia and arthralgia associated with EP demonstrate substantial resolution with risankizumab [147].

Palmoplantar Psoriasis

Palmoplantar psoriasis (PPP) describes plaque psoriasis present over the palms and soles. This variant of psoriasis is quite difficult to treat, often causing higher levels of impairment in life quality, along with psychological, physical and occupational repercussions [148]. PPP has been estimated to occur in 10.1–76% in patients with psoriasis, and risankizumab has shown to bring about almost complete clearance of PPP after the second dose (by week 6), with significant improvement in the functional QoL [149–151].

Caldarola et al. [152], in their real-life series, propounded risankizumab to be highly effective in the management of PPP, with an incredible celerity of action. Palmoplantar (pp) PASI90 responses were seen in 18.7%, 62.2%, 75% and 81.2% of patients at weeks 4, 16, 28 and 52, respectively, with ppPASI 100 responses being 12.5%, 56.2%, 68.7% and 75% at the same time points.

In another report, efficacy of risankizumab in PPP recalcitrant to adalimumab was outlined [153].

Nail Psoriasis

Nail psoriasis (NP) is seen in 10–82% of psoriasis patients and is often difficult to treat. In 5–10% of cases, NP can be the only presentation of the disease. NP is often associated with pain, impaired finger mobility/function and loss of manual dexterity [28, 154, 155].

AlAjlan et al. [156] reported risankizumab to be highly effective in a 20-year-old male with NP who had been unresponsive to adalimumab. Within 12 weeks of risankizumab treatment, there was 70% subjective improvement of the affected fingernails.

In another publication, following treatment with risankizumab, complete resolution of NP was observed by week 16, highlighting its rapid onset of action [157].

Further, in a placebo-controlled, double-blind trial, risankizumab treatment resulted in significant improvements of the mean Nail Psoriasis Severity Index (mNAPSI) from 18.1 to 9.8 at baseline and 24 weeks, respectively [158]. Besides, in all reports, the safety profile of risankizumab was acceptable. However, in order to verify these preliminary findings, long-term studies with larger sample sizes are mandated.

Generalized Pustular Psoriasis

GPP is a distinctive variant of psoriasis that is very difficult to treat. As therapy for GPP is often protracted, selection of an effective drug with a favourable toxicity profile becomes mandatory. Gene expression profiling of skin biopsies from GPP have demonstrated higher expression of IL-36α, IL-36γ and IL-1β, with lower expression of IFNγ and IL-17A than plaque psoriasis [159]. Owing to this feature, currently the anti-IL-36 drug spesolimab has been approved by the FDA for its management.

Risankizumab has elucidated rapid and substantial clearance of lesions in GPP. This is linked to its antagonistic property against IL-23, acting at an earlier stage of the inflammatory cascade, interfering with T-cell activation and inhibiting the expression of pro-inflammatory cytokines such as IL-17 [160]. Currently, there exist only case reports that highlight the efficacy of risankizumab in GPP [161–164].

Psoriatic Arthropathy

PsA is a chronic, systemic inflammatory disease characterised by diverse clinical manifestations that include arthritis, enthesitis, dactylitis, axial involvement and skin and/or nail psoriasis [9]. In a randomized double-blind phase 3 trial, risankizumab was found to be safe and effective in treating PsA [165, 166].

Hidradenitis Suppurativa

HS is a debilitating disease of the apocrine glands presenting as painful, recurrent nodules, abscesses, sinus tracts and fistulas typically affecting the axilla, inguinal folds and gluteal/perianal areas [167]. Till date, there exists 1 RCT studying the efficacy and safety of risankizumab in patients with moderate-to-severe HS [168]. In this RCT, 243 patients were enrolled who were divided into 3 groups: group A (n = 82), group B (n = 80) and group C (n = 81) to receive placebo, risankizumab (180 mg) and risankizumab (360 mg), respectively at weeks 0, 1, 2, 4 and 12. The primary end point of this study was the achievement of HS clinical response (HiSCR) at week 16, which however, was not met at the end of the allotted time frame, owing to which the study was terminated early. Besides, in the open-label period of this trial, 77% of the participants discontinued due to the study's premature termination [168]. Remaining available data assessing the efficacy of risankizumab in HS comprise a case series of six patients, a series of two patients, and two case reports [169–172].

It is hypothesized that inflammation in HS is caused by abnormal Notch signalling [173]. These signals induce differentiation of outer hair root sheath cells that are destroyed easily and release keratins, which in turn triggers activation of macrophages via Toll-like receptors. This consequently activates dendritic cells, facilitating release of IL-23 that activates Th17 cells and subsequently disturbs the existent homeostasis between Th17 cells and regulatory T cells (Tregs) [173, 174]. By antagonizing IL-23, risankizumab restores this imbalance and suppresses inflammation.

Pyoderma Gangrenosum

PG is a rare neutrophilic dermatosis presenting as painful ulceration along with pathological abundance of neutrophils, in the absence of infection. PG is often resistant to various forms of treatment. IL-23, a cytokine implicated in neutrophilic diseases, has shown promise as a potential target in the management of PG. [175] Additionally, IL-23 plays an essential role in bolstering Th17 cells, resulting in IL-17 production, that further boosts neutrophilic recruitment, setting up a relentlessly progressive inflammatory cycle [174]. Risankizumab's role in PG is based on its potential to antagonize IL-23.

Burgdorf et al. [175] were the first to demonstrate profitability of risankizumab in a 59-year-old female with PG who had been unresponsive to prednisolone, cyclosporine, methotrexate, azathioprine, infliximab and adalimumab. Following four doses of risankizumab, significant improvement was obtained, despite the discontinuation of other immunosuppressants.

In another report, risankizumab outlined success in the management of PG caused by secukinumab in a 68-year-old patient who had coexistent psoriasis [176].

As there exist only two case reports of risankizumab for PG, the need for RCTs to confirm these observations becomes essential.

Atopic Dermatitis

AD is a common, chronic inflammatory skin disease with varied clinical presentations. Although certain systemic therapies (e.g., dupilumab, upadacitinib) address the needs of some patients with moderate-to-severe AD, there still exists a need for short- and long-term safe and efficacious treatments for AD [177].

A phase 2, multicentre, randomized, double-blind placebo-controlled trial utilizing risankizumab (150 mg and 300 mg dosing) as monotherapy versus placebo in adults and adolescents with moderate-to-severe AD failed to demonstrate a statistically significant reduction of the Eczema Area Severity Index (EASI) over the placebo group at week 16. However though, the average daily Worst Pruritus Numeric rating scale value delineated reduction in both risankizumab (150 mg and 300 mg; 13.6% and 15.2%, respectively) groups by ≥4 points from baseline at week 16 when compared to the placebo group (0%) [178]. Although risankizumab was well tolerated, it failed to outline any therapeutic benefit, making future studies necessary for risankizumab in AD.

Pityriasis Rubra Pilaris

PRP is a disorder of keratinization presenting as generalized papulosquamous pruritic eruptions and palmoplantar keratoderma [179]. Since the role of IL-23-Th17 axis has been identified in PRP, IL-23 blockers have been utilized for this dermatosis [180]. However, results with risankizumab in PRP have been mixed, requiring large-scale studies to confirm its use in PRP [180–183].

Alopecia Areata

Beneficial effects of risankizumab have been described in a 35-year-old man with alopecia universalis who was primarily prescribed risankizumab for psoriasis. Within 4 weeks of treatment, significant improvement of alopecia areata was seen, with replacement of yellow dots by vellus hair on trichoscopy, and reduction of inflammatory cells around hair follicles, and new vellus hairs on reflectance confocal microscopy [184].

Adverse Effects

Most frequent adverse effects with risankizumab reported through clinical trials are upper respiratory tract infections, nasopharyngitis, headache and arthralgia [134, 185, 186].

Potential risks related to risankizumab as per the European Medicines Agency (EMA) include serious infections, major adverse cardiac events (MACEs), malignancies and serious hypersensitivity reactions, varying in incidence from 1.67% to 15% in different reports, with fatal outcomes being reported in 8.2% of cases, as signalled in EudraVigilance [187–189]. Most serious infections related to risankizumab involve the respiratory tract and range from 0.9% to 1% in most studies [166, 190, 191].

According to EMA, caution needs to be exercised while using risankizumab in patients with chronic infections, history of recurrent infections and known risk factors for infections. Moreover, risankizumab therapy should not be started with an existent clinically active infection; commencement of therapy being only after infection resolves or is adequately treated [192]. As IL-23 has a potential role against tuberculosis (TB), risankizumab does carry risk of TB activation [193]. However, in an RCT, despite lack of prophylaxis in a small number of patients with latent TB, no active TB developed following 55 weeks of risankizumab therapy [194]. Interestingly, analogous results were demonstrated in real-world settings [188]. In another report, despite the non-administration of anti-TB prophylaxis in a patient with prior history of properly treated active TB and a current positive QuantiFERON-TB gold test, there was no reactivation of TB after a mean 9.3 months of follow-up, even after initiation of risankizumab therapy [195]. Even so, despite these preliminary findings, the need for a consensus on the usefulness and interpretation of *Mycobacterium tuberculosis* screening in these subset of patients needs to be arrived at.

Malignancies reported following risankizumab treatment include lung cancer, squamous cell carcinoma, prostate cancer, diffuse large B-cell lymphoma and IgA myeloma. Besides, in psoriatic patients, there is increased risk of developing non-melanoma skin cancer (NMSC), particularly in those who have received early systemic therapy or phototherapy, although reasons for this increased risk remain to be determined [196]. In a recent analysis of long-term phase I–III clinical trials though, it was observed that risankizumab's use did not expand the risk of malignancies over that already affiliated with psoriasis pathophysiology. Furthermore, in this study, basal cell carcinoma and squamous cell carcinoma were reported in 23 and 14 patients, respectively, but lymphoma and other hematological malignancies were not detected [197]. Nevertheless, it becomes mandatory to evaluate each patient for the risk of malignancies, both before and during treatment with risankizumab.

MACEs represent another serious adverse event with risankizumab. Besides, an enhanced risk for myocardial infarction, cardiovascular mortality as well as increased risk for stroke has been delineated in patients with psoriasis [198, 199], not only due to the higher prevalence of metabolic syndrome but also secondary to chronic systemic and cutaneous inflammation [200]. It has been observed that MACEs account for 10.9% of serious toxicities with risankizumab, with MI being most important [201]. The reason for MACEs with risankizumab is currently unexplained.

Neurologic side effects like epilepsy, schizophrenia aggravation, polyradiculopathy, polyneuropathy, motor ataxia, obnubilation, depression and motor ataxia, though reported with risankizumab, have not produced alarming signals [202].

Another adverse effect of concern reported is liver cirrhosis [203].

All the same, risankizumab is relatively safe, with incidence of serious events being quite low, and following appropriate monitoring, chances of adverse events can be considerably minimized.

Drug Monitoring

Baseline

- Routine blood tests: complete blood counts (CBC), liver function test (LFT), renal function test (RFT), CRP, ESR, serum electrolytes.
- Varicella antibody status should be clarified, and vaccination considered in appropriate patients.
- Screening for tuberculosis: chest X-ray and interferon-gamma release assay.
- Hepatitis B and C and HIV tests.
- Pregnancy test needs to be done in females where pregnancy is a possibility.

Ongoing

- Routine blood tests including CBC, urea, electrolytes, LFTs, CRP, and ESR need to be done every 4–6 months.
- Retesting for hepatitis and HIV needs consideration if clinically indicated.
- Patients must be monitored clinically for development of severe infections (including TB), jaundice, malignancy, noninfectious pneumonia, posterior reversible encephalopathy syndrome or serious skin conditions like exfoliative dermatitis. Patients should be encouraged to report any concerning symptoms.
- Clinical monitoring for efficacy should be carried out using disease-specific measuring systems for psoriasis, psoriatic arthritis and inflammatory bowel disease.
- There are experimental data to suggest that monitoring serum drug levels may be beneficial during ustekinumab treatment, but this is not the current standard for care.

Availability and Administration

It is available as a colourless to yellow, and clear to slightly opalescent solution, in a prefilled syringe containing 90 mg/ml or 150 mg/ml. Further, it is also available in a prefilled pen containing 150 mg/ml. It needs to be stored at 2° to 8 °C, protected from light until use and should not be shaken. It needs to be kept out of the refrigerator 30 min prior to injection.

Injection sites include front of thighs, lower abdomen (except for a 2-inch area around the umbilicus) or back of the arms (if administered by another person) and must not be erythematous, indurated, scaly or affected by psoriasis. It is administered at weeks 0 and 4 and then every 12 weeks thereafter.

Pregnancy

Based on animal studies, risankizumab does cross the placenta with the possibility of foetal losses and neonatal deaths in monkeys [204]. Currently, limited data exist for the use of risankizumab in psoriasis in pregnant women and is therefore not recommended during pregnancy. Utilizing contraceptive methods during treatment and for a minimum of 21 weeks after its completion is recommended [192]. In a phase 2 open-label extension study wherein the long-term efficacy of risankizumab was assessed for Crohn's disease, three pregnancies were reported of which foetal defects were encountered in one, requiring abortion, with the other two being uneventful [205].

Lactation

Till date, no information is available for the use of risankizumab in lactation. As it has a large molecular weight (146,000 Da), the amount in breast milk is likely to be scant. It is largely destroyed in the infants' gut making absorption unlikely. However, until more data is available, caution needs to be exercised here. Waiting for at least 2 weeks postpartum is essential to minimize transfer to the infant [98, 208, 209].

Paediatric

No clinical trials are available currently for risankizumab's utility/safety in paediatric psoriasis. However, because of its high compliance and safety, it can be considered a useful drug for childhood psoriasis [135].

Geriatric

Clinical trials and real-world studies have demonstrated risankizumab to be safe and effective in the management of psoriasis in patients aged ≥65 years [113, 210].

Future Direction

For off-label dermatologic indications related to risankizumab, more RCTs are needed to strengthen its use further. Besides, the role of other non-biologics in combination with risankizumab to achieve synergistic responses remain an avenue to explore. Another area open for investigation especially in countries like ours is the evaluation of drug efficacy with modified dosing schedules using longer spaced intervals, with the aim of reducing financial burden on patients.

Conclusion

Risankizumab is a newer IL-23 antagonist used for psoriasis and PsA that has demonstrated considerable efficacy and safety for the same. However, currently in India, the associated high cost proves to be a major barrier for its incorporation in regular day-to-day therapeutics.

Tildrakizumab: Introduction

Tildrakizumab is a high-affinity humanized monoclonal IgG kappa IL-23p19 antibody [206]. It is the second IL-23p19inhibitor to be approved by the FDA (in 2018) for the treatment of moderate-to-severe chronic plaque psoriasis in adults (who are candidates for systemic therapy/phototherapy), after guselkumab.

Pharmacokinetics

Following subcutaneous (SC) injection, bioavailability of tildrakizumab is ~73–80%, with a $t_{1/2}$ of approximately 20.2–28.2 days, and a volume of distribution of 10.8 litres. Drug clearance occurs via catabolic pathways after degradation into small peptides and amino acids. Excretion of tildrakizumab is most likely via the renal route [207].

Mechanism of Action

Tildrakizumab's mechanism of action is represented in Fig. 37.2 [208–210].

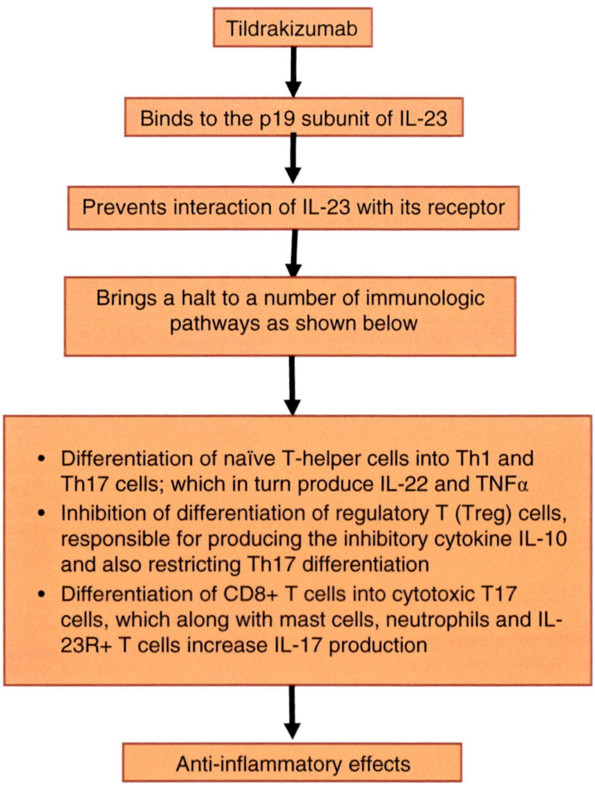

Fig. 37.2 Mechanism of action of tildrakizumab

Indications

FDA Approved

- Moderate to severe plaque psoriasis.

Off-Label

- Psoriatic arthropathy.
- Pyoderma gangrenosum (PG).
- Lichen planus (LP).
- Alopecia areata (AA).
- Pityriasis rubra pilaris (PRP).
- Vitiligo.
- Lupus erythematosus tumidus.

Contraindications

Absolute

- Hypersensitivity to tildrakizumab.

Relative

- PUVA sessions being received.
- Premalignant conditions.
- Optic neuritis.
- Multiple sclerosis.
- Congestive cardiac failure.
- Concurrent use of live vaccines.
- Marked elevated levels of hepatic transaminases.

Clinical Uses: Psoriasis

Plaque Psoriasis

Tildrakizumab's antagonistic effect on IL-23p19 determines its role in the management of psoriasis, aiding rapid clinical benefit along with histologic improvement [211].

Blockade of IL-23 additionally impedes functioning of pathogenic Th17 cells [212], restores Treg cell function [213], hinders production of IL-23 and downregulates tissue resident memory T cells [214].

Moreover, as tildrakizumab minimizes clonal expansion of cutaneous Th17 cells, and inhibits upstream cytokines, its effects are prolonged despite wider spaced dosing schedules when compared to other biologic drugs with clinical responses maintained up to 36 weeks following last administration [215].

Furthermore, tildrakizumab acts against intestinal Th17 cells, thereby protecting against development of obesity and metabolic diseases. Owing to this contribution, tildrakizumab can be considered the biologic of choice in psoriatic patients with metabolic syndrome. Also, it is safe and well tolerated for up to 5 years of treatment, with no apparent dose-related differences in adverse effects [216].

Interestingly, tildrakizumab has a very low incidence of drug discontinuation following untoward effects, with specifically low rates of severe infections and major adverse cardiovascular events (MACEs), no discernible increased risk of malignancies (including non-melanoma skin cancers), even if more data is required to corroborate an absence of association [217]. Besides, even in cases of relapse, tildrakizumab can be reinstituted with no decline in its efficacy and tolerability [218]. These facets can be attributed to an overall higher cumulative probability of drug survival (defined as the duration of time a patient remains under a specific therapy, from the day of first administration to the point in time when treatment is discontinued [219]) for tildrakizumab, owing to its antagonistic effect on tissue resident-memory T cells, and simultaneous ability to maintain levels of regulatory T cells [220, 221]. It is speculated that by direct blockade of the IL-23 pathway, long-term efficacy of tildrakizumab is influenced, along with an increased propensity for drug survival [220]. Nevertheless, more studies become essential to better understand this interplay and the likely overall consequence on disease pathophysiology.

Currently, no direct head-to-head comparative clinical trials evaluating the efficacy/safety of tildrakizumab with IL-17 and other IL-23 antagonists exist, and all inferences are based on data from systematic reviews/network meta-analysis, with the onset of action of tildrakizumab (5.6–5.7 weeks) being slower than brodalumab (2.1–2.6 weeks), ixekizumab (2.2–2.3 weeks), secukinumab (3.0–4.3 weeks) and guselkumab (3.8 weeks), and PASI 75 scores demonstrating tildrakizumab to be superior to ustekinumab but inferior to brodalumab, ixekizumab, secukinumab and risankizumab, along with comparable toxicity profiles [117, 222–224]. However, as the number of studies included for tildrakizumab is low, caution needs to be exercised while interpreting these conclusions.

Various studies have elaborated the utility of tildrakizumab for moderate-to-severe chronic plaque psoriasis [217, 225–227].

Palmoplantar Psoriasis (Non-pustular)

Profitability of tildrakizumab in palmoplantar psoriasis (PPP) was first described by Gambardella et al. [228] in a 35-year-old man with elevated hepatic transaminases and a positive anamnesis for ulcerative colitis. After 8 weeks of administration of tildrakizumab (100 mg SC at weeks 0 and 4 and then every 12 weeks), almost complete clinical response was obtained, which was maintained at 6 months of follow-up.

This was reiterated in two case series of seven patients with PPP. In both reports, the drug was well tolerated, with an impressive celerity of action and a remarkable improvement in symptoms as well as quality of life (QoL) within 12–16 weeks of treatment with tildrakizumab [229, 230].

Palmoplantar Pustulosis

Complete clearance of palmoplantar pustulosis within 3 months of tildrakizumab therapy (100 mg SC at weeks 0 and 4 and every 12 weekly) was observed in a 69-year-old lady who had failed to respond to cyclosporine, apremilast, prednisone, phototherapy and topical steroids. As she was later diagnosed with carcinoma lung, tildrakizumab was stopped, and topical steroids was continued as monotherapy, with no further recurrence of pustular lesions, thereby establishing the long-lasting effects of tildrakizumab [231].

Scalp Psoriasis

Scalp psoriasis (SP) presents as circumscribed, erythematous and scaly plaques commonly advancing beyond the hairline to involve the postauricular region and proximal part of the forehead. Because of its apparent nature, it has a significant impact on the QoL of patients.

A post hoc analysis of reSURFACE 1 studied the favourable profile of tildrakizumab (label dosing) on SP in patients with moderate to severe chronic plaque psoriasis. At 28 weeks, in all patients, the PASI head (PASIh) component scores had tremendously reduced, with 21.5% of patients delineating a PASIh score of 0 [232].

A case series of 6 patients highlighted reduction of the Psoriasis Severity Scalp Index (PSSI) score by 83.4% at week 4, 95% at week 12 and 92.5% at week 28 following treatment with tildrakizumab [229].

Besides, tildrakizumab was well tolerated, without any major adverse reaction [229, 232].

Nail Psoriasis

NP is one of the most difficult-to-treat variants of psoriasis. In 5–10% of cases, it has an isolated manifestation, lacking any form of cutaneous involvement [233]. Besides, nail involvement in psoriasis often portents the onset of PsA, making it essential for clinicians to begin early treatment in all cases of NP so that long-term outcomes can be improved [234].

In terms of data evaluating the efficacy of tildrakizumab in NP, no randomized controlled trials (RCTs) are currently available. Nevertheless, some real-life experiences do suggest tildrakizumab to be a plausible treatment option for the same.

Ismail et al. [235] reported successful outcome with tildrakizumab (label dosing) in a 40-year-old male with NP and PsA that had been recalcitrant to treatment with topical/intralesional steroids and systemic methotrexate.

Simpson and colleagues [236] reiterated the benefit of tildrakizumab in two cases of resistant NP (to conventional anti-psoriasis treatment).

Patient 1 (a 63-year-old female) had isolated NP, predominantly affecting the toenails with a baseline Modified Nail Psoriasis Severity Index (mNAPSI) of 44. Following 6 months of treatment with tildrakizumab, the mNAPSI had come down to 13, and after 12 months, the mNAPSI score became 8 (with a total score reduction of 81.8%). Besides, DLQI improved from 16 (at baseline) to 3 (after 1 year).

The second patient (a 53-year-old male) had NP, SP and PsA. Following tildrakizumab treatment, mNAPSI improved from 56 (baseline) to 7 (after 12 months), and DLQI reduced from 19 to 8 in the given time period.

Similar findings were corroborated in two real-life retrospective studies with tildrakizumab, with the NAPSI score reducing from 48.4 (baseline) to 15.7 (week 28) in one study, and the mNAPSI plummeting by 90% (at week 20 from baseline) in the other [229, 237].

Additionally, in all reports, a good safety profile with tildrakizumab was documented.

However, in order to verify these preliminary findings, long-term studies with larger sample sizes are mandated.

Genital Psoriasis

Genital psoriasis (GP) is commonly encountered in patients with inverse psoriasis and less frequently in those with plaque psoriasis. In some patients, GP may be the only presentation observed. In men, glans penis is the site commonly affected, whereas vulvar involvement is primarily seen in females. Because of involvement of genitals, problems associated with sexual function potentially impair QoL of these patients.

In a series of seven patients with GP, tildrakizumab (label dosing) resulted in almost complete remission after 28 weeks of treatment, with the Static Physician's Global Assessment of Genitalia (SPGA-G) score decreasing by 93.9% and all patients tolerating the drug well [229].

Psoriatic Arthritis

Psoriatic arthritis (PsA) is a disorder in which immune abnormalities strongly characterize its development. Reduction of Treg cells has been distinctly identified in these patients, along with nail fold capillary abnormalities, such as nail fold bleeding and enlarged capillaries, both being cardinal risk factors in determining progression to PsA [238]. Tildrakizumab precisely targets both these facets, helping restoration of the number of Treg cells and amelioration of nail fold capillary abnormalities [238]. Further, it is considered that IL-23 induces osteoclastogenesis and osteoclast-mediated activation of nuclear factor of activated T cells and in this way promotes joint degeneration. By antagonizing IL-23, and the associated kinase signalling system, tildrakizumab circumvents further progression of joint destruction [239, 240].

Buononato et al. [241] reported tildrakizumab to be a valuable therapeutic option in two patients suffering from PsA.

The first patient was a 45-year-old male with a 10-year history of PsA in whom methotrexate and secukinumab could not be continued due to drug toxicity.

In the second patient (a 56-year-old female), PsA had been present for 15 years that was unresponsive to methotrexate, and adalimumab had precipitated cutaneous adverse effects.

In both patients, tildrakizumab (label dosing) helped in controlling PsA without the occurrence of any adverse events.

A study from the United States emphasized the utility of tildrakizumab in PsA employing various dosing schedules. A total of 391 patients were randomized into five groups to receive tildrakizumab.

Group 1: Tildrakizumab 200 mg every 4 weeks (Q4w).
Group 2: Tildrakizumab 200 mg Q12w.
Group 3: Tildrakizumab 100 mg Q12w.
Group 4: Tildrakizumab 20 mg Q12w.
Group 5: Placebo Q4w.

At 24 weeks, the American College of Rheumatology Criteria (ACR) 20 response was witnessed in 79.5%, 77.2%, 71.4%, 73.1% and 50.6% in groups 1, 2, 3, 4 and 5, respectively, and minimal disease activity was observed in 33.3%, 34.2%, 28.6%, 19.2% and 6.3% in groups 1, 2, 3, 4 and 5, respectively. Further, it was seen that improvement in swollen joint count in 66 joints (SJC66) was greater for patients receiving tildrakizumab 200 mg Q4w, but not Q12w, and improvement in tender joint count in 68 joints (TJC68) and Health Assessment Questionnaire-Disability Index (HAQ-DI) was greater for patients receiving tildrakizumab 200 mg Q12w, but not Q4w, relative to placebo-treated patients. Moreover, responses were maintained through week 52, with no deaths being encountered. Serious treatment emergent adverse events (TEAE) were observed in 9 patients, with only one having to discontinue treatment. However, despite improvement of arthritis in these patients, tildrakizumab failed to demonstrate any positive effect regarding dactylitis and enthesitis. Besides, dosing tildrakizumab (200 mg) at Q4w was not consistently superior to the Q12w dosing [242].

Hidradenitis Suppurativa

HS is a chronic and recurrent inflammatory disease of the pilosebaceous follicles in postpubertal individuals, characterized by deep-seated, painful, inflamed lesions involving the apocrine gland-bearing areas. Till date, there exist no clinical trials or large-scale studies for the use of tildrakizumab in HS. On literature search, in two case series and two case reports, the use of tildrakizumab in HS was elaborated [243–246]. Because of overexpression of IL-23 in lesions of HS, as well as increased serum levels of IL-23 in these patients, tildrakizumab is effective in the treatment of HS [247].

Pyoderma Gangrenosum

PG is a rare autoimmune neutrophilic dermatosis, clinically characterized by intensely painful, rapidly growing ulcers, associated with suppuration and undermined irregular edges [248].

Tildrakizumab has been used in PG owing to its antagonistic effects on IL-23 and Th17 cell recruitment, involved in the pathogenesis of PG. However, it needs to be stated that there is no gold standard therapy for PG, and more evidence is needed to establish a standardized approach [249]. Besides, tildrakizumab has a secondary inhibitory effect on staphylococcal biofilm colonies in PG that exacerbate chronic infection, trigger Th1/Th17 responses and have a negative impact on wound healing [250].

John and Sinclair [251] reported complete healing of penile PG with tildrakizumab in a 69-year-old man refractory to treatment with prednisolone and cyclosporine.

Another publication reiterated tildrakizumab to be effective in 85-year-old women with ulcerating PG of the left leg, who did not achieve satisfactory results with cyclosporine and systemic steroids, with dapsone resulting in emergent severe tremors. Tildrakizumab (100 mg) was administered every 8 weekly initially and then every 6 weekly after the initial loading dose at weeks 0 and 4, along with oral antibiotics, pentoxifylline and appropriate wound care. Within 6 months of this regimen, adequate re-epithelialization was noticed [252].

Combination therapy with tildrakizumab and ustekinumab was shown to be effective in a case of recalcitrant PG by Sheriff et al. [253]

In none of the above reports were any untoward events accounted. Based on the above reports, tildrakizumab does have a place in the therapeutic ladder of PG. Nevertheless, more studies are needed to promote this observation.

Alopecia Areata

AA is an autoimmune disease associated with non-scarring alopecia. Recent evidence outlines involvement of IL-23 in the pathogenesis of AA. Also, Janus kinase 2 has been revealed to be an intracellular mediator of IL-23 cell surface receptor binding, thereby allowing cogitation of tildrakizumab in the therapeutic discourse of AA [254, 255].

However, in a pilot study on nine patients with chronic AA (who had failed previous treatments that included oral prednisolone, tofacitinib, azathioprine, contact sensitizers and intralesional steroids), tildrakizumab (label dosing) was only able to demonstrate a partial response in two patients, with no response in the remaining seven patients. Besides, mild toxicities like upper respiratory tract infection and acne were encountered in two patients, with one being a partial responder to tildrakizumab [256].

More RCTs are warranted with tildrakizumab currently for its use in chronic AA.

Vitiligo

Vitiligo is an autoimmune disease associated with cutaneous/mucosal depigmentation. When extensive, it profoundly affects patient QoL. As IL-23 levels have been described to be striking higher in vitiligo patients, it can serve as a potential therapeutic target for the same [257].

The propitious effect of tildrakizumab (label dosing) in a 63-year-old male with rapidly progressive vitiligo was reported by Jerjen et al. [258] Within 16 weeks of therapy initiation, significant subjective and objective improvement was observed that continued with subsequent dosing of tildrakizumab. After 1 year of treatment, 90% re-pigmentation of affected areas was documented and DLQI improved from 9 to 4. Besides, no side effects were encountered.

Despite this finding, there is a small subset of patients who have developed de novo vitiligo following the use of ustekinumab (an IL-12/23 antagonist) for other diseases, and this aspect needs to be kept in mind [259].

Nonetheless, tremendous improvement with tildrakizumab shown in the above report does hold promise in the treatment of generalized vitiligo.

Lupus Erythematosus Tumidus

Lupus erythematosus tumidus (LET) is a rare variant of chronic LE, characterized by non-scarring, erythematous, oedematous plaques in photo-exposed areas. Human and animal studies have shown IL-23 to play a vital role in the pathogenesis of LE, and therefore, IL-23 blockers may be advantageous here [260].

Tildrakizumab (100 mg, label dosing) demonstrated significant improvement in a 39-year-old male with LET following two doses that was unresponsive to methotrexate, hydroxychloroquine and intralesional triamcinolone acetonide. With consequent doses of tildrakizumab, improvement was sustained and convincing, with no adverse effects [261].

Lichen Planus

LP is the most typical and best characterized idiopathic lichenoid dermatosis with diverse clinical manifestations. IL-23 is markedly elevated in LP lesions. Tildrakizumab, by antagonizing IL-23, suppresses Th17/Tc17 cells, and consequently Th1 cells in LP, and facilitates lesional regression [262]. There have been reports on the use of tildrakizumab in oral LP, LP pemphigoids, lichen planopilaris (LPP) and genital LP [263–266].

Although few reports have highlighted tildrakizumab to be effective in LP, more robust, prospective clinical trials are warranted to further substantiate these findings.

Pityriasis Rubra Pilaris

PRP is a papulosquamous disorder, often recalcitrant to conventional therapies.

Licata and colleagues [267] reported tildrakizumab to be effective in a 59-year-old man with PRP in whom acitretin was ineffective, with methotrexate and IL-17 antagonists being contraindicated. Following the third dose of tildrakizumab, complete clinical response was obtained.

Another report demonstrated rapid improvement of erythrodermic PRP in two patients, following treatment with tildrakizumab [268].

The role of IL23/17 axis has been suggested in the pathogenesis of PRP, and this could possibly be the reason for the efficacy of tildrakizumab in PRP [269].

Adverse Effects

Common reactions include nasopharyngitis, upper respiratory tract infection, headache, infection site reaction and fatigue [270, 271].

A rare though serious complication of tildrakizumab is upper airway obstruction. [271]

Drug Monitoring [270]

Baseline

- Complete blood count/hemogram.
- Erythrocyte sedimentation rate.
- C-reactive protein.

- Liver function test.
- Renal function test.
- Serum electrolytes.
- Screening for hepatitis and human immunodeficiency virus.
- Chest X-ray.
- Tuberculin skin testing or QuantiFERON gold test.
- Pregnancy test in females of childbearing age.
- Serology for varicella zoster and measles (if clinically indicated).
- Urinalysis.

Ongoing Monitoring

- Evaluation of response to treatment is measurable by respective assessment scores, that is, PASI and DLQI at 3 months initially and subsequently every 6 months.
- A complete blood count and hemogram needs to be repeated at 3 months and then every 6 months.
- Liver and renal function tests, electrolytes and urinalysis need similar evaluation.

Use in Specific Populations

Pregnancy

Limited available data with tildrakizumab use in pregnant women are insufficient to inform its risk related to development outcomes in babies. As human IgG is known to cross the placental barrier, tildrakizumab may be transferred from the mother to foetus [270].

A report of 14 human pregnancies exposed to tildrakizumab did not find birth defects. Besides, animal studies also did not reveal an increase in birth defects with exposure to tildrakizumab [272].

Nevertheless, pregnant patients should use contraceptive measures when treated with tildrakizumab, until more data becomes available [273].

Lactation

Tildrakizumab has not been studied during breastfeeding. Tildrakizumab is a very large protein (molecular weight of 147,000 Da), so not very much of it is expected to pass into breast milk.

Furthermore, as tildrakizumab is likely to get partially destroyed in the infant's gastrointestinal tract, absorption by the infant is probably minimal. Some professional guidelines state that the drug can be used during lactation [274].

Until more data is available, tildrakizumab should be cautiously used during lactation. Waiting for at least 2 weeks postpartum to resume therapy may minimize chances of transfer to the infant [100].

Paediatric Use

Currently, the safety and effectiveness of tildrakizumab in paediatric patients (<18 years of age) have not been established [272].

Geriatric Use

Tildrakizumab has been associated with long-term control of psoriasis, with a favourable safety profile in patients more than 65 years of age, even in those with associated comorbidities and co-medications [275]. However, more confirmatory studies are desirable to better understand the profile of tildrakizumab in this population.

Drug Interactions

Live Vaccines

Use of live vaccines needs to be avoided in patients getting treatment with tildrakizumab [270].

Cytochrome (CY) P450 Substrates

Tildrakizumab does not have a discernible effect on CYP metabolism in patients with psoriasis. However, in rheumatoid arthritis, potential drug-drug interactions may occur owing to the much greater extent of systemic inflammation in rheumatoid arthritis when compared to psoriasis [276].

Availability and Administration

Tildrakizumab is available as prefilled, single-dose 1 ml syringes, containing 100 mg of the drug for SC administration. It should only be administered by a healthcare provider. Schedule of administration is at 0, 4 and then every 12 weeks.

If a dose is missed, the next dose needs to be given as soon as possible.

Before injection, the prefilled syringe needs to be removed from the refrigerator (non-freezer compartment) and kept at room temperature for 30 min. The needle cover should not be pulled off until ready for injection.

Also, the syringe needs to be inspected for any particulate matter and discoloration prior to administration, and if detected, then it should not be used. Presence of air bubbles is not a contraindication for tildrakizumab's use.

Sites for injection need to be clear with no erythema, induration, bruise or disease. Injection sites include abdomen, thighs and upper arm [270].

Conclusion

Tildrakizumab has proven to be a valuable drug in the management of psoriasis. Apart from its efficacy for this indication, the use of tildrakizumab in HS, PG, PRP, LP and vitiligo has further expanded its dermatologic horizon. Further, its wider spaced dosing schedule offers an added advantage over other biologics, along with sustained long-lasting effects and an acceptable safety profile.

References

1. Markham A. Guselkumab: First Global Approval. Drugs. 2017;77(13):1487–92.
2. Tran L, Yao Z, Xu Z, Vermeulen A. Population pharmacokinetics analysis of guselkumab in healthy subjects and patients with psoriatic arthritis, plaque psoriasis and palmoplantar pustulosis. Br J Clin Pharmacol. 2022;88(10):4481–93.
3. Data on File. Guselkumab. CCDS. Janssen Research & Development, LLC. EDMS-ERI-111962822. US-SRSM-4518. 2023.
4. Wilson NJ, Boniface K, Chan JR, BS MK, Blumenschein WM, Mattson JD, et al. Development, cytokine profile and function of human interleukin 17–producing helper T cells. Nat Immunol. 2007;8(9):950–7.
5. MJ MG, Bak-Jensen KS, Chen Y, Tato CM, Blumenschein W, McClanahan T, et al. TGF-β and IL-6 drive the production of IL-17 and IL-10 by T cells and restrain TH-17 cell–mediated pathology. Nat Immunol. 2007;8(12):1390–7.
6. Jeon C, Sekhon S, Yan D, Afifi L, Nakamura M, Bhutani T. Monoclonal antibodies inhibiting IL-12, −23, and −17 for the treatment of psoriasis. Hum Vacc Immunother. 2017;13:2247–59.
7. Ciric B, El-behi M, Cabrera R, Zhang GX, Rostami A. IL-23 drives pathogenic IL-17-producing CD8+ T cells. J Immunol. 2009;182:5296–305.
8. Lin AM, Rubin CJ, Khandpur R, Wang JY, Riblett M, Yalavarthi S, et al. Mast cells and neutrophils release IL-17 through extracellular trap formation in psoriasis. J Immunol. 2011;187:490–500.
9. Gooderham MJ, Papp KA, Lynde CW. Shifting the focus—the primary role of IL −23 in psoriasis and other inflammatory disorders. J Eur Acad Dermatol Venereol. 2018;32:1111–9.
10. Hawkes JE, Yan BY, Chan TC, Krueger JG. Discovery of the IL-23/IL-17 signaling pathway and the treatment of psoriasis. J Immunol. 2018;201:1605–13.
11. Chan TC, Hawkes JE, Krueger JG. Interleukin 23 in the skin: role in psoriasis pathogenesis and selective interleukin 23 blockade as treatment. Ther Adv Chron Dis. 2018;9:111–9.
12. Yang K, Oak ASW, Elewski BE. Use of IL-23 inhibitors for the treatment of plaque psoriasis and psoriatic arthritis: A comprehensive review. Am J Clin Dermatol. 2021;22:173–92.
13. Sofen H, Smith S, Matheson RT, Leonardi CL, Calderon C, Brodmerkel C, et al. Guselkumab (an IL-23–specific mAb) demonstrates clinical and molecular response in patients with moderate-to-severe psoriasis. J Allerg Clin Immunol. 2014;133:1032–40.

14. Martini E, Wikén M, Cheuk S, Gallais Sérézal I, Baharom F, Ståhle M, et al. Dynamic changes in resident and infiltrating epidermal dendritic cells in active and resolved psoriasis. J Invest Dermatol. 2017;137:865–73.
15. Fotiadou C, Lazaridou E, Sotiriou E, Ioannides D. Targeting IL-23 in psoriasis: current perspectives. Psoriasis (Auckl). 2018;8:1–5.
16. Blauvelt A, Papp KA, Griffiths CEM, Randazzo B, Wasfi Y, Shen YK, et al. Efficacy and safety of guselkumab, an anti-interleukin-23 monoclonal antibody, compared with adalimumab for the continuous treatment of patients with moderate to severe psoriasis: results from the phase III, double-blinded, placebo- and active comparator–controlled VOYAGE 1 trial. J Amer Acad Dermatol. 2017;76:405–17.
17. Langley RG, Tsai T-F, Flavin S, Song M, Randazzo B, Wasfi Y, et al. Efficacy and safety of guselkumab in patients with psoriasis who have an inadequate response to ustekinumab: results of the randomized, double-blind, phase III NAVIGATE trial. Br J Dermatol. 2018;178:114–23.
18. Reich K, Armstrong AW, Langley RG, Flavin S, Randazzo B, Li S, et al. Guselkumab versus secukinumab for the treatment of moderate-to-severe psoriasis (ECLIPSE): results from a phase 3, randomised controlled trial. Lancet. 2019;394(10201):831–9.
19. Du Jardin K, Lopez P, Lange M, McCool R, Naval S, Quickert S. A systematic literature review and bucher indirect comparison: Tildrakizumab versus Guselkumab. J Health Econ Outcomes Res. 2020:123–9.
20. Griffiths CEM, Papp KA, Song M, Miller M, You Y, Shen YK, et al. Continuous treatment with guselkumab maintains clinical responses through 4 years in patients with moderate-to-severe psoriasis: results from VOYAGE 1. J Dermatolog Treat. 2022;33:848–56.
21. Ohtsuki M, Kubo H, Morishima H, Goto R, Zheng R, Nakagawa H. Guselkumab, an anti-interleukin-23 monoclonal antibody, for the treatment of moderate to severe plaque-type psoriasis in Japanese patients: efficacy and safety results from a phase 3, randomized, double-blind, placebo-controlled study. J Dermatol. 2018;45:1053–62.
22. Hall SL, Haidari W, Feldman SR. Resolution of Guttate psoriasis plaques after one-time Administration of Guselkumab. J Drugs Dermatol. 2019;18:822–3.
23. Bartholomew E, Chung BY, Davis M, Yeroushalmi S, Chung M, Hakimi M, et al. Rapid remission of sunburn-induced Guttate psoriasis with Guselkumab. Dermatol Ther (Heidelb). 2023;13:2473–8.
24. Schwarz A, Bhardwaj R, Aragane Y, Mahnke K, Riemann H, Metze D, et al. Ultraviolet-B-induced apoptosis of keratinocytes: evidence for partial involvement of tumor necrosis factor-α in the formation of sunburn cells. J Invest Dermatol. 1995;104:922–7.
25. McGonagle D, Tan AL, Benjamin M. The nail as a musculoskeletal appendage—implications for an improved understanding of the link between psoriasis and arthritis. Dermatology. 2009;218:97–102.
26. Kassir M, Kircik L, Weinberg J, Fatima F, Yamauchi P, Lotti T, et al. Treatment of nail psoriasis. J Drugs Dermatol. 2022;21:146–50.
27. Egeberg A, See K, Garrelts A, Burge R. Epidemiology of psoriasis in hard-to-treat body locations: data from the Danish skin cohort. BMC Dermatol. 2020;20:3.
28. Langley RG, Daudén E. Treatment and Management of Psoriasis with nail involvement: A focus on biologic therapy. Dermatology. 2010;221:29–42.
29. Kaeley GS, Eder L, Aydin SZ, Rich P, Bakewell CJ. Nail psoriasis: diagnosis, assessment, treatment options, and unmet clinical needs. J Rheumatol. 2021;48:1208–20.
30. Temiz SA, Özer İ, Ataseven A, Dursun R, Uyar M. The effect of smoking on the psoriasis: is it related to nail involvement? Dermatol Ther. 2020;33:e13960.
31. Schwarz CW, Loft N, Rasmussen MK, Nissen CV, Dam TN, Ajgeiy KK, et al. Predictors of response to biologics in patients with moderate-to-severe psoriasis: A Danish Nationwide cohort study. Acta Derm Venereol. 2021;101:adv00579.
32. Pirro F, Caldarola G, Chiricozzi A, Burlando M, Mariani M, Parodi A, et al. Impact of body mass index on the efficacy of biological therapies in patients with psoriasis: A real-world study. Clin Drug Investig. 2021;41:917–25.

33. Gerdes S, Bräu B, Hoffmann M, Korge B, Mortazawi D, Wiemers F, et al. Real-world effectiveness of guselkumab in patients with psoriasis: health-related quality of life and efficacy data from the noninterventional, prospective, German multicenter PERSIST trial. J Dermatol. 2021;48:1854–62.
34. Foley P, Gordon K, Griffiths CEM, Wasfi Y, Randazzo B, Song M, et al. Efficacy of Guselkumab compared with adalimumab and placebo for psoriasis in specific body regions: A secondary analysis of 2 randomized clinical trials. JAMA Dermatol. 2018;154:676.
35. Gerdes S, Asadullah K, Hoffmann M, Korge B, Mortazawi D, Wegner S, et al. Real-world evidence from the non-interventional, prospective, German multicentre PERSIST study of patients with psoriasis after 1 year of treatment with guselkumab. J Eur Acad Dermatol Venereol. 2022;36:1568–77.
36. Jo SJ, Huang Y, Tsai T, Kim BS, Reich K, Saadoun C, et al. Efficacy of guselkumab in difficult-to-treat psoriasis regions: data from VOYAGE 1 and VOYAGE 2 Asian subpopulations. J Dermatol. 2023;50:1180–9.
37. Blauvelt A, Leonardi C, Elewski B, Crowley JJ, Guenther LC, Gooderham M, et al. A head-to-head comparison of ixekizumab vs. guselkumab in patients with moderate-to-severe plaque psoriasis: 24-week efficacy and safety results from a randomized, double-blinded trial. Br J Dermatol. 2021;184:1047–58.
38. Farley E, Masrour S, McKey J, Menter A. Palmoplantar psoriasis: A phenotypical and clinical review with introduction of a new quality-of-life assessment tool. J Am Acad Dermatol. 2009;60:1024–31.
39. Raposo I, Torres T. Palmoplantar psoriasis and palmoplantar Pustulosis: current treatment and future prospects. Am J Clin Dermatol. 2016;17:349–58.
40. Passeron T, Carrascosa JM, Warren RB, Pinter A, Romanelli M, Gorecki P, et al. A phase IIIb, multicentre, interventional, randomised, placebo-controlled clinical trial investigating the efficacy and safety of Guselkumab for the treatment of nonpustular palmoplantar psoriasis (G-PLUS). Dermatol Ther. 2023;2023:1–14.
41. Brunasso AMG, Massone C. Psoriasis and palmoplantar pustulosis: an endless debate? J Eur Acad Dermatol Venereol. 2017;31:e335–7.
42. Terui T, Kobayashi S, Okubo Y, Murakami M, Hirose K, Kubo H. Efficacy and safety of Guselkumab, an anti–interleukin 23 monoclonal antibody, for palmoplantar Pustulosis: A randomized clinical trial. JAMA Dermatol. 2018;154:309–16.
43. Terui T, Kobayashi S, Okubo Y, Murakami M, Zheng R, Morishima H, et al. Efficacy and safety of Guselkumab in Japanese patients with palmoplantar Pustulosis: A phase 3 randomized clinical trial. JAMA Dermatol. 2019;155:1153–61.
44. Okubo Y, Morishima H, Zheng R, Terui T. Sustained efficacy and safety of guselkumab in patients with palmoplantar pustulosis through 1.5 years in a randomized phase 3 study. J Dermatol. 2021;48:1838–53.
45. Morita A, Chen Y, Leung MWL, Kawashima N, Terui T. Effect of guselkumab on serum biomarkers in Japanese palmoplantar pustulosis patients in a randomized phase 3 study. JEADV Clin Pract. 2023;2:59–72.
46. Girolomoni G, Strohal R, Puig L, Bachelez H, Barker J, Boehncke WH, et al. The role of IL −23 and the IL-23/TH17 immune axis in the pathogenesis and treatment of psoriasis. J Eur Acad Dermatol Venereol. 2017;31:1616–26.
47. Bridgewood C, Watad A, Russell T, Palmer TM, Marzo-Ortega H, Khan A, et al. Identification of myeloid cells in the human enthesis as the main source of local IL-23 production. Ann Rheum Dis. 2019;78:929–33.
48. Lee Y. The role of interleukin-17 in bone metabolism and inflammatory skeletal diseases. BMB Rep. 2013;46:479–83.
49. Murphy CA, Langrish CL, Chen Y, Blumenschein W, McClanahan T, Kastelein RA, et al. Divergent pro- and Antiinflammatory roles for IL-23 and IL-12 in joint autoimmune inflammation. J Exp Med. 2003;198:1951–7.

50. Schurich A, Raine C, Morris V, Ciurtin C. The role of IL-12/23 in T cell–related chronic inflammation: implications of immunodeficiency and therapeutic blockade. Rheumatology. 2018;57:246–54.
51. Kopp T, Lenz P, Bello-Fernandez C, Kastelein RA, Kupper TS, Stingl G. IL-23 production by Cosecretion of endogenous p19 and transgenic p40 in keratin 14/p40 transgenic mice: evidence for enhanced cutaneous immunity. J Immunol. 2003;170:5438–44.
52. Deodhar A, Gottlieb AB, Boehncke WH, Dong B, Wang Y, Zhuang Y, et al. Efficacy and safety of guselkumab in patients with active psoriatic arthritis: a randomised, double-blind, placebo-controlled, phase 2 study. Lancet. 2018;391:2213–24.
53. Mease PJ, Gladman DD, Deodhar A, McGonagle DG, Nash P, Boehncke WH, et al. Impact of guselkumab, an interleukin-23 p19 subunit inhibitor, on enthesitis and dactylitis in patients with moderate to severe psoriatic arthritis: results from a randomised, placebo-controlled, phase II study. RMD Open. 2020;6:e001217.
54. Mease PJ, Rahman P, Gottlieb AB, Kollmeier AP, Hsia EC, Xu XL, et al. Guselkumab in biologic-naive patients with active psoriatic arthritis (DISCOVER-2): a double-blind, randomised, placebo-controlled phase 3 trial. Lancet. 2020;395:1126–36.
55. Deodhar A, Helliwell PS, Boehncke WH, Kollmeier AP, Hsia EC, Subramanian RA, et al. Guselkumab in patients with active psoriatic arthritis who were biologic-naive or had previously received TNFα inhibitor treatment (DISCOVER-1): a double-blind, randomised, placebo-controlled phase 3 trial. Lancet. 2020;395:1115–25.
56. Kelly G, Sweeney CM, Tobin A, Kirby B. Hidradenitis suppurativa: the role of immune dysregulation. Int J Dermatol. 2014;53:1186–96.
57. Schlapbach C, Hänni T, Yawalkar N, Hunger RE. Expression of the IL-23/Th17 pathway in lesions of hidradenitis suppurativa. J Am Acad Dermatol. 2011;65:790–8.
58. Littman DR, Rudensky AY. Th17 and regulatory T cells in mediating and restraining inflammation. Cell. 2010;140:845–58.
59. Cole S, Murray J, Simpson C, Okoye R, Tyson K, Griffiths M, et al. Interleukin (IL)-12 and IL-18 synergize to promote MAIT cell IL-17A and IL-17F production independently of IL-23 signaling. Front Immunol. 2020;11:585134.
60. Dudink K, Bouwman K, Chen Y, DePrimo SE, Munoz-Elias EJ, Aarts P, et al. Guselkumab for hidradenitis suppurativa: a phase II, open-label, mode-of-action study. Br J Dermatol. 2023;188:601–9.
61. Kimball AB, Podda M, Alavi A, Miller M, Shen Y, Li S, et al. Guselkumab for the treatment of patients with moderate-to-severe hidradenitis suppurativa: A phase 2 randomized study. J Eur Acad Dermatol Venereol. 2023;37:2098–108.
62. Casseres RG, Kahn JS, Her MJ, Rosmarin D. Guselkumab in the treatment of hidradenitis suppurativa: A retrospective chart review. J Am Acad Dermatol. 2019;81:265–7.
63. Montero-Vilchez T, Martinez-Lopez A, Salvador-Rodriguez L, Arias-Santiago S, Molina-Leyva A. The use of guselkumab 100 mg every 4 weeks on patients with hidradenitis suppurativa and a literature review. Dermatol Ther. 2020;33:e13456.
64. Kearney N, Byrne N, Kirby B, Hughes R. Successful use of guselkumab in the treatment of severe hidradenitis suppurativa. Clin Exp Dermatol. 2020;45:618–9.
65. Kovacs M, Podda M. Guselkumab in the treatment of severe hidradenitis suppurativa. J Eur Acad Dermatol Venereol. 2019;33:e140–1.
66. Martora F, Fabbrocini G, Marasca C, Battista T, Megna M. Paradoxical hidradenitis suppurativa induced by adalimumab biosimilar successfully treated with guselkumab in a patient with psoriasis. Comment on 'Paradoxical hidradenitis suppurativa due to anti-interleukin-1 agents for mevalonate kinase deficiency successfully treated with the addition of ustekinumab.'. Clin Exp Dermatol. 2023;48:701–3.
67. Garcia-Melendo C, Vilarrasa E, Cubiró X, Bittencourt F, Puig L. Sequential paradoxical psoriasiform reaction and sacroiliitis following adalimumab treatment of hidradenitis suppurativa, successfully treated with guselkumab. Dermatol Ther. 2020;33:e14180.

68. Burzi L, Repetto F, Ramondetta A, Rozzo G, Licciardello M, Ribero S, et al. Guselkumab in the treatment of severe hidradenitis suppurativa, a promising role? Dermatol Ther. 2021;34:e14930.
69. Croitoru DO, Seigel K, Nathanielsz N, Elsawi R, Silverberg MS, Piguet V, et al. Treatment of severe hidradenitis Suppurativa and Fistulizing Crohn's disease with Guselkumab. J Eur Acad Dermatol Venereol. 2022;36:e563–5.
70. Berman HS, Villa NM, Shi VY, Hsiao JL. Guselkumab in the treatment of concomitant hidradenitis suppurativa, psoriasis, and Crohn's disease. J Dermatol Treat. 2021;32:261–3.
71. Jørgensen AR, Holm JG, Thomsen SF. Guselkumab for hidradenitis suppurativa in a patient with concomitant Crohn's disease: report and systematic literature review of effectiveness and safety. Clin Case Rep. 2020;8:2873–6.
72. George C, Deroide F, Rustin M. Pyoderma gangrenosum – a guide to diagnosis and management. Clin Med (Lond). 2019;19:224–8.
73. Yamanaka K. New treatment of pyoderma gangrenosum and hidradenitis suppurativa: a review. J Dermatol. 2023:1346-8138.17031.
74. Baier C, Barak O. Guselkumab as a treatment option for recalcitrant pyoderma gangrenosum. JAAD Case Rep. 2021;8:43–6.
75. Reese AM, Erickson K, Reed KB, Ortega-Loayza AG. Modified dose of guselkumab for treatment of pyoderma gangrenosum. JAAD Case Rep. 2022;21:38–42.
76. Villaverde Piñeiro L, Loureiro Martínez M, Cachafeiro Pin AI. Tratamiento del pioderma gangrenoso con guselkumab en condiciones diferentes a las autorizadas en la ficha técnica. Med Clín. 2023;161:226–7.
77. Wang D, Chong VCL, Chong WS, Oon HH. A review on Pityriasis Rubra pilaris. Am J Clin Dermatol. 2018;19:377–90.
78. Feldmeyer L, Mylonas A, Demaria O, Mennella A, Yawalkar N, Laffitte E, et al. Interleukin 23–helper T cell 17 Axis as a treatment target for Pityriasis Rubra pilaris. JAMA Dermatol. 2017;153:304–8.
79. Kannan AK, Su Z, Gauvin DM, Paulsboe SE, Duggan R, Lasko LM, et al. IL-23 induces regulatory T cell plasticity with implications for inflammatory skin diseases. Sci Rep. 2019;9:17675.
80. Pilz AC, Seiringer P, Biedermann T, Eyerich K. Treatment of Pityriasis Rubra pilaris with Guselkumab. JAMA Dermatol. 2019;155:1424–6.
81. Nagai H, Jimbo H, Matsuura S, Tatsuoka S, Shiraki E, Nishigori C. Successful treatment of pityriasis rubra pilaris with guselkumab: serum CCL20 as a potential marker for the disease activity. Dermatol Ther. 2020;33:e14403.
82. Nishimura M, Kondo M, Habe K, Hayashi A, Yamanaka K. Successful treatment with cyclosporine and guselkumab for pityriasis rubra pilaris. Clin Case Rep. 2022;10:e6413.
83. Langrish CL, Chen Y, Blumenschein WM, Mattson J, Basham B, Sedgwick JD, et al. IL-23 drives a pathogenic T cell population that induces autoimmune inflammation. J Exp Med. 2005;201:233–40.
84. McGeachy MJ, Chen Y, Tato CM, Laurence A, Joyce-Shaikh B, Blumenschein WM, et al. The interleukin 23 receptor is essential for the terminal differentiation of interleukin 17–producing effector T helper cells in vivo. Nat Immunol 2009;10:314–324.
85. Wang R, Hasnain SZ, Tong H, Das I, Che-Hao Chen A, Oancea I, et al. Neutralizing IL-23 is superior to blocking IL-17 in suppressing intestinal inflammation in a spontaneous murine colitis model. Inflamm Bowel Dis. 2015;21:973–84.
86. Solimani F, Pollmann R, Schmidt T, Schmidt A, Zheng X, Savai R, et al. Therapeutic targeting of Th17/Tc17 cells leads to clinical improvement of lichen planus. Front Immunol. 2019;10:1808.
87. Murgia RD, Gross GP. Stewart-Treves syndrome [internet]. In: StatPearls. Treasure Island (FL): StatPearls Publishing; 2023 [cited 2023 Dec 27]. Available from: http://www.ncbi.nlm.nih.gov/books/NBK507833/

88. Nardinocchi L, Sonego G, Passarelli F, Avitabile S, Scarponi C, Failla CM, et al. Interleukin-17 and interleukin-22 promote tumor progression in human nonmelanoma skin cancer. Eur J Immunol. 2015;45(3):922–31.
89. Sheng S, Zhang J, Ai J, Hao X, Luan R. Aberrant expression of IL-23/IL-23R in patients with breast cancer and its clinical significance. Mol Med Rep. 2018;17:4639–44.
90. Nie W, Yu T, Sang Y, Gao X. Tumor-promoting effect of IL-23 in mammary cancer mediated by infiltration of M2 macrophages and neutrophils in tumor microenvironment. Biochem Biophys Res Commun. 2017;482:1400–6.
91. Van Esbeen L, Roquet-Gravy PP. Improvement of Stewart-Treves angiosarcoma through interleukin 23p19 inhibition. JAAD Case Rep. 2021;17:84–6.
92. Product Information: Tremfya (guselkumab) solution for injection. Janssen Inc. Toronto, ON Accessed November 10, 2017. https://pdf.hres.ca/dpd_pm/00042101.PDF.
93. Burlando M, Capurro N, Herzum A, Cozzani E, Parodi A. Guselkumab-associated bullous pemphigoid in a psoriasis patient: A case report and review of the literature. Dermatol Ther. 2022;35:e15207.
94. Martora F, Annunziata MC, Guerriero L, Battista T, Potestio L, Megna M. Guselkumab-induced vitiligo in a patient with psoriatic arthritis. JAAD Case Rep. 2023;41:46–8.
95. Le Guern A, Alkeraye S, Vermersch-Langlin A, Coupe P, Vonarx M. Bullous pemphigoid during ustekinumab therapy. JAAD Case Rep. 2015;1:359–60.
96. Frisoli ML, Essien K, Harris JE. Vitiligo: mechanisms of pathogenesis and treatment. Ann Rev Immunol. 2020;38:621–48.
97. Guselkumab (Tremfya®) [Internet]. In: Mother to baby | fact sheets. Brentwood (TN): Organization of Teratology Information Specialists (OTIS); 1994 [cited 2023 Dec 27]. Available from: http://www.ncbi.nlm.nih.gov/books/NBK582737/
98. Stratigakis A, Paty D, Zou P, Zhao Z, Li Y, Zhang T. A regression approach for assessing large molecular drug concentration in breast milk. Reproduction and Breeding. 2023;3:199–207.
99. Anderson PO. Monoclonal antibodies during breastfeeding. Breastfeed Med. 2021;16:591–3.
100. Krysko KM, Dobson R, Alroughani R, Amato MP, Bove R, Ciplea AI, et al. Family planning considerations in people with multiple sclerosis. Lancet Neurol. 2023;22:350–66.
101. Kim SR, Kibbi N, Craiglow BG. Guselkumab for the treatment of severe refractory psoriasis in a pediatric patient. JAAD Case Rep. 2019;5:552–4.
102. Song EJ, Whitman P, Samsel J. The use of ustekinumab and guselkumab in a pediatric psoriasis patient with active hepatitis B infection. JAAD Case Rep. 2021;8:37–9.
103. Ruggiero A, Fabbrocini G, Cinelli E, Ocampo Garza SS, Camela E, Megna M. Anti-interleukin-23 for psoriasis in elderly patients: guselkumab, risankizumab and tildrakizumab in real-world practice. Clin Exp Dermatol. 2022;47:561–7.
104. Chiricozzi A, Gisondi P, Bellinato F, Girolomoni G. Immune response to vaccination in patients with psoriasis treated with systemic therapies. Vaccines (Basel). 2020;8:769.
105. Zhu Y, Xu Y, Zhuang Y, Piantone A, Shu C, Chen D, et al. Evaluating potential disease-mediated protein-drug interactions in patients with moderate-to-severe plaque psoriasis receiving subcutaneous Guselkumab. Clin Transl Sci. 2020;13:1217–26.
106. Singh S, Kroe-Barrett RR, Canada KA, Zhu X, Sepulveda E, Wu H, et al. Selective targeting of the IL23 pathway: generation and characterization of a novel high-affinity humanized anti-IL23A antibody. MAbs. 2015;7:778–91.
107. Blair HA. Risankizumab: a review in moderate to severe plaque psoriasis. Drugs. 2020;80:1235–45.
108. Pang Y, Khatri A, Suleiman AA, Othman AA. Clinical pharmacokinetics and pharmacodynamics of risankizumab in psoriasis patients. Clin Pharmacokinet. 2020;59:311–26.
109. Rendon A, Schäkel K. Psoriasis pathogenesis and treatment. Int J Mol Sci. 2019;20:1475.
110. Kim J, Krueger JG. Highly effective new treatments for psoriasis target the IL-23/type 17 T cell autoimmune axis. Annu Rev Med. 2017;68:255–69.
111. Puig L. The role of IL 23 in the treatment of psoriasis. Exp Rev Clin Immunol. 2017;13:525–34.
112. Megna M, Potestio L, Ruggiero A, Camela E, Fabbrocini G. Risankizumab treatment in psoriasis patients who failed anti-IL17: a 52-week real-life study. Dermatol Ther. 2022;35:e15524.

113. Gordon KB, Strober B, Lebwohl M, Augustin M, Blauvelt A, Poulin Y, et al. Efficacy and safety of risankizumab in moderate-to-severe plaque psoriasis (UltIMMa-1 and UltIMMa-2): results from two double-blind, randomised, placebo-controlled and ustekinumab-controlled phase 3 trials. Lancet. 2018;392:650–61.
114. Rentz AM, Skalicky AM, Burslem K, Becker K, Kaschinski D, Esser D, et al. The content validity of the PSS in patients with plaque psoriasis. J Patient Rep Outcomes. 2017;1:1–4.
115. Reich K, Gooderham M, Thaçi D, Crowley JJ, Ryan C, Krueger JG, et al. Risankizumab compared with adalimumab in patients with moderate-to-severe plaque psoriasis (IMMvent): a randomised, double-blind, active-comparator-controlled phase 3 trial. Lancet. 2019;394:576–86.
116. Warren RB, Blauvelt A, Poulin Y, Beeck S, Kelly M, Wu T, et al. Efficacy and safety of risankizumab vs. secukinumab in patients with moderate-to-severe plaque psoriasis (IMMerge): results from a phase III, randomized, open-label, efficacy–assessor-blinded clinical trial. Br J Dermatol. 2021;184:50–9.
117. Shi J, Xu J, Chen Y. A network meta-analysis for the comparison of efficacy and safety of interleukin (IL)-23 targeted drugs in the treatment of moderate to severe psoriasis. Dermatol Ther. 2020;33:e13802.
118. Ruggiero A, Fabbrocini G, Cinelli E, Megna M. Real world practice indirect comparison between guselkumab and risankizumab: results from an Italian retrospective study. Dermatol Ther. 2022;35:e15214.
119. Ruggiero A, Fabbrocini G, Cinelli E, Megna M. Guselkumab and risankizumab for psoriasis: a 44-week indirect real-life comparison. J Am Acad Dermatol. 2021;85:1028–30.
120. Dawoud NM, El Badawy MB, Al Eid HS, Abdel Fattah MM. Risankizumab effectiveness and safety in psoriasis patients who failed other biologics: real-life case series. Indian J Dermatol Venereol Leprol. 2022;88:235–40.
121. Singh S, Singh S, Thangaswamy A, Thangaraju P, Varthya SB. Efficacy and safety of Risankizumab in moderate to severe psoriasis: A systematic review and meta-analysis. Dermatol Ther. 2021;34:e14487.
122. Mastorino L, Dapavo P, Susca S, Cariti C, Siliquini N, Verrone A, et al. Drug survival and clinical effectiveness of secukinumab, ixekizumab, brodalumab, guselkumab, risankizumab, tildrakizumab for psoriasis treatment. J Dtsch Dermatol Ges. 2024;22:34–42.
123. Megna M, Fabbrocini G, Ruggiero A, Cinelli E. Efficacy and safety of risankizumab in psoriasis patients who failed anti-IL-17, anti-12/23 and/or anti IL-23: preliminary data of a real-life 16-week retrospective study. Dermatol Ther. 2020;33:e14144.
124. Bonifati C, Morrone A, Cristaudo A, Graceffa D. Effectiveness of anti-interleukin 23 biologic drugs in psoriasis patients who failed anti-interleukin 17 regimens. A real-life experience. Dermatol Ther. 2021;34:e14584.
125. Mastorino L, Castelli F, Stroppiana E, Verrone A, Ortoncelli M, Susca S, et al. Risankizumab shows faster response in bio naïve than in bio-experienced psoriatic patients. J Eur Acad Dermatol Venereol. 2022;36:e838–41.
126. Borroni RG, Malagoli P, Gargiulo L, Valenti M, Pavia G, Facheris P, et al. Real-life effectiveness and safety of Risankizumab in moderate-to-severe plaque psoriasis: A 40-week multicentric retrospective study. Acta Derm Venereol. 2021;101:adv00605.
127. Mastorino L, Susca S, Megna M, Siliquini N, Quaglino P, Ortoncelli M, et al. Risankizumab shows high efficacy and maintenance in improvement of response until week 52. Dermatol Ther. 2022;35:e15378.
128. Hendrix N, Ollendorf DA, Chapman RH, Loos A, Liu S, Kumar V, et al. Cost-effectiveness of targeted pharmacotherapy for moderate to severe plaque psoriasis. J Manag Care Spec Pharm. 2018;24:1210–7.
129. Megna M, Balato A, Napolitano M, Gallo L, Caso F, Costa L, Balato N, et al. Psoriatic disease treatment nowadays: unmet needs among the "jungle of biologic drugs and small molecules". Clin Rheumatol. 2018;37:1739–41.

130. Ruiz-Villaverde R, Ayén-Rodriguez A, Llamas-Molina JM, Ruiz-Carrascosa JC. Risankizumab as a promising therapeutic approach in obese patients. Dermatol Ther. 2020;33:e13323.
131. Gkalpakiotis S, Cetkovska P, Arenberger P, Dolezal T, Arenbergerova M, Velackova B, et al. Risankizumab for the treatment of moderate-to-severe psoriasis: real-life multicenter experience from The Czech Republic. Dermatol Ther (Heidelb). 2021;11:1345–55.
132. Ruiz-Villaverde R, Ruiz-Carrascosa JC, Galán-Gutierrez M, Armario-Hita JC. Risankizumab: A pilot study of short-term effectiveness and safety in real clinical practice. Dermatol Ther. 2021;34:e14711.
133. Hansel K, Zangrilli A, Bianchi L, Peris K, Chiricozzi A, Offidani A, et al. A 52-week update of a multicentre real-life experience on effectiveness and safety of risankizumab in psoriasis. J Eur Acad Dermatol Venereol. 2022;36:e111–3.
134. Megna M, Cinelli E, Gallo L, Camela E, Ruggiero A, Fabbrocini G. Risankizumab in real life: preliminary results of efficacy and safety in psoriasis during a 16-week period. Arch Dermatol Res. 2022;314:619–23.
135. Ruggiero A, Portarapillo A, Megna M, Patruno C, Napolitano M. Management strategies for pediatric moderate-to-severe plaque psoriasis: spotlight on biologics. Pediatric Health Med Ther. 2023;14:435–51.
136. Caldarola G, Zangrilli A, Bernardini N, Bavetta M, De Simone C, Graceffa D, et al. Risankizumab for the treatment of moderate-to-severe psoriasis: A multicenter, retrospective, 1-year real-life study. Dermatol Ther. 2022;35:e15489.
137. Meeuwis KA, de Hullu JA, Massuger LF, van de Kerkhof PC, van Rossum MM. Genital psoriasis: A systematic literature review on this hidden skin disease. Acta Derm Venereol. 2011;91:5–11.
138. American Academy of Dermatology Work Group, Menter A, Korman NJ, Elmets CA, Feldman SR, Gelfand JM, et al. Guidelines of care for the management of psoriasis and psoriatic arthritis: section 6. Guidelines of care for the treatment of psoriasis and psoriatic arthritis: case-based presentations and evidence-based conclusions. J Am Acad Dermatol. 2011;65:137–74.
139. Guenther L, Potts Bleakman A, Weisman J, Poulin Y, Spelman L, Burge R, et al. Ixekizumab results in persistent clinical improvement in moderate-to-severe genital psoriasis during a 52 week, randomized, placebo-controlled, phase 3 clinical trial. Acta Derm Venereol. 2020;100:adv00006.
140. Merola JF, Ghislain PD, Dauendorffer JN, Potts Bleakman A, Brnabic AJM, Burge R, et al. Ixekizumab improves secondary lesional signs, pain and sexual health in patients with moderate-to-severe genital psoriasis. J Eur Acad Dermatol Venereol. 2020;34:1257–62.
141. Sotiriou E, Bakirtzi K, Papadimitriou I, Tsentemeidou A, Eftychidou P, Eleftheriadis V, et al. A head-to-head comparison of risankizumab and ixekizumab for genital psoriasis: a real-life, 24-week, prospective study. J Eur Acad Dermatol Venereol. 2022;36:e359–61.
142. Shao S, Wang G, Maverakis E, Gudjonsson JE. Targeted treatment for Erythrodermic psoriasis: rationale and recent advances. Drugs. 2020;80:525–34.
143. Stinco G, Errichetti E. Erythrodermic psoriasis: current and future role of biologicals. BioDrugs. 2015;29:91–101.
144. Rosenbach M, Hsu S, Korman NJ, Lebwohl MG, Young M, Bebo BF Jr, et al. Treatment of erythrodermic psoriasis: from the medical board of the National Psoriasis Foundation. J Am Acad Dermatol. 2010;62:655–62.
145. Moy AP, Murali M, Kroshinsky D, Duncan LM, Nazarian RM. Immunologic overlap of helper T-cell subtypes 17 and 22 in Erythrodermic psoriasis and atopic dermatitis. JAMA Dermatol. 2015;151:753–60.
146. McKeage K, Duggan S. Risankizumab: First Global Approval. Drugs. 2019;79:893–900.
147. Alajlan A, Madani A, Qadoumi TA, Aljaloud A, Alessa M. Erythrodermic psoriasis managed with Risankizumab. Case Rep Dermatol. 2022;14:219–24.

148. Pettey AA, Balkrishnan R, Rapp SR, Fleischer AB, Feldman SR. Patients with palmoplantar psoriasis have more physical disability and discomfort than patients with other forms of psoriasis: implications for clinical practice. J Am Acad Dermatol. 2003;49:271–5.
149. Timotijević ZS, Trajković G, Jankovic J, Relić M, Đorić D, Vukićević D, et al. How frequently does palmoplantar psoriasis affect the palms and/or soles? A systematic review and meta-analysis. Postepy Dermatol Alergol. 2019;36:595–603.
150. Al Muqrin AM, Alghamdi AA, AlShaalan ZM. Rapid response of palmoplantar psoriasis to Risankizumab: A case report. Clin Cosmet Investig Dermatol. 2022;15:2129–32.
151. Calabrese L, Caldarola G, Peris K, DE Simone C. Severe and resistant palmar psoriasis successfully treated with risankizumab. Ital J Dermatol Venerol. 2022;157:118–9.
152. Caldarola G, Zangrilli A, Palmisano G, Bavetta M, Moretta G, Pagnanelli G, et al. Effectiveness of risankizumab in the treatment of palmoplantar psoriasis: a 52-week Italian real-life experience. Drugs Context. 2023;12:2023-1-8.
153. Alajlan AM, Qadoumi TA. Palmoplantar psoriasis successfully treated with Risankizumab. Cureus. 2021;13:e17434.
154. Rachakonda TD, Schupp CW, Armstrong AW. Psoriasis prevalence among adults in the United States. J Am Acad Dermatol. 2014;70:512–6.
155. Ortonne JP, Baran R, Corvest M, Schmitt C, Voisard JJ, Taieb C. Development and validation of nail psoriasis quality of life scale (NPQ10). J Eur Acad Dermatol Venereol. 2010;24:22–7.
156. AlAjlan A, Qasim R, AlTassan F, Qadoumi T, AlKaff T. A case of nail psoriasis improved with treatment by risankizumab. Oxf Med Case Rep. 2022;11:397–9.
157. Orsini D, Pacifico A, Iacovelli P, Frascione P, De Simone P, Assorgi C, et al. Rapidly and successful improvement of nail psoriasis with risankizumab. Clin Case Rep. 2023;11:e8035.
158. Kristensen LE, Soliman AM, Papp K, Merola JF, Barcomb L, Wang Z, et al. Effects of risankizumab on nail psoriasis in patients with active psoriatic arthritis: results from KEEPsAKE 1. J Eur Acad Dermatol Venereol. 2022;36:e389–92.
159. Cai Y, Xue F, Quan C, Qu M, Liu N, Zhang Y, et al. A critical role of the IL-1β-IL-1R signaling pathway in skin inflammation and psoriasis pathogenesis. J Invest Dermatol. 2019;139:146–56.
160. Avallone G, Maronese CA, Murgia G, Carrera CG, Mastorino L, Roccuzzo G, et al. Interleukin-17 vs. Interleukin-23 inhibitors in pustular and Erythrodermic psoriasis: A retrospective, multicentre cohort study. J Clin Med. 2023;12:1662.
161. Song EJ. Generalized pustular psoriasis treated with Risankizumab. Cutis. 2023;111:96–8.
162. May Lee M, Fantini C, Mori E, Feliciani C, Satolli F. Rapid response of generalized pustular psoriasis to treatment with risankizumab. A therapeutic option for a difficult-to-treat disease. Ital J Dermatol Venerol. 2023;158:377–8.
163. Hermann AE, Weis SE. Complete clearance of pustular psoriasis after A single dose of Risankizumab. HCA Healthc J Med. 2023;4:209–13.
164. Yamanaka K, Okubo Y, Yasuda I, Saito N, Messina I, Morita A. Efficacy and safety of risankizumab in Japanese patients with generalized pustular psoriasis or erythrodermic psoriasis: primary analysis and 180-week follow-up results from the phase 3, multicenter IMMspire study. J Dermatol. 2023;50:195–202.
165. Orbai AM, de Wit M, Mease P, Shea JA, Gossec L, Leung YY, et al. International patient and physician consensus on a psoriatic arthritis core outcome set for clinical trials. Ann Rheum Dis. 2017;76:673–80.
166. Kristensen LE, Keiserman M, Papp K, McCasland L, White D, Lu W, et al. Efficacy and safety of risankizumab for active psoriatic arthritis: 24-week results from the randomised, double-blind, phase 3 KEEPsAKE 1 trial. Ann Rheum Dis. 2022;81:225–31.
167. Saunte DML, Jemec GBE. Hidradenitis Suppurativa: advances in diagnosis and treatment. JAMA. 2017;318:2019–32.
168. Kimball AB, Prens EP, Passeron T, Maverakis E, Turchin I, Beeck S, et al. Efficacy and safety of Risankizumab for the treatment of hidradenitis Suppurativa: A phase 2, randomized, placebo-controlled trial. Dermatol Ther (Heidelb). 2023;13:1099–111.

169. Repetto F, Burzi L, Ribero S, Quaglino P, Dapavo P. Efficacy and safety of Risankizumab in hidradenitis Suppurativa: A case series. Acta Derm Venereol. 2022;102:adv00780.
170. Licata G, Gambardella A, Buononato D, De Rosa A, Calabrese G, Pellerone S, et al. A case of moderate hidradenitis suppurativa and psoriasis successfully treated with risankizumab. Int J Dermatol. 2022;61:e126–9.
171. Caposiena Caro RD, Pensa C, Lambiase S, Candi E, Bianchi L. Risankizumab effectiveness in a recalcitrant case of hidradenitis suppurativa after anti-TNF and anti-interleukin-17 failures. Dermatol Ther. 2021;34:e15116.
172. Marques E, Arenberger P, Smetanová A, Gkalpakiotis S, Zimová D, Arenbergerová M. Successful treatment of recalcitrant hidradenitis suppurativa with risankizumab after failure of anti-tumour necrosis factor alpha. Br J Dermatol. 2021;184:966–7.
173. Ali N, Zirak B, Rodriguez RS, Pauli ML, Truong HA, Lai K, et al. Regulatory T cells in skin facilitate epithelial stem cell differentiation. Cell. 2017;169:1119–1129.e11.
174. Yamanaka K. New treatment of pyoderma gangrenosum and hidradenitis suppurativa: A review. J Dermatol. 2024;51:172–9.
175. Burgdorf B, Schlott S, Ivanov IH, Dissemond J. Successful treatment of a refractory pyoderma gangrenosum with risankizumab. Int Wound J. 2020;17:1086–8.
176. Orita A, Hoshina D, Hirosaki K. Pyoderma gangrenosum caused by secukinumab successfully treated with risankizumab: a case report and literature review. Clin Exp Dermatol. 2022;47:1372–4.
177. Weidinger S, Beck LA, Bieber T, Kabashima K, Irvine AD. Atopic dermatitis. Nat Rev Dis Primers. 2018;4:1.
178. Tyring SK, Rich P, Tada Y, Beeck S, Messina I, Liu J, et al. Risankizumab in patients with moderate-to-severe atopic dermatitis: A phase 2, randomized, double-blind, placebo-controlled study. Dermatol Ther (Heidelb). 2023;13:595–608.
179. Kromer C, Sabat R, Celis D, Mössner R. Systemic therapies of pityriasis rubra pilaris: a systematic review. J Dtsch Dermatol Ges. 2019;17:243–59.
180. Duarte B, Paiva Lopes MJ. Response to: 'successful treatment of refractory extensive pityriasis rubra pilaris with risankizumab'. Br J Dermatol. 2021;185:235–6.
181. Ricar J, Cetkovska P. Successful treatment of refractory extensive pityriasis rubra pilaris with risankizumab. Br J Dermatol. 2021;184:e148.
182. Fouarge AL, Cuvelier M, Roquet-Gravy C, de Montjoye L, Baeck M. Successful treatment of pityriasis rubra pilaris with risankizumab, a IL-23/p19 antagonist. J Eur Acad Dermatol Venereol. 2023;37:e106–9.
183. Balestri R, Magnano M, Girardelli CR, Rech G. Is risankizumab effective in the treatment of pityriasis rubra pilaris? Dermatol Ther. 2021;34:e15112.
184. Martora F, Villani A, Ocampo-Garza SS, Fabbrocini G, Megna M. Alopecia universalis improvement following risankizumab in a psoriasis patient. J Eur Acad Dermatol Venereol. 2022;36:e543–5.
185. Ohtsuki M, Fujita H, Watanabe M, Suzaki K, Flack M, Huang X, et al. Efficacy and safety of risankizumab in Japanese patients with moderate to severe plaque psoriasis: results from the SustaIMM phase 2/3 trial. J Dermatol. 2019;46:686–94.
186. Papp KA, de Vente S, Zeng J, Flack M, Padilla B, Tyring SK. Long-term safety and efficacy of Risankizumab in patients with moderate-to-severe chronic plaque psoriasis: results from a phase 2 open-label extension trial. Dermatol Ther (Heidelb). 2021;11:487–97.
187. Papp KA, Blauvelt A, Bukhalo M, Gooderham M, Krueger JG, Lacour JP, et al. Risankizumab versus Ustekinumab for Moderate-to-Severe Plaque Psoriasis. N Engl J Med. 2017;376:1551–60.
188. Ruggiero A, Megna M, Fabbrocini G, Ocampo-Garza SS. Anti-IL23 biologic therapies in the treatment of psoriasis: real-world experience versus clinical trials data. Immunol Res. 2023;71:328–55.
189. EudraVigilence. Available online. https://www.ema.europa.eu/en/human-regulatory/research-development/pharmacovigilance/eudravigilance. Accessed 14 Mar 2023.

190. Östör A, Van den Bosch F, Papp K, Asnal C, Blanco R, Aelion J, et al. Efficacy and safety of risankizumab for active psoriatic arthritis: 24-week results from the randomised, double-blind, phase 3 KEEPsAKE 2 trial. Ann Rheum Dis. 2022;81:351–8.
191. Östör A, Van den Bosch F, Papp K, Asnal C, Blanco R, Aelion J, et al. Efficacy and safety of risankizumab for active psoriatic arthritis: 52-week results from the KEEPsAKE 2 study. Rheumatology (Oxford). 2023;62:2122–9.
192. Summary of product characteristics. Available online:https://www.ema.europa.eu/en/documents/productinformation/skyrizi-epar-product-information-en.pdf. Accessed 14 Mar 2023.
193. Huang YW, Tsai TF. A drug safety evaluation of risankizumab for psoriasis. Expert Opin Drug Saf. 2020;19:395–402.
194. Blauvelt A, Leonardi CL, Gooderham M, Papp KA, Philipp S, Wu JJ, et al. Efficacy and safety of continuous Risankizumab therapy vs treatment withdrawal in patients with moderate to severe plaque psoriasis: A phase 3 randomized clinical trial. JAMA Dermatol. 2020;156:649–58.
195. Mastorino L, Dapavo P, Trunfio M, Avallone G, Rubatto M, Calcagno A, et al. Risk of reactivation of latent tuberculosis in psoriasis patients on biologic therapies: A retrospective cohort from a tertiary Care Centre in Northern Italy. Acta Derm Venereol. 2022;102:adv00821.
196. Geller S, Xu H, Lebwohl M, Nardone B, Lacouture ME, Kheterpal M. Malignancy risk and recurrence with psoriasis and its treatments: A concise update. Am J Clin Dermatol. 2018;19:363–75.
197. Butrón-Bris B, Daudén E, Rodríguez-Jiménez P. Psoriasis therapy and skin cancer: A review. Life (Basel). 2021;11:1109.
198. Armstrong EJ, Harskamp CT, Armstrong AW. Psoriasis and major adverse cardiovascular events: a systematic review and meta-analysis of observational studies. J Am Heart Assoc. 2013;2:e000062.
199. Polachek A, Touma Z, Anderson M, Eder L. Risk of cardiovascular morbidity in patients with psoriatic arthritis: A meta-analysis of observational studies. Arthritis Care Res (Hoboken). 2017;69:67–74.
200. Maradit-Kremers H, Dierkhising RA, Crowson CS, Icen M, Ernste FC, McEvoy MT. Risk and predictors of cardiovascular disease in psoriasis: a population-based study. Int J Dermatol. 2013;52:32–40.
201. Calapai F, Ammendolia I, Cardia L, Currò M, Calapai G, Esposito E, et al. Pharmacovigilance of Risankizumab in the treatment of psoriasis and arthritic psoriasis: real-world data from EudraVigilance database. Pharmaceutics. 2023;15:1933.
202. Woods RH. Potential cerebrovascular accident signal for risankizumab: A disproportionality analysis of the FDA adverse event reporting system (FAERS). Br J Clin Pharmacol. 2023;89:2386–95.
203. Shu Y, Chen J, Ding Y, Zhang Q. Adverse events with risankizumab in the real world: post-marketing pharmacovigilance assessment of the FDA adverse event reporting system. Front Immunol. 2023;14:1169735.
204. Yeung J, Gooderham MJ, Grewal P, Hong CH, Lansang P, Papp KA, et al. Management of Plaque Psoriasis with biologic therapies in women of child-bearing potential consensus paper. J Cutan Med Surg. 2020;24:3S–14S.
205. Ferrante M, Feagan BG, Panés J, Baert F, Louis E, Dewit O, et al. Long-term safety and efficacy of Risankizumab treatment in patients with Crohn's disease: results from the phase 2 open-label extension study. J Crohns Colitis. 2021;15:2001–10.
206. Beck KM, Sanchez IM, Yang EJ, Liao W. Profile of tildrakizumab-asmn in the treatment of moderate to severe plaque psoriasis: evidence to date. Psoriasis. 2018;8:49–58.
207. Markham A. Tildrakizumab: First global approval. Drug. 2018;78:845–9.
208. Di Meglio P, Nestle FO. The role of IL-23 in the immunopathogenesis of psoriasis. F1000 Biol Rep. 2010;2:40.
209. Tang C, Chen S, Qian H, Huang W. Interleukin 23: as a drug target for autoimmune inflammatory diseases. Immunology. 2012;135:112–24.

210. Duvallet E, Semerano L, Assier E, Falgarone G, Boissier MC. Interlekin-23: a key cytokine in inflammatory diseases. Ann Med. 2011;43:503–11.
211. Jeon C, Sekhon S, Yan D, SahilSekhon AL, Nakamura M, Bhutani T. Monoclonal antibodies inhibiting IL-12, −23, and −17 for the treatment of psoriasis. Hum Vaccin Immunother. 2017;13:2247–59.
212. Gooderham MJ, Papp KA, Lynde CW. Shifting the focus- the primary role of IL-23 in psoriasis and other inflammatory disorders. J EurAcadDermatolVenerol. 2018;32:1111–9.
213. Puig L. The role of IL-23 in the treatment of psoriasis. Expert Rev ClinImmunol. 2017;13:525–34.
214. Mehta H, Mashiko S, Angsana J, Rubio M, Hsieh YM, Maari C, et al. Differential changes in inflammatory mononuclear phagocytic and T- cell profiles within psoriatic skin during treatment with guselkumab vs. secukinumab. J Invest Dermatol. 2021;141:1707–18.e9.
215. Naslund-Koch C, Zachariae C, Skov L. Tildrakizumab: an evidence- based review of its use in the treatment of moderate to severe chronic plaque psoriasis. Ther Clin Risk Manag. 2020;16:903–16.
216. Martins LMS, Perez MM, Pereira CA, Costa FRC, Dias MS, Tostes RC, et al. Interleukin-23 promotes intestinal T helper type 17 immunity and ameliorates obesity- associated metabolic syndrome in a murine high- fat diet model. Immunology. 2018;154:624–36.
217. Thaci D, Piaserico S, Warren RB, Gupta AK, Cantrell W, Draelos Z, et al. Five year efficacy and safety of tildrakizumab in patients with moderate-to-severe psoriasis who respond at week 28: pooled analyses of two randomized phase III clinical trials (reSURFACE 1 and reSURFACE 2). Br J Dermatol. 2021;185:323–34.
218. Kimball AB, Papp KA, Reich K, Gooderham M, Li Q, Cichanowitz N, et al. Efficacy and safety of tildrakizumab for plaque psoriasis with continuous dosing, treatment interruption, dose adjustments and switching from etanercept: results from phase III studies. Br J Dermatol. 2020;182:1359–68.
219. Costanzo A, Malara G, Pelucchi C, Fatiga F, Barbera G, Franchi A, et al. Effectiveness end points real world studies on biological therapies in psoriasis: systemic review with focus on drug survival. Dermatology. 2018;234:1–12.
220. Torres T, Puig L, Vender R, Yeung J, Carrascosa JM, Piaserico S, et al. Drug survival of interleukin (IL)-17 and IL-23 inhibitors for the treatment of psoriasis: A retrospective multicountry, multicentric cohort study. Am J Clin Dermatol. 2022;23:891–904.
221. Nedoszytko B, Lange M, Sokolowska-Wojdylo M, Renke J, Trzonkowski P, Sobjanek M, et al. The role of regulatory T cells and genes involved in their differentiation in pathogenesis of selected inflammatory and neoplastic skin diseases. Part II. The Treg role in skin disease pathogenesis. Postepy Dermatol Alergol. 2017;34:405–17.
222. Crowley JJ, Warren RB, Cather JC. Safety of selective IL-23p19 inhibitors for the treatment of psoriasis. J Eur Acad Dermatol Venereol. 2019;33:1676–84.
223. Egeberg A, Anderson YMF, Halling-Overgaard AS, Alignahi E, Thyssen JP, Burge R, et al. Systematic review on rapidity of onset of action for interleukin-17 and interleukin-23 inhibitors for psoriasis. J Eur Acad Dermatol Venereol. 2020;34:39–46.
224. Sbidan E, Chaimani A, Garcia-Doval I, Do G, Hua C, Mazaud C, et al. Systemic pharmacological treatments for chronic plaque psoriasis: a network meta-analysis. Cochrane Database Syst Rev. 2017;12:CD011535.
225. Papp K, Thaci D, Reich K, Riedl E, Langley RG, Krueger JG, et al. Tildrakizumab (MK-3222), an anti-interleukin-23p19 monoclonal antibody, improves psoriasis in a phase IIb randomized placebo-controlled trial. Br J Dermatol. 2015;173:930–9.
226. Reich K, Papp KA, Blauvelt A, Tyring SK, Sinclair R, Thaci D, et al. Tildrakizumab versus placebo or etanercept for chronic plaque psoriasis (reSURFACE 1 and reSURFACE 2): results from two randomised controlled, phase 3 trials. Lancet. 2017;390:276–88.
227. Ruggiero A, Fabbrocicni G, Cacciapuoti S, Potestio L, Gallo L, Megna M. Tildrakizumab for the treatment of moderate-to-severe psoriasis: results from 52 weeks real-life retrospective study. ClinCosmet Invest Dermatol. 2023;16:529–36.

228. Gambardella A, Licata G, Tancredi V, Calabrese G, DE Rosa A, Alfano R, et al. A case of refractory palmoplantar psoriasis treated with tildrakizumab. Ital J Dermatol Venereol. 2022;157:379–80.
229. Galluzzo M, Talamonti M, Cioni A, Maffei V, Shumak RG, Tofani L, et al. Efficacy of Tildrakizumab for the treatment of difficult-to-treat areas: scalp, nail, palmoplantar and genital psoriasis. J Clin Med. 2022;11:2631.
230. Ariasi C, Licata G, Romano C, Bettolini L, Mezzana S, Maione V, et al. Real- life effectiveness of tildrakizumab in chronic palmoplantar psoriasis. A case series of 7 patients with 28 weeks of follow up. Clin Dermatol J. 2023;8:000299.
231. Del Campo DC. Successful use of Tildrakizumab for treatment of palmoplantar Pustulosis: A case report. J Drugs Dermatol. 2021;20:1117–9.
232. Menter MA, Murakawa GJ, Glover H, Mendelsohn AM, Parno J, Rozzo SJ, et al. Clearance of head and neck involvement in plaque psoriasis with tildrakizumab treatment in the phase 3 reSURFACE 1 study. J Eur Acad Dermatol Venereol. 2020;34:e803–5.
233. Langley RG, Dauden E. Treatment and management of psoriasis with nail involvement: a focus on biologic therapy. Dermatology. 2010;221(Suppl 1):29–42.
234. Girolomoni G, Griffiths CE, Krueger J, Nestle FO, Nicolas JF, et al. Early intervention in psoriasis and immune-mediated inflammatory diseases: A hypothesis paper. J Dermatolog Treat. 2015;26:103–12.
235. Ismail FF, May J, Moi J, Sinclair R. Clinical improvement in psoriatic nail disease and psoriatic arthritis with tildrakizumab treatment. Dermatol Ther. 2020;33:e13216.
236. Simpson K, Low ZM, Howard A, Kern JS. Successful management of treatment resistant nail psoriasis with tildrakizumab. Australas J Dermatol. 2021;62:390–3.
237. Brunasso A. Nail psoriasis improvement during Tildrakizumab therapy: A real-life experience. J Drugs Dermatol. 2022;21:914–6.
238. Fukasawa T, Yamashita T, Enomoto A, Norimatsu Y, Toyama S, Yoshizaki-Ogawa A, et al. The optimal use of tildrakizumab in the elderly via improvement of Treg function and its preventive effect of psoriatic arthritis. Front Immunol. 2023;14:1286251.
239. Shin HS, Sarin R, Dixit N, Wu J, Gershwin E, Bowman EP, et al. Crosstalk among IL-23 and DNAX activating protein of 12 kDa-dependent pathways promotes osteoclastogenesis. J Immunol. 2015;194:316–24.
240. Adamopoulos IE, Tessmer M, Chao CC, Adda S, Gorman D, Petro M, et al. IL-23 is critical for induction of arthritis, osteoclast formation, and maintenance of bone mass. J Immunol. 2011;187:951–9.
241. Buononato D, Licata G, Gambardella A, De Rosa A, Calabrese G, Argenziano G. Tildrakizumab: successful response in two patients with psoriatic arthritis. Dermatol Pract Concept. 2022;12:e2022049.
242. Mease PJ, Chohan S, Fructuoso FJG, Luggen ME, Rahman P, Raychaudhuri SP, et al. Efficacy and safety of tildrakizumab in patients with active psoriatic arthritis: results of a randomised, double-blind, placebo-controlled, multiple-dose, 52-week phase IIb study. Ann Rheum Dis. 2021;0:1–11.
243. Kok Y, Nicolopoulos J, Howard A, Dolianitis C, et al. Tildrakizumab in the treatment of moderate-to-severe hidradenitis suppurativa. Australas J Dermatol. 2020;61:e488–90.
244. Kok Y, Nicolopoulos J, Dolianitis C. Tildrakizumab as a potential long-term therapeutic agent for severe hidradenitis Suppurativa: A 15 months experience of an Australian institution. Australas J Dermatol. 2021;62:e313–6.
245. Kok Y, Nicolopoulos J, Varigos G, Howard A, Dolianitis C. Tildrakizumab in the treatment of PASH syndrome: A potential novel therapeutic target. Australas J Dermatol. 2020;6:e373–4.
246. Damsin T. A case of concurrent psoriasis and HidradenitisSuppurativa successfully treated with Tildrakizumab. DermatolTher. 2023;13:1611–5.
247. Frew JW. In search of therapeutic biomarkers to interleukin-23 antagonism in hidradenitis suppurativa. Br J Dermatol. 2023;188:588–9.

248. Xu A, Balgobind A, Strunk A, Garg A, Alloo A. Prevalence estimates for pyoderma gangrenosum in the United States: an age- and sex-adjusted population analysis. J Am Acad Dermatol. 2020;83:425–9.
249. McKenzie F, Cash D, Gupta A, Cummings LW, Ortega-Loayza AG. Biologic and small-molecule medications in the management of pyoderma gangrenosum. J Dermatolog Treat. 2019;30:264–76.
250. Prabhakara R, Harro JM, Leid JG, Keegan AD, Prior ML, Shirtliff ME. Suppression of the inflammatory immune response prevents the development of chronic biofilm infection due to methicillin-resistant Staphylococcus aureus. Infect Immun. 2011;79:5010–8.
251. John JM, Sinclair RD. Tildrakizumab for treatment of refractory pyoderma gangrenosum of the penis and polymyalgia rheumatica: killing two birds with one stone. Australas J Dermatol. 2020;61:170–1.
252. Leow LJ, Zubrzycki N. Recalcitrant ulcerative pyoderma Gangrenosum of the leg responsive to Tildrakizumab: A case report. Clin Cosmet Investig Dermatol. 2022;15:1729–36.
253. Sheriff TM, Murrell DF. Ustekinumab and tildrakizumab in pyoderma gangrenosum. Australas J Dermatol. 2021;62:114–5.
254. Bloch Y, Bouchareychas L, Merceron R, Składanowska K, Van den Bossche L, Detry S, et al. Structural activation of pro-inflammatory human cytokine IL-23 by cognate IL-23 receptor enables recruitment of the shared receptor IL-12Rβ1. Immunity. 2018;48:45–58.
255. Bernardini N, Skroza N, Tolino E, Mambrin A, Anzalone A, Balduzzi V, et al. IL-17 and its role in inflammatory, autoimmune, and oncological skin diseases: state of art. Int J Dermatol. 2020;59:406–11.
256. Kerkemeyer KLS, Sinclair R. Treatment of chronic alopecia areata with tildrakizumab: an open-label pilot study. Int J Dermatol. 2020;59:e136–7.
257. Vaccaro M, Cannavo SP, Imbesi S, Cristani M, Barbuzza O, Tigano V, et al. Increased serum levels of IL-23 circulating in patients with non- segmental generalized vitiligo. Int J Dermatol. 2015;54:672–4.
258. Jerjen R, Moodley A, Sinclair R. Repigmentation of acrofacial vitiligo with subcutaneous tildrakizumab. Australas J Dermatol. 2020;61:e446–8.
259. Mery-Bossard L, Bagny K, Chaby G, Khemis A, Maccari F, Marotte H, et al. New-onset vitiligo and progression of pre-existing vitiligo during treatment with biological agents in chronic inflammatory diseases. J Eur Acad Dermatol Venereol. 2017;31:181–6.
260. Leng RX, Pan HF, Chen GM, Wang C, Qin WZ, Chen LL, et al. IL-23: a promising therapeutic target for systemic lupus erythematosus. Arch Med Res. 2010;41:221–5.
261. Ismail FF, Sinclair RD, Pinczewski J. Refractory lupus erythematosus tumidus responsive to tildrakizumab. Dermatol Ther. 2019;32:e13070.
262. Lu R, Zeng X, Han Q, Lin M, Long L, Dan H, et al. Overexpression and selectively regulatory roles of IL-23/IL-17 axis in the lesions of oral lichen planus. Mediat Inflamm. 2014;2014:701094.
263. Ismail FF, Sinclair R. Clinical healing of erosive oral lichen planus with tildrakizumab implicates the interleukin-23/interleukin-17 pathway in the pathogenesis of lichen planus. Australas J Dermatol. 2020;61:e244–5.
264. Kherlopian A, Fischer G. Disease remission of refractory vulvovaginal and gingival lichen planus with tildrakizumab. Australas J Dermatol. 2021;62:246–7.
265. Kerkemeyer KL, Pinczewski J, Sinclair R. Successful treatment of recalcitrant lichen planus pemphigoides with tildrakizumab. Australas J Dermatol. 2020;61:e366–8.
266. De Carvalho L, Meah N, Wall D, Sinclair R. Recalcitrant lichen planopilaris and frontal fibrosing alopecia responding to tildrakizumab. Dermatol Ther. 2020;33:e13694.
267. Licata G, Gambardella A, Calabrese G, Pagluica F, Alfano R, Argenzianzo G. Refractory type I pityriasis rubra pilaris treated with tildrakizumab. Clin Exp Dermatol. 2021;46:1594–5.
268. Villa-Gonzalez JM, Gonzalez-Hermosa MR, Atxutegi-Ayestaran X, Nieto JAR, Garcia JG, Elgezua OL. Rapid response of erythrodermic pityriasis rubra pilaris to tildrakizumab. Clin Exp Dermatol. 2023:llad352. https://doi.org/10.1093/ced/llad352. [online ahead of print]

269. Feldmeyer L, Mylonas A, Demaria O, Mennella A, Yawalkar N, Laffitte E, et al. Interleukin 23-helper T cell axis as a treatment target for pityriasis rubra pilaris. JAMA Dermatol. 2017;153:304–8.
270. Merck and Co. ILUMYA™ (Tildrakizumab- asmn) Injection. U.S. Approval: 2018. Carlow:Merck and Co.
271. Khalilieh S, Hodsman P, Xu C, Tzontcheva A, Glasgow S, Montgomery D. Pharmacokinetics of Tildrakizumab (MK-3222), an anti-IL-23 monoclonal antibody, after intravenous or subcutaneous Administration in Healthy Subjects. Basic ClinPharmacolToxicol. 2018;123:294–300.
272. Mother To Baby | Fact Sheets [Internet]. Brentwood (TN): Organization of Teratology Information Specialists (OTIS); 1994. Tildrakizumab (Ilumya®) 2021 Apr 1. Available from: https://www.ncbi.nlm.nih.gov/books/NBK582978/
273. Haycraft K, DiRuggiero D, Rozzo SJ, Mendelsohn AM, Bhutani T. Outcomes of pregnancies from the tildrakizumab phase I-III clinical development programme. Br J Dermatol. 2020;183:184–6.
274. Smith CH, Yiu ZZN, Bale T, Burden AD, Coates LC, Edwards W, British Association of Dermatologists' Clinical Standards Unit, et al. British Association of Dermatologists guidelines for biologic therapy for psoriasis 2020: a rapid update. Br J Dermatol. 2020;183:628–37.
275. Ter Haar ELM, Van Den Reek JMPA, Gaarn Du Jardin K, Barbero-Castillo A, De Jong EMGJ, Lubeek SFK. Efficacy and safety of Tildrakizumab in older patients: pooled analyses of two randomized phase III clinical trials (reSURFACE 1 and reSURFACE 2) through 244 weeks. Acta Derm Venereol. 2023;103:adv17752.
276. Khalilieh S, Hussain A, Montgomery D, Levine V, Shaw PM, Bodrug I, et al. Effect of tildrakizumab (MK-3222), a high affinity, selective anti-IL23p19 monoclonal antibody, on cytochrome P450 metabolism in subjects with moderate to severe psoriasis. Br J Clin Pharmacol. 2018;84:2292–302.

Dupilumab

38

Introduction

Dupilumab is a fully human monoclonal IgG4 antibody, which in dermatology has been approved by the US Food and Drug Administration (FDA) for the treatment of moderate-to-severe atopic dermatitis (AD) in adults/paediatric patients (>6 months of age) and prurigo nodularis (PN) [1, 2]. Besides, it has also shown efficacy in various off-label dermatologic conditions.

Pharmacokinetics

Following a 600 mg subcutaneous (SC) injection of dupilumab, maximum serum concentrations are attained within 7 days, with steady-state concentrations available by week 16. Bioavailability of dupilumab is 64% and its $t_{1/2}$ ranges from 11.7 to 20.5 days [3, 4]. Being a human monoclonal IgG4 antibody, degradation of dupilumab occurs via catabolic pathways into small peptides similar to endogenous IgG. It is considered that following degradation, elimination occurs via the renal route [3].

Administration and Dosing

Dupilumab is administered subcutaneously. The recommended dose is 300 mg every fortnight after an initial loading dose of 600 mg (given as two 300 mg injections at different sites) [3]. However, some studies suggest weekly administration of 300 mg of dupilumab to be equally or even more effective than the current approved dosing schedule [5, 6].

A. K. Bubna, *Therapeutics in Dermatology - Essentials for Clinical Practice*, https://doi.org/10.1007/978-981-95-3791-4_38

Indications

FDA Approved

- Atopic dermatitis (AD).
- Prurigo nodularis (PN).

Off-Label

- Chronic hand eczema.
- Allergic contact dermatitis.
- Alopecia areata.
- Chronic urticaria.
- Bullous pemphigoid.
- Pemphigoid gestationis.
- Brunsting-Perry pemphigoid.
- Epidermolysis bullosa pruriginosa.
- Grover's disease.
- Hailey-Hailey disease.
- Pemphigus vulgaris.
- Lichen planus.
- Kimura's disease.
- Reactive perforating collagenosis.
- Lichen amyloidosis.
- Eosinophilic annular erythema.
- Chronic pruritus.
- Chronic actinic dermatitis.
- Cutaneous T-cell lymphoma.
- Wells' syndrome.
- Keloid/hypertrophic scars.
- Granuloma annulare.
- Hyper-IgE syndrome.
- Hidradenitis suppurativa.
- Neurofibromatosis.
- IPEX syndrome.
- Netherton syndrome.
- Papuloerythroderma of Ofuji.
- Recalcitrant palmoplantar pustulosis.
- Hyper-eosinophilic syndrome.
- Lamellar ichthyosis.
- Graft versus host disease.
- Trichothiodystrophy.

Contraindications

Absolute

- Hypersensitivity to dupilumab.

Relative

- Keratitis and conjunctivitis.
- Eosinophilic conditions.
- Helminth infections.
- Concurrent use of live vaccines.

Clinical Uses

Atopic Dermatitis

Profitability of dupilumab in AD was first exemplified in a robust, early-phase, development program by Beck et al. [7] At 12 weeks, 85% of dupilumab-treated patients achieved 50% reduction of the Eczema Area Severity Index (EASI) score compared to 35% in the placebo group ($p < 0.001$). Similarly, the pruritus Numeric Rating Scale (NRS) score reduced by 55.7% for dupilumab-treated patients, compared with 15.1% for the placebo group.

A larger, dose-ranging trial of 380 patients using five dupilumab dosing schedules with one placebo showed 300 mg weekly and biweekly dosing to be more effective than the 300 mg monthly, 200 mg biweekly and 100 mg monthly dosing schedules, with percentage reduction of the EASI being 73.7%, 68%, 64%, 65% and 45%, respectively. The placebo arm on the other hand depicted reduction of the EASI score by 18.1% ($p < 0.0001$) [8].

Dupilumab's efficacy in AD was further corroborated by two phase III studies: SOLO-1 and SOLO-2. In both programs, 1379 adult patients with moderate-to-severe AD were randomized to receive placebo or a 600 mg loading dose of dupilumab, followed by weekly or biweekly injections of dupilumab. In SOLO-1, Investigator's Global Assessment (IGA) score of 0 or 1 with a 2-point or greater improvement was reached by 37% in the weekly cohort, and 38% in the fortnightly cohort, with EASI-75 responses being achieved by 52% and 51% in both groups, respectively. In the placebo group, IGA score was sustained by 10%, and EASI-75 response was seen in 15% of the patients. In SOLO-2, both dupilumab groups achieved a 36% IGA response, with EASI-75 responses observed in 48% of patients receiving weekly dupilumab and 44% of patients receiving fortnightly dupilumab. The placebo group on the other hand demonstrated IGA and EASI-75 responses in 8% and12% of patients, respectively [4].

An additional phase III trial, CHRONOS, analysed concomitant topical corticosteroid (TCS) along with dupilumab versus placebo, over 52 weeks in moderate-to-severe AD. The EASI-75 response was obtained by week 16 and sustained through 1 year in 64% of patients treated with dupilumab (300 mg weekly) plus a TCS and in 65% of patients receiving dupilumab (300 mg fortnightly) plus a TCS. In the placebo group, the EASI-75 response at 1 year was reported in 22% of patients [9]. Other findings revealed through this study included fewer AD flares in both dupilumab groups (13% and 14% in those receiving it weekly and fortnightly, respectively, compared with 41% of those treated with placebo), reduction in TCS and systemic rescue therapy with 33.7% (weekly dupilumab) and 30.1% (fortnightly dupilumab) of topical and systemic medication free days versus 23.7% in the placebo group ($p < 0.0001$), statistically significant improvement in the pruritus NRS score at week 2 in the dupilumab plus TCS groups versus placebo, with improvements maintained through week 52, and parallel improvement in health-related quality of life (HR-QoL) and least square mean reduction from baseline in the Dermatology Life Quality Index (DLQI) scores of each group, along with statistically significant benefit in both dupilumab-treated groups ($p < 0.0001$) [9].

Moreover, the safety profile of dupilumab according to these trials (SOLO-1, SOLO-2 and CHRONOS) was comparable to placebo, with discontinuation rates being lower overall for dupilumab versus placebo (3% vs 8%, respectively).

Mechanism of action of dupilumab in AD is described in Fig. 38.1 [7, 10]. Dupilumab also significantly decreases serum levels of the chemokine CCL17, a key regulator of Th2-mediated immunity that is a specific and objective marker of AD disease activity [11].

Prurigo Nodularis

PN is a chronic cutaneous disorder presenting as multiple pruritic nodules particularly involving the trunk and extensor surfaces of the extremities. In 50% of cases, an atopic predisposition is present [12]. Although the pathogenic mechanism underlying PN is not clearly elucidated, an emerging role of Th2 signalling is suggested. Increased expression of phosphorylated signal transducer and activator of transcription (STAT) 6 (a key transcription factor mediating Th2 signalling), as well as upregulation of interleukin (IL)-31, IL-4 and IL-13 in PN-affected skin, majorly contributes towards the intense pruritus accounted in PN by activating sensory neuronal pathways following direct stimulation of Th2 inflammatory factor receptors in the sensory neurons of the dorsal root ganglia [13–15]. Dupilumab by binding to IL-4Rα (types I and II) and IL-13Rα1 receptors antagonizes Th2 cell-mediated inflammatory responses and blocks significant abnormal interactions and dysfunction between immune cells and neuronal circuits that drive the itch-scratch cycle in PN [7, 16].

Till date, around 120 PN patients with successful outcomes following dupilumab therapy (label dosing) in individual reports and case series have been reported [16–36]. Pruritus is generally the first symptom to respond in PN, followed by

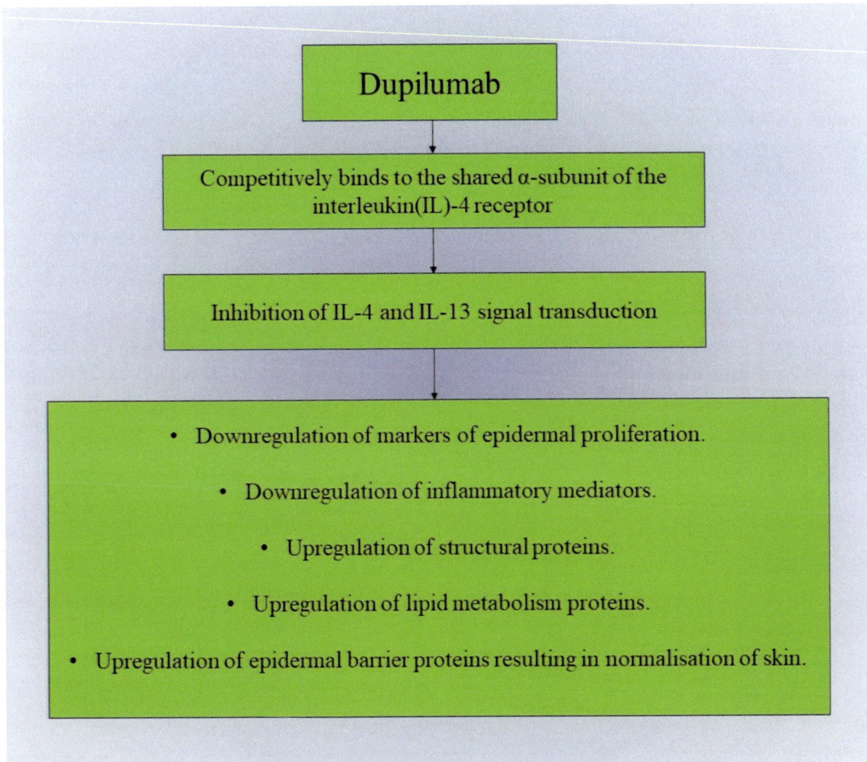

Fig. 38.1 Mechanism of action of dupilumab in atopic dermatitis

nodular regression. Besides, latency periods for the reduction of pruritus and clinical manifestations of PN vary from patient to patient. Further in atopics with PN, a faster response is obtained, although final outcomes in atopics and nonatopics are similar [7, 17].

In a systematic review by Husein-ElAhmed et al. [37], the authors concluded that following dupilumab therapy, complete remission can be expected if by 8 weeks patients observe clinical improvement and a 50% reduction of lesions on the NRS. Conversely, if amelioration of lesions occurs after 12 weeks and a 50% reduction of lesions is not achieved, obtaining a complete clinical response is unlikely.

Chronic Hand Eczema

In chronic hand eczema (CHE), clinical manifestations are diverse and pose diagnostic/therapeutic challenges. Further, the debilitating quality of CHE profoundly affects the QoL of patients [38]. Frequent phenotypes observed include dyshidrotic (vesicular) and hyperkeratotic/fissured hand eczema, allergic contact dermatitis and irritant contact dermatitis [39]. As IL-4R is highly elevated in CHE skin, IL-4/IL-13 may have a role in the pathophysiology of CHE, similar to that observed in AD. This imbrication of CHE and AD transcriptomes outlines the efficacy of dupilumab in CHE [40]. Currently, utility of dupilumab in CHE has been majorly demonstrated in case reports/case series, with two prospective observational studies and one retrospective review highlighting the same. [41–54]

Allergic Contact Dermatitis

Allergic contact dermatitis (ACD) is commonly seen in patients with AD, suggesting a type IV hypersensitivity reaction, associated with defective skin barrier function. Although Th1 and Th17 cells are traditionally considered the primary effector cells in ACD, recent studies have demonstrated cytokine responses to be hapten specific in ACD, with additional elaboration of Th2 and Th22 responses, depending on the involved allergen [55]. Besides, after prolonged/repeated allergen exposure in ACD, a predominant Th2 response is elicited [56].

The role of IL-4 in ACD has been substantiated by IL-4 knockout mice to contact allergens like oxazolone, characterized by Th2_mediated sensitization [57]. In addition, immunochemical analysis in ACD patients have revealed IL-4 receptor α-chain immunoreactivity and > five-fold increase in IL-4 mRNA levels, thereby concluding IL-4 and IL-13 as important cytokines in ACD [58, 59]. By targeting IL-4, dupilumab can reduce symptoms in this subset of patients. Moreover, as barrier function improves in patients with AD following dupilumab therapy, patients' susceptibility to allergens further reduce [60]. Besides, even in ACD not associated with AD, dupilumab maybe effective following failed immunosuppressive therapies [61].

Dupilumab has been particularly beneficial in ACD secondary to fragrances, balsam of Peru, sesquiterpene lactones, nickel, glues, textile, rubber, dyes, cosmetic preservatives and home care products [62–67]. Further, in systemic allergic dermatitis (SAD), namely, balsam and nickel allergy syndrome, where ACD remains uncontrolled despite prudent contact allergen avoidance, dupilumab has proven to be an efficacious solution [68]. However, even when on dupilumab, localized flares of ACD have been reported, necessitating simultaneous allergen avoidance. Additionally, in patients experiencing good clinical response with dupilumab, a trial of reexposure to contact allergens needs to be considered, and though dupilumab is effective in some cases of ACD, clinicians need to be aware that patients may not achieve complete clinical improvement and may benefit from shorter intervals/longer duration of follow-up, use of standardized assessments to monitor for clinical improvement and continued allergen avoidance [69]. Another point to consider is the occurrence of false-negative patch test reactions and recall dermatitis at patch test sites in patients on dupilumab for ACD. For this, repeat patch testing is warranted once dupilumab is discontinued. Moreover, patch testing in patients on dupilumab should always be interpreted with caution [70]. Currently, literature emphasizing the utility of dupilumab is limited to case reports/series with the need for RCTs to provide more evidence in this regard.

Alopecia Areata

Alopecia areata (AA) is an inflammatory non-scarring alopecia commonly encountered by dermatologists. Despite its increased prevalence, therapeutic outcomes of AA remain limited. Based on the fact that AA and AD demonstrate common inflammatory signalling pathways (including Th2 overactivation and upregulation of IL-4 and IL-13), the role of dupilumab in AA has been proposed [71, 72]. However, antagonistic Th2 effects by dupilumab results in dysregulation (either up- or down-regulation) of Th1/Th17 responses, causing a cytokine shift that eventually determines whether dupilumab will precipitate or remit AA [73]. Moreover, in patients with severe AD and AA, where massive release of interferon (IFN)-α is involved, control of AD is sufficient to allow resolution of AA with dupilumab. Conversely, in patients without preexisting AA in AD, dupilumab therapy heralds an immune shifting that paradoxically precipitates AA, mediated by autoreactive CD8+ T cells [74]. In addition, it is seen that reduction in serum levels of thymus and activation related chemokine (TARC) is associated with hair regrowth in AA, whereas elevation of TARC levels exacerbate AA following treatment with dupilumab [75]. Furthermore, blockade of IL-4 and IL-13 by dupilumab disrupts the interleukin milieu in sebaceous glands, resulting in sebaceous gland atrophy and non-scarring alopecia [76], which histologically does not express features of AA, suggesting dupilumab-induced non-scarring alopecia to be an AA-like drug reaction [77]. Interestingly, Stander et al. [78] have postulated that dupilumab neither induces nor improves AA, with the observed association being random, owing to high rates of spontaneous remission and IFN signature characterization in AA. Nevertheless, as reports exemplify both precipitation and alleviation of AA post-dupilumab therapy, studying them becomes essential [73, 75, 76, 78–90].

Chronic Urticaria

Chronic urticaria is a mast cell (MC)-mediated disease presenting as wheals, angioedema or both and lasting for >6 weeks. Although current management guidelines recommend a stepwise approach, beginning with antihistamine therapy and gradually escalating its dose, some patients remain refractory to the usual treatment guidelines that include omalizumab and cyclosporine [91]. Dupilumab is of particular value in those chronic urticaria patients who are unresponsive to omalizumab, in both chronic spontaneous urticaria (CSU) and chronic inducible urticaria [92–102].

Th2 inflammation dominates urticaria pathogenesis, wherein IL-4 and IL-5 stimulate the production of IgE antibodies that subsequently bind to the FcεRI, and promote MC degranulation. Further, IL-4 augments FcεRI cell surface expression, FcεRI α-specific mRNA and FcεRI-mediated histamine release. In addition, following long-term exposure, IL-4 alters human skin MCs by strengthening MC numbers and intensifying the processes associated with allergic inflammation. By blocking both IL-4 and IL-13, dupilumab halts the class switching of B-cell immunoglobulins towards IgE and ameliorates symptoms and signs associated with urticaria [97, 103–105].

In two RCTs that studied the efficacy of dupilumab in CSU for omalizumab-naïve patients (n = 138) and omalizumab intolerant/incomplete responders (n = 108), it was seen that in the omalizumab-naïve group, there was an 8.5 points higher reduction in the urticaria activity score over 7 days (UAS7) ($p = 0.0003$), as well as greater reduction of pruritus and wheals at week 24 (31.4% of patients), whereas in the omalizumab refractory group, the UAS7 score had reduced to zero in 13% of patients treated, and improvement in itch and hives severity demonstrated only a marginal statistical significance based on health authority hierarchy [106]. Apart from the above RCTs, remaining data for dupilumab in chronic urticaria are limited to case reports/series [93–98, 101, 102].

Bullous Pemphigoid

Bullous pemphigoid (BP) is the most common autoimmune subepidermal blistering disease of the skin, affecting all age groups, though most commonly encountered in the elderly [107]. Two target antigens, BP180 and BP230, are involved in blister formation in BP. Additionally, type 2 pro-inflammatory cytokines, namely, IL-4 and IL-13, have been detected in blister fluid/skin biopsies of BP patients, and increased levels of IgE and peripheral eosinophilia correlate with disease activity [108, 109]. Dupilumab in BP directly blocks IL-13 and IL-4 and indirectly downregulates IgE secretion and eosinophilic activity by inhibiting preactivated B-cell proliferation, directing human B lymphocytes to switch to IgG4, and plummeting eosinophilic chemotaxis and Th2-associated chemokine activity without significant modulation of Th1-associated genes [110, 111]. Besides, dupilumab reduces peripheral itch sensory neuronal signalling by antagonizing IL-4 and IL-13 and reducing IL-31 secretion from eosinophils and is of particular value in BP [112].

Dupilumab is effective in new/relapsed cases of BP, requiring at least 16–20 weeks to demonstrate disease clearance (defined as absence of both bulla and pruritus) or satisfactory response (defined as documented clinical improvement and patients desire to continue dupilumab) [113, 114]. Generally within 5 weeks, the consolidation phase (time at which no new lesions have developed for a minimum of 2 weeks and approximately 80% of lesions have healed) ends, with significant improvements being witnessed after 8 weeks of treatment initiation [114]. Pruritus is the first symptom to improve (as early as 1 week) majorly improving the patient's QoL [115]. Furthermore, dupilumab enables amelioration of blistering and intractable pruritus in those BP patients refractory to systemic glucocorticoids, multiple immunosuppressants, omalizumab, intravenous immunoglobins (IVIG), rituximab and plasmapheresis [116, 117]. Moreover, dupilumab can be combined with systemic glucocorticoids, azathioprine, mycophenolate mofetil (MMF), methotrexate, IVIG and rituximab to treat BP, enabling faster steroid taper, quicker dose reduction and subsequent stoppage of immunosuppressants [107, 113, 114, 116–119]. Interestingly, Yang et al. [120] demonstrated combination of dupilumab and low-dose glucocorticoids (0.4 mg/kg/day methylprednisolone) to be effective/safe in treating BP, allowing the cumulative dose of methylprednisolone to be >50% less than the conventional regimen and offering an added steroid-sparing advantage.

In addition, dupilumab delineates efficacy/safety in treating immune checkpoint inhibitor (ICI)-induced BP. Of the ICIs that induce BP, dupilumab has been effective against nivolumab and pembrolizumab [121, 122]. As traditional therapies like azathioprine and MMF are relatively contraindicated in these patients due to their concurrent malignancies, dupilumab serves as a valuable alternative because of lower rates associated with immunosuppression [122]. Cessation of new blister formation is usually evident by 1–2 months, following dupilumab treatment in these cases [121, 122]. Besides, dupilumab is safe as well as effective in elderly individuals and adolescents with refractory BP [107, 113–119]. Even so, as dupilumab has minimal immunosuppressive effects, it can be safely used in patients with tuberculosis and hepatitis C [115, 123]. In BP presently, the dose of dupilumab has not been standardized. In most patients, the AD dosing is employed. However, in patients not showing satisfactory responses, the dose can be augmented by 300 mg weekly or 600 mg every other week. This up dosing has been associated with clinical remission with no apparent adverse reactions [113, 120].

Furthermore, dupilumab's favourable discourse has been observed in BP variants like vesicular pemphigoid, erythrodermic pemphigoid and pemphigoid nodularis [123–125]. Currently, the utility of dupilumab in BP is only exemplified in case reports/series, with the need of RCTs to strengthen each observation [107, 113–120].

Pemphigoid Gestationis

Pemphigoid gestationis (PG) is a dermatosis of pregnancy presenting in the second and third trimester. Despite spontaneous improvement during late pregnancy, relapses during the time of delivery are typical. Recurrence in successive pregnancies is frequent, occasionally having an earlier onset that may pose the risk of prematurity and growth restriction for the foetus [126]. Owing to clinical and pathogenic similarities of PG and BP, dupilumab's utility in PG is considered.

Dupilumab (label dosing) in an anecdotal report demonstrated improvement of pruritus and bullous lesions in a 30-year-old woman with PG (20 weeks of gestation), along with prednisolone. Besides, following delivery, there was no recurrence in the postpartum period, and within 3 months, BP-180 antibodies had negativized. Even so, following the loading dose of dupilumab, only two maintenance doses were sufficient to control the disease. Moreover, no untoward events were witnessed in the mother and neonate [127].

Brunsting-Perry Pemphigoid

Brunsting-Perry Pemphigoid (BPP) is a clinical subtype of cicatricial pemphigoid (CP) without mucous membrane involvement, characterized clinically by subepidermal blisters, erosions, haemorrhagic crusts and atrophic scars confined to the head, neck and upper trunk [128]. Dupilumab outlined favourable effects in two patients with BPP, unresponsive to conventional therapy (that included systemic steroids, MMF, methotrexate, dapsone, doxycycline, nicotinamide and rituximab). Rapid improvement and clearance of lesions were observed after the completion of three doses of dupilumab [129, 130]. As pathogenesis in BPP comprises lymphocytosis, eosinophilia, elevated levels of basement membrane IgG and tissue scarring/fibrosis, the role of dupilumab in BPP has been propounded [129].

Epidermolysis Bullosa Pruriginosa

Epidermolysis bullosa pruriginosa (EBP) is a rare clinical subtype of autosomal dominant (or less commonly recessive) dystrophic epidermolysis bullosa (DEB). In addition to usual manifestations of DEB like skin fragility (secondary to trauma), milia and nail dystrophy, EBP presents with severe pruritus, prurigo nodularis and lichen simplex chronicus-like lesions, often complicating the clinical diagnosis [131]. Proposed mechanism of dupilumab in EBP is blockade of IL-4Rα-induced sensitization of sensory neurons to pruritogens, thereby interrupting the itch-scratch cycle, a critical component in the recovery of lesions in EBP [14]. However, expressions of IL-4 and IL-13 in EBP remain to be investigated. Nevertheless, as dupilumab has been successful in the treatment of a variety of pruritic diseases, dupilumab may be considered a good choice in EBP [132]. At present, only case reports/series have elaborated the usefulness of dupilumab in EBP, with RCTs being needed to strengthen these findings [132–135].

Grover's Disease

Grover's disease (GD) is an inflammatory immune disorder presenting as flesh-coloured to erythematous, oedematous papules, and/or papulovesicles, commonly involving the trunk and proximal extremities of middle-aged men [136]. Apart from its idiopathic occurrence, GD has been reported following conventional chemotherapy, ICI therapy, recombinant human IL-4 therapy and ipilimumab (anti-CTLA-4 monoclonal antibody) therapy [137–140]. The pathophysiology of GD is yet to be elucidated, though some reports suggest an overexpression of IL-4 to play a role [141]. Furthermore, with increasing age, the Th1/Th2 system is skewed towards a Th2-inflammation profile, with enhanced nonspecific B-cell activation and IgE antibody production [142, 143]. Based on these postulations, dupilumab has been employed in the treatment of GD. Currently, two individual reports and a case series of three patients have elaborated dupilumab's contribution in GD [144–146]. In all, within 12–14 weeks of dupilumab treatment, complete regression of dermatologic signs and pruritus was observed, without the occurrence of any untoward event.

Hailey-Hailey Disease

Hailey-Hailey disease (HHD) is an autosomal dominant genodermatosis principally characterized by flaccid blisters and malodorous erosions involving intertriginous areas, often accompanied by chronic pruritus. Mutations in the ATP2C1 gene is responsible for defective keratinocyte cell-to-cell adhesion leading to acantholysis [147]. Although not indicated for HHD, few reports have delineated dupilumab to be effective for the same [148–151]. As the mechanism of dupilumab in HHD is unclear, it is proposed that blockade of IL-4 and IL-13 may interfere with the agonistic effects of the cytokine CCL26 on CCR3, thereby preventing activation and chemotaxis of eosinophils, basophils and Th2 lymphocytes, with subsequent inhibition of intracellular calcium release [152]. Right now, the optimal dose and frequency of dupilumab in HHD is not known, and some patients may benefit with more frequent injections.

Pemphigus Vulgaris

Pemphigus vulgaris (PV) is an intraepidermal immunobullous disorder targeting desmosomal adhesion proteins, desmoglein (Dsg) 1 and Dsg 3 [153]. Although systemic glucocorticoids remain the first-line therapy for PV, requirement for high dosage and long-term usage often herald untoward events. Moreover, other immunosuppressive drugs like rituximab, azathioprine, MMF, cyclophosphamide and methotrexate are not viable options in patients with an underlying infection.

Presently, the utility of dupilumab in PV has been exemplified in two case reports [154, 155]. In the first report (35-year-old male), the patient had PV along with pulmonary Kochs and was on antitubercular therapy. As an underlying sepsis was suspected, the dose of methylprednisolone (40 mg/day) could not be increased and dupilumab (label dosing) was added to the therapeutic regimen, along with antibiotics and low-dose IVIG (15 gms for 4 days). The above combination resulted in regression of lesions with the Pemphigus Disease Area Index (PDAI) decreasing from 97 to 42 after 45 days of treatment, along with reduction of blood IgE levels and eosinophil count [154]. The second report delineated dupilumab (label dosing) monotherapy to be effective in PV following failed treatment with systemic steroids. Within 4 weeks, marked improvement was noticed, but as fledgeling oral lesions continued erupting within days before the next dose, weekly dupilumab (300 mg) injections were given that resulted in healing of all lesions by 6 weeks [155].

In acute PV, higher concentrations of serum IgE and IgG4 antibodies are seen along with IgE epidermal deposits. As Th2 cells assist formation of IgG1 and IgG4 antibodies against Dsgs, dupilumab's role in PV is postulated. By antagonizing IL-4, dupilumab affects IgE-related signalling via IL-4 on Th2 cells and ameliorates the pathogenic cascade [156, 157]. RCTs with dupilumab in PV become essential to strengthen its utility for this indication.

Lichen Planus

Profitability of dupilumab in lichen planus (LP) has been expounded in a 52-year-old man who had been unresponsive to systemic corticosteroids and acitretin. Following 3 months of treatment with dupilumab (label dosing), remarkable improvement in lesions was observed and his NRS itch intensity plummeted from 9/10 to 1/10 [158]. In another report, dupilumab (label dosing) promoted rapid resolution of widespread cutaneous LP and generalized pruritus in a 92-year-old female following 2 months of treatment [159].

The role of Th2 cells and Th2-related chemokines has been proposed in the pathogenesis of LP, with elevated levels of IL-6, that consequently increases IL-4. By inhibiting IL-4, dupilumab decreases subsequent effector cell function that can have value in LP [160–162]. Nonetheless, more studies are essential to substantiate this concept further.

Lichen Planus Pemphigoids

Lichen planus pemphigoids (LPP) is a rare autoimmune immunobullous disorder with overlapping clinical features between LP and BP. As lichenoid lesions typically precede bulla formation, it is suggested that epitope spreading following lichenoid inflammation and subsequent antibody formation against basement membrane zone (BMZ) proteins are responsible for the lesional phenotype of LPP [163]. Dupilumab decreases inflammation by modulating the signalling of two key cytokines, IL-4 and IL-13, responsible for dysregulating the Th2 cell pathway towards BP180 NC16A (the target autoantibody in LPP) and in this way may help in bringing about disease remission [164].

Literature search revealed two case reports describing the beneficial effects of dupilumab in LPP. In one report (an 18-year-old male), dupilumab (label dosing) monotherapy was employed owing to patients concerns regarding treatment with steroids and MMF. After 15 weeks of dupilumab treatment, patient achieved complete clinical remission. Moreover, following 4 months of treatment cessation, patient remained lesion free [164]. In the other report (69-year-old man), dupilumab (label dosing) along with prednisolone (50 mg/day) was used for LPP with rapid improvement of lesions in 3 days and 90% clearance by 2 months, along with normalization of the eosinophil percentage and serum anti-BP180NC16A IgG levels [165].

Kimura's Disease

Kimura's disease (KD) is a rare, idiopathic benign condition characterized by localized lymphoid proliferation mainly involving the head and neck regions. The Th2 pathway is involved in the pathogenesis of KD, with elevated expression of IL-4, IL-5 and IL-13 mRNA in peripheral blood mononuclear cells in patients with KD

[166, 167]. Recent evidence has highlighted the existence of CD4 + GATA3+ T cells in the affected lymph nodes of KD patients that, following stimulation by IL-4 and IL-5, synthesize IgE with subsequent eosinophil aggregation [168, 169]. Inhibition of IL-4 with dupilumab effectively reduces tumour mass by substantial reduction of eosinophils within the tumour. Besides, this action of dupilumab is independent of IgE. Current literature describing the role of dupilumab in KD is confined to case reports, wherein dupilumab monotherapy as well as its combination with surgical excision following therapeutic failure with systemic corticosteroids, tetracycline and omalizumab has been employed. In all reports, improvement was demonstrated within a period of 2–16 months, with no recurrence at follow-up. Moreover, dupilumab maintained acceptable levels of safety and tolerability [170–175].

Chronic Pruritus

Chronic pruritus (CP), though a common symptom of dermatologic and systemic medical disorders, can arise even in the absence of a well-defined rash or systemic disease, when it is referred to as chronic pruritus of unknown origin (CPUO). Regardless of its origin, CP markedly impairs the QoL of patients and needs to be appropriately managed. Often, CP can be refractory to various therapies that include topical/systemic CS, antihistamines, antidepressants, opioid antagonists, cannabinoids and anticonvulsants [176].

In CPUO, itch lasts >6 weeks, with recent studies outlining Th2 cytokines like IL-4, IL-13 and IL-31 in being instrumental for promoting pruritus via effects on sensory neurons. By blocking IL-4 and IL-13, dupilumab suppresses neuronal hypersensitivity, thereby alleviating itching [14]. Besides, by decreasing the production of IL-31 from Th2 cells, dupilumab further promotes improvement of CPUO [177].

In several reports, the efficacy of dupilumab in CPUO has been demonstrated utilizing numeric scales, including a series of 15 patients wherein the mean itch NRS score reduced by 7 points (SD 1.9) [178], and a series of 6 patients outlining a mean reduction of 8.75 points (SD 1.26) for the same [179]. In Zhai et al.'s case series, the mean NRS itch intensity reduced from 9.6 at baseline to 3.2 at 12 weeks [180], and in another series, within 4 weeks of dupilumab therapy, highly satisfactory reduction of CPUO was noted, allowing drug withdrawal, with persistence of the improved status at 20 weeks of follow-up [181]. Interestingly, of all the reported patients, only one had coexistent AD.

Moreover, dupilumab's effectiveness has been outlined in six cases of uraemic pruritus (UP) [180, 182]. Silverberg and Brieva in their report elucidated significant improvement of UP in a 45-year-old patient diagnosed with polycystic kidney disease. After 6 months of dupilumab treatment, there was marked improvement in the average pruritus NRS score and DLQI by 6 and 11 points, respectively [182].

Further, in an anecdotal report, dupilumab delineated profitability in the treatment of brachioradial pruritus in a 53-year-old woman with history of fibromyalgia and bulging cervical disc. Within 3 months of dupilumab therapy, there was 95% improvement of itching [183]. Additionally, dupilumab's effectiveness in recalcitrant anal and genital pruritus has been elaborated in an isolated report. Following 1 month of dupilumab therapy, there was 95% resolution of itching, and physical examination revealed complete clearance of perianal dermatitis [184]. Interestingly, in a 5-year-old girl with TTC7A mutation, dupilumab (100 mg SC every 2 weekly) was successful in controlling pruritus as early as few days following the first injection, with no relapse of pruritus at 1 year of follow-up [185].

Chronic Actinic Dermatitis

Chronic actinic dermatitis (CAD) is an immune-mediated photodermatosis characterized by persistent pruritic eczematous plaques involving the sun-exposed sites. Pathogenesis of CAD involves a delayed hypersensitivity reaction to antigens developed in patient's skin following molecular alteration, secondary to stimulation by UV rays. The acute phase of CAD is characterized by Th2 overactivation, whereas in the chronic stage apart from active Th1 responses, Th2 responses are sustained. Besides, UV irritation suppresses Th1 cells and enhances antigen presentation capacity of Th2 cells resulting in a Th1/Th2 disbalance [186]. Further in CAD, UVB-induced CD3+, CD4+ and CD8- regulatory T cells mediate their suppressive effects by releasing IL-4 and IL-10 [187]. It is suggested that dupilumab particularly interacts with Th2-mediated inflammatory pathways in CAD to bring about disease control.

Five publications have reported the treatment of 11 patients with CAD using dupilumab (label dosing). All patients had failed to appropriately respond to at least one line of previous therapy such as TCS, methotrexate, MMF, azathioprine, apremilast, hydroxychloroquine and cyclosporine. Besides, all patients tolerated dupilumab therapy well. Of the 11 patients, conjunctivitis developed in 3 patients, facial erythema in 1 and diffuse pigmentation in 1. However, apart from the patient who developed facial redness, dupilumab therapy continued in others [188–192].

Cutaneous T-Cell Lymphoma

Mycosis fungoides (MF) is the most common variant of cutaneous T-cell lymphoma (CTCL) and Sezary syndrome (SS) is the erythrodermic variant of MF. A predominant Th2 cytokine milieu, similar to AD consisting of IL-4, IL-5, IL-10 and IL-13, is observed in MF. Besides, MF and SS may often masquerade as adult-onset AD, and SS has been reported in patients with AD during the disease course [193, 194]. Theoretically, owing to the Th2 cytokine profile, dupilumab may be effective in MF/SS. However, the efficacy of dupilumab in CTCL has demonstrated failure in most reports with exacerbation of existing lesions and development of new lesions [195–201], Moreover, despite initial improvement with dupilumab, subsequent worsening and disease progression with potentially fatal outcomes of MF/SS has been observed. The initial improvement seen may be following transient blockade of Th2 inflammation, with shifting to a Th1 tumour-suppressive effect via IFNα secretion [193], but as disease progresses, tumour cells escape dupilumab targeting and resistant clones emerge, making CTCL cells immune to IL-4 and IL-13 blockade [193, 201].

Although few reports have shown dupilumab to be effective in MF/SS, long-term data are lacking, and dupilumab cannot be used as a general drug for MF/SS because there exists no clarity regarding which cases would benefit from dupilumab without worsening. Lazaridou et al. [202], in their series of two patients, highlighted dupilumab to be effective in one patient (55-year-old-male) resulting in improvement of pruritus and partial remission of MF after 4 months of follow-up. Mollanazar et al. [203] demonstrated dupilumab to be a highly effective adjunct drug in bringing about dramatic improvement of AD and CTCL in a 68-year-old man where comprehensive multimodality therapy (with bexarotene, IFNα, IFNγ, narrow-band UVB irradiation and extracorporeal photopheresis [ECP]) for 6 months resulted only in partial remission. Steck et al. [204] reported marked improvement of skin symptoms after addition of dupilumab to ECP in a 74-year-old woman with SS.

Nevertheless, as of now, given the potential of dupilumab to deteriorate MF/SS, its use in CTCL can only be implemented in selective situations.

Wells' Syndrome

Wells' syndrome (WS) is an eosinophilic inflammatory disorder whose pathogenesis is poorly understood and is clinically characterized by recurrent cutaneous lesions of variable latency. Overexpression of IL-4/IL-13 is observed in hypereosinophilic syndromes, which go on to stimulate the recruitment and growth of eosinophils via IgE production, and differentiation of B cells. Further, these activated eosinophils promote release of pre-formed IL-4/IL-13 that potentiate Th2 immune responses [205].

By directly/indirectly inhibiting eosinophil-associated Th2 inflammatory cascades (through an unknown mechanism), dupilumab may be efficacious in WS. Currently, there are two case reports elaborating the benefits of dupilumab in WS [206, 207]. In the first report (52-year-old woman), after an initial lesional flare at 4 weeks following dupilumab therapy (label dosing), lesions eventually completely resolved by 6 months [206]. In the second patient (80-year-old woman), dupilumab (400 mg loading dose and then 200 mg q2w) along with dapsone (100 mg/day) eventuated in almost complete clinical remission within 5 weeks of treatment [207]. Besides, no adverse events were encountered in both reports.

Keloids and Hypertrophic Scars

Keloids and hypertrophic scars (HTS) represent an increased connective tissue response to meagre injury. Both keloids and HTS are benign, well-demarcated fibrotic growths; only that keloids extend beyond the original margins of the defect, whereas HTS remain confined to the original defect. Elevated expression of IL-4/IL-13 receptors in keloids, as well as increased production of IL-4/IL-13 in chronic lesional and non-lesional keloidal skin, provides the basis for dupilumab's implementation in the management of keloids. Furthermore, enhanced levels of IL-13/IL-4 potentiates TGF-β signalling in keloidal fibroblasts and promotes fibrosis via periostin, which again is considerably suppressed by dupilumab [208, 209].

Till date, two reports have elaborated the utility of dupilumab in keloids [210, 211]. In the first report (a 53-year-old male, with two keloids and concurrent AD), within 7 months of dupilumab therapy, complete disappearance of the smaller keloid and shrinkage of ~50% of the larger keloid were noted, with visibility of normal skin lines [210]. In the second patient (37-year-old woman), though there was no reduction of keloidal size following 3 months of dupilumab treatment, there was near complete absence of her incapacitating symptoms, and she was now able to perform her routine delay activates without any discomfort [211]. Despite the above positive reports, a shared decision-making is essential to employ dupilumab for keloids, owing to high costs involved, and optimal duration of treatment still needing elucidation. Besides, nonresponsiveness of dupilumab in keloids have also been outlined, making appropriate patient selection critical [212, 213].

For HTS, an isolated report demonstrated dupilumab to considerably alleviate the symptomology and size of lesions after 10 months of therapy. However, as little is known about the cytokine involvement in HTS, more research becomes essential for the same [214].

Granuloma Annulare

Granuloma annulare (GA) is a therapeutically challenging necrobiotic disorder. Although Th1 cytokine levels are generally raised in GA, overexpression of the Th2 axis has been recently propounded. By blocking Th2 cytokines, dupilumab may help in the regression of GA in selected patients [215].

In a recent report of a 74-year-old woman with GA, where potent topical steroids, oral antibiotics, hydroxychloroquine, methotrexate, niacinamide, allopurinol and adalimumab had failed, dupilumab (label dosing) demonstrated complete clearance of most lesions at 4-week follow-up and significant reduction of erythema and induration in the other lesions, which was maintained at 3 months. Based on this anecdotal report, it needs to be contemplated whether dupilumab can duplicate the efficacious results produced by TNFα blockers in GA or whether it should be reserved in those GA cases where anti-TNFα therapy has failed [216].

Reactive Perforating Collagenosis

Reactive perforating collagenosis (RPC) is the most common acquired perforating disorder (APD). Although its pathogenesis remains undefined, repeated scratching secondary to intense pruritus constitutes an integral pathogenic trigger for RPC. In APD, IL-4, IL-13 and IL-31 act as regulators of chronic itch. In addition, IL-4 promotes neuronal hypersensitivity to other strong pruritogens like histamine, IL-31 and cytokine-thymic stromal lymphopoietin [217]. Owing to dupilumab's antipruritic properties, the rationale for its use in APD has been suggested. Besides, when pruritus is reduced, skin trauma eventually decreases, preventing further disease progression.

Ying et al. recently reported complete clearance of RPC after 3 months of dupilumab in two elderly AD patients [218]. This was followed by two individual reports reiterating similar findings. In one report, a nearly complete response was seen after 12 months of dupilumab therapy, whereas in the other, pruritus cleared completely after 2 weeks with gradual amelioration of lesions by 10 weeks of dupilumab therapy [219, 220].

Lichen Amyloidosis

Lichen amyloidosis (LA) is the most common form of primary cutaneous amyloidosis and is often resistant to various forms of therapy. Previous studies elucidate the role of IL-31 for the intense pruritus seen in LA. Besides, IL-13 expression has been detected in keratinocytes and dermal infiltrates of LA lesions [221, 222]. By directly blocking IL-13 and IL-4 signalling in sensory neurons and inhibiting Th2 cells from producing IL-31 (a potent itch inciter), dupilumab helps in alleviating pruritus in LA that eventuates in ultimate resolution of skin lesions [222]. Profitability of dupilumab in LA has been elaborated in two-case reports. Within 2–4 weeks of treatment, dramatic improvement of pruritus was noticed, and by 3 months, papular lesions of LA steadily flattened and reduced in size and number [222, 223].

Eosinophilic Annular Erythema

Eosinophilic annular erythema (EAE) is a chronic inflammatory disorder presenting as annular erythematous plaques and tissue eosinophilia and is marked by its refractoriness to most treatments. EAE results following various triggers that lead to IL-5 release and increased eosinophilic chemotaxis. These activated eosinophils produce IL-4 and IL-13 that facilitate disease persistence. By blocking IL-4/IL-13, dupilumab plummets eosinophil activity, and eventual reduction of eosinophil-related cytokines and IgE [224]. Presently, dupilumab's efficacy in EAC has been described in two-case reports with favourable results. In both reports, rapid and complete remission of lesions was obtained after the second injection of dupilumab with sustained remission at 5–6 months of follow-up [224, 225].

Netherton's Syndrome

Netherton's syndrome (NS) is a rare autosomal recessive genetic disorder characterized by a triad of congenital ichthyosis, trichorrhexis invaginata and severe atopy. Treatment options for NS are mostly symptomatic and publications regarding the efficacy of biologicals in NS is scarce. Deficiency of LEKTI (a serine protease inhibitor) in NS impairs the cutaneous barrier, thereby triggering percutaneous allergen sensitization and overproduction of Th2 cytokines [226]. Besides, increased IL-4 production in T-cell subsets induces B-cell proliferation and IgE production [169]. Following antagonism of IL-4Rα by dupilumab, gradual decline of IL-6/IL-8 is observed (with normal levels of IL-4 and IL-5 remaining). Owing to reduced IL-6 levels, B-cell induction and IgE secretion in NS plummet and decreased IL-8 levels promotes reduced dermal neutrophilic chemotaxis, thus alleviating cutaneous inflammation [227]. As of now, dupilumab's utility in NS is confined to case reports/series with improvements visible by 2 weeks to 10 months of therapy. Besides, dupilumab has been well tolerated by patients, with drug discontinuation in two patients being secondary to suboptimal responses rather than drug-related toxicity [228–238].

Papuloerythroderma of Ofuji

Papuloerythroderma of Ofuji (PEO) is a distinct dermatologic entity commonly affecting elderly males and presenting as confluent papules with characteristic sparing of skin folds. Th2 cells are characteristically involved in the pathogenesis of PEO along with elevation in serum TARC levels. TARC is a Th2-type chemokine that attracts CC chemokine receptor-4-positive cells and is a useful clinical biomarker for PEO [239]. As PEO is a Th2-mediated disease, dupilumab has expressed profitability in its management. In three-case reports from Japan, dupilumab (label dosing) was effective in bringing about remission of PEO within 2–4 months of treatment [240–242]. Despite these positive preliminary findings, RCTs become mandatory to substantiate these results further.

Hidradenitis Suppurativa

Hidradenitis suppurativa (HS) is a disorder of the pilosebaceous apparatus commonly involving the intertriginous sites and, if extensive, can be debilitating. Expression of enzymes generating sphingomyelins and ceramide is significantly reduced in HS lesional skin, whereas there is an increased expression of enzymes converting ceramide to galactosyl ceramide and gangliosides [243]. Dupilumab's propitious effects in HS may be linked with its ability to alter the sphingolipid metabolism [244]. Current medical literature elaborates two case reports on dupilumab's utility for HS. Both patients (50–/43-year-old males) had Hurley stage 2 disease. In one patient following 4 months of dupilumab (label dosing) therapy, Hidradenitis Suppurativa Clinical Response (HiSCR) was obtained, whereas in the other patient after 4 months of dupilumab therapy, DLQI reduced to 3 from 25. Besides, both patients tolerated the drug with no adverse events being reported [244, 245].

Hyperimmunoglobulin E Syndrome

Hyperimmunoglobulin E syndrome (HIES) is a rare immunodeficiency syndrome presenting as atopic dermatitis, recurrent cutaneous/pulmonary infections and high serum IgE levels. Clinically and mechanistically eczema in HIES largely overlaps with AD. Heterozygous mutations in STAT3 gene are responsible for majority cases of HIES, although other genetic mutations are also encountered. These mutations impair IFNγ production and IL-10 signal transduction, resulting in an unbalanced IL-4 state. Besides, there is reduction in T-cell receptor signalling along with dysfunction of regulatory T cells with eventual Th2 cell expansion [246]. Dupilumab's inhibitory effects on IL-4 and IL-13 signalling may explain its efficacy in HIES. Literature search revealed 12 patients with HIES who were treated with dupilumab. Of them, seven had mutations of STAT-3, three of DOCK8 and one with ZNF391. Pruritus and skin lesions completely resolved in 10 patients, and in 2 patients, partial remission was obtained. In all patients, substantial improvement of eczema and pruritus were evident as early as 1–2 months of therapy with dupilumab, along with sustained maintenance as treatment progressed [247–257].

Neurofibromatosis

In an isolated report, dupilumab's effectiveness in reducing the size and swelling of neurofibromas in a patient with type 1 neurofibromatosis (NF-1) who had been primarily started with dupilumab for AD was discovered as a collateral finding. Furthermore, after 16 weeks, besides complete remission of AD, there was no progression of NF-1 [258]. The inhibitory effect of dupilumab on neurofibromas may be linked to the interference of IL-4/IL-13 binding to type 1 and type 2 receptors expressed on mast cells and fibroblasts. In this way, excessive production of collagen is halted, thereby inhibiting neurofibroma development [169]. Despite this promising report, need for more clinical trials become mandatory to substantiate the utility of dupilumab for this indication.

IPEX Syndrome

Immune dysregulation, polyendocrinopathy, enteropathy, X-linked (IPEX) syndrome is an X-linked condition. An anecdotal report of a 2-month-old boy with IPEX syndrome described dupilumab (200 mg SC every 4 weeks) to be effective in bringing about improvement of pruritus and almost complete resolution of dermatitis following 3 months of therapy, without the development of additional autoimmune disorders [259]. Because of FOXP3 mutations in IPEX syndrome, an alteration in the function of regulatory T cells occurs that skews the immune system towards a Th2 predominance, explaining the propitious effects of dupilumab in this scenario [259]. More clinical reports however are needed to confirm dupilumab's efficacy for IPEX syndrome.

Recalcitrant Palmoplantar Pustulosis

In a report by Smith et al. [260], dupilumab (label dosing) demonstrated efficacy for the treatment of recalcitrant palmoplantar pustulosis (PPP) in a 60-year-old smoker woman, who had been unresponsive to various topical agents as well as dapsone, acitretin, apremilast and secukinumab. Within 30 days of treatment, pustules, pruritus, hyperkeratotic scales and erythema resolved with residual hyperpigmentation. In PPP, a complex Th2/Th17 cell activation pattern has been identified with prominent Th2 signature in skin samples and Th-17 skewed inflammation in blood samples. Besides, CD4+ T cells in the skin and peripheral blood co-express Th17 and Th2 markers, suggesting a Th17-to-Th2 plasticity [261]. Based on these postulations, dupilumab may be beneficial in PPP owing to the skewed Th2 pattern.

Hyper-Eosinophilic Syndrome

Hyper-eosinophilic syndrome (HES) are rare disorders defined by persistent peripheral eosinophilia (absolute eosinophil count >$1.5x10^9$/L), plus evidence of organ involvement [262]. These disorders are very difficult to treat, requiring immunomodulators that have substantial side effects. With the emergence of biologicals, an alternative treatment modality becomes available in the management of HES [262, 263].

Dupilumab may benefit a subset of patients of HES, owing to its ability to antagonize IL-4 and IL-13 signalling. A total of 11 patients with HES, 7 of which with cutaneous manifestations, were treated with dupilumab following failure with systemic steroids. Of the 7 patients, 5 reported varied levels of improvement of skin lesions. In all patients, dupilumab was dosed as per the standard AD schedule along with other concomitant drugs that included hydroxyurea, gabapentin and tapering systemic steroids. Improvement of dermatologic lesions were evident by 4–7 weeks of treatment initiation. Besides, all patients tolerated dupilumab, without the occurrence of any major adverse event [262–264].

Lamellar Ichthyosis

Lamellar ichthyosis (LI) is a rare autosomal recessive cornification disorder with a variable genetic inheritance pattern. Of late, an association of AD with LI has been iterated. Dupilumab (label dosing) was found to be effective in treating a 22-year-old male with LI and AD, with marked clinical improvement after 3 months of drug initiation [265]. The exact mechanism for the activity of dupilumab in LI still requires elucidation.

Graft Versus Host Disease

Graft versus host disease (GVHD) is one of the most severe complications of allogenic hematopoietic stem cell transplantation (HSCT) and often presents as a multiorgan disease with cutaneous features being the first to manifest. In two case series consisting of four paediatric patients, dupilumab was successful in treating AD like GVHD following HSCT that was recalcitrant to conventional therapies [266, 267]. Although the pathogenesis of AD-like GVHD is not clearly delineated, research suggests that it may involve a Th2 response as evidenced by increased levels of eosinophils, IgE, Th2 cells and regulatory T cells in some patients, [268] thereby accounting for dupilumab's promising response. Nevertheless, more research is essential to appropriately outline dupilumab's role for GVHD.

Food Allergy

Dupilumab was effective in allowing a 30-year-old woman with severe AD to tolerate canned corn and pistachios that had induced anaphylactic shock and generalized urticaria, respectively, earlier on. Dupilumab's effect may be secondary to its inhibitory action on IL-4/IL-13 signalling, reducing the recruitment of MCs at the intestinal level and diminishing the clinical expression of food allergy [269]. However, RCTs need to be undertaken to further substantiate this finding.

Trichothiodystrophy

Gruber et al. [270] delineated dupilumab to be effective in an 8-year-old boy with trichothiodystrophy (TTD) that was unresponsive to topical glucocorticoids/tacrolimus (0.03%), ceramides and vitis vinifera seed oil, as well as systemic antihistamines. Within 3 months of dupilumab treatment, ichthyosis, eczema and pruritus, all significantly subsided and after 1 year of dupilumab therapy, patient's skin appeared almost normal. Although the eczema in TTD has not been characterized in detail, it is most likely that a Th2-driven inflammation is responsible, thus making dupilumab helpful here.

Adverse Effects

Nasopharyngitis, upper respiratory tract infection, injection site reactions, skin infections and conjunctivitis are the most common adverse reactions associated with dupilumab, which is mild to moderate in nature [4, 9]. Interestingly, trials with dupilumab for asthma and nasal polyposis have not reported any increased incidence of conjunctivitis; therefore, conjunctivitis may be a risk related to an underlying AD pathogenesis and not specifically to dupilumab itself [4]. The safety profile of dupilumab can therefore be adjudged as favourable and consistent, both as monotherapy and in combination with TCS for AD. Nevertheless, long-term data is needed to fully determine dupilumab's safety and tolerability.

Use in Pregnancy and Lactation

Since IgG antibodies can cross the placenta, possibility of dupilumab's transmission from the mother to foetus exists. In several case reports where dupilumab was discontinued a few weeks after conception, it did not demonstrate any foetal harm. However, more research is mandated to analyse the harmful effects of dupilumab used continually during pregnancy [271].

It is unknown whether dupilumab is excreted in breast milk or systemic absorption occurs after ingestion. Given the large size of dupilumab, its amount in breast milk is expected to be low. Further, as it gets destroyed in the infant's digestive tract, its absorption is unlikely. Nevertheless, it is crucial to assess the importance of breast milk, along with the mother's medical indication and urgency for dupilumab use [271].

Future Direction

As dupilumab's propensity to cause immunosuppression is considerably low compared to other biologicals, its utility in vesiculobullous disorders as monotherapy as well as in combination with systemic CS and conventional immunosuppressive drugs needs scrupulous evaluation. RCTs done in this regard can enable outlining a valid protocol regarding dosing schedules and duration of dupilumab therapy for these disorders. Further, owing to the risk of infections associated with systemic CS and the usual immunosuppressive agents for vesiculobullous disorders, the therapeutic discourse is often interrupted and does not have a smooth progression. In these situations, dupilumab can prove to be advantageous. However, more evidence is required to confirm these postulations.

Conclusion

Though primarily used for AD, dupilumab has been found to be useful in a number of off-label dermatologic indications. Besides, with a favourable safety profile, and an established and efficient clinical use for a broad range of populations, dupilumab holds promise as a newer treatment option for a plethora of dermatologic conditions. With numerous clinical trials ongoing, the author expects dupilumab's usage in dermatology to expand in the near future.

References

1. Gooderham MJ, Hong HC, Eshtiaghi P, Papp KA. Dupilumab: a review of its use in the treatment of atopic dermatitis. J Am Acad Dermatol. 2018 Mar;78(3 Suppl 1):S28–36.
2. Dupixent(dupilumab) approved by FDA as the first and only treatment indicated for prurigo nodularis. Available at: http://www.sanofi.com/en/media-room/press-releases/2022/2022-09-28-22-05-26-2524764.

3. DUPIXENT® [package insert]. Tarrytown, NY: Regeneron Pharmaceuticals;2017.
4. Simpson EL, Bieber T, Guttman-Yassky E, Beck LA, Blauvelt A, Cork MJ, et al. Two phase 3 trials of Dupilumab versus placebo in atopic dermatitis. N Engl J Med. 2016;375:2335–48.
5. Worm M, Simpson EL, Thaçi D, Bissonnette R, Lacour JP, Beissert S, et al. Efficacy and safety of multiple Dupilumab dose regimens after initial successful treatment in patients with atopic dermatitis: a randomized clinical trial. JAMA Dermatol. 2020;156:131–43.
6. Tofte SJ, Papp K, Sadick N, Bohnert K, Simpson E, Thaçi D, et al. Efficacy and safety of dupilumab for the treatment of moderate-to-severe atopic dermatitis in adults: a pooled analysis of two phase 2 clinical trials. J Am Assoc Nurse Pract. 2018;30:529–41.
7. Beck LA, Thaçi D, Hamilton JD, Graham NM, Bieber T, Rocklin R, et al. Dupilumab treatment in adults with moderate-to-severe atopic dermatitis. N Engl J Med. 2014;371:130–9.
8. Thaçi D, Simpson EL, Beck LA, Bieber T, Blauvelt A, Papp K, et al. Efficacy and safety of dupilumab in adults with moderate-to-severe atopic dermatitis inadequately controlled by topical treatments: a randomised, placebo-controlled, dose-ranging phase 2b trial. Lancet. 2016;387:40–52.
9. Blauvelt A, de Bruin-Weller M, Gooderham M, Cather JC, Weisman J, Pariser D, et al. Long-term management of moderate-to-severe atopic dermatitis with dupilumab and concomitant topical corticosteroids (LIBERTY AD CHRONOS): a 1-year, randomised, double-blinded, placebo-controlled, phase 3 trial. Lancet. 2017;389:2287–303.
10. Hamilton JD, Suárez-Fariñas M, Dhingra N, Cardinale I, Li X, Kostic A, et al. Dupilumab improves the molecular signature in skin of patients with moderate-to-severe atopic dermatitis. J Allergy Clin Immunol. 2014;134:1293–300.
11. Kakinuma T, Nakamura K, Wakugawa M, Mitsui H, Tada Y, Saeki H, et al. Thymus and activation-regulated chemokine in atopic dermatitis: serum thymus and activation-regulated chemokine level is closely related with disease activity. J Allergy Clin Immunol. 2001;107:535–41.
12. Zeidler C, Tsianakas A, Pereira M, Ständer H, Yosipovitch G, Ständer S. Chronic Prurigo of nodular type: a review. Acta Derm Venereol. 2018;98:173–9.
13. Fukushi S, Yamasaki K, Aiba S. Nuclear localization of activated STAT6 and STAT3 in epidermis of prurigo nodularis. Br J Dermatol. 2011;165:990–6.
14. Oetjen LK, Mack MR, Feng J, Whelan TM, Niu H, Guo CJ, et al. Sensory neurons co-opt classical immune signaling pathways to mediate chronic itch. Cell. 2017;171:217–228.e13.
15. Oetjen L, Kim B. Interactions of the immune and sensory nervous systems in atopy. FEBS. 2018;285:3138–51.
16. Calugareanu A, Jachiet M, Tauber M, Nosbaum A, Aubin F, Misery L, et al. Effectiveness and safety of dupilumab for the treatment of prurigo nodularis in a French multicenter adult cohort of 16 patients. J Eur Acad Dermatol Venereol. 2020;34:e74–6.
17. Chiricozzi A, Maurelli M, Gori N, Argenziano G, De Simone C, Calabrese G, et al. Dupilumab improves clinical manifestations, symptoms, and quality of life in adult patients with chronic nodular prurigo. J Am Acad Dermatol. 2020;83:39–45.
18. Ferrucci S, Tavecchio S, Berti E, Angileri L. Dupilumab and prurigo nodularis-like phenotype in atopic dermatitis: our experience of efficacy. J Dermatolog Treat. 2021;32:453–4.
19. Tilotta G, Pistone G, Caruso P, Gurreri R, Castelli E, Curiale S, et al. Our experience with prurigo nodularis treated with dupilumab. J Eur Acad Dermatol Venereol. 2021;35:e285–7.
20. Napolitano M, Fabbrocini G, Scalvenzi M, Nisticò SP, Dastoli S, Patruno C. Effectiveness of Dupilumab for the treatment of generalized Prurigo Nodularis phenotype of adult atopic dermatitis. Dermatitis. 2020;31:81–4.
21. Tavecchio S, Angileri L, Pozzo Giuffrida F, Germiniasi F, Marzano AV, Ferrucci S. Efficacy of Dupilumab on different phenotypes of atopic dermatitis: one-year experience of 221 patients. J Clin Med. 2020;9:2684.
22. Reynolds MT, Dinehart SM, Anderson KR, Gorelick J. Treatment of recalcitrant Prurigo Nodularis with Dupilumab. SKIN The Journal of Cutaneous Medicine. 2020;4:279–83.
23. Beck KM, Yang EJ, Sekhon S, Bhutani T, Liao W. Dupilumab treatment for generalized Prurigo Nodularis. JAMA Dermatol. 2019;155:118–20.

24. Holm JG, Agner T, Sand C, Thomsen SF. Dupilumab for prurigo nodularis: case series and review of the literature. Dermatol Ther. 2020;33:e13222.
25. Almustafa ZZ, Weller K, Autenrieth J, Maurer M, Metz M. Dupilumab in treatment of chronic Prurigo: a case series and literature review. Acta Derm Venereol. 2019;99:905–6.
26. Calugareanu A, Jachiet M, Lepelletier C, De Masson A, Rybojad M, Bagot M, et al. Dramatic improvement of generalized prurigo nodularis with dupilumab. J Eur Acad Dermatol Venereol. 2019;33:e303–4.
27. Mitsuyama S, Higuchi T. Effectiveness of dupilumab for chronic prurigo in elderly patients with atopic dermatitis. An Bras Dermatol. 2023;98:86–9.
28. Giura MT, Viola R, Fierro MT, Ribero S, Ortoncelli M. Efficacy of dupilumab in prurigo nodularis in elderly patient. Dermatol Ther. 2020;33:e13201.
29. Romano C. Safety and effectiveness of Dupilumab in Prurigo Nodularis. J Investig Allergol Clin Immunol. 2021;31:162–3.
30. Bloomstein JD, Hawkes JE. Simultaneous treatment of Samter triad and prurigo nodularis with dupilumab. JAAD Case Rep. 2021;18:20–2.
31. Criado PR, Pincelli TP, Criado RFJ. Dupilumab as a useful treatment option for prurigo nodularis in an elderly patient with atopic diathesis. Int J Dermatol. 2020;59:e358–61.
32. Tanis R, Ferenczi K, Payette M. Dupilumab treatment for Prurigo Nodularis and Pruritis. J Drugs Dermatol. 2019;18:940–2.
33. Fachler T, Maria Faitataziadou S, Molho-Pessach V. Dupilumab for pediatric prurigo nodularis: A case report. Pediatr Dermatol. 2021;38:334–5.
34. Liu T, Bai J, Wang S, Ying S, Li S, Qiao J, et al. Effectiveness of Dupilumab for an elderly patient with Prurigo Nodularis who was refractory and contradicted to traditional therapy. J Asthma Allergy. 2021;14:175–8.
35. Wieser JK, Mercurio MG, Somers K. Resolution of treatment-refractory Prurigo Nodularis with Dupilumab: a case series. Cureus. 2020;12:e8737.
36. Kovács B, Rose E, Kuznik N, Shimanovich I, Zillikens D, Ludwig RJ, et al. Dupilumab for treatment-refractory prurigo nodularis. J Dtsch Dermatol Ges. 2020;18:618–24.
37. Husein-ElAhmed H, Steinhoff M. Dupilumab in prurigo nodularis: a systematic review of current evidence and analysis of predictive factors to response. J Dermatolog Treat. 2022;33:1547–53.
38. Coenraads PJ. Hand eczema. N Engl J Med. 2012;367:1829–37.
39. Veien NK, Hattel T, Laurberg G. Hand eczema: causes, course, and prognosis I. Contact Derm. 2008;58:330–4.
40. Voorberg AN, Niehues H, Oosterhaven JAF, Romeijn GLE, van Vlijmen-Willems IMJJ, van Erp PEJ, et al. Vesicular hand eczema transcriptome analysis provides insights into its pathophysiology. Exp Dermatol. 2021;30:1775–86.
41. Weins AB, Biedermann T, Eyerich K, Moeckel S, Schnopp C. Successful treatment of recalcitrant dyshidrotic eczema with dupilumab in a child. J Dtsch Dermatol Ges. 2019;17:1165–7.
42. Gan H, Gao YD. Occupational chronic hand dermatitis in hospital environment successfully treated with Dupilumab: a case report. Iran J Allergy Asthma Immunol. 2022;21:484–7.
43. Zhu GA, Honari G, Ko JM, Chiou AS, Chen JK. Dupilumab for occupational irritant hand dermatitis in a nonatopic individual: a case report. JAAD Case Rep. 2020;6:296–8.
44. Nanda S, Nagrani N, MacQuhae F, Nichols A. A case of complete resolution of severe plantar dyshidrotic eczema with Dupilumab. J Drugs Dermatol. 2019;18:211–2.
45. Oosterhaven JAF, Romeijn GLE, Schuttelaar MLA. Dupilumab treatment of very severe refractory atopic hand eczema. JAMA Dermatol. 2018;154:969–70.
46. Halling AS, Zachariae C, Thyssen JP. Severe treatment-resistant acute and recurrent vesicular chronic hand eczema successfully treated with dupilumab. Contact Derm. 2020;83:37–8.
47. Zirwas MJ. Dupilumab for hand eczema. J Am Acad Dermatol. 2018;79:167–9.
48. Gall RA, Peters JD, Brinker AJ. Two cases of recalcitrant dyshidrotic eczema treated with Dupilumab. J Drugs Dermatol. 2021;20:558–9.
49. Weston GK, Hooper J, Strober BE. Dupilumab in the treatment of Dyshidrosis: a report of two cases. J Drugs Dermatol. 2018;17:355–6.

50. Loman L, Diercks GFH, Schuttelaar MLA. Three cases of non-atopic hyperkeratotic hand eczema treated with dupilumab. Contact Derm. 2021;84:124–7.
51. Waldman RA, DeWane ME, Sloan B, Grant-Kels JM, Lu J. Dupilumab for the treatment of dyshidrotic eczema in 15 consecutive patients. J Am Acad Dermatol. 2020;82:1251–2.
52. Oosterhaven JAF, Voorberg AN, Romeijn GLE, de Bruin-Weller MS, Schuttelaar MLA. Effect of dupilumab on hand eczema in patients with atopic dermatitis: an observational study. J Dermatol. 2019;46:680–5.
53. Voorberg AN, Romeijn GLE, de Bruin-Weller MS, Schuttelaar MLA. The long-term effect of dupilumab on chronic hand eczema in patients with moderate to severe atopic dermatitis-52-week results from the Dutch BioDay registry. Contact Derm. 2022;87:185–91.
54. Lee N, Chipalkatti N, Zancanaro P, Kachuk C, Dumont N, Rosmarin D. A retrospective review of Dupilumab for hand dermatitis. Dermatology. 2019;235:187–8.
55. Muñoz-Bellido FJ, Moreno E, Dávila I. Dupilumab: a review of present indications and off-label uses. J Investig Allergol Clin Immunol. 2022;32:97–115.
56. Kitagaki H, Ono N, Hayakawa K, Kitazawa T, Watanabe K, Shiohara T. Repeated elicitation of contact hypersensitivity induces a shift in cutaneous cytokine milieu from a T helper cell type 1 to a T helper cell type 2 profile. J Immunol. 1997;159:2484–91.
57. Dieli F, Sireci G, Scirè E, Salerno A, Bellavia A. Impaired contact hypersensitivity to trinitrochlorobenzene in interleukin-4-deficient mice. Immunology. 1999;98:71–9.
58. Rowe A, Bunker CB. Interleukin-4 and the interleukin-4 receptor in allergic contact dermatitis. Contact Derm. 1998;38:36–9.
59. Neis MM, Peters B, Dreuw A, Wenzel J, Bieber T, Mauch C, et al. Enhanced expression levels of IL-31 correlate with IL-4 and IL-13 in atopic and allergic contact dermatitis. J Allergy Clin Immunol. 2006;118:930–7.
60. Chipalkatti N, Lee N, Zancanaro P, Dumont N, Kachuk C, Rosmarin D. A retrospective review of dupilumab for atopic dermatitis patients with allergic contact dermatitis. J Am Acad Dermatol. 2019;80:1166–7.
61. Joshi SR, Khan DA. Effective use of Dupilumab in managing systemic allergic contact dermatitis. Dermatitis. 2018;29:282–4.
62. Goldminz AM, Scheinman PL. A case series of dupilumab-treated allergic contact dermatitis patients. Dermatol Ther. 2018;31:e12701.
63. Ruge IF, Skov L, Zachariae C, Thyssen JP. Dupilumab treatment in two patients with severe allergic contact dermatitis caused by sesquiterpene lactones. Contact Derm. 2020;83:137–9.
64. Slodownik D, Levi A, Lapidoth M, Moshe S. Occupational chronic contact dermatitis successfully treated with Dupilumab: a case series. Dermatology. 2022;238:1073–5.
65. Jo CE, Mufti A, Sachdeva M, Pratt M, Yeung J. Effect of dupilumab on allergic contact dermatitis and patch testing. J Am Acad Dermatol. 2021;84:1772–6.
66. Zhu GA, Chen JK, Chiou A, Ko J, Honari G. Repeat patch testing in a patient with allergic contact dermatitis improved on dupilumab. JAAD Case Rep. 2019;5:336–8.
67. Machler BC, Sung CT, Darwin E, Jacob SE. Dupilumab use in allergic contact dermatitis. J Am Acad Dermatol. 2019;80:280–281.e1.
68. Jacob SE, Sung CT, Machler BC. Dupilumab for systemic allergy syndrome with dermatitis. Dermatitis. 2019;30:164–7.
69. Stout M, Silverberg JI. Variable impact of dupilumab on patch testing results and allergic contact dermatitis in adults with atopic dermatitis. J Am Acad Dermatol. 2019;81:157–62.
70. Collantes-Rodríguez C, Jiménez-Gallo D, Ossorio-García L, Villegas-Romero I, Linares-Barrios M. Recall dermatitis at patch test sites in an atopic dermatitis patient treated with dupilumab. Contact Derm. 2019;80:69–70.
71. Andersen YM, Egeberg A, Gislason GH, Skov L, Thyssen JP. Autoimmune diseases in adults with atopic dermatitis. J Am Acad Dermatol. 2017;76:274–280.e1.
72. Renert-Yuval Y, Guttman-Yassky E. The changing landscape of alopecia Areata: the therapeutic paradigm. Adv Ther. 2017;34:1594–609.
73. Kulkarni M, Rohan CA, Travers JB, Serrao R. Long-term efficacy of Dupilumab in alopecia Areata. Am J Case Rep. 2022;23:e936488.

74. Sibbald C. Alopecia Areata: an updated review for 2023. J Cutan Med Surg. 2023;27:241–59.
75. Fukuyama M, Kinoshita-Ise M, Mizukawa Y, Ohyama M. Two-sided influence of dupilumab on alopecia areata co-existing with severe atopic dermatitis: a case series and literature review. J Cut Immunol Allergy. 2023;6:13–7.
76. Flanagan K, Sperling L, Lin J. Drug-induced alopecia after dupilumab therapy. JAAD Case Rep. 2018;5:54–6.
77. Maloney NJ, Worswick S, Cheng K. Development of alopecia in patients treated with dupilumab. Dermatol Ther. 2019;32:e12869.
78. Ständer S, Trense Y, Thaçi D, Ludwig RJ. Alopecia areata development in atopic dermatitis patients treated with dupilumab. J Eur Acad Dermatol Venereol. 2020;34:e612–3.
79. Alotaibi L, Alfawzan A, Alharthi R, Al Sheikh A. Improvement of atopic dermatitis and alopecia universalis with dupilumab. Dermatol Rep. 2021;14:9359.
80. Szekely S, Vaccari D, Salmaso R, Belloni-Fortina A, Alaibac M. Onset of Schamberg disease and resolution of alopecia Areata during treatment of atopic dermatitis with Dupilumab. J Investig Allergol Clin Immunol. 2021;31:65–6.
81. Babino G, Fulgione E, D'Ambra I, Calabrese G, Alfano R, Argenziano G. Rapid hair regrowth induced by dupilumab in a patient affected by alopecia totalis of 28 years' duration: clinical and dermoscopic features. Dermatol Ther. 2020;33:e13582.
82. Flanagan KE, Pupo Wiss IM, Pathoulas JT, Walker CJ, Senna MM. Dupilumab-induced psoriasis in a patient with atopic dermatitis and alopecia totalis: a case report and literature review. Dermatol Ther. 2022;35:e15255.
83. Cho SK, Craiglow BG. Dupilumab for the treatment of alopecia areata in children with atopic dermatitis. JAAD Case Rep. 2021;16:82–5.
84. Ludriksone L, Elsner P, Schliemann S. Simultaneous effectiveness of dupilumab in atopic dermatitis and alopecia areata in two patients. J Dtsch Dermatol Ges. 2019;17:1278–80.
85. Harada K, Irisawa R, Ito T, Uchiyama M, Tsuboi R. The effectiveness of dupilumab in patients with alopecia areata who have atopic dermatitis: a case series of seven patients. Br J Dermatol. 2020;183:396–7.
86. Kanda N, Koto M, Hoashi T, Saeki H. Case of alopecia areata during dupilumab treatment for atopic dermatitis. J Dermatol. 2019;46:e332–3.
87. Gallo R, Trave I, Parodi A. Massive acute alopecia of the scalp in a patient treated with Dupilumab. Acta Derm Venereol. 2020 Jun;100:adv00191.
88. Mitchell K, Levitt J. Alopecia areata after dupilumab for atopic dermatitis. JAAD Case Rep. 2018;4:143–4.
89. Barroso-García B, Rial MJ, Molina A, Sastre J. Alopecia Areata in severe atopic dermatitis treated with Dupilumab. J Investig Allergol Clin Immunol. 2018;28:420–1.
90. Guttman-Yassky E, Renert-Yuval Y, Bares J, Chima M, Hawkes JE, Gilleaudeau P, et al. Phase 2a randomized clinical trial of dupilumab (anti-IL-4Rα) for alopecia areata patients. Allergy. 2022;77:897–906.
91. Zuberbier T, Abdul Latiff AH, Abuzakouk M, Aquilina S, Asero R, Baker D, et al. The international EAACI/GA²LEN/EuroGuiDerm/APAAACI guideline for the definition, classification, diagnosis, and management of urticaria. Allergy. 2022;77:734–66.
92. Staubach P, Peveling-Oberhag A, Lang BM, Zimmer S, Sohn A, Mann C. Severe chronic spontaneous urticaria in children – treatment options according to the guidelines and beyond – a 10 years review. J Dermatolog Treat. 2022;33:1119–22.
93. Ferrucci S, Benzecry V, Berti E, Asero R. Rapid disappearance of both severe atopic dermatitis and cold urticaria following dupilumab treatment. Clin Exp Dermatol. 2020;45:345–6.
94. Sun Y, Lin SY, Lan CE. Dupilumab as a rescue therapy for a chronic urticaria patient who showed secondary failure to omalizumab. Kaohsiung J Med Sci. 2022;38:610–1.
95. Goodman B, Jariwala S. Dupilumab as a novel therapy to treat adrenergic urticaria. Ann Allergy Asthma Immunol. 2021;126:205–6.
96. Zhu C, Fok JS, Lin L, Su H, Maurer M. Complete response to dupilumab in a patient with chronic spontaneous urticaria who did not tolerate omalizumab. JAAD Case Rep. 2022;32:109–12.

97. Sirufo MM, Catalogna A, Raggiunti M, De Pietro F, Ginaldi L, De Martinis M. Cholinergic Urticaria, an effective and safe "off label" use of Dupilumab: a case report with literature review. Clin Cosmet Investig Dermatol. 2022;15:253–60.
98. Puxkandl V, Hoetzenecker W, Altrichter S. Case report: severe chronic spontaneous urticaria successfully treated with omalizumab and dupilumab. Allergol Select. 2023;7:17–9.
99. Holm JG, Sørensen JA, Thomsen SF. Concurrent use of omalizumab and dupilumab in a 47-year-old woman with chronic spontaneous urticaria and atopic dermatitis. Int J Dermatol. 2022;61:e173–4.
100. Abadeh A, Lee JK. Long-term follow-up of patients treated with dupilumab for chronic spontaneous urticaria: a case report. SAGE Open Med Case Rep. 2022;10:2050313X221117702.
101. Lee JK, Simpson RS. Dupilumab as a novel therapy for difficult to treat chronic spontaneous urticaria. J Allergy Clin Immunol Pract. 2019;7:1659–1661.e1.
102. Marchal V, Reguiai Z. Efficacity of dupilumab in severe idiopathic cold urticaria: a case report. J Dermatolog Treat. 2023;34:2182620.
103. JJ ML, Baker B, Ryan JJ. Mast cell production and response to IL-4 and IL-13. Cytokine. 2015;75:57–61.
104. Babina M, Guhl S, Artuc M, Zuberbier T. IL-4 and human skin mast cells revisited: reinforcement of a pro-allergic phenotype upon prolonged exposure. Arch Dermatol Res. 2016;308:665–70.
105. Garcovich S, Maurelli M, Gisondi P, Peris K, Yosipovitch G, Girolomoni G. Pruritus as a distinctive feature of type 2 inflammation. Vaccines (Basel). 2021;9:303.
106. Maurer M, Casale TB, Saini SS, Ben-Shoshan M, Giménez-Arnau AM, Bernstein JA, et al. Dupilumab in patients with chronic spontaneous urticaria (LIBERTY-CSU CUPID): two randomized, double-blind, placebo-controlled, phase 3 trials. J Allergy Clin Immunol. 2024:S0091-674900196-9.
107. Zhang Y, Xu Q, Chen L, Chen J, Zhang J, Zou Y, Gong T, Ji C. Efficacy and safety of Dupilumab in moderate-to-severe bullous pemphigoid. Front Immunol. 2021;12:738907.
108. Daniel BS, Murrell DF. Review of autoimmune blistering diseases: the pemphigoid diseases. J Eur Acad Dermatol Venereol. 2019;33:1685–94.
109. Teraki Y, Hotta T, Shiohara T. Skin-homing interleukin-4 and -13-producing cells contribute to bullous pemphigoid: remission of disease is associated with increased frequency of interleukin-10-producing cells. J Invest Dermatol. 2001;117:1097–102.
110. Messingham KN, Holahan HM, Frydman AS, Fullenkamp C, Srikantha R, Fairley JA. Human eosinophils express the high affinity IgE receptor, FcεRI, in bullous pemphigoid. PLoS One. 2014;9:e107725.
111. Günther C, Wozel G, Meurer M, Pfeiffer C. Up-regulation of CCL11 and CCL26 is associated with activated eosinophils in bullous pemphigoid. Clin Exp Immunol. 2011;166:145–53.
112. Hashimoto T, Kursewicz CD, Fayne RA, Nanda S, Shah SM, Nattkemper L, et al. Pathophysiologic mechanisms of itch in bullous pemphigoid. J Am Acad Dermatol. 2020;83:53–62.
113. Abdat R, Waldman RA, de Bedout V, Czernik A, Mcleod M, King B, et al. Dupilumab as a novel therapy for bullous pemphigoid: a multicenter case series. J Am Acad Dermatol. 2020;83:46–52.
114. Zhang X, Man X, Tang Z, Dai R, Shen Y. Dupilumab as a novel therapy for bullous pemphigoid. Int J Dermatol. 2023;62:e263–6.
115. Kaye A, Gordon SC, Deverapalli SC, Her MJ, Rosmarin D. Dupilumab for the treatment of recalcitrant bullous pemphigoid. JAMA Dermatol. 2018;154:1225–6.
116. Seidman JS, Eichenfield DZ, Orme CM. Dupilumab for bullous pemphigoid with intractable pruritus. Dermatol Online J. 2019;25:13030/qt25q9w6r9.
117. Zhou AE, Shao K, Ferenczi K, Adalsteinsson JA. Recalcitrant bullous pemphigoid responsive to dupilumab in an adolescent patient. JAAD Case Rep. 2022;29:149–51.
118. Seyed Jafari SM, Feldmeyer L, Bossart S, Simon D, Schlapbach C, Borradori L. Case report: combination of Omalizumab and Dupilumab for recalcitrant bullous pemphigoid. Front Immunol. 2021;11:611549.

119. Saleh M, Reedy M, Torok H, Weaver J. Successful treatment of bullous pemphigoid with dupilumab: a case and brief review of the literature. Dermatol Online J. 2021;27:13030/qt0dv3f9h6.
120. Yang J, Gao H, Zhang Z, Tang C, Chen Z, Wang L, et al. Dupilumab combined with low-dose systemic steroid therapy improves efficacy and safety for bullous pemphigoid. Dermatol Ther. 2022;35:e15648.
121. Klepper EM, Robinson HN. Dupilumab for the treatment of nivolumab-induced bullous pemphigoid: a case report and review of the literature. Dermatol Online J. 2021;27:6.
122. Pop SR, Strock D, Smith RJ. Dupilumab for the treatment of pembrolizumab-induced bullous pemphigoid: a case report. Dermatol Ther. 2022;35:e15623.
123. Shan Y, Zuo YG. A successful case of vesicular pemphigoid concurrent with pulmonary tuberculosis with dupilumab. Dermatol Ther. 2022;35:e15330.
124. Bal A, Sorensen A, Ondreyco SM. Nonbullous erythrodermic pemphigoid with florid lymphadenopathy, response to dupilumab. JAAD Case Rep. 2021;17:58–60.
125. Jendoubi F, Bost C, Tournier E, Paul C, Konstantinou MP. Severe pemphigoid nodularis successfully treated with dupilumab. Dermatol Ther. 2022;35:e15727.
126. Mascaró JM Jr, Lecha M, Mascaró JM. Fetal morbidity in herpes gestationis. Arch Dermatol. 1995;131:1209–10.
127. Riquelme-Mc Loughlin C, Mascaró JM Jr. Treatment of pemphigoid gestationis with dupilumab. Clin Exp Dermatol. 2021;46:1578–9.
128. Brunsting LA, Perry HO. Benign pemphigoid; a report of seven cases with chronic, scarring, herpetiform plaques about the head and neck. AMA Arch Derm. 1957;75:489–501.
129. Blum FR, Sigmon JR. Successful treatment of Brunsting-Perry pemphigoid with dupilumab. JAAD Case Rep. 2021;10:107–9.
130. Raef HS, Elmariah SB. Successful treatment of Brunsting-Perry Cicatricial pemphigoid with Dupilumab. J Drugs Dermatol. 2021;20:1113–5.
131. Mellerio JE, Ashton GH, Mohammedi R, Lyon CC, Kirby B, Harman KE, et al. Allelic heterogeneity of dominant and recessive COL7A1 mutations underlying epidermolysis bullosa pruriginosa. J Invest Dermatol. 1999;112:984–7.
132. Wang Y, Zhou M, Zhang L, Zheng S, Hong Y, Gao XH. Amelioration of dystrophic epidermolysis bullosa pruriginosa symptoms with dupilumab: a case report. Dermatol Ther. 2021;34:e15130.
133. Shehadeh W, Sarig O, Bar J, Sprecher E, Samuelov L. Treatment of epidermolysis bullosa pruriginosa-associated pruritus with dupilumab. Br J Dermatol. 2020;182:1495–7.
134. Clawson RC, Duran SF, Pariser RJ. Epidermolysis bullosa pruriginosa responding to dupilumab. JAAD Case Rep. 2021;16:69–71.
135. Zhou AG, Little AJ, Antaya RJ. Epidermolysis bullosa pruriginosa treated with dupilumab. Pediatr Dermatol. 2021;38:526–7.
136. Aldana PC, Khachemoune A. Grover disease: review of subtypes with a focus on management options. Int J Dermatol. 2020;59:543–50.
137. Beer J, Rosenbach M. Grover disease associated with chemotherapy: review of potential pathophysiology, current treatments, and future directions. J Drugs Dermatol. 2020;19:1056–64.
138. Chen WS, Tetzlaff MT, Diwan H, Jahan-Tigh R, Diab A, Nelson K, et al. Suprabasal acantholytic dermatologic toxicities associated checkpoint inhibitor therapy: a spectrum of immune reactions from paraneoplastic pemphigus-like to Grover-like lesions. J Cutan Pathol. 2018;45:764–73.
139. Mahler SJ, De Villez RL, Pulitzer DR. Transient acantholytic dermatosis induced by recombinant human interleukin 4. J Am Acad Dermatol. 1993;29:206–9.
140. Munoz J, Guillot B, Girard C, Dereure O, Du-Thanh A. First report of ipilimumab-induced Grover disease. Br J Dermatol. 2014;171:1236–7.
141. Sehra S, Yao Y, Howell MD, Nguyen ET, Kansas GS, Leung DY, et al. IL-4 regulates skin homeostasis and the predisposition toward allergic skin inflammation. J Immunol. 2010;184:3186–90.

142. De Martinis M, Sirufo MM, Viscido A, Ginaldi L. Food Allergies and Ageing. Int J Mol Sci. 2019;20:5580.
143. Alberti S, Cevenini E, Ostan R, Capri M, Salvioli S, Bucci L, et al. Age-dependent modifications of type 1 and type 2 cytokines within virgin and memory CD4+ T cells in humans. Mech Ageing Dev. 2006;127:560–6.
144. Barei F, Torretta S, Morini N, Ferrucci S. A case of Grover disease treated with Dupilumab: just serendipity or a future perspective? Dermatol Ther. 2022;35:e15429.
145. Shelton E, Doolittle C, Shinohara MM, Thompson JA, Moshiri AS. Can't handle the itch? Refractory immunotherapy-related transient acantholytic dermatosis: prompt resolution with dupilumab. JAAD Case Rep. 2022;22:31–3.
146. Butler DC, Kollhoff A, Berger T. Treatment of Grover disease with Dupilumab. JAMA Dermatol. 2021;157:353–6.
147. Hu Z, Bonifas JM, Beech J, Bench G, Shigihara T, Ogawa H, et al. Mutations in ATP2C1, encoding a calcium pump, cause Hailey-Hailey disease. Nat Genet. 2000;24:61–5.
148. Alzahrani N, Grossman-Kranseler J, Swali R, Fiumara K, Zancanaro P, Tyring S, et al. Hailey-Hailey disease treated with dupilumab: a case series. Br J Dermatol. 2021;185:680–2.
149. Alamon-Reig F, Serra-García L, Bosch-Amate X, Riquelme-Mc Loughlin C, Mascaró JM Jr. Dupilumab in Hailey-Hailey disease: a case series. J Eur Acad Dermatol Venereol. 2022;36:e776–9.
150. Licata G, Buononato D, Calabrese G, Gambardella A, Briatico G, Pagliuca F, et al. A case of Hailey-Hailey disease successfully treated with dupilumab. Int J Dermatol. 2022;61:1427–8.
151. Caldeira MB, Pestana M, Duarte B. Successful treatment of Hailey-Hailey disease with Dupilumab. Actas Dermosifiliogr. 2023;114:914–5.
152. Petkovic V, Moghini C, Paoletti S, Uguccioni M, Gerber B. Eotaxin-3/CCL26 is a natural antagonist for CC chemokine receptors 1 and 5. A human chemokine with a regulatory role. J Biol Chem. 2004;279:23357–63.
153. Schmidt E, Kasperkiewicz M, Joly P. Pemphigus. Lancet. 2019;394:882–94.
154. Chen S, Zhan S, Hua C, Tang Y, Cheng H. A novel combined use of Dupilumab for treatment of aggressive refractory pemphigus vulgaris complicated with pulmonary tuberculosis: a case report and the RNA-seq analysis. Front Immunol. 2022;13:825796.
155. Moore AY, Hurley K. Dupilumab monotherapy suppresses recalcitrant pemphigus vulgaris. JAAD Case Rep. 2022;31:16–8.
156. Nagel A, Lang A, Engel D, Podstawa E, Hunzelmann N, de Pita O, et al. Clinical activity of pemphigus vulgaris relates to IgE autoantibodies against desmoglein 3. Clin Immunol. 2010;134:320–30.
157. Eming R, Hennerici T, Bäcklund J, Feliciani C, Visconti KC, Willenborg S, et al. Pathogenic IgG antibodies against desmoglein 3 in pemphigus vulgaris are regulated by HLA-DRB1*04:02-restricted T cells. J Immunol. 2014;193:4391–9.
158. Pousti BT, Jin A, Sklovar L, Savage KT, Zhai LL, Mollanazar NK, et al. Dupilumab for the treatment of lichen planus. Cutis. 2021;107:E8–E10.
159. Kazemi S, Murphrey M, Hawkes JE. Rapid resolution of widespread cutaneous lichen planus and generalized pruritus in an elderly patient following treatment with dupilumab. JAAD Case Rep. 2022;30:108–10.
160. Yamauchi M, Moriyama M, Hayashida JN, Maehara T, Ishiguro N, Kubota K, et al. Myeloid dendritic cells stimulated by thymic stromal lymphopoietin promote Th2 immune responses and the pathogenesis of oral lichen planus. PLoS One. 2017;12:e0173017.
161. Piccinni MP, Lombardelli L, Logiodice F, Tesi D, Kullolli O, Biagiotti R, et al. Potential pathogenetic role of Th17, Th0, and Th2 cells in erosive and reticular oral lichen planus. Oral Dis. 2014;20:212–8.
162. Kidd P. Th1/Th2 balance: the hypothesis, its limitations, and implications for health and disease. Altern Med Rev. 2003;8:223–46.
163. Hübner F, Langan EA, Recke A. Lichen planus Pemphigoides: from lichenoid inflammation to autoantibody-mediated blistering. Front Immunol. 2019;10:1389.

164. Ch'en PY, Song EJ. Lichen planus pemphigoides successfully treated with dupilumab. JAAD Case Rep. 2022;31:56–8.
165. Li SZ, Xie YH, Wang SH, Fang RY, Jin HZ, Zuo YG. Case report: successful treatment of non-bullous lichen planus pemphigoides with dupilumab. Front Med. 2022;9:1023458.
166. Katagiri K, Itami S, Hatano Y, Yamaguchi T, Takayasu S. In vivo expression of IL-4, IL-5, IL-13 and IFN-gamma mRNAs in peripheral blood mononuclear cells and effect of cyclosporin a in a patient with Kimura's disease. Br J Dermatol. 1997;137:972–7.
167. Nonaka M, Sakitani E, Ono E, Yamamura Y, Seo Y, Shibata N, Pawankar R, Yoshihara T. Basophils are increased and express increased levels of interleukin-4 in the parotid lesions of Kimura disease. Asia Pac Allergy. 2017;7:221–6.
168. Maehara T, Munemura R, Shimizu M, Kakizoe N, Kaneko N, Murakami Y, et al. Tissue-infiltrating immune cells contribute to understanding the pathogenesis of Kimura disease: a case-report. Medicine (Baltimore). 2019;98:e18300.
169. Gandhi NA, Bennett BL, Graham NM, Pirozzi G, Stahl N, Yancopoulos GD. Targeting key proximal drivers of type 2 inflammation in disease. Nat Rev Drug Discov. 2016;15:35–50.
170. Bellinato F, Mastrosimini MG, Querzoli G, Gisondi P, Girolomoni G. Dupilumab for recalcitrant Kimura disease. Dermatol Ther. 2022;35:e15674.
171. Huang HY, Yang CY, Yao WT, Chen YF, Yu CM, Tung KY, Tsai MF. Kimura disease of the thigh treated with surgical excision and Dupilumab. Ann Plast Surg. 2022;88(1s Suppl 1):S110–3.
172. Suga K, Kiuchi M, Kageyama T, Kokubo K, Tanaka S, Iwata A, et al. Single-cell RNA sequencing of peripheral blood mononuclear cells from Kimura disease patient successfully treated with dupilumab. Allergol Int. 2023;72:610–3.
173. Yang B, Yu H, Jia M, Yao W, Diao R, Li B, et al. Successful treatment of dupilumab in Kimura disease independent of IgE: a case report with literature review. Front Immunol. 2022;13:1084879.
174. Teraki Y, Terao A. Treatment of Kimura disease with Dupilumab. JAMA Dermatol. 2022;158:329–30.
175. Shang BS, Hsiao CH, Tsao TF, Liao YY, Lin WL, Lee WI, et al. Clinical effects of dupilumab: a novel treatment for Kimura disease. Immun Inflamm Dis. 2023;11:e1084.
176. Kim BS, Berger TG, Yosipovitch G. Chronic pruritus of unknown origin (CPUO): uniform nomenclature and diagnosis as a pathway to standardized understanding and treatment. J Am Acad Dermatol. 2019;81:1223–4.
177. Gangemi S, Quartuccio S, Casciaro M, Trapani G, Minciullo PL, Imbalzano E. Interleukin 31 and skin diseases: a systematic review. Allergy Asthma Proc. 2017;38:401–8.
178. Jeon J, Wang F, Badic A, Kim BS. Treatment of patients with chronic pruritus of unknown origin with dupilumab. J Dermatolog Treat. 2022;33:1754–7.
179. Edmonds N, Noland M, Flowers RH. Six cases of refractory pruritus and histologic dermal hypersensitivity reaction successfully treated with dupilumab. JAAD Case Rep. 2021;19:28–33.
180. Zhai LL, Savage KT, Qiu CC, Jin A, Valdes-Rodriguez R, Mollanazar NK. Chronic pruritus responding to Dupilumab-a case series. Medicines (Basel). 2019;6:72.
181. Stanger R, Rivera-Oyola R, Lebwohl M. Dupilumab as a treatment for generalized idiopathic pruritus: a report of two cases. Br J Dermatol. 2020;182:1494–5.
182. Silverberg JI, Brieva J. A successful case of dupilumab treatment for severe uremic pruritus. JAAD Case Rep. 2019;5:339–41.
183. Abel MK, Ashbaugh AG, Stone HF, Murase JE. The use of dupilumab for the treatment of recalcitrant brachioradial pruritus. JAAD Case Rep. 2021;10:69–71.
184. Yang EJ, Murase JE. Recalcitrant anal and genital pruritus treated with dupilumab. Int J Womens Dermatol. 2018;4:223–6.
185. Alipour Tehrany Y, Marois L, Colmant C, Marchand V, Kokta V, Coulombe J, et al. Refractory pruritus responds to dupilumab in a patient with TTC7A mutation. JAAD Case Rep. 2020;8:9–12.

186. Ulrich C, Schmook T, Sachse MM, Sterry W, Stockfleth E. Comparative epidemiology and pathogenic factors for nonmelanoma skin cancer in organ transplant patients. Dermatol Surg. 2004;30:622–7.
187. Rivas JM, Ullrich SE. The role of IL-4, IL-10, and TNF-alpha in the immune suppression induced by ultraviolet radiation. J Leukoc Biol. 1994;56:769–75.
188. Verma L, Pratt M. A case report of therapeutically challenging chronic actinic dermatitis. SAGE Open Med Case Rep. 2019;7:2050313X19845235.
189. Patel N, Konda S, Lim HW. Dupilumab for the treatment of chronic actinic dermatitis. Photodermatol Photoimmunol Photomed. 2020;36:398–400.
190. Chen J, Li H, Zhu H. Successful treatment of chronic actinic dermatitis with Dupilumab: a case report and review of the literature. Clin Cosmet Investig Dermatol. 2021;14:1913–7.
191. Chen JC, Lian CH. Chronic actinic dermatitis in an old adult significantly improved by dupilumab. Photodermatol Photoimmunol Photomed. 2022;38:176–7.
192. Ali K, Wu L, Lou H, Zhong J, Qiu Y, Da J, et al. Clearance of chronic actinic dermatitis with Dupilumab therapy in Chinese patients: a case series. Front Med (Lausanne). 2022;9:803692.
193. Krejsgaard T, Lindahl LM, Mongan NP, Wasik MA, Litvinov IV, Iversen L, et al. Malignant inflammation in cutaneous T-cell lymphoma-a hostile takeover. Semin Immunopathol. 2017;39:269–82.
194. Sokołowska-Wojdyło M, Barańska-Rybak W, Cegielska A, Trzeciak M, Lugowska-Umer H, Gniadecki R. Atopic dermatitis-like pre-Sézary syndrome: role of immunosuppression. Acta Derm Venereol. 2011;91:574–7.
195. Newsom M, Hrin ML, Hamid RN, Strowd LC, Ahn C, Jorizzo JL, et al. Two cases of mycosis fungoides diagnosed after treatment non-response to dupilumab. Dermatol Online J. 2021;27:13030/qt1133121d.
196. Chiba T, Nagai T, Osada SI, Manabe M. Diagnosis of mycosis Fungoides following Administration of Dupilumab for misdiagnosed atopic dermatitis. Acta Derm Venereol. 2019;99:818–9.
197. Tran J, Morris L, Vu A, Duvic M. Development of Sézary syndrome following the administration of dupilumab. Dermatol Online J. 2020;26:13030/qt1m67z8sb.
198. Miyashiro D, Vivarelli AG, Gonçalves F, Cury-Martins J, Sanches JA. Progression of mycosis fungoides after treatment with dupilumab: a case report. Dermatol Ther. 2020;33:e13880.
199. Umemoto N, Demitsu T, Otaki K, Matsumoto T, Takazawa M, Yamada A, et al. Dupilumab therapy in Sézary syndrome misdiagnosed as atopic dermatitis: a case report. J Dermatol. 2020;47:e356–7.
200. Hashimoto M, Miyagaki T, Komaki R, Takeuchi S, Kadono T. Development of nodular lesions after Dupilumab therapy in Erythrodermic mycosis Fungoides with Interleukin-13 receptor alpha2 expression. Acta Derm Venereol. 2022;102:adv00766.
201. Espinosa ML, Nguyen MT, Aguirre AS, Martinez-Escala ME, Kim J, Walker CJ, et al. Progression of cutaneous T-cell lymphoma after dupilumab: case review of 7 patients. J Am Acad Dermatol. 2020;83:197–9.
202. Lazaridou I, Ram-Wolff C, Bouaziz JD, Bégon E, Battistella M, Rivet J, et al. Dupilumab treatment in two patients with cutaneous T-cell lymphomas. Acta Derm Venereol. 2020;100:adv00271.
203. Mollanazar NK, Savage KT, Pousti BT, Jariwala N, Del Guzzo C, Haun P, et al. Cutaneous T-cell lymphoma and concomitant atopic dermatitis responding to dupilumab. Cutis. 2020;106:131–2.
204. Steck O, Bertschi NL, Luther F, van den Berg J, Winkel DJ, Holbro A, et al. Rapid and sustained control of itch and reduction in Th2 bias by dupilumab in a patient with Sézary syndrome. J Eur Acad Dermatol Venereol. 2021;35:1331–7.
205. Spencer LA, Weller PF. Eosinophils and Th2 immunity: contemporary insights. Immunol Cell Biol. 2010;88:250–6.
206. Traidl S, Angela Y, Kapp A, Suhling H, Schacht V, Werfel T. Dupilumab in eosinophilic cellulitis (Wells' syndrome) – case report of a potential new treatment option. J Dtsch Dermatol Ges. 2021;19:1653–5.

207. Kirven RM, Plotner AN. Wells syndrome successfully treated with dupilumab. Int J Dermatol. 2023;62:e454–5.
208. Jumper N, Hodgkinson T, Paus R, Bayat A. Site-specific gene expression profiling as a novel strategy for unravelling keloid disease pathobiology. PLoS One. 2017;12:e0172955.
209. Maeda D, Kubo T, Kiya K, Kawai K, Matsuzaki S, Kobayashi D, et al. Periostin is induced by IL-4/IL-13 in dermal fibroblasts and promotes RhoA/ROCK pathway-mediated TGF-β1 secretion in abnormal scar formation. J Plast Surg Hand Surg. 2019;53:288–94.
210. Diaz A, Tan K, He H, Xu H, Cueto I, Pavel Ab, et al. Keloid lesions show increased IL-4/IL-13 signaling and respond to Th2-targeting dupilumab therapy. J Eur Acad Dermatol Venereol. 2020;34:e161–4.
211. Wong AJS, Song EJ. Dupilumab as an adjuvant treatment for keloid-associated symptoms. JAAD Case Rep. 2021;13:73–4.
212. Tirgan MH, Uitto J. Lack of efficacy of dupilumab in the treatment of keloid disorder. J Eur Acad Dermatol Venereol. 2022;36:e120–2.
213. Luk K, Fakhoury J, Ozog D. Nonresponse and progression of diffuse keloids to Dupilumab therapy. J Drugs Dermatol. 2022;21:197–9.
214. Peterson DM, Damsky WE, Vesely MD. Treatment of lichen sclerosis and hypertrophic scars with dupilumab. JAAD Case Rep. 2022;23:76–8.
215. Min MS, Wu J, He H, Sanz-Cabanillas JL, Del Duca E, Zhang N, et al. Granuloma annulare skin profile shows activation of T-helper cell type 1, T-helper cell type 2, and Janus kinase pathways. J Am Acad Dermatol. 2020;83:63–70.
216. Song EJ, Bezecny J, Farrer S. Recalcitrant generalized granuloma annulare treated successfully with dupilumab. JAAD Case Rep. 2020;7:1–2.
217. Erickson S, Heul AV, Kim BS. New and emerging treatments for inflammatory itch. Ann Allergy Asthma Immunol. 2021;126:13–20.
218. Ying Y, Shuang C, Zhen-Ying Z. Dupilumab may be an alternative option in the treatment of acquired reactive perforating collagenosis combined with AD. Immun Inflamm Dis. 2022;10:e574.
219. Gil-Lianes J, Riquelme-Mc Loughlin C, Mascaró JM Jr. Reactive perforating collagenosis successfully treated with dupilumab. Australas J Dermatol. 2022;63:398–400.
220. Alsebayel MM, Alzaid T, Alobaida SA. Dupilumab in acquired perforating dermatosis: a potential new treatment. JAAD Case Rep. 2022;28:34–6.
221. He A, Zampella JG, Kwatra SG. Interleukin-31 receptor and pruritus associated with primary localized cutaneous amyloidosis. Br J Dermatol. 2016;175:433.
222. Aoki K, Ohyama M, Mizukawa Y. A case of lichen amyloidosis associated with atopic dermatitis successfully treated with dupilumab: a case report and literature review. Dermatol Ther. 2021;34:e15005.
223. Humeda Y, Beasley J, Calder K. Clinical resolution of generalized lichen amyloidosis with dupilumab: a new alternative therapy. Dermatol Online J. 2020;26:13030/qt64s0s466.
224. Maione V, Caravello S, Cozzi C, Venturini M, Incardona P, Frassi M, et al. Refractory eosinophilic annular erythema treated successfully with dupilumab. J Dtsch Dermatol Ges. 2020;18:1031–2.
225. Gordon SC, Robinson SN, Abudu M, Her M, Deverapalli S, Levin A, et al. Eosinophilic annular erythema treated with dupilumab. Pediatr Dermatol. 2018;35:e255–6.
226. Petrova E, Hovnanian A. Advances in understanding of Netherton syndrome and therapeutic implications. Expert Opin Orphan Drugs. 2020;8:455–87.
227. Matsushima K, Yang D, Oppenheim JJ. Interleukin-8: An evolving chemokine. Cytokine. 2022;153:155828.
228. Steuei AB, Cohen DE. Successful treatment of Netherton's syndrome with dupilumab. JAMA Dermatol. 2020;156:350–1.
229. Andreasen TH, Karstensen HG, Duno M, Lei U, Zachariae C, Thyssen JP. Successful treatment with dupilumab of an adult with Netherton syndrome. Clin Exp Dermatol. 2020;45:915–7.
230. Aktas M, Salman A, Apti Sengun O, Comert Ozer E, Hosgoren Tekin S, Akin Cakici O, et al. Netherton syndrome: temporary response to dupilumab. Pediatr Dermatol. 2020;37:1210–1.

231. Süßmuth K, Traupe H, Loser K, Ständer S, Kessel C, Wittkowski H, et al. Response to dupilumab in two children with Netherton syndrome: improvement of pruritus and scaling. J Eur Acad Dermatol Venereol. 2021;35:e152–5.
232. Murase C, Takeichi T, Taki T, Yoshikawa T, Suzuki A, Ogi T, et al. Successful dupilumab treatment for ichthyotic and atopic features of Netherton syndrome. J Dermatol Sci. 2021;102:126–9.
233. Inaba Y, Kanazawa N, Muraoka K, Yariyama A, Kawaguchi A, Kunimoto K, et al. Dupilumab improves pruritus in Netherton syndrome: a case study. Children (Basel). 2022;9:310.
234. Ragamin A, Nouwen AEM, Dalm VASH, van Mierlo MMF, Lincke CR, Pasmans SGMA. Treatment experiences with intravenous immunoglobulins, Ixekizumab, Dupilumab, and Anakinra in Netherton syndrome: a case series. Dermatology. 2023;239:72–80.
235. Galdo G, Fania L. A Netherton syndrome case report: response to dupilumab treatment. Dermatol Ther. 2022;35:e15862.
236. Wang J, Yu L, Zhang S, Wang C, Li Z, Li M, Zhang S. Successful treatment of Netherton syndrome with dupilumab: a case report and review of the literature. J Dermatol. 2022;49:165–7.
237. Martin-García C, Godoy E, Cabrera A, Cañueto J, Muñoz-Bellido FJ, Perez-Pazos J, et al. Report of two sisters with Netherton syndrome successfully treated with dupilumab and review of the literature. Int J Immunopathol Pharmacol. 2023;37:3946320231172881.
238. Yan S, Wu X, Jiang J, Yu S, Fang X, Yang H, et al. Dupilumab improves clinical symptoms in children with Netherton syndrome by suppressing Th2-mediated inflammation. Front Immunol. 2022;13:1054422.
239. Imai T, Baba M, Nishimura M, Kakizaki M, Takagi S, Yoshie O. The T cell-directed CC chemokine TARC is a highly specific biological ligand for CC chemokine receptor 4. J Biol Chem. 1997;272:15036–42.
240. Komatsu-Fujii T, Nonoyama S, Ogawa M, Fukumoto T, Tanabe H. Rapid effects of dupilumab treatment on papuloerythroderma of Ofuji. J Eur Acad Dermatol Venereol. 2020;34:e739–41.
241. Teraki Y, Taguchi R, Takamura S, Fukuda T. Use of Dupilumab in the treatment of Papuloerythroderma of Ofuji. JAMA Dermatol. 2019;155:979–80.
242. Mizuno A, Habe K, Matsushima Y, Kondo M, Yamanaka K. A case of Papuloerythroderma successfully treated with Dupilumab. Case Rep Dermatol. 2022;14:117–22.
243. Dany M, Elston D. Gene expression of sphingolipid metabolism pathways is altered in hidradenitis suppurativa. J Am Acad Dermatol. 2017;77:268–273.e6.
244. Gambardella A, Calabrese G, Di Brizzi EV, Alfano R, Argenziano G. A case of atopic dermatitis and hidradenitis Suppurativa successfully treated with Dupilumab. J Eur Acad Dermatol Venereol. 2020;34:e284–6.
245. Molinelli E, Sapigni C, Simonetti O, Radi G, Gambini D, Maurizi A, et al. Successfully and safety use of dupilumab in the management of severe atopic dermatitis and concomitant moderate-to-severe hidradenitis suppurativa. Dermatol Ther. 2022;35:e15645.
246. Al-Shaikhly T, Ochs HD. Hyper IgE syndromes: clinical and molecular characteristics. Immunol Cell Biol. 2019;97:368–79.
247. Lévy R, Béziat V, Barbieux C, Puel A, Bourrat E, Casanova JL, et al. Efficacy of Dupilumab for controlling severe atopic dermatitis in a patient with hyper-IgE syndrome. J Clin Immunol. 2020;40:418–20.
248. Nihal A, Comstock JR, Holland KE, Singh AM, Seroogy CM, Arkin LM. Clearance of atypical cutaneous manifestations of hyper-IgE syndrome with dupilumab. Pediatr Dermatol. 2022;39:940–2.
249. Matucci-Cerinic C, Viglizzo G, Pastorino C, Corcione A, Prigione I, Bocca P, et al. Remission of eczema and recovery of Th1 polarization following treatment with Dupilumab in STAT3 hyper IgE syndrome. Pediatr Allergy Immunol. 2022;33:e13770.
250. Wang HJ, Yang TT, Lan CE. Dupilumab treatment of eczema in a child with STAT3 hyperimmunoglobulin E syndrome. J Eur Acad Dermatol Venereol. 2022;36:e367–9.
251. Gracia-Darder I, Pons De Ves J, Reyero Cortina M, Martín-Santiago A. Patient with atopic dermatitis, hyper IgE syndrome and ulcerative colitis, treated successfully with dupilumab during pregnancy. Dermatol Ther. 2022;35:e15237.

252. Lu CW, Lee WI, Chung WH. Dupilumab for STAT3-hyper-IgE syndrome with refractory intestinal complication. Pediatrics. 2021;148:e2021050351.
253. Dixit C, Thatayatikom A, Pappa H, Knutsen AP. Treatment of severe atopic dermatitis and eosinophilic esophagitis with dupilumab in a 14-year-old boy with autosomal dominant hyper-IgE syndrome. J Allergy Clin Immunol Pract. 2021;9:4167–9.
254. Su CJ, Tseng HC. Treatment efficacy of dupilumab in a hyper-immunoglobulin E syndrome patient with severe atopic dermatitis. JAAD Case Rep. 2021;11:60–2.
255. Sogkas G, Hirsch S, Jablonka A, Witte T, Schmidt RE, Atschekzei F. Dupilumab to treat severe atopic dermatitis in autosomal dominant hyper-IgE syndrome. Clin Immunol. 2020;215:108452.
256. Joshi TP, Anvari S, Gupta MR, Davis CM, Hajjar J. Case report: Dupilumab successfully controls severe eczema in a child with elevated IgE levels and recurrent skin infections. Front Pediatr. 2021;9:646997.
257. Ollech A, Mashiah J, Lev A, Simon AJ, Somech R, Adam E, et al. Treatment options for DOCK8 deficiency-related severe dermatitis. J Dermatol. 2021;48:1386–93.
258. Chello C, Sernicola A, Paolino G, Grieco T. Effects of dupilumab in type 1 neurofibromatosis coexisting with severe atopic dermatitis. An Bras Dermatol. 2021;96:638–40.
259. Maher MC, Hall EM, Horii KA. Generalized eczematous dermatitis and pruritus responsive to dupilumab in a patient with immune dysregulation, polyendocrinopathy, enteropathy, X-linked (IPEX) syndrome. Pediatr Dermatol. 2021;38:1370–1.
260. Smith HD, Montoya L, De Benedetto A. Recalcitrant palmoplantar pustulosis controlled with dupilumab. JAAD Case Rep. 2023;35:33–7.
261. McCluskey D, Benzian-Olsson N, Mahil SK, Hassi NK, Wohnhaas CT, APRICOT and PLUM study team, et al. Single-cell analysis implicates T_H17-to-TH2 cell plasticity in the pathogenesis of palmoplantar pustulosis. J Allergy Clin Immunol. 2022;150:882–93.
262. Wieser JK, Kuehn GJ, Prezzano JC, Cusick EH, Stiegler JD, Scott GA, et al. Improvement in a patient with hypereosinophilic syndrome after initiation of dupilumab treatment. JAAD Case Rep. 2020;6:292–5.
263. Chen MM, Roufosse F, Wang SA, Verstovsek S, Durrani SR, Rothenberg ME, et al. An international, retrospective study of off-label biologic use in the treatment of Hypereosinophilic syndromes. J Allergy Clin Immunol Pract. 2022;10:1217–1228.e3.
264. Du X, Chen Y, Chang J, Sun X, Zhang Y, Zhang M, Maurer M, Li Y, Zhao Z, Tong X. Dupilumab as a novel steroid-sparing treatment for hypereosinophilic syndrome. JAAD Case Rep. 2022;29:106–9.
265. Binkhonain FK, Aldokhayel S, BinJadeed H, Madani A. Successful treatment of an adult with atopic dermatitis and lamellar ichthyosis using Dupilumab. Biologics. 2022;16:85–8.
266. Larijani M, Zarowin D, Wohlschlaeger A, Perman MJ, Treat JR. Atopic dermatitis-like graft-versus-host disease treated with dupilumab. Pediatr Dermatol. 2023;40:320–2.
267. Belmesk L, Hatami A, Powell J, Kokta V, Coulombe J. Successful use of dupilumab in recalcitrant pediatric atopic dermatitis-like graft-versus-host disease: a case series. JAAD Case Rep. 2023;44:11–6.
268. Li K, Mu Z, Wen G, Zhao Y, Cong X, Zhang J. Increased regulatory T cells and eosinophils characterize atopic dermatitis-like graft-versus-host disease compared with lichen planus-like graft-versus-host disease. J Am Acad Dermatol. 2020;83:824–31.
269. Rial MJ, Barroso B, Sastre J. Dupilumab for treatment of food allergy. J Allergy Clin Immunol Pract. 2019;7:673–4.
270. Gruber R, Zschocke A, Zellner H, Schmuth M. Successful treatment of trichothiodystrophy with dupilumab. Clin Exp Dermatol. 2021;46:1381–3.
271. Bosma AL, Gerbens LAA, Middelkamp-Hup MA, Spuls PI. Paternal and maternal use of dupilumab in patients with atopic dermatitis: a case series. Clin Exp Dermatol. 2021;46:1089–92.

Omalizumab

39

Introduction

Omalizumab is a murine-derived recombinant humanized IgG1 monoclonal antibody acting against human immunoglobin E (IgE) [1]. It was approved by the US Food and Drug Administration (FDA) in 2014 for the treatment of chronic spontaneous urticaria (CSU) unresponsive to H1 antihistamines. Besides, omalizumab has been found to be beneficial in a number of other off-label indications that include atopic dermatitis (AD), bullous pemphigoid (BP), hyper-IgE syndrome (HIES), mastocytosis and Kimura's disease (KD) [2].

Pharmacokinetics

After subcutaneous (SC) injection, omalizumab is absorbed with an average bioavailability of 62%. It undergoes slow absorption, reaching peak serum concentrations by approximately 1 week. At doses greater than 0.5 mg/kg, the pharmacokinetics of omalizumab is linear, exhibiting a serum $t_{1/2}$ of around 26 days. Clearance of omalizumab involves IgG clearance processes, as well as clearance via specific binding, and formation of complexes with its target IgE ligand. Hepatic elimination of IgG includes degradation in the liver reticuloendothelial system and endothelial cells. Besides, intact IgG is also excreted in the bile [3].

Indications

FDA Approved

- Chronic spontaneous urticaria.

A. K. Bubna, *Therapeutics in Dermatology - Essentials for Clinical Practice*,
https://doi.org/10.1007/978-981-95-3791-4_39

Off-Label

- Atopic dermatitis (AD).
- Bullous pemphigoid (BP).
- Hyper-IgE syndrome (HIES).
- Mastocytosis.
- Kimura's disease (KD).

Contraindications

- Drug hypersensitivity.

Clinical Uses

Chronic Spontaneous Urticaria

CSU is defined as itchy wheals that last for at least 6 weeks and cannot be associated with any apparent exogenous trigger [4]. Although the recommended first-line management of CSU consists of nonsedating H1 blockers, a substantial proportion of patients demonstrate poor responsiveness to these drugs, even after dose escalation (up to 4 times) or addition of H2 antagonists and leukotriene receptor inhibitors [5]. In such patients, oral corticosteroids and cyclosporine are often administered to control symptoms. However, owing to the toxicity profile of these drugs, alternative agents with acceptable levels of tolerability/safety become essential [6, 7].

Omalizumab is effective in the management of CSU and also exhibits a favourable toxicity profile. It interacts with the Cε3 domain of IgE on membranes of mast cells (MCs), basophils, eosinophils and lymphocytes, preventing both FcεRI and FcεRII from attaching to IgE, thereby plummeting release of inflammatory mediators, along with reduction in the surface expression of FcεRI receptors, particularly in MCs and basophils [8]. Further, details regarding the mechanism of action of omalizumab in CSU is highlighted in Fig. 39.1 [9, 10].

Based on three high-quality randomized controlled trials (RCTs), omalizumab was approved by the US FDA at doses of 150 mg/300 mg every 4 weeks for the management of CSU [11–13].

Omalizumab is effective in around 85% of its recipients, with clinical effects being observed either within 3–5 days following the first dose in 70% of patients (the so-called early/fast responders) or after 3–4 months of treatment in 15% of patients (the so-called late/slow responders). In others, omalizumab fails to demonstrate clinical efficacy [14].

A possible IgE-mediated auto-allergic pathogenesis specific for self-proteins may well be a plausible explanation regarding the expeditious response to omalizumab in some patients with CSU [15, 16]. In contrast, the basis for the late/slow responder category in relation to omalizumab is not clearly denoted. It is suggested

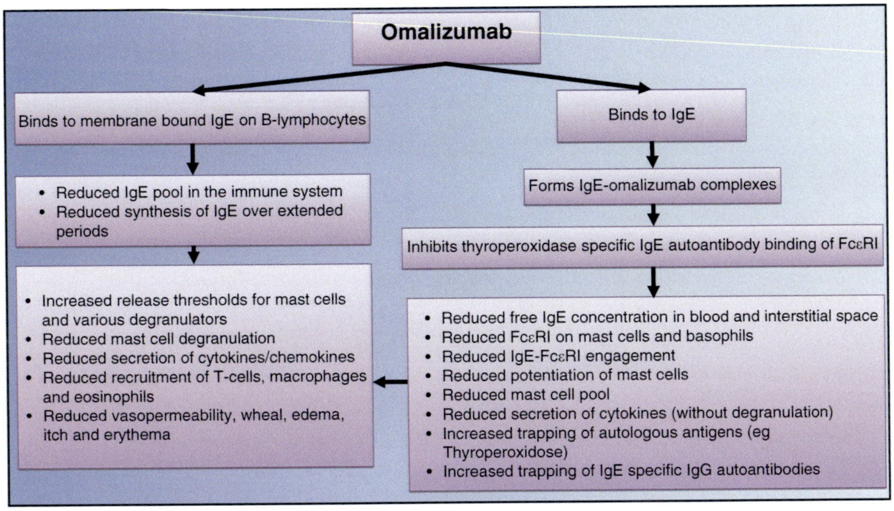

Fig. 39.1 Details of the mechanism of omalizumab's action in chronic spontaneous urticaria

that in this subset of patients, an IgG-mediated autoimmune process capable of activating basophils and MCs via high-affinity IgE receptors both directly (by IgE-anti-FcεRI) and indirectly (by IgG directed against receptor-bound IgE) is involved, making omalizumab rely upon the downregulation of IgE receptors to accomplish its effects, an action requiring some months for completion [17–19]. Besides, omalizumab has the ability to bind IgE fixed to FcεRI and subsequently detach them, eventuating in receptor downregulation, which may hold significance in patients delineating slow responses with omalizumab [20]. In addition, the contemporary existence of IgE- and IgG-mediated autoimmunity (specifically opposing the FcεRI) may also facilitate a delayed clinical outcome with omalizumab [21].

Predictive markers associated with poor responsiveness to omalizumab in CSU include low IgE levels [22], basopenia [23], eosinopenia [24], positive autologous serum skin test [25, 26], positive basophil activation test [25] and past treatment with cyclosporine [27]. Interestingly, a connection between CSU, obesity and omalizumab resistance has been described [28]. In obese individuals, elevated expression of pro-inflammatory cytokines and C-reactive protein, along with the potential of adipokines to activate MCs, aggravates the clinical severity of CSU [29–31]. Besides, elevated levels of complement 3 in patients with metabolic syndrome delineates a positive correlation with the severity of CSU and omalizumab resistance, reflecting an ongoing low-grade inflammation in this population [32, 33]. It therefore becomes essential to appropriately screen patients prior to initiating treatment with omalizumab.

In around 30% of CSU patients, there is failure to respond to the approved dosing regimens of omalizumab, and the dose or the frequency of omalizumab may need escalation. Generally, the dose is increased to 450 mg or 600 mg every 4 weeks in case of insufficient responses following five doses of omalizumab. If still adequate control of CSU is not obtained after three doses of 600 mg, then the frequency of omalizumab is escalated to 600 mg every 2 weeks for two consecutive doses [34]. However, the 2 weekly therapeutic approach with 600 mg of omalizumab is rarely applied in CSU and is more regularly used in the management of asthma patients. [35] Moreover, changing the schedule from 300 mg/4 weekly to 150 mg/2 weekly has also shown to be effective in cases unresponsive to the 4 weekly dosing intervals, although there is still no consensus on this subject [36].

The duration of therapy with omalizumab for CSU is yet to be standardized as per the EAACI guidelines, and weaning can be contemplated once remission is achieved [37]. This can be done by reducing the frequency of administration or decreasing the dosage. The injection interval is gradually spaced by 1 week (q5w) to 4 weeks (q8w) once urticaria is controlled. If the patient is in remission with the q8w schedule for 8 weeks and tapering, then omalizumab can be stopped [38, 39].

Furthermore, retreatment with omalizumab in cases of relapses following treatment cessation is associated with rapid remission of CSU, without any reduction in its efficacy. However, in some patients, greater number of doses may be required. Previous studies have delineated that omalizumab treatment does not lead to the development of measurable levels of anti-omalizumab antibodies, and this may be the reason for its efficacy in relapses of CSU [40]. Besides, during the entire course of omalizumab therapy, combining H1 antihistamines is helpful [41].

To summarize, (a) omalizumab is not the first-line agent for CSU, (b) it may not be effective as monotherapy alone, (c) combining H1 blockers with omalizumab plays a synergistic role and (d) omalizumab helps to prevent long-term side effects associated with systemic glucocorticoids.

Inducible Urticarias

Solar Urticaria

Solar urticaria (SU) is a rare IgE-mediated photodermatosis characterized by wheals following exposure to UV or visible light. In susceptible individuals, solar exposure results in activation of an unidentified chromophore that supposedly binds to IgE on MCs, eventuating degranulation [42]. Although H1 antihistamines, phototherapy and sun protection form the crux of SU management, the role of omalizumab in SU has been propounded. Interestingly, the efficacy of omalizumab in SU is found to be mixed, with therapeutic success in some and therapeutic failure in others [43–49].

Cold Urticaria

Cold urticaria (CU) is an inducible urticaria occurring following contact with cold water, cold air or cold surfaces. It accounts for 3% of cases of chronic urticaria and can precipitate angioedema of the upper airways following inhalation of cold air, mandating emergency care and management [50]. Currently, the beneficial effects of omalizumab in cold urticaria are limited to case reports and small case series [45, 51–53].

Boyce reported omalizumab (375 mg SC every 2weekly) to be effective in a 12-year-old girl with CU refractory to H1 antihistamines (even after dose escalation) and montelukast. Following the second injection itself, the patient was able to tolerate cold liquids (with mild palatal pruritus), and after 5 months of continuous treatment, patient was in complete remission, along with a negative ice cube test [51]. Similarly, Metz et al. [45] described complete control of symptoms in a 19-year-old boy with cold contact urticaria after the first injection of omalizumab (150 mg SC/month).

In a French case series of three patients, the profitability of omalizumab (300 mg SC every 2 weeks for 2 months) in H1 antihistamine and montelukast-resistant CU was further exemplified. Of the three patients, one patient remained symptom-free after the last injection of omalizumab even at 16 months of follow-up and did not require further treatment. In the remaining two, there was relapse of CU after 1 month and 4 months of cessation of omalizumab therapy, which after the subsequent injection of omalizumab resolved and was maintained at 2 months for one patient and 5 months for the other [52].

However, in the publication by Brodska and Schmid-Grendelmeier, conflicting results with regard to omalizumab were obtained in their series of two patients. One (53-year-old woman) reported significant improvement of symptoms after the first injection of omalizumab (300 mg SC given every month) with complete symptom control after 4 months of therapy, whereas in the other (30-year-old lady), insufficient efficacy with omalizumab (similar dosing) was observed [53].

Despite the beneficial effects of omalizumab in CU, there exist a subset of patients who may not be completely responsive to omalizumab. Besides, the exact mechanism of omalizumab in cold urticaria requires proper elucidation.

Heat Contact Urticaria

Heat contact urticaria (HCU) is a rare variant of physical urticaria that is often refractory to treatment. The role of omalizumab in HCU has been elaborated in only two reports till date, with different therapeutic outcomes in both.

In the first (42-year-old male), omalizumab (dosed at 300 mg and 450 mg SC alternatively every 2 weekly) was successful in bringing about considerable improvement of lesions after the second dose, with superior responses after the 450 mg dosing. Besides, following the fourth dose, patient was almost completely free of symptoms and could reconvene his professional duties with ease [54].

In the second (63-year-old female) however, only minor improvement was witnessed with omalizumab (300 mg every 2 weeks) even after 2 months, with subsequent treatment termination [45]. The exact therapeutic mechanism of omalizumab in HCU still remains unclear, and controlled studies become essential to clarify the active principle, as well as the optimal dose and duration of treatment with omalizumab in HCU.

Cholinergic Urticaria

Cholinergic urticaria (ChU) is a type of physical urticaria characterized by pin-sized wheals with surrounding erythema provoked following an increase in the core body temperature. Although the exact pathogenesis of ChU remains unclear, it is speculated that IgE may have a prominent role. [55] Beneficial effects of omalizumab in ChU have been elucidated in two patients, with both outlining significant improvement following two doses of omalizumab [56, 57].

Symptomatic Dermographism

Symptomatic dermographism (SD) is the most common physical urticaria encountered, with greatest incidence observed in young adults. Pruritus in SD is generally disproportionately severe compared to whealing and has a nocturnal preponderance [58]. The response to omalizumab in SD has been mixed, with dosages ranging from 150 to 300 mg/month. In two patients, complete remission was observed after the first injection of omalizumab, whereas another patient was unresponsive to omalizumab therapy [45, 59]. The specific role of omalizumab in SD still needs elucidation.

Delayed Pressure Urticaria

Delayed pressure urticaria (DPU) presents with whealing of skin at sites of sustained pressure applied to the skin after a delay of 30 min to 9 h, but usually 4–8 h, and lasts for 12–72 h. Wheals frequently occur under tight clothing, on hands after manual work, on the buttocks and lower back after sitting and the feet after walking. Lesions may be pruritic but are often tender or painful, especially on the scalp and soles, and may be accompanied by malaise, flu-like symptoms, myalgia and arthralgia [58].

Literature search revealed omalizumab to be effective in bringing about complete symptom control of DPU in two patients (one receiving 150 mg/2 weekly and the other 150 mg/month), who were unresponsive to H1 antihistamines (even after 2- to six-fold dose escalation) and montelukast [45, 60]. As IgE signalling via basophils is involved in the pathogenesis of DPU, omalizumab therapy has been utilized for the same [60].

Atopic Dermatitis

Atopic dermatitis (AD) is a multifactorial disorder with a chronic and relapsing course. Although the diagnosis of AD is straightforward, its management remains challenging [61]. Prominent expression of FcεRI on MCs and mononuclear antigen presenting cells has been identified in patients with AD [62, 63]. Furthermore, increased levels of serum L-selectin (a marker for leukocyte activation) and elevated circulating activated T cells correlate with AD disease activity [64]. Additionally, pronounced expression of thymic stromal lymphopoietin (TSLP) and IL-9 (an epithelial cell-derived cytokine) in keratinocytes of AD-affected skin is reported to play a major role in the pathogenesis of AD by stimulating secretion of Th2-cell attracting chemokines like thymus and activation regulated chemokine (TARC) and chemokine [C-C motif] ligand 17 (CCL17) that activate dendritic cells (DCs), facilitating expression of OX40 ligand (OX40L) on its surface, which in turn interacts with OX40 on the membranes of naïve T-helper cells, eventuating in Th2 proliferation and cytokine production [65–67]. Besides, TSLP also acts on MCs and natural killer cells, amplifying the production of Th2 cytokines [68].

Omalizumab apart from effectively reducing free IgE levels also plummets levels of TSLP, TARC, OX40L and IL-9 and in this way effectively diminishes Th2 polarization. Moreover, an increase in IL-10 (an anti-inflammatory cytokine) is detected in atopic skin following omalizumab therapy. By abrogating IgE from binding to FcεRI on MCs, omalizumab inactivates these cells, resulting in reduction of various components that constitute the allergic response cycle in AD (as described above) [65–68].

Studies utilizing omalizumab for AD have delineated conflicting results and is likely that only a subset of patients benefit from anti-IgE therapy [69–76].

Bullous Pemphigoid

Bullous pemphigoid (BP) is the most common autoimmune subepidermal blistering disease that presents clinically as pruritic urticarial plaques, tense vesicles and bullae. Although IgG is the autoantibody predominating in the plasma and skin of BP patients, many of them also have IgE autoantibodies against type XVII collagen that demonstrate pathogenic properties [77–79]. Furthermore, it is observed that IgE autoantibodies targeting the NC16A domain of BP180 protein can reproduce urticarial lesions encountered in early lesions of BP, due to which omalizumab may have a role in BP therapeutics [80, 81].

As the exact mechanism of action of omalizumab in BP is unknown, rationale for its use in this disorder is based on the following observations: (a) elevated levels of IgE in most untreated BP patients [79, 82], (b) reduction in free IgE levels within hours after the first dose of omalizumab [83] and (c) the presence of numerous eosinophils and MCs in the inflammatory infiltrate of BP (along with their close association and activation related to IgE autoantibodies) [84, 85]. Thus, the ideal candidate to receive omalizumab in BP would be a patient with intensely pruritic generalized urticarial and bullous lesions, having blood eosinophilia, and recalcitrant to systemic glucocorticoids and immunosuppressive drugs [80].

As there are no specific guidelines till date regarding the use of omalizumab in BP, no standardized dosing regimen is available currently. Published reports have utilized dosages ranging from 300 mg SC every 2 weeks or 4 weeks to 375 mg SC every 2 weeks or 4 weeks to 100 mg SC every 2 weekly (for an infant with BP) for BP. [77, 86–88].

Based on the above reports, although omalizumab is effective as monotherapy in some patients, in others, concomitant use of systemic corticosteroids and immunosuppressive agents are needed to obtain disease remission. Moreover, combing omalizumab with conventional immunosuppressive drugs allows faster taper and subsequent stoppage of these medications, thereby ensuring a better safety profile. Because omalizumab only prevents IgE from binding to MCs and basophils without directly antagonizing the effects of IgE produced by binding to BP180 on the surface of keratinocytes, and as IgG autoantibodies in BP are not targeted by omalizumab, persistence of residual disease in some patients on omalizumab monotherapy can be explained. Therefore ideally, combination therapy with omalizumab in BP would be preferable to obtain quicker and effective responses [77, 86–88].

Mastocytosis

Mastocytosis is a rare acquired condition characterized by excessive accumulation of MCs in skin and other tissues. Whereas cutaneous mastocytosis (CM) remains confined to the skin, systemic mastocytosis (SM) involves extracutaneous organs, with or without skin involvement. Omalizumab is effective in both CM and SM. Although the exact mechanism of omalizumab in mastocytosis is not determined, it is proposed that by decreasing the activity of MCs, omalizumab reduces symptoms resulting as a consequence of the elevated MC profile [89]. Omalizumab is less likely to affect MC turnover but facilitates reduction of free serum IgE levels, downregulates FCεRI on MCs and increases the threshold above which MC activation is triggered, and in this way helps ameliorating symptoms of mastocytosis [90, 91].

Various reports have elucidated omalizumab to be effective in the treatment of mastocytosis. [89, 92–100]

Urticarial Vasculitis

Urticarial vasculitis (UrV) is a small vessel vasculitis characterized by inflamed erythematous patches resembling urticaria but persist for more than 24 h. Though there are no prospective clinical studies outlining the efficacy of omalizumab in UrV, few case reports have highlighted its benefits for this indication. In all the above patients, omalizumab was administered following unsuccessful treatments with systemic glucocorticoids and conventional immunosuppressives. The dosage of omalizumab ranged from 300 mg SC every 2/4 weekly to 150 mg SC every month, with remission of symptoms observed as early as 1 month, along with favourable tolerability [101–105]. The precise mechanism of action of omalizumab in UrV is still under speculation, and its efficacy in hypocomplementemic/normocomplementemic vasculitis needs appropriate elucidation [105].

Toxic Epidermal Necrolysis

Toxic epidermal necrolysis (TEN) is a severe mucocutaneous reaction related to drugs, characterized by blistering and epithelial sloughing. In an anecdotal report, omalizumab (300 mg SC single dose) was found to be an effective adjunct along with methylprednisolone (500 mg for 3 days) pulse for treating TEN (secondary to levofloxacin) in a 74-year-old woman. Interestingly, laboratory analysis delineated an eight-fold increase of eosinophil cationic peptide in the blister fluid of this patient, thereby delineating a close relationship between immunologic reactions in the pathogenesis of TEN, which may explain the utility of omalizumab. Nevertheless, more studies are needed to investigate whether Th2-mediated inflammation does indeed have a role in altering the cytokine profile in TEN [106].

Netherton Syndrome

Netherton syndrome (NS) is a rare autosomal recessive disorder characterized by a triad of ichthyosiform erythroderma, atopic manifestations and trichorrhexis invaginata. In an isolated report, omalizumab (400 mg/kg for 4 months) along with pulse prednisolone (250 mg once a week for 4 weeks) was effective in bringing about clinical improvement that was evident following 2 weeks of treatment initiation. Besides, after 4 months, levels of IgE, IgG, CRP, IL-4, IL-5, IL-1β and IL-17A demonstrated significant reduction. Although the exact mechanism of omalizumab in NS is not yet propounded, an association between omalizumab and the Th2 inflammatory cascade has been proposed [107].

Kimura's Disease

Kimura's disease (KD) is a chronic inflammatory disease presenting as painless subcutaneous head and neck swelling, eosinophilia and elevated serum IgE levels. The efficacy of omalizumab in KD is currently limited to case reports, with the need for RCTs to strengthen each observation.

In all reports, omalizumab (300 mg SC every 2 weeks) was effective in reducing the size of the tumorous lesions, as well as peripheral blood eosinophil and basophil counts after 4 months of therapy [108, 109]. It is postulated that inhibition in the expression of FcεRI on basophils and consequent suppression of histamine release may have an important bearing with regard to the therapeutic benefit of omalizumab in KD [108]. Nevertheless, further research to confirm these preliminary findings becomes essential.

Hyper-IgE Syndrome

Hyper-IgE syndrome (HIES) is a rare primary immunodeficiency disorder characterized by recurrent staphylococcal cutaneous abscesses, recurrent pneumonia and increased levels of serum IgE [110]. In a report from Thailand, the propitious effects of omalizumab (300 mg SC every 2 weeks) were described in a 32-year-old patient with HIES who had failed therapy with topical/systemic glucocorticoids and topical tacrolimus. Within 1 month of omalizumab therapy, notable improvement was seen, allowing gradual reduction and subsequent discontinuation of systemic steroids [111]. In another publication, complete remission of severe recalcitrant eczematous dermatitis was obtained within 3 months of starting treatment with omalizumab (450 mg SC every 2 weeks) in a 26-year-old woman. Furthermore, the patient remained symptom free 6 months after discontinuing omalizumab, thereby delineating the long-lasting efficacy of omalizumab [112]. Postulated mechanisms of omalizumab in HIES include reduction of serum IgE levels, blockade of MC degranulation and subsequent histamine release following IgE stimulation [111, 112].

Eosinophilic Granulomatosis with Polyangiitis

Eosinophilic granulomatosis with polyangiitis (EGPA) is a rare systemic small-vessel vasculitis associated with asthma and blood/tissue eosinophilia [113]. Data evaluating the efficacy of omalizumab in EGPA have been mixed, with some reports suggesting omalizumab to be effective in active disease [114–117], whereas others highlighting a temporal association between the development of EGPA and the use of omalizumab [118–121]. Because of these findings, the use of omalizumab in EGPA has been considerably hindered. In a retrospective study on 17 adults with EGPA who had received omalizumab (300 mg SC every 4 weeks or 2 weekly), all demonstrated prompt and sustained improvement of asthma and/or sinonasal manifestations. However, the criteria for complete remission as per the EULAR recommendation (i.e., using prednisolone at a dose of $\leq$7.5 mg/day to control systemic manifestations) was observed in only six patients. Besides, in four patients, despite therapy with omalizumab, there was a flare, warranting drug discontinuation. Furthermore, the efficacy of omalizumab on vasculitic manifestations could not be assessed owing to the low Birmingham Vasculitis Activity Score (BVAS) at the start of the study. Moreover, relapses observed were attributed to vasculitis as the underlying pathology, exacerbated following prednisolone taper, rather than a direct effect of omalizumab. It therefore becomes essential to properly analyse the benefit/risk ratio individually in all patients prior to initiating omalizumab treatment for EGPA [122].

Adverse Effects

Although omalizumab generally demonstrates excellent safety, there are some important adverse effects (AEs) that need to be noted while prescribing it [123].

Common

Most commonly observed adverse effects associated with omalizumab include injection site reactions (45%), viral infection (23%), URTI (20%), pruritus (16%), headache (15%) and pharyngitis (11%) [124].

Immune System Effects and Hypersensitivity Reactions

These include anaphylaxis, urticaria, serum sickness-like syndrome (SSLS) and EGPA [40, 125, 126].

Anaphylaxis

The incidence of anaphylaxis in the "all-controlled-studies" populations was rare (omalizumab 0.14%, control 0.07%) [40].

Based on an estimated exposure of 57,300 patients from June 1, 2003 to December 31, 2006, 124 cases of anaphylaxis were linked to omalizumab (reporting proportion 0.2%) [127]. Furthermore, within these 124 patients, 24% had a previous history of anaphylaxis. The incidence of anaphylaxis occurring after the first, second and third or subsequent omalizumab injections was reported in 39%, 19% and 10% of patients, respectively. The reported time to onset ranged from ≤30 min (35%) to >1 day (5%), with hospitalization being necessary in 15% of cases [127].

An observation period of 2 h for the first three injections and 30 min for subsequent injections, and providing patients with epinephrine, is therefore recommended in all patients receiving omalizumab injection [128].

Urticaria

Currently, there exists only one publication reporting the occurrence of paradoxical urticaria in 47-year-old women with severe asthma, who was receiving omalizumab (600 mg every 4 weeks for 12 months). The hypothesis suggested for this antinomy was the immunologic activation of MCs following binding of omalizumab to the cell surface FcR receptors [125].

Serum Sickness-like Syndrome

The occurrence of SSLS has been reported in patients with MC activation disease (MCAD) receiving omalizumab, who have regular adrenal function. SSLS occurs within 3–10 days in these patients and eventually resolves within 1 week, after the circulating immune complexes have cleared. If symptoms do not resolve within this time frame, then treatment with omalizumab needs to be stopped, and treatment with systemic glucocorticoids (prednisolone 20–40 mg on 2 consecutive days) needs to be started to stop SSLS [40, 129, 130]. Although omalizumab is well tolerated, transient mild-to-moderate MC mediator-induced symptoms occurring within several hours following injection have been observed, suggesting potential activation of MCs superseding the desired pharmacologic effects of omalizumab [131].

Eosinophilic Granulomatosis with Polyangiitis

Published case reports have described reduction in the dose of oral glucocorticoids prior to the emergence of symptoms of EGPA, and related correspondences have supported the hypothesis that steroid dose titration rather than omalizumab is to be the likely reason for this observation [132–134]. Nevertheless, current omalizumab EU label under "special warnings and special precautions for use" advices physicians to be alert regarding the development of marked eosinophilia, vasculitis rash, worsening of pulmonary symptoms, cardiac complications and/or neuropathy following its administration [135].

Malignant Neoplasia

Despite there being some mention of malignancy risk associated with IgE, pooled analysis of phase 1 through 4 clinical trials conducted in 2012 revealed no clear association between the risk of malignancy in randomized, double-blind, placebo-controlled trials following omalizumab treatment [136]. In another report, the crude rates for malignancies including non-melanoma skin cancers were 6.2 and 6.3 per 1000 person-years in omalizumab-treated and placebo-treated cohorts, respectively. The most common cancers detected were skin, breast and prostate cancers, although the study size and follow-up were insufficient to detect a meaningful increase in the incidence for individual cancer types. Furthermore, subgroup analysis reiterated the poor association of omalizumab with malignancy progression [137]. Overall, there is no documented increase in carcinogenic risk in long-term-treated patients. Besides, evidence suggests that the reduction of IgE by omalizumab is not extremely low to alter the immune system related to the malignancy itself [138].

Parasitic Infestations

There is a theoretical possibility of an increased susceptibility to helminth infestation following omalizumab treatment as production of IgE serves as an immune effector mechanism against helminths [139]. In a 52-week randomized placebo-controlled trial on 137 patients, it was found that in high-risk patients, the number of patients developing one or more geohelminth infestation was slightly more with omalizumab (50%) than placebo (41%). However, severity of the infestation and response to anti-helminthic treatment were unaltered by omalizumab [140].

Thrombocytopenia

In preclinical studies, reduction in platelet counts was observed in juvenile cynomolgus monkeys receiving omalizumab doses 3.7- to 20-fold greater than the highest recommended dose in humans. However, no difference was found between patients treated with omalizumab and the control group in terms of development of thrombocytopenia in clinical studies (70.7% and 65.7%, respectively) [141]. However, immune thrombocytopenia has been reported in a 13-year-old patient treated with omalizumab for severe asthma [142].

Use in Special Populations

Pregnancy

Omalizumab can cross the placenta and is largely transferred to the foetus, with an omalizumab cord/maternal serum concentration ratio of 2.3 [143]. Considering the very long elimination $t_{1/2}$ of omalizumab (26 days), neonatal exposure to omalizumab would be expected to persist for weeks after birth. However, based on preclinical studies, no maternal toxicity, embryo toxicity or teratogenicity were observed, except neonatal thrombocytopenia in primates [144]. Experience in pregnant woman is based on case reports and on the Xolair Pregnancy Registry (EXPECT) study that enrolled 230 pregnancies and concluded no apparent increase of major congenital malformations among women treated with omalizumab [145]. Nevertheless, though the usage of omalizumab appears safe in pregnancy, the risk-benefit ratio needs to be adequately assessed prior to its prescription as neonates will be exposed to omalizumab weeks after birth.

Lactation

As omalizumab is a large molecule, the amount present in breast milk is likely to be low. Besides, as omalizumab is expected to get destroyed in the infant's gastrointestinal tract, chances of absorption are minimal. Therefore, use of omalizumab in lactating women is permissible [146].

Paediatric

Currently, omalizumab is approved for the management of CSU in patients ≥12 years of age and for asthma patients ≥6 years [147].

Geriatric

Omalizumab is found to be well tolerated and effective in treating elderly patients with CSU, refractory to nonsedative H1 antihistamines [148].

Drug Interactions

Concomitant use of ACE inhibitors in CSU may reduce the efficacy of omalizumab [149]. Although simultaneous use of omalizumab with immunotherapy was avoided earlier, a recent study indicated that this combination can be safely administered [150].

Availability, Administration and Dosing

Omalizumab injection is available as single-dose (150 mg/ml and 300 mg/ml) pre-filled syringes.

It is dosed as 150 mg/300 mg SC every 4 weekly.

It shows a Clarity/Opalescence ≤30 NTU (Ph.Eur.) and Color ≤ BY5. It needs to be stored at 2° to 8 °C, protected from light until use and should not be shaken. It needs to be kept out of the refrigerator 20 min prior to injection.

Injection sites include front of thighs, lower abdomen (except for a 2-inch area around the umbilicus) or back of the arms (if administered by another person).

Drug Monitoring

Owing to the risk of anaphylaxis, the need to closely observe patients 2–3 h after administration of omalizumab (which is administered only by a physician/healthcare professional) becomes mandatory. Furthermore, clinicians administering omalizumab should be prepared and trained to manage any episode of anaphylaxis encountered following omalizumab, with ready availability of resuscitation equipment [151]. Interestingly, no specific monitoring of any laboratory parameter is required while prescribing omalizumab.

Future Direction

The use of omalizumab as a steroid-sparing agent needs further exploration specifically in blistering disorders and urticarial vasculitis, with the aim of reducing immunosuppressive effects of systemic glucocorticoids and other conventional drugs, bringing about quicker disease remission, along with superior safety and tolerability.

Conclusion

In dermatology, apart from its use in CSU, omalizumab has proven to be beneficial in other off-label conditions. Furthermore, owing to minimal immunosuppression associated with omalizumab, it can be safely used for prolonged periods under medical supervision. Unfortunately, the high cost prevents its incorporation in regular day-to-day therapeutics in developing countries like India.

References

1. Easthope S, Jarvis B. Omalizumab. Drugs. 2001;61:253–60.
2. Chia JC, Mydlarski PR. Dermatologic uses of omalizumabtitle. J Dermatolog Treat. 2017;28:332–7.

3. McCormack PL. Omalizumab: a review of its use in patients with chronic spontaneous urticaria. Drugs. 2014;74:1693–9.
4. Greaves MW. Chronic urticaria. N Engl J Med. 1995;332:1767–72. [Erratum in: N Engl J Med 1995;333:1091]
5. Kaplan AP. Urticaria and angioedema. In: Wolf K, Goldsmith LA, Katz S, Gilchrist BA, Paller AS, Leffell DJ, editors. Fitzpatricks dermatology in general medicine. 7th ed. New York: McGraw Hill Publishing; 2007. p. 330–43.
6. Kaplan AP. Clinical practice. Chronic urticaria and angioedema. N Engl J Med. 2002;346:175–9.
7. Toubi E, Blant A, Kessel A, Golan TD. Low-dose cyclosporin a in the treatment of severe chronic idiopathic urticaria. Allergy. 1997;52:312–6.
8. Maurer M, Altrichter S, Bieber T, Biedermann T, Bräutigam M, Seyfried S, et al. Efficacy and safety of omalizumab in patients with chronic urticaria who exhibit IgE against thyroperoxidase. J Allergy Clin Immunol. 2011;128:202–209.e5.
9. Chang TW, Chen C, Lin CJ, Metz M, Church MK, Maurer M. The potential pharmacologic mechanisms of omalizumab in patients with chronic spontaneous urticaria. J Allergy Clin Immunol. 2015;135:337–42.
10. Mankad VS, Burks AW. Omalizumab: other indications and unanswered questions. Clin Rev Allergy Immunol. 2005;29:17–30.
11. Maurer M, Rosén K, Hsieh HJ, Saini S, Grattan C, Gimenéz-Arnau A, et al. Omalizumab for the treatment of chronic idiopathic or spontaneous urticaria. N Engl J Med. 2013;368:924–35.
12. Kaplan A, Ledford D, Ashby M, Canvin J, Zazzali JL, Conner E, et al. Omalizumab in patients with symptomatic chronic idiopathic/spontaneous urticaria despite standard combination therapy. J Allergy Clin Immunol. 2013;132:101–9.
13. Saini SS, Bindslev-Jensen C, Maurer M, Grob JJ, Bülbül Baskan E, Bradley MS, et al. Efficacy and Safety of Omalizumab in Patients with Chronic Idiopathic/Spontaneous Urticaria who Remain Symptomatic on H1 Antihistamines: A Randomized, Placebo-Controlled Study. J Invest Dermatol. 2015;135:925. Erratum for: J Invest Dermatol. 2015;135:67–75
14. Asero R. Chronic spontaneous urticaria treated with omalizumab: what differentiates early from late responders? Eur Ann Allergy Clin Immunol. 2021;53:47–8.
15. Schmetzer O, Lakin E, Topal FA, Preusse P, Freier D, Church MK, et al. IL-24 is a common and specific autoantigen of IgE in patients with chronic spontaneous urticaria. J Allergy Clin Immunol. 2018;142:876–82.
16. Cugno M, Asero R, Ferrucci S, Lorini M, Carbonelli V, Tedeschi A, et al. Elevated IgE to tissue factor and thyroglobulin are abated by omalizumab in chronic spontaneous urticaria. Allergy. 2018;73:2408–11.
17. Grattan CE, Francis DM, Hide M, Greaves MW. Detection of circulating histamine releasing autoantibodies with functional properties of anti-IgE in chronic urticaria. Clin Exp Allergy. 1991;21:695–704.
18. Hide M, Francis DM, Grattan CE, Hakimi J, Kochan JP, Greaves MW. Autoantibodies against the high-affinity IgE receptor as a cause of histamine release in chronic urticaria. N Engl J Med. 1993;328:1599–604.
19. Kaplan AP, Giménez-Arnau AM, Saini SS. Mechanisms of action that contribute to efficacy of omalizumab in chronic spontaneous urticaria. Allergy. 2017;72:519–33.
20. Maggi L, Rossettini B, Montaini G, Matucci A, Vultaggio A, Mazzoni A, et al. Omalizumab dampens type 2 inflammation in a group of long-term treated asthma patients and detaches IgE from FcεRI. Eur J Immunol. 2018;48:2005–14.
21. Asero R, Marzano AV, Ferrucci S, Lorini M, Carbonelli V, Cugno M. Co-occurrence of IgE and IgG autoantibodies in patients with chronic spontaneous urticaria. Clin Exp Immunol. 2020;200:242–9.
22. Straesser MD, Oliver E, Palacios T, Kyin T, Patrie J, Borish L, et al. Serum IgE as an immunological marker to predict response to omalizumab treatment in symptomatic chronic urticaria. J Allergy Clin Immunol Pract. 2018;6:1386–1388.e1.

23. Kolkhir P, Church MK, Altrichter S, Skov PS, Hawro T, Frischbutter S, Metz M, et al. Eosinopenia, in chronic spontaneous Urticaria, is associated with high disease activity, autoimmunity, and poor response to treatment. J Allergy Clin Immunol Pract. 2020;8:318–325.e5.
24. Deza G, Bertolín-Colilla M, Pujol RM, Curto-Barredo L, Soto D, García M, et al. Basophil FcεRI expression in chronic spontaneous Urticaria: a potential immunological predictor of response to Omalizumab therapy. Acta Derm Venereol. 2017;97:698–704.
25. Gericke J, Metz M, Ohanyan T, Weller K, Altrichter S, Skov PS, et al. Serum autoreactivity predicts time to response to omalizumab therapy in chronic spontaneous urticaria. J Allergy Clin Immunol. 2017;139:1059–1061.e1.
26. Nettis E, Cegolon L, Di Leo E, Lodi Rizzini F, Detoraki A, Canonica GW, et al. Omalizumab in chronic spontaneous urticaria: Efficacy, safety, predictors of treatment outcome, and time to response. Ann Allergy Asthma Immunol. 2018;121:474–8. Erratum in: Ann Allergy Asthma Immunol. 2018;121:749
27. Mustari AP, Bishnoi A, Kumaran MS. Biologicals in the treatment of chronic urticaria: a narrative review. Indian Dermatol Online J. 2023;14:9–20.
28. Magen E, Chikovani T, Waitman DA, Kahan NR. Factors related to omalizumab resistance in chronic spontaneous urticaria. Allergy Asthma Proc. 2019;40:273–8.
29. Devaraj S, Rosenson RS, Jialal I. Metabolic syndrome: an appraisal of the pro-inflammatory and procoagulant status. Endocrinol Metab Clin N Am. 2004;33:431–53.
30. Chaldakov GN, Fiore M, Ghenev PI, Beltowski J, Rančić G, Tunçel N, et al. Triactome: neuro-immune-adipose interactions. Implication in vascular biology. Front Immunol. 2014;5:130.
31. Kaplan A. Inflammation in chronic urticaria is not limited to the consequences of mast cell (or basophil) degranulation. Clin Exp Allergy. 2010;40:834–5.
32. Ye YM, Jin HJ, Hwang EK, Nam YH, Kim JH, Shin YS, et al. Co-existence of chronic urticaria and metabolic syndrome: clinical implications. Acta Derm Venereol. 2013;93:156–60.
33. Ritchie RF, Palomaki GE, Neveux LM, Navolotskaia O, Ledue TB, Craig WY. Reference distributions for complement proteins C3 and C4: a practical, simple and clinically relevant approach in a large cohort. J Clin Lab Anal. 2004;18:1–8.
34. Curto-Barredo L, Spertino J, Figueras-Nart I, Expósito-Serrano V, Guilabert A, Melé-Ninot G, et al. Omalizumab updosing allows disease activity control in patients with refractory chronic spontaneous urticaria. Br J Dermatol. 2018;179:210–2.
35. Alizadeh Aghdam M, van den Broek F, Rijken F, Knulst AC, Röckmann H. High-dose omalizumab use in patients with chronic spontaneous urticaria. J Allergy Clin Immunol Pract. 2020;8:1426–1427.e1.
36. Türk M, Kocatürk E, Cüre K, Yılmaz İ. Two-week intervals during omalizumab treatment may provide better symptom control in selected patients with chronic urticaria. J Allergy Clin Immunol Pract. 2018;6:1389–90.
37. Zuberbier T, Abdul Latiff AH, Abuzakouk M, Aquilina S, Asero R, Baker D, et al. The international EAACI/GA²LEN/EuroGuiDerm/APAAACI guideline for the definition, classification, diagnosis, and management of urticaria. Allergy. 2022;77:734–66.
38. Türk M, Carneiro-Leão L, Kolkhir P, Bonnekoh H, Buttgereit T, Maurer M. How to treat patients with chronic spontaneous Urticaria with Omalizumab: questions and answers. J Allergy Clin Immunol Pract. 2020;8:113–24.
39. Zhao Z, Cai T, Chen H, Chen L, Chen Y, Gao X, et al. Expert consensus on the use of omalizumab in chronic urticaria in China. World Allergy Organ J. 2021;14:100610.
40. Corren J, Casale TB, Lanier B, Buhl R, Holgate S, Jimenez P. Safety and tolerability of omalizumab. Clin Exp Allergy. 2009;39:788–97.
41. Metz M, Ohanyan T, Church MK, Maurer M. Retreatment with omalizumab results in rapid remission in chronic spontaneous and inducible urticaria. JAMA Dermatol. 2014;150:288–90.
42. Schauder S. Lichturtikaria [Solar urticaria]. Hautarzt. 2003;54:952–8.
43. Güzelbey O, Ardelean E, Magerl M, Zuberbier T, Maurer M, Metz M. Successful treatment of solar urticaria with anti-immunoglobulin E therapy. Allergy. 2008;63:1563–5.
44. Waibel KH, Reese DA, Hamilton RG, Devillez RL. Partial improvement of solar urticaria after omalizumab. J Allergy Clin Immunol. 2010;125:490–1.

45. Metz M, Altrichter S, Ardelean E, et al. Anti-immunoglobulin E treatment of patients with recalcitrant physical urticaria. Int Arch Allergy Immunol. 2011;154:177–80.
46. Aubin F, Avenel-Audran M, Jeanmougin M, Adamski H, Peyron JL, Marguery MC, et al. Omalizumab in patients with severe and refractory solar urticaria: a phase II multicentric study. J Am Acad Dermatol. 2016;74:574–5.
47. Zimmer S, Peveling-Oberhag A, Weber A, Gilfert T, Rady-Pizarro U, Staubach P. Unique coexistence of cold and solar urticaria and its efficient treatment. Br J Dermatol. 2016;174:1150–2.
48. Müller S, Schempp CM, Jakob T. Failure of omalizumab in the treatment of solar urticaria. J Eur Acad Dermatol Venereol. 2016;30:524–5.
49. Duchini G, Bäumler W, Bircher AJ, Scherer K. Failure of omalizumab (Xolair®) in the treatment of a case of solar urticaria caused by ultraviolet a and visible light. Photodermatol Photoimmunol Photomed. 2011;27:336–7.
50. Buss YL, Sticherling M. Cold urticaria; disease course and outcome--an investigation of 85 patients before and after therapy. Br J Dermatol. 2005;153:440–1.
51. Boyce JA. Successful treatment of cold-induced urticaria/anaphylaxis with anti-IgE. J Allergy Clin Immunol. 2006;117:1415–8.
52. Le Moing A, Bécourt C, Pape E, Dejobert Y, Delaporte E, Staumont-Sallé D. Effective treatment of idiopathic chronic cold urticaria with omalizumab: report of 3 cases. J Am Acad Dermatol. 2013;69:e99–101.
53. Brodská P, Schmid-Grendelmeier P. Treatment of severe cold contact urticaria with omalizumab: case reports. Case Rep Dermatol. 2012;4:275–80.
54. Bullerkotte U, Wieczorek D, Kapp A, Wedi B. Effective treatment of refractory severe heat urticaria with omalizumab. Allergy. 2010;65:931–2.
55. Murphy GM, Greaves MW, Zollman PE, Winkelmann RK. Cholinergic urticaria, passive transfer experiments from human to monkey. Dermatologica. 1988;177:338–40.
56. Metz M, Bergmann P, Zuberbier T, Maurer M. Successful treatment of cholinergic urticaria with anti-immunoglobulin E therapy. Allergy. 2008;63:247–9.
57. Kutlu A, Tanoglu A, Ozturk S. Healing effects of omalizumab in a patient with cholinergic urticaria associated severe dyspeptic complaints. Chin Med J. 2015;128:1559–60.
58. Grattan CEH, Marsland AM. Urticaria. In: Griffiths C, Barker J, Bleiker T, Chalmers R, Creamer D, editors. Rook's textbook of dermatology. 9th ed. Sussex: Wiley Blackwell; 2016. p. 42.1–42.18.
59. Vieira Dos Santos R, Locks Bidese B, Rabello de Souza J, Maurer M. Effects of omalizumab in a patient with three types of chronic urticaria. Br J Dermatol. 2014;170:469–71.
60. Bindslev-Jensen C, Skov PS. Efficacy of omalizumab in delayed pressure urticaria: a case report. Allergy. 2010;65:138–9.
61. Boguniewicz M, Leung DY. 10. Atopic dermatitis. J Allergy Clin Immunol. 2006;117:S475–80.
62. Stingl G. IgE-mediated, fc(epsilon)RI-dependent allergen presentation: a pathogenetic factor in atopic dermatitis? J Am Acad Dermatol. 2001;45:S17–20.
63. Leung DY, Schneeberger EE, Siraganian RP, Geha RS, Bhan AK. The presence of IgE on macrophages and dendritic cells infiltrating into the skin lesion of atopic dermatitis. Clin Immunol Immunopathol. 1987;42:328–37.
64. Hirata T, Furie BC, Furie B. P-, E-, and L-selectin mediate migration of activated CD8+ T lymphocytes into inflamed skin. J Immunol. 2002;169:4307–13.
65. Soumelis V, Reche PA, Kanzler H, Yuan W, Edward G, Homey B, et al. Human epithelial cells trigger dendritic cell mediated allergic inflammation by producing TSLP. Nat Immunol. 2002;3:673–80.
66. Corrigan CJ, Jayaratnam A, Wang Y, Liu Y, de Waal Malefyt R, Meng Q, et al. Early production of thymic stromal lymphopoietin precedes infiltration of dendritic cells expressing its receptor in allergen-induced late phase cutaneous responses in atopic subjects. Allergy. 2009;64:1014–22.

67. Sismanopoulos N, Delivanis DA, Alysandratos KD, Angelidou A, Vasiadi M, Therianou A, et al. IL-9 induces VEGF secretion from human MCs and IL-9/IL-9 receptor genes are overexpressed in atopic dermatitis. PLoS One. 2012;7:e33271.
68. Liu YJ, Soumelis V, Watanabe N, Ito T, Wang YH, Malefyt RW, et al. TSLP: an epithelial cell cytokine that regulates T cell differentiation by conditioning dendritic cell maturation. Annu Rev Immunol. 2007;25:193–219.
69. Forman SB, Garrett AB. Success of omalizumab as monotherapy in adult atopic dermatitis: case report and discussion of the high-affinity immunoglobulin E receptor. FcepsilonRI Cutis. 2007;80:38–40.
70. Barrios JL, Paradis L, Desroches A. Efficacy of Omalizumab therapy in a case of severe atopic dermatitis. Allergy, Asthma & Clin Immunol. 2011;7(Suppl 2):A33.
71. Krathen RA, Hsu S. Failure of omalizumab for treatment of severe adult atopic dermatitis. J Am Acad Dermatol. 2005;53:338–40.
72. Sheinkopf LE, Rafi AW, Do LT KRM, Klaustermeyer WB. Efficacy of omalizumab in the treatment of atopic dermatitis: a pilot study. Allergy Asthma Proc. 2008;29:530–7.
73. Lane JE, Cheyney JM, Lane TN, Kent DE, Cohen DJ. Treatment of recalcitrant atopic dermatitis with omalizumab. J Am Acad Dermatol. 2006;54:68–72.
74. Hotze M, Baurecht H, Rodríguez E, Chapman-Rothe N, Ollert M, Fölster-Holst R, et al. Increased efficacy of omalizumab in atopic dermatitis patients with wild-type filaggrin status and higher serum levels of phosphatidylcholines. Allergy. 2014;69:132–5.
75. Iyengar SR, Hoyte EG, Loza A, Bonaccorso S, Chiang D, Umetsu DT, et al. Immunologic effects of omalizumab in children with severe refractory atopic dermatitis: a randomized, placebo-controlled clinical trial. Int Arch Allergy Immunol. 2013;162:89–93.
76. Vigo PG, Girgis KR, Pfuetze BL, Critchlow ME, Fisher J, Hussain I. Efficacy of anti-IgE therapy in patients with atopic dermatitis. J Am Acad Dermatol. 2006;55:168–70.
77. Fairley JA, Baum CL, Brandt DS, Messingham KA. Pathogenicity of IgE in autoimmunity: successful treatment of bullous pemphigoid with omalizumab. J Allergy Clin Immunol. 2009;123:704–5.
78. Zone JJ, Taylor T, Hull C, Schmidt L, Meyer L. IgE basement membrane zone antibodies induce eosinophil infiltration and histological blisters in engrafted human skin on SCID mice. J Invest Dermatol. 2007;127:1167–74.
79. Dimson OG, Giudice GJ, Fu CL, Van den Bergh F, Warren SJ, Janson MM, et al. Identification of a potential effector function for IgE autoantibodies in the organ-specific autoimmune disease bullous pemphigoid. J Invest Dermatol. 2003;120:784–8.
80. Fairley JA, Burnett CT, Fu CL, Larson DL, Fleming MG, Giudice GJ. A pathogenic role for IgE in autoimmunity: bullous pemphigoid IgE reproduces the early phase of lesion development in human skin grafted to nu/nu mice. J Invest Dermatol. 2007;127:2605–11.
81. Christophoridis S, Büdinger L, Borradori L, Hunziker T, Merk HF, Hertl M. IgG, IgA and IgE autoantibodies against the ectodomain of BP180 in patients with bullous and cicatricial pemphigoid and linear IgA bullous dermatosis. Br J Dermatol. 2000;143:349–55.
82. Arbesman CE, Wypych JI, Reisman RE, Beutner EH. IgE levels in sera of patients with pemphigus or bullous pemphigoid. Arch Dermatol. 1974;110:378–81.
83. Djukanović R, Wilson SJ, Kraft M, Jarjour NN, Steel M, Chung KF, et al. Effects of treatment with anti-immunoglobulin E antibody omalizumab on airway inflammation in allergic asthma. Am J Respir Crit Care Med. 2004;170:583–93.
84. Wintroub BU, Mihm MC Jr, Goetzl EJ, Soter NA, Austen KF. Morphologic and functional evidence for release of mast-cell products in bullous pemphigoid. N Engl J Med. 1978;298:417–21.
85. Stone KD, Prussin C, Metcalfe DD. IgE, MCs, basophils, and eosinophils. J Allergy Clin Immunol. 2010;125:S73–80.
86. Yu KK, Crew AB, Messingham KA, Fairley JA, Woodley DT. Omalizumab therapy for bullous pemphigoid. J Am Acad Dermatol. 2014;71:468–74.
87. London VA, Kim GH, Fairley JA, Woodley DT. Successful treatment of bullous pemphigoid with omalizumab. Arch Dermatol. 2012;148:1241–3.

88. Dufour C, Souillet AL, Chaneliere C, Jouen F, Bodemer C, Jullien D, et al. Successful management of severe infant bullous pemphigoid with omalizumab. Br J Dermatol. 2012;166:1140–2.
89. Lieberoth S, Thomsen SF. Cutaneous and gastrointestinal symptoms in two patients with systemic mastocytosis successfully treated with omalizumab. Case Rep Med. 2015;2015:903541.
90. Milgrom H, Fick RB Jr, Su JQ, Reimann JD, Bush RK, Watrous ML, Metzger WJ. Treatment of allergic asthma with monoclonal anti-IgE antibody. rhuMAb-E25 study group. N Engl J Med. 1999;341:1966–73.
91. Beck LA, Marcotte GV, MacGlashan D, Togias A, Saini S. Omalizumab-induced reductions in mast cell Fce psilon RI expression and function. J Allergy Clin Immunol. 2004 Sep;114(3):527–30.
92. Siebenhaar F, Kühn W, Zuberbier T, Maurer M. Successful treatment of cutaneous mastocytosis and Ménière disease with anti-IgE therapy. J Allergy Clin Immunol. 2007;120:213–5.
93. Matito A, Azaña JM, Torrelo A, Alvarez-Twose I. Cutaneous Mastocytosis in adults and children: new classification and prognostic factors. Immunol Allergy Clin N Am. 2018;38:351–63.
94. Sokol KC, Ghazi A, Kelly BC, Grant JA. Omalizumab as a desensitizing agent and treatment in mastocytosis: a review of the literature and case report. J Allergy Clin Immunol Pract. 2014;2:266–70.
95. Douglass JA, Carroll K, Voskamp A, Bourke P, Wei A, O'Hehir RE. Omalizumab is effective in treating systemic mastocytosis in a nonatopic patient. Allergy. 2010;65:926–7.
96. Kibsgaard L, Skjold T, Deleuran M, Vestergaard C. Omalizumab induced remission of idiopathic anaphylaxis in a patient suffering from indolent systemic mastocytosis. Acta Derm Venereol. 2014;94:363–4.
97. Paraskevopoulos G, Sifnaios E, Christodoulopoulos K, Mantopoulou F, Papakonstantis M, Sabaziotis D. Successful treatment of mastocytic anaphylactic episodes with reduction of skin MCs after anti-IgE therapy. Eur Ann Allergy Clin Immunol. 2013;45:52–5.
98. Pitt TJ, Cisneros N, Kalicinsky C, Becker AB. Successful treatment of idiopathic anaphylaxis in an adolescent. J Allergy Clin Immunol. 2010;126:415–6.
99. Kontou-Fili K, Filis CI, Voulgari C, Panayiotidis PG. Omalizumab monotherapy for bee sting and unprovoked "anaphylaxis" in a patient with systemic mastocytosis and undetectable specific IgE. Ann Allergy Asthma Immunol. 2010;104:537–9.
100. Carter MC, Robyn JA, Bressler PB, Walker JC, Shapiro GG, Metcalfe DD. Omalizumab for the treatment of unprovoked anaphylaxis in patients with systemic mastocytosis. J Allergy Clin Immunol. 2007;119:1550–1.
101. Del Pozo MER, Saenz NPM, Vera JG, Tiro JL. Vasculitic urticaria treated with omalizumab. Case Rep World Allergy Org J. 2012;5(supplement 2):S106.
102. Varricchi G, Detoraki A, Liccardo B, et al. Efficacy of omalizumab in the treatment of urticaria-vasculitis associated to Churg-Strauss syndrome: a case report. World Allergy Organ J. 2012;5(supplement 2):S89–90.
103. Díez LS, Tamayo LM, Cardona R. Omalizumab: therapeutic option in chronic spontaneous urticaria difficult to control with associated vasculitis, report of three cases. Biomedica. 2013;33:503–12.
104. Sussman G, Hébert J, Barron C, Bian J, Caron-Guay RM, Laflamme S, et al. Real-life experiences with omalizumab for the treatment of chronic urticaria. Ann Allergy Asthma Immunol. 2014;112:170–4.
105. Ghazanfar MN, Thomsen SF. Omalizumab for urticarial Vasculitis: case report and review of the literature. Case Rep Dermatol Med. 2015;2015:576893.
106. Uzun R, Yalcin AD, Celik B, Bulut T, Yalcin AN. Levofloxacin induced toxic epidermal necrolysis: successful therapy with Omalizumab (anti-IgE) and pulse prednisolone. Am J Case Rep. 2016;17:666–71.
107. Yalcin AD. A case of Netherton syndrome: successful treatment with omalizumab and pulse prednisolone and its effects on cytokines and immunoglobulin levels. Immunopharmacol Immunotoxicol. 2016;38:162–6.

108. Nonaka M, Sakitani E, Yoshihara T. Anti-IgE therapy to Kimura's disease: a pilot study. Auris Nasus Larynx. 2014;41:384–8.
109. Ao S, Huang G, Tang X, Zhu Z, Han J, Wang F, Zhai W. Anti-immunoglobulin E provides an additional therapy to conventional steroids for Kimura's disease. J Dermatol. 2024;51:602–6.
110. Ohameje NU, Loveless JW, Saini SS. Atopic dermatitis or hyper-IgE syndrome? Allergy Asthma Proc. 2006;27:289–91.
111. Chularojanamontri L, Wimoolchart S, Tuchinda P, Kulthanan K, Kiewjoy N. Role of omalizumab in a patient with hyper-IgE syndrome and review dermatologic manifestations. Asian Pac J Allergy Immunol. 2009;27:233–6.
112. Bard S, Paravisini A, Avilés-Izquierdo JA, Fernandez-Cruz E, Sánchez-Ramón S. Eczematous dermatitis in the setting of hyper-IgE syndrome successfully treated with omalizumab. Arch Dermatol. 2008;144:1662–3.
113. Jennette JC. Overview of the 2012 revised international Chapel Hill consensus conference nomenclature of vasculitides. Clin Exp Nephrol. 2013;17:603–6.
114. Latorre M, Baldini C, Seccia V, Notarstefano C, Della Rossa A, Tani C, et al. Omalizumab: a novel steroid sparing agent in eosinophilic granulomatosis with polyangiitis? Clin Exp Rheumatol. 2013;31:S91–2.
115. Pabst S, Tiyerili V, Grohé C. Apparent response to anti-IgE therapy in two patients with refractory "forme fruste" of Churg-Strauss syndrome. Thorax. 2008;63:747–8.
116. Iglesias E, Camacho Lovillo M, Delgado Pecellín I, Lirola Cruz MJ, Falcón Neyra MD, Salazar Quero JC, et al. Successful management of Churg-Strauss syndrome using omalizumab as adjuvant immunomodulatory therapy: first documented pediatric case. Pediatr Pulmonol. 2014;49:E78–81.
117. Spina MF, Miadonna A. Role of omalizumab and steroids in Churg-Strauss syndrome. J Allergy Clin Immunol. 2009;124:600–1.
118. Puéchal X, Rivereau P, Vinchon F. Churg-Strauss syndrome associated with omalizumab. Eur J Intern Med. 2008;19:364–6.
119. Bargagli E, Madioni C, Olivieri C, Penza F, Rottoli P. Churg-Strauss vasculitis in a patient treated with omalizumab. J Asthma. 2008;45:115–6.
120. Wechsler ME, Wong DA, Miller MK, Lawrence-Miyasaki L. Churg-Strauss syndrome in patients treated with omalizumab. Chest. 2009;136:507–18.
121. Cisneros C, Segrelles G, Herráez L, Gonzalez A, Girón R. Churg-Strauss syndrome in a patient treated with omalizumab. J Investig Allergol Clin Immunol. 2013;23:515–6.
122. Jachiet M, Samson M, Cottin V, Kahn JE, Le Guenno G, Bonniaud P, et al. Anti-IgE monoclonal antibody (Omalizumab) in refractory and relapsing eosinophilic granulomatosis with Polyangiitis (Churg-Strauss): data on seventeen patients. Arthritis Rheumatol. 2016;68:2274–82.
123. Kumar C, Zito PM. Omalizumab. [Updated 2023 Aug 17]. In: StatPearls [Internet]. Treasure Island (FL): StatPearls Publishing; 2024. Available from: https://www.ncbi.nlm.nih.gov/books/NBK545183/.
124. Plosker GL, Keam SJ. Omalizumab: a review of its use in the treatment of allergic asthma. BioDrugs. 2008;22:189–204.
125. Fougerousse AC, Badaoui A. Omalizumab-induced paradoxical urticaria responsive to dupilumab. Ann Dermatol Venereol. 2023;150:302–3.
126. Molderings GJ, Dumoulin FL, Homann J, Sido B, Textor J, Mücke M, et al. Adrenal insufficiency is a contraindication for omalizumab therapy in mast cell activation disease: risk for serum sickness. Naunyn Schmiedeberg's Arch Pharmacol. 2020;393:1573–80.
127. Limb SL, Starke PR, Lee CE, Chowdhury BA. Delayed onset and protracted progression of anaphylaxis after omalizumab administration in patients with asthma. J Allergy Clin Immunol. 2007;120:1378–81.
128. Cox L, Platts-Mills TA, Finegold I, Schwartz LB, Simons FE, Wallace DV, et al. American Academy of Allergy, Asthma & Immunology/American College of Allergy, asthma and immunology joint task force report on omalizumab-associated anaphylaxis. J Allergy Clin Immunol. 2007;120:1373–7.

129. Stokes J. Anti-IgE treatment for disorders other than asthma. Front Med (Lausanne). 2017;4:152.
130. Broesby-Olsen S, Vestergaard H, Mortz CG, Jensen B, Havelund T, Hermann AP, Mastocytosis Centre Odense University Hospital (MastOUH), et al. Omalizumab prevents anaphylaxis and improves symptoms in systemic mastocytosis: efficacy and safety observations. Allergy. 2018;73:230–8.
131. Molderings GJ, Raithel M, Kratz F, Azemar M, Haenisch B, Harzer S, Homann J. Omalizumab treatment of systemic mast cell activation disease: experiences from four cases. Intern Med. 2011;50:611–5.
132. Ruppert AM, Averous G, Stanciu D, Deroide N, Riehm S, Poindron V, et al. Development of Churg-Strauss syndrome with controlled asthma during omalizumab treatment. J Allergy Clin Immunol. 2008;121:253–4.
133. Bargagli E, Rottoli P. Omalizumab treatment associated with Churg-Strauss vasculitis. Int Arch Allergy Immunol. 2008;145:268.
134. Giavina-Bianchi P, Agondi R, Kalil J. One year administration of anti-IgE to a patient with Churg-Strauss syndrome. Int Arch Allergy Immunol. 2008;146:176.
135. European Medicines Agency (EMEA): Omalizumab (Xolair®) full prescribing information (EU). 2007. http://www.emea.europaeu/humandocs/PDFs/EPAR/Xolair/H-606-PI-en.pdf. Accessed 8 Apr 2008.
136. Busse W, Buhl R, Fernandez Vidaurre C, Blogg M, Zhu J, Eisner MD, Canvin J. Omalizumab and the risk of malignancy: results from a pooled analysis. J Allergy Clin Immunol. 2012;129:983–9.e6.
137. Long A, Rahmaoui A, Rothman KJ, Guinan E, Eisner M, Bradley MS, et al. Incidence of malignancy in patients with moderate-to-severe asthma treated with or without omalizumab. J Allergy Clin Immunol. 2014;134:560–567.e4.
138. Bagnasco D, Canevari RF, Del Giacco S, Ferrucci S, Pigatto P, Castelnuovo P, et al. Omalizumab and cancer risk: current evidence in allergic asthma, chronic urticaria, and chronic rhinosinusitis with nasal polyps. World Allergy Organ J. 2022;15:100721.
139. Jarrett EE, Miller HR. Production and activities of IgE in helminth infection. Prog Allergy. 1982;31:178–233.
140. Cruz AA, Lima F, Sarinho E, Ayre G, Martin C, Fox H, et al. Safety of anti-immunoglobulin E therapy with omalizumab in allergic patients at risk of geohelminth infection. Clin Exp Allergy. 2007;37:197–207.
141. Öztop N, Demır S, Beyaz Ş, Tüzer ÖC, Çolakoğlu B, Büyüköztürk S, Gelıncık A. Omalizumab in practice: ten-year experience of a tertiary referral allergy Centre. Asthma Allergy Immunol. 2022;20:36–47.
142. Lopez-Rodriguez JA, Santos FL. Trombocitopenia por omalizumab [Thrombocytopenia due to omalizumab]. An Pediatr (Barc). 2014;80:413–4.
143. Saito J, Yakuwa N, Sandaiji N, Uno C, Yagishita S, Suzuki T, et al. Omalizumab concentrations in pregnancy and lactation: a case study. J Allergy Clin Immunol Pract. 2020;8:3603–4.
144. Majou D, Moreira B, Martin C, Chhun S, Treluyer JM, Tsatsaris V, et al. Safety of Omalizumab during pregnancy and breast-feeding with assessment of placental transfer: a case report. Allergy Asthma Immunol Res. 2021;13:515–6.
145. Namazy JA, Blais L, Andrews EB, Scheuerle AE, Cabana MD, Thorp JM, et al. Pregnancy outcomes in the omalizumab pregnancy registry and a disease-matched comparator cohort. J Allergy Clin Immunol. 2020;145:528–536.e1.
146. Drugs and Lactation Database (LactMed®) [Internet]. National Institute of Child Health and Human Development, Bethesda (MD). Nov 15, 2023. Omalizumab.
147. Yu L, Zhang H, Pan J, Ye L. Pediatric usage of Omalizumab: a promising one. World Allergy Organ J. 2021;14:100614.
148. Nettis E, Cegolon L, Di Leo E, Canonica WG, Detoraki A, Italian OCUReL Study Group. Omalizumab in elderly patients with chronic spontaneous urticaria: an Italian real-life experience. Ann Allergy Asthma Immunol. 2018;120:318–23.

149. Asero R. ACE inhibitors may interfere with omalizumab in chronic spontaneous urticaria. J Eur Acad Dermatol Venereol. 2017;31:e358–9.
150. Dantzer JA, Wood RA. Update on omalizumab in allergen immunotherapy. Curr Opin Allergy Clin Immunol. 2021;21:559–68.
151. Kim HL, Leigh R, Becker A. Omalizumab: practical considerations regarding the risk of anaphylaxis. Allergy Asthma Clin Immunol. 2010;6:32.

40 Rituximab

Introduction

Rituximab (RTX) is a specific mouse and human chimeric monoclonal antibody. It is an immunoglobulin G1 (IgG1) kappa monoclonal antibody composed of a murine variable region (Fab portion) that is fused onto a human constant region (Fc portion) that targets the CD20 antigen present on pre-B, immature and mature B cells.

Mechanism of Action

Mechanism of action of rituximab is described in Fig. 40.1.

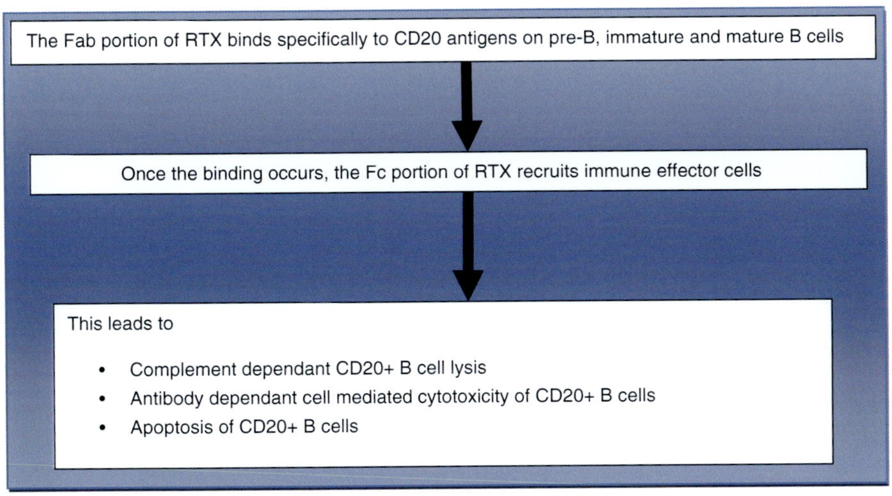

Fig. 40.1 Mechanism of action of rituximab

A. K. Bubna, *Therapeutics in Dermatology - Essentials for Clinical Practice*,
https://doi.org/10.1007/978-981-95-3791-4_40

Besides, as CD20 is not expressed on pro-B cells, plasmablasts and plasma cells, depletion of B-cell subpopulation is transient and does not affect immunoglobulin synthesis. It is further observed that regeneration of B cells occurs within 6–12 months following therapy, and serum immunoglobulins are not significantly reduced [1, 2]. This can account for relapses as B cells regenerate.

Pharmacokinetics

RTX is administered as an intravenous (IV) infusion. Following lymphoma protocol, RTX is detectable in serum of patients even after 3–6 months of completion of therapy. The median terminal elimination half-life of RTX is 22 days (range from 6.1 to 52 days). No formal studies have been conducted to examine the effects of either hepatic or renal impairment on the pharmacokinetics of RTX.

Indications [3, 4]

FDA Approved

- Relapsing and refractory follicular lymphoma (non-Hodgkin's type).
- Rheumatoid arthritis.
- Pemphigus group of disorders (US FDA approval was obtained on June 2018).

Off-Label

Autoimmune Vesiculobullous Disorders

- Mucous membrane pemphigoid (MMP).
- Bullous pemphigoid (BP).

Connective tissue disorders

- Dermatomyositis.
- Cutaneous lupus erythematosus.
- Systemic sclerosis.

Vasculitis

- Wegener's granulomatosis.
- Churg-Strauss syndrome.
- Microscopic polyangiitis.
- *Graft* versus *host disease.*
- *Atopic dermatitis.*
- *Primary cutaneous B-cell lymphoma.*

Others

- Melanoma.
- Kimura's disease.
- Schnitzler's syndrome.
- Intravascular large B-cell lymphoma.

Contraindications

- Hypersensitivity to the drug.
- Hypersensitivity to murine proteins.
- Severe heart failure.
- HIV infection with CD4+ counts less than 250/μl.

Pregnancy Prescribing Status: Category 'C'.

Clinical Uses

Dosage and Administration of RTX for FDA-Approved Indications

- Non-Hodgkin's lymphoma: RTX 375 mg/m^2 is administered as an IV infusion once a week, with four infusions over a month. It can be used either as monotherapy or combined with other chemotherapy regimens like the cyclophosphamide, hydroxydaunorubicin, oncovin and prednisolone (CHOP) regimen.
- Rheumatoid arthritis: RTX 1 gm is administered as an IV infusion. Two infusions, one on day 1 and the other on day 15, are given [5, 6].

Pemphigus

RTX was first used by Heizmann et al. [7] for paraneoplastic pemphigus with a successful outcome. Subsequently, RTX has been utilized by many dermatologists for the same.

Indications of RTX in Pemphigus [8–12]

- Patients who have failed to respond adequately to conventional therapy.
- Patients in whom corticosteroids or other immunosuppressives are contraindicated or are causing severe adverse reactions necessitating discontinuation of the drug.
- Patients who relapse after conventional therapy for pemphigus.
- Approved as a first-line therapy for pemphigus.

Treatment Protocols Followed in Pemphigus

- **Lymphoma protocol**: This is the most commonly followed protocol in pemphigus. Here, 375/m^2 of RTX is administered per week for 4 weeks [13, 14].

- **Rheumatoid arthritis protocol**: This protocol is now being increasingly followed by most dermatologists. Two doses, 1gm each, of RTX is administered at an interval of 15 days. This regimen is economic to the patient due to less number of infusions involved. [10]
- **Combination therapy**: RTX is combined with IVIG, dexamethasone pulse or immunoadsorption [15, 16]. Rheumatoid arthritis protocol is followed here.
- Long-term therapy with regular infusions of RTX every 4 or 12 weeks following the induction phase of RTX infusion [9].
- **Low-dose RTX:** Two doses of 500 mg each of RTX are administered at an interval of 15 days. This can be followed up with one injection of 500 mg, once in 6 months, or if there is a relapse.

Premedication

The patient is premedicated with:

- Injection hydrocortisone 100 mg IV stat.
- Injection pheniramine maleate 22.75 mg IV stat.
- Tablet paracetamol 500 mg PO, 30 min prior to RTX infusion.

Rituximab Infusion

Infusion protocol for rituximab is described in Fig. 40.2.

Subsequent infusions are administered at 100 mg/h, and the rate increased by 50 mg/h every 30 min till a maximum infusion rate of 400 mg/h is obtained.

It would be easier to infuse with an infusion pump:

- 30 ml/h for half-hour (15 ml)
- 60 ml/h for half hour (30 ml)
- 90 ml/h till infusion is over (455 ml, 5 h)
- Total infusion period is 6 h.

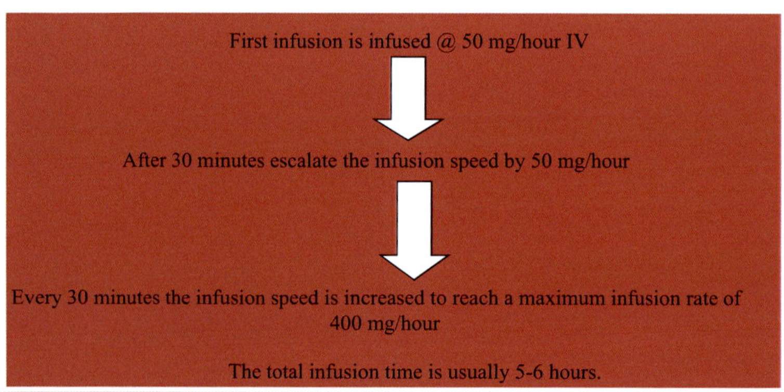

Fig. 40.2 Infusion protocol for rituximab

Eming et al. [17] have demonstrated RTX in pemphigus vulgaris to work by depleting autoreactive T cells and downregulating desmoglein-3-specific CD4+ Th cells.

In India, however, the cost of the drug may pose an important drawback in patient management. As pemphigus is not a neoplastic disease, it has been suggested that lower doses of RTX (500 mg given at 2 weeks interval) could also suffice without compromising on the efficacy and at the same time maintaining a better safety profile [18]. Gupta et al. [19], in a study conducted on refractory pemphigus, utilized RTX in the lower dosing schedule, as described above. In those cases where satisfactory results were not obtained, two additional doses of RTX were administered after 6 months in the similar dosing pattern. Complete remission was seen in 82% of their patients. In the remaining 18 patients, maintenance therapy with low-dose steroids, either 5 mg once daily or on alternate days, or on cyclophosphamide 50 mg or azathioprine 50 mg daily, was continued with no relapses. Kanwar et al. [20] have compared two doses of 1 gm given 2 weeks apart and 2 doses of 500 mg given 2 weeks apart. They concluded that no statistically significant difference in clinical outcomes or relapse rates was seen in both regimens.

Londhe et al. [21] have used a modified dosing of the lymphoma protocol wherein the fourth dose of RTX was administered 3 months after the third dose, with an efficacious result. Apart from improvement of cutaneous lesions, they also demonstrated an 82.8% fall in the mean antibody levels of desmoglein-3 in these patients.

Therefore, it would be worthwhile to point out that the optimal dose of RTX in pemphigus has not been clearly determined with modifications in its dosing schedule being continuously contemplated by various authors, in order to reduce the cost and interval of dosing, without compromising on the therapeutic efficacy of RTX.

In most cases, duration of remission after RTX therapy is 2 years. Moreover, when RTX is readministered during relapses, its safety and therapeutic benefits are still maintained [22]. Long-term follow-up is therefore mandatory to determine the appropriate dosing for pemphigus patients [18]. Dosing can also be individualized based on patient requirement.

Mucous Membrane Pemphigoid (MMP)

MMP is a rare and orphan disease. The estimated incidence is 1 case per million individuals in the general population [23]. Owing to its rarity, literature on the use of RTX in MMP is limited. Le-Roux Villet et al. [24], in their study on 25 patients with refractory MMP, demonstrated RTX to be a valuable therapeutic agent for MMP, administered according to the lymphoma protocol. Within 3 months of the first RTX cycle, complete response was seen for both ocular and extraocular manifestations in 68% of patients. In 20% of patients, a second cycle of RTX was required to obtain complete clinical remission. However, in the remaining 12% of patients, owing to complications related to RTX, therapy had to be discontinued. Of note, in the 88% of patients who developed complete clinical remission, there was a relapse in 40% of patients within 4 months of completion of the treatment, thereby suggesting that effects of RTX in MMP are short lived. In the above study, concomitant immunotherapy with dapsone and sulfasalazine was also utilized.

There have been six more case reports highlighting the use of RTX, using the lymphoma protocol in MMP. In all patients, RTX was used because of unresponsiveness of the disease to conventional regimens. Also, concomitant immunosuppressive treatment was continued [25–29]. In one patient, four additional infusions of RTX ($375/m^2$) had to be given every 3 months as maintenance therapy [29]. Of these six cases, three demonstrated reasonable stabilization of conjunctival scarring [25, 26, 29], one had partial response [28] and one became totally blind [27]. Optimum response was seen in the cutaneous component of the disease. It has been therefore postulated that the principal response of RTX is obtained during the phase of active inflammation, owing to its ability to destroy pathogenic B cells and eliminating pathogenic antibodies while simultaneously influencing the inflammatory processes by its effects on T cells [17, 30]. Consequently, if scarring occurs, then the response demonstrated by RTX is poor. Therefore, the onus of initiating therapy with RTX rests with the treating clinician, and it becomes his obligation to carefully assess the extent and severity of the disease, evaluate lesions and blister formation and compare active inflammation versus irreversible scarring [31]. Once the clinician arrives at a concrete conclusion, he can begin therapy with RTX for MMP, based on his discretion. It needs to be emphasized that mortality caused by septicaemia in patients treated with RTX for many autoimmune diseases has been reported [2, 32]. This becomes an alarming concern in patients of MMP where mortality from the disease is limited, even though morbidity and sequel of scarring are considerably disabling and serious [33].

Dermatomyositis

Dermatomyositis (DM) is a systemic autoimmune disease that primarily affects the muscles, skin and lungs and is associated with considerable morbidity.

There is substantial evidence suggesting the role of B lymphocytes in its pathogenesis. Moreover, muscle biopsy specimens exhibit a predominance of perivascular B cells and up to 40% of DM patients have detectable myositis-specific autoantibodies [34, 35].

RTX has been utilized in treating both adult and juvenile DM.

In the study by Cooper et al. [36], with RTX on four children for recalcitrant juvenile DM, utilizing the standard lymphoma protocol, three reported clinical improvement, with the fourth patient demonstrating progression of the disease. Of these, one patient who was positive for anti-Mi-2 demonstrated a dramatic response to two cycles of RTX given at an interval of 1 year. Along with RTX, this patient also received weekly methotrexate. This excellent response can be explained by the presence of a strong B-cell-driven component in the disease of this patient, depicted by the presence of myositis-specific autoantibody, anti-Mi-2.

In adult DM also, RTX has demonstrated good results. Levine [37] has expressed that both muscle symptoms and cutaneous signs improve following RTX administration according to the lymphoma protocol. However, in a pilot study conducted by Chung et al. [38], it was only myositis that revealed improvement, with cutaneous manifestations exhibiting meagre changes. In this study, the rheumatoid arthritis protocol was advocated though. This differential efficacy for skin and muscle disease can be explained by the fact that skin inflammation is predominantly characterized by CD4+ T cells rather than B cells [39, 40]. However, there are reports of the beneficial effects of RTX on cutaneous manifestations of DM as well [37, 41].

Cutaneous Lupus Erythematosus (CLE)

According to the SLICC (Systemic Lupus International Collaborating Clinics) classification criteria for systemic lupus erythematosus (SLE), mucocutaneous manifestations include acute cutaneous lupus erythematosus (ACLE), subacute cutaneous lupus erythematosus (SCLE) and chronic cutaneous lupus erythematosus (CCLE), oral ulcers and non-scarring alopecia [42].

First-line therapy in CLE is generally initiated with antimalarials and oral or topical glucocorticoids. In cases that are unresponsive to the above agents, immunosuppressives like azathioprine, mycophenolate mofetil, cyclophosphamide and methotrexate are employed for patient management. However, till date, there exist no reliable evidence to conclude an optimal therapeutic regimen for CLE [43, 44]. Now, the question arises: Where actually does RTX fit in this scenario? RTX has been introduced in those patients who are unresponsive or intolerant to standard conventional treatment. It is proven that CD20+ B cells play an important role in the pathogenesis of SLE and SCLE. Apart from being an antigen presenter, B cells produce autoantibodies and are responsible for secreting a number of inflammatory cytokines that enhance inflammation [45, 46]. As RTX plays an antagonistic role against these B cells, it may be of value in these patients.

It is further observed that RTX is more valuable in patients with ACLE and SCLE and in patients with nonspecific cutaneous lesions in SLE. In contrast, the role of RTX in CCLE is limited. This can be attributed to CD8+ cytotoxic T cells rather than B cells being involved in the pathogenesis of CCLE, particularly in the scarring and disseminated variant of discoid lupus erythematosus (DLE) [47, 48].

There are various reports describing the successful use of RTX in CLE. Both lymphoma and rheumatoid arthritis protocols have been utilized with equal efficacy [49–52]. Marks et al. [53] have utilized a modified protocol wherein 2 weekly infusions of 750 mg/m^2 of RTX were administered with good results. In most patients, in the abovementioned studies, oral prednisolone in a dose less than 15 mg and oral antimalarials were continued as maintenance therapy. Duration of remission in most patients after the first cycle of RTX was around 10 months. After administration of the second cycle, the period of remission extended up to 18 months.

Vasculitis

RTX has been utilized in treating ANCA-associated vasculitis (AAV) [54]. The rationale behind using RTX in AAV is secondary to the finding that B-cell targeted therapy reduce ANCA levels and in this way block disease pathogenesis [55, 56]. Further, it is witnessed that levels of B cells in the circulation have positive correlation to disease activity, thereby when levels of B cells come down, activity of the disease is halted [57]. RTX is usually used in those cases that are refractory to conventional therapy or in those cases where cyclophosphamide is contraindicated. Both lymphoma and rheumatoid arthritis protocols have been followed in patients with AAV, and both have been equally effective. Further, maintenance dosing of 1 gm RTX once in 4–6 months have been used for relapses [58].

Retro-orbital disease in Wegener's granulomatosis is usually refractory to treatment, which has demonstrated response to RTX. However, more than one treatment course is generally needed before a therapeutic response is evident [59].

Graft Versus Host Disease (GVHD)

Teshima et al. [60] have utilized RTX according to the lymphoma protocol in seven patients following hematopoietic stem cell transplantation. Following 1 year of treatment, partial response was seen in three patients, three patients had stable disease and in the remaining one patient, the disease was progressive. It was therefore concluded that RTX is mainly effective in those cases of steroid refractory GVHD that is not advanced, and if manifestations involving the skin, eye and fascia are severe, the role of RTX in this scenario is minimal.

Atopic Dermatitis (AD)

Though T cells are the prime players in the pathogenesis of AD, B cells too have a role. RTX administered according to the rheumatoid arthritis protocol has demonstrated significant improvement both clinically and histologically along with slight reduction in the level of IgE. These effects are evident within 1–2 months of initiating treatment with RTX. It must be remembered, however, that RTX should only be reserved for refractory severe cases of AD [61, 62].

Melanoma

Schlaak et al. [63] have used intralesional injections of RTX along with low-dose systemic dacarbazine therapy for melanoma. Long-lasting remission of tumour lesions was demonstrated by RTX. Furthermore, RTX helped reducing the melanoma serum marker S-100 to physiological levels and potentiated a switch of serum cytokines from a T helper-2 to a pro-inflammatory T helper-1 cell profile. Therefore, targeting minor subsets of CD20+ melanoma sustaining cells does have a role in inducing regression of chemotherapy refractory melanoma.

Primary Cutaneous B-Cell Lymphoma (PCBCL)

Generally, treatment of CBCL is straightforward with a combination of antibiotics, topical or intralesional corticosteroids and/or localized radiotherapy. In case lesions are diffuse, then systemic or intralesional interferons can be considered an alternative in PCBCL. Only in aggressive forms of PCBCL does RTX have a role, which too at present is in the evolving phase. RTX has been utilized both intralesionally (10 mg/lesion) [64] and systemically for PCBCL. In systemic therapy, apart from the usual four dosages at weekly intervals, in a selected subset of patients, six dosages of RTX were administered in the study by Valencak et al. [65] In their study, it was found that 87.5% of patients achieved complete clinical resolution, making them postulate that RTX monotherapy can result in a high rate of durable remission, comparable to radiotherapy. Similarly, responses seen with intralesional RTX have been satisfactory. Further, combining RTX with anthracycline containing chemotherapies can be more effective [66].

Special Considerations

Rituximab in Paediatric Population

It has been stated that the use of RTX in children is not recommended owing to limited clinical experience in this age group [8]. However, there have been a few reports of recalcitrant pemphigus wherein RTX had to be used to obtain clinical remission. In majority of patients, the lymphoma protocol was followed [67–70], except for the case of Kanwar et al. [71], who used RTX at a dose of 375 mg/m^2 BSA, two doses 15 days apart. In all cases, good clinical remission was obtained. No serious infections were encountered in all patients, except for one patient wherein bacteraemia secondary to the central venous port was the cause. With all data available, it would be prudent to conclude that RTX can be a good alternative therapy in recalcitrant cases of childhood pemphigus. However, long-term prospective studies, with an adequate sample size for RTX in childhood pemphigus, are required to determine its safety and efficacy.

Rituximab in Pemphigus Patients with Viral Hepatitis

In patients with HCV, it has been largely concluded that there is no evidence that RTX therapy accelerates the course of HCV infection [72]. However, the 2008

American College of Rheumatology guidelines recommend that RTX is contraindicated in Child-Pugh class B and C chronic HCV infection [73]. Therefore, the decision to treat such patients should be individualized, along with active involvement of the hepatologist or gastroenterologist. Though the use of RTX is contraindicated in HCV, RTX paradoxically can be used as a therapeutic modality for the treatment of HCV-associated rheumatic diseases including cryoglobulinaemic vasculitis [74]. Kanwar et al. [75] have treated two HCV pemphigus patients with RTX using the rheumatoid arthritis protocol. One had partial remission, and the other showed complete remission. The patient who had partial remission was further administered two more cycles of RTX. Besides, none of the patients delineated deranged hepatic parameters.

For HBV infections, various studies and case series have clearly established the risk of worsening/reactivation of undetected chronic HBV infection following RTX administration [76]. The current European Association for the Study of the Liver (EASL) guidelines state that patients with active hepatitis B (HBsAg + and/or HBV-DNA +) must undergo preemptive antiviral treatment before starting RTX [77]. EASL recommends prophylactic lamivudine for patients with low baseline HBV-DNA levels (< 2000 IU/ml) when a finite and short duration of immunosuppression is scheduled. In patients with a high baseline HBV-DNA levels (>2000 IU/ml) and/or those patients likely to receive a prolonged duration of immunosuppression, entecavir and tenofovir are recommended [77]. Antiviral treatment must be continued for at least 1 year after stopping RTX to prevent late reactivation of the virus.

The third patient of Kanwar et al. [75] was an active carrier of HBV with progressive derangement of liver function tests while on steroids and azathioprine. The patient was administered lamivudine by the hepatologist with progressive improvement in her liver function tests and viral load. Following this, RTX was administered adhering to the EASL guidelines, with no worsening of viral hepatitis.

Therefore, RTX can be given in pemphigus patients with hepatitis provided appropriate monitoring and EASL guidelines are followed, along with good collaboration with the hepatologist, when regular treatment modalities have failed.

Adverse Effects

Cutaneous

- Frequent but not so serious: night sweats, skin rash, urticaria, pruritus.
- Serious side effects: paraneoplastic pemphigus, Steven-Johnson syndrome, lichenoid dermatitis, toxic epidermal necrolysis, serum sickness, vasculitis, novel delayed pro-inflammatory syndrome occurring at or near completion of a 4-week intense course of RTX [78].

Non-cutaneous

- Fatal infusion reactions usually in the first infusion.
- Tumour lysis syndrome.
- Hepatitis B reactivation with related fulminant hepatitis.
- Severe life-threatening cardiac arrhythmias.
- Cytopenia.
- Rarely, progressive multifocal leukoencephalopathy.

Monitoring Guidelines

Baseline

- Complete hemogram.
- Liver function tests.
- Renal function tests.
- Chest X-ray.
- Mantoux test.
- HRCT chest (when indicated).
- Screening test for HBsAg, anti HBc, anti HCV, and HIV 1 and 2.
- ECG and echocardiography.
- Baseline IgG levels (as there is an increased risk of severe infections with RTX if IgG is low and is therefore recommended by some authors).

Drug Interactions

Cisplatin: associated with nephrotoxicity.

Management of Adverse Reactions Secondary to Rituximab

- If an infusion reaction develops, then discontinue treatment.
- Administer hydrocortisone and antihistamines again.
- After 30 min, consider reinfusion with RTX.

  In the following conditions, RTX should be discontinued:

- Severe infections.
- Anaphylaxis in those patients who do not tolerate mouse proteins.
- Pregnancy.

Conclusion

RTX has proven to be a substantial boon for dermatologists in difficult-to-treat cases of pemphigus. With its horizons expanding in dermatology, and with better information regarding its efficacy and safety profile, RTX has now become an approved first-line therapy for pemphigus.

References

1. Sundharam J. Anti CD20 monoclonal antibody(rituximab) in the treatment of pemphigus. Indian J Dermatol Venereol Leprol. 2006;72:173–4.
2. Gurcan HM, Keskin DB, Stern JN, Nitzberg MA, Shekhani H, Ahmed AR. A review of the current use of rituximab in autoimmune diseases. Int Immunopharmacol. 2009;9:10–25.
3. Rituxan [package insert]. South San Francisco: Genentech, Inc; 2008.
4. Callen JP. Complications and adverse reactions in the use of newer biological agents. Semin Cutan Med Surg. 2007;26:6–14.
5. Cohen SB, Emery P, Greenwald MW, Dougados M, Furie RA, Genovese MC, et al. Rituximab for rheumatoid arthritis refractory to anti tumor necrosis factor therapy: results of a multicentre, randomized, double blind, placebo-controlled, phase III trial evaluating primary efficacy and safety at twenty four weeks. Arthritis Rheum. 2006;54:2793–806.
6. Emery P, Fleischmann R, Filipowicz-Sosnowka A, Schechtman J, Szczepanski L, Kavanaugh A, et al. The efficacy and safety of rituximab in patients with active rheumatoid arthritis despite methotrexate treatment: results of a phase IIB randomized, double blind, placebo controlled, dose ranging trial. Arthritis Rheum. 2006;54:1390–400.
7. Heizmann M, Itin P, Wernli M, Borradori L, Bargetzi MJ. Successful treatment of paraneoplastic pemphigus in follicular NHL with rituximab: a report in a case and review of treatment for paraneoplastic pemphigus in NHL and CLL. Am J Hematol. 2001;66:142–4.
8. Hertl M, Zillikens D, Borradori L, Burckhard H, Eming R, Engert A, et al. Recommendations for the use of rituximab (anti CD20 antibody) in the treatment of autoimmune bullous skin disease. J Dtsch Dermatol Ges. 2008;6:366–73.
9. Schmidt E, Brocker EB, Goebeler M. Rituximab in treatment of resistant autoimmune blistering skin disorders. Clin Rev Allergy Immunol. 2008;34:56–64.
10. Matasukura S, Knowles SR, Walsh S, et al. Effect of single cycle alternative dosing regimen rituximab for recalcitrant pemphigus. A case series of 9 patients. Arch Dermatol. 2012;148:734–9.
11. Craythorne EE, Mufti G, AW DV. Rituximab used as a first line single agent in the treatment of pemphigus vulgaris. J Am Acad Dermatol. 2011;65:1064–5.
12. Schmidt E, Goebeler M, Zillikens D. Rituximab in severe pemphigus. Ann N Y Acad Sci. 2009;1173:683–91.
13. Cianchini G, Corona R, Frezzolini A, Ruffelli M, Didona B, Puddu P. Treatment of severe pemphigus with rituximab: report of 12 cases and a review of the literature. Arch Dermatol. 2007;143:1033–8.
14. Goh MS, McCormack C, Dinh HV, Welsh B, Foley P, Prince HM. Rituximab in the adjuvant treatment of pemphigus vulgaris: a prospective open label pilot study in five patients. Br J Dermatol. 2007;156:990–6.
15. Ahmed AR, Spigelman Z, Cavacini LA, Posner MR. Treatment of pemphigus vulgaris rituximab and intravenous immune globulin. N Engl J Med. 2006;355:1772–9.
16. Kasperkiewicz M, Shimanovich I, Meier M, Schumacher N, Westermann L, Kramer J, et al. Treatment of severe pemphigus with a combination of immunoadsorption, rituximab, pulsed dexamethasone and azathioprine/mycophenolate mofetil: a pilot study of 23 patients. Br J Dermatol. 2012;166:154–60.

17. Eming R, Nagel R, Wolff-Franke S, Podstawa E, Debus D, Hertl M. Rituximab exerts a dual effect in pemphigus vulgaris. J Invest Dermatol. 2008;128:2850–8.
18. Hovarth B, Huizinga J, Pas HH, Mulder AB, Jonkman MF. Low dose rituximab is effective in pemphigus. Br J Dermatol. 2012;166:405–12.
19. Gupta J, Raval RC, Shah AN, Solanki RB, Patel DD, Shah KB, et al. Low dose rituximab as an adjuvant therapy in pemphigus. Indian J Dermatol Venereol Leprol. 2017;83:317–25.
20. Kanwar AJ, Vinay K, Sawatkar GU, Dogra S, Minz RW, Shear NH, et al. Clinical and immunological outcomes of high and low dose rituximab treatments in patients with pemphigus: a randomized comparative observer blinded study. Br J Dermatol. 2014;170:1341–9.
21. Londhe PJ, Kalyanpad Y, Khopkar US. Intermediate doses of rituximab used as an adjuvant therapy in refractory pemphigus. Indian J Dermatol Venereol Leprol. 2014;80:300–5.
22. Kasperkiewicz M, Shimanovich I, Ludwig RJ, Rose C, Zillikens D, Schmidt E. Rituximab for treatment refractory pemphigus and pemphigoid. A case series of 17 patients. J Am Acad Dermatol. 2011;65:552–8.
23. Kirtsching G, Murrell D, Wojnarowska F, Khumalo N. Interventions for mucous membrane pemphigoid/cicatricial pemphigoid and epidermolysis bullosa acquisita: a systematic literature review. Arch Dermatol. 2002;138:380–4.
24. Le-Roux Villet C, Prost-Squarcioni C, Alexandre M, Caux F, Pascal F, Doan S, et al. Rituximab for patients with refractory mucous membrane pemphigoid. Arch Dermatol. 2011;147:843–9.
25. Wollina U, Koch A. Rituximab therapy for recalcitrant bullous dermatoses. J Dermatol Case Rep. 2008;29:4–7.
26. Schumann T, Schmidt E, Booker N, et al. Successful treatment of mucous membrane pemphigoid with the anti-CD20 antibody rituximab. Acta Dermatol Venereol. 2009;89:101–2.
27. Schmidt E, Seitz CS, Benoit S, Bröcker EB, Goebeler M. Rituximab in autoimmune bullous disease: mixed responses and adverse effects. Br J Dermatol. 2007;156:352–6.
28. Lourari S, Herve C, Doffoel-Hantz V, Meyer N, Bulai-Livideanu C, Viraben R, et al. Bullous and mucous membrane pemphigoid show a mixed response to rituximab: experience in seven patients. J Eur Acad Dermatol Venereol. 2010;25:1238–40.
29. Taverna JA, Lerner A, Bhawan J, Demierre MF. Successful adjuvant treatment of recalcitrant mucous membrane pemphigoid with anti CD20 antibody rituximab. J Drugs Dermatol. 2007;6:731–2.
30. Nagel A, Hertl M, Eming R. B cell directed therapy for inflammatory skin diseases. J Invest Dermatol. 2009;129:289–301.
31. Knudson RM, Kalaaji AN, Bruce AJ. The management of mucous membrane pemphigoid and pemphigus. Dermatol Ther. 2010;23:268–80.
32. Cooper N, Arnold DM. The effect of rituximab on humoral and cell mediated immunity and infection in the treatment of autoimmune diseases. Br J Haematol. 2010;149:3–13.
33. Chan LS. Ocular and oral mucous membrane pemphigoid (cicatricial pemphigoid). Clin Dermatol. 2012;30:34–7.
34. Botet JC, Grau JM, Casademont J, Urbano-Márquez A, Rozman C. Characterization of mononuclear exudates in idiopathic inflammatory myopathies. Virchows Arch A Pathol Anat Histopathol. 1988;412:371–4.
35. Sarkar K, Miller FW. Autoantibodies as predictive and diagnostic markers of idiopathic inflammatory myopathies. Autoimmunity. 2004;37:291–4.
36. Cooper MA, Willingham DL, Brown DE, French AR, Shih FF, White AJ. Rituximab for the treatment of juvenile dermatomyositis. Arthritis Rheum. 2007;56:3107–11.
37. Levine TD. Rituximab in the treatment of dermatomyositis. Arthritis Rheum. 2005;52:601–7.
38. Chung L, Genovese MC, Fiorentino DF. A pilot trial of rituximab in the treatment of patients with dermatomyositis. Arch Dermatol. 2007;143:763–7.
39. Hausmann G, Herrero C, Cid MC, Casademont J, Lecha M, Mascaró JM. Immunopathologic study of skin lesions in dermatomyositis. J Am Acad Dermatol. 1991;25:225–30.
40. Caproni M, Torclua D, Cardinali C, Volpi W, Del Bianco E, D'Agata A, et al. Infiltrating cells, related cytokines and chemokine receptors in lesional skin of patients with dermatomyositis. Br J Dermatol. 2004;151:784–91.

41. Dinh HV, McCormack C, Hall S, Prince HM. Rituximab for the treatment of skin manifestations of dermatomyositis: a report of 3 cases. J Am Acad Dermatol. 2007;56:148–53.
42. Werth VP. Cutaneous lupus: insights into pathogenesis and disease classification. Bull N Y U Hosp Jt Dis. 2007;65:200–4.
43. Kuhn A, Ruland V, Bonsmann G. Cutaneous lupus erythematosus: update of therapeutic options part I. J Am Acad Dermatol. 2011;65:e179–93.
44. Jessop S, Whitelaw DA, Delamere FM. Drugs for discoid lupus erythematosus. Cochrane Database Syst Rev. 2009:CD002954.
45. Kind P, Lipsky PE, Sontheimer RD. Circulating T and B cell abnormalities in cutaneous lupus erythematosus. J Invest Dermatol. 1986;86:235–9.
46. Batista FD, Harwood NE. The who, how and where of antigen presentation to B cells. Nat Rev Immunol. 2009;9:15–27.
47. Wenzel J, Zahn S, Tuting T. Pathogenesis of cutaneous lupus erythematosus: common and different features in distinct subsets. Lupus. 2010;19:1020–8.
48. Hofmann SC, Leandro MJ, Morris SD, Isenberg DA. Effects of rituximab based B cell depletion therapy on skin manifestations of lupus erythematosus—report of 17 cases and review of literature. Lupus. 2013;22:932–9.
49. Risselada AP, Kallenberg CG. Therapy resistant lupus skin disease successfully treated with rituximab. Rheumatology(Oxford). 2006;45:915–6.
50. Uthman I, Taher A, Abbas O, Menassa J, Ghosn S. Successful treatment of refractory skin manifestations of systemic lupus erythematosus with rituximab. Report of a case. Dermatology. 2008;216:257–9.
51. McArdle A, Baker JF. A case of refractory lupus erythematosus profundus responsive to rituximab [case report]. Clin Rheumatol. 2009;28:745–6.
52. Kieu V, O'Brien T, Yap LM, Baker C, Foley P, Mason G, et al. Refractory subacute cutaneous lupus erythematosus successfully treated with rituximab. Australas J Dermatol. 2009;50:202–6.
53. Marks SD, Patey S, Brogan PA et al. B lymphocyte depletion therapy in children with refractory systemic lupus erythematosus. Arhtritis Rheum 2005;52:3168–3174, Arthritis Rheum.
54. Rhee EP, Laliberte KA, Niles JL. Rituximab as maintenance therapy for anti-neutrophilic cytoplasmic antibody associated vasculitis. Clin J Am Soc Nephrol. 2010;5:1394–400.
55. Xiao H, Heernga P, Hu P, Liu Z, Zhao M, Aratani Y, et al. Antineutrophilic cytoplasmic autoantibodies specific for myeloperoxidase cause glomerulonephritis and vasculitis in mice. J Clin Invest. 2002;110:955–63.
56. Specks U, Fervenza FC, McDonald TJ, Hogan MC. Response to Wegner's granulomatosis to anti CD20 chimeric monoclonal antibody therapy. Arthritis Rheum. 2001;44:2836–40.
57. Popa ER, Stegeman CA, Bos NA, Kallenberg CG, Tervaert JW. Differential B and T cell activation in Wegner's granulomatosis. J Allergy Clin Immunol. 1999;103:885–94.
58. Jones RB, Ferraro AJ, Chaudhry AN, Brogan P, Salama AD, Smith KG, et al. A muticentric survey of rituximab therapy for refractory antineutrophil cytoplasmic antibody associated vasculitis. Arthritis Rheum. 2009;60:2156–68.
59. Martinez Del Pero M, Chaudhry A, Jones RB, Sivasothy P, Jani P, Jayne D. B cell depletion with rituximab for refractory head and neck Wegner's granulomatosis: a cohort study. Clin Otolaryngol. 2009;34:328–35.
60. Teshima T, Nagafuji K, Henzan H, Miyamura K, Takase K, Hidaka M, et al. Rituximab for the treatment of corticosteroid refractory chronic graft versus host disease. Int J Hematol. 2009;90:253–60.
61. Simon D, Hosli S, Kostylina G, Yawalkar N, Simon HU. Anti CD20(rituximab) treatment improves atopic eczema. J Allergy Immunol. 2008;121:122–8.
62. Simon D, Simon HU. New drug targets in atopic dermatitis. Chem Immunol Allergy. 2102;96:126–31.
63. Schlaak M, Schmidt P, Bongard C, Kurschat P, Mauch C, Abken H. Regression of metastatic melanoma in a patient by antibody targeting of cancer stem cells. Oncotarget. 2012;3:22–30.

64. Penate Y, Hernandez-Machin B, Perez-Mendez LI, Santiago F, Rosales B, Servitje O, et al. Intralesional rituximab in the treatment of indolent primary cutaneous B cell lymphomas: an epidemiological observational multicentric study. The Spanish working group on cutaneous lymphoma. Br J Dermatol. 2012;167:174–9.
65. Valencak J, Weihsengruber F, Rappersberger K, Trautinger F, Chott A, Streubel B, et al. Rituximab monotherapy for primary cutaneous B cell lymphoma: response and follow up in 16 patients. Ann Oncol. 2009;20:326–30.
66. Grange F, Beylot-Barry M, Courville P, Maubec E, Bagot M, Vergier B, et al. Primary cutaneous diffuse large B cell lymphoma leg type. Clinicopathologic features and prognostic analysis in 60 cases. Arch Dermatol. 2007;143:1144–50.
67. Connelly EA, Aber C, Kleiner G, Nousari C, Charles C, Schachner LA. Generalized erythrodermic pemphigus foliaceous in a child and its successful response to rituximab treatment. Pediatr Dermatol. 2007;24:172–6.
68. Kong HH, Prose NS, Ware RE, Hall RP. successful treatment of refractory childhood pemphigus vulgaris with anti-CD20 monoclonal antibody(rituximab). Pediatr Dermatol. 2005;22:461–4.
69. Schmidt E, Herzog S, Brocker EB, Zillikens D, Goebeler M. Long standing remission of recalcitrant juvenile pemphigus vulgaris after adjuvant therapy with rituximab. Br J Dermatol. 2005;153:449–51.
70. Fuertes I, Guilabert a, Mascaro JM Jr, Iranzo P. Rituximab in childhood pemphigus vulgaris: a long term follow up case and review of the literature. Dermatology. 2010;221:13–6.
71. Kanwar AJ, Sawatkar GU, Vinay K, Hashimoto T. Childhood pemphigus vulgaris successfully treated with rituximab. Indian J Dermatol Venereol Leprol. 2012;78:632–4.
72. Ferri C, Govoni M, Calabrese L. The A, B, Cs of viral hepatitis in the biologic era. Curr Opin Rheumatol. 2010;22:443–50.
73. Saag KG, Teng GG, Patkar NM, Anuntiyo J, Finney C, Curtis JR, et al. American college of rheumatology 2008 recommendations for the use of non-biologic and biologic disease modifying anti-rheumatic drugs in rheumatoid arthritis. Arthritis Rheum. 2008;59:762–84.
74. Ferri C, Cacoub P, Mazzaro C, Roccatello D, Scaini P, Sebastiani M, et al. Treatment with rituximab in patients with mixed cryoglobulinemia syndrome: results of a multicentre cohort study and review of the literature. Autoimmun Rev. 2011;11:48–55.
75. Kanwar AJ, Vinay K, Heelan K, Walsh S, Shear NH, et al. Use of rituximab in pemphigus patients with chronic viral hepatitis. Report of 3 cases. Indian J Dermatol Venereol Leprol. 2014;80:422–6.
76. Hay AE, Meyer RM. Hepatitis B, rituximab, screening and prophylaxis. Effectiveness and cost effectiveness. J Clin Oncol. 2012;30:3155–7.
77. European association for the study of the liver. EASL clinical practice guidelines. Management of chronic hepatitis B virus infection. J Hepatol. 2012;57:167–85.
78. Buda-Okreglok EM, Drabick JJ, Delany NR. Pro-inflammatory syndrome mimicking rheumatoid arthritis in a patient with Waldenstorm's macroglobulinemia treated with rituximab. Ann Hematol. 2004;83:117–9.

Anakinra

41

Introduction

Anakinra (AK) is an IL-1 receptor antagonist which has been approved for the management of joint disease of rheumatoid arthritis. It is a non-glycosylated version of human IL-1 receptor antagonist prepared from cultures of genetically modified *E. coli*, using recombinant DNA technology. It consists of 153 amino acids and has a molecular weight of 17.3 kDa. It differs from native human IL-1 receptor antagonists in that it has the addition of a single methionine residue on its amino terminus [1].

Mechanism of Action

AK competitively binds with IL-1 receptors and in this way downregulates inflammation.

Pharmacokinetics

After subcutaneous injection, AK has a bioavailability of 95% in healthy adults. Peak plasma concentrations of AK are attained within 3–7 h of subcutaneous injection. The $t_{1/2}$ of AK is 4–6 h [2]. AK undergoes endogenous proteolysis, with minimal hepatic metabolism. Excretion of AK occurs via the renal route [2].

Indications

FDA Approved

- Rheumatoid arthritis
- Plaque psoriasis

A. K. Bubna, *Therapeutics in Dermatology - Essentials for Clinical Practice*,
https://doi.org/10.1007/978-981-95-3791-4_41

Off-Label

- Schnitzler's syndrome
- Cryopyrin-associated periodic syndrome
- DIRA (deficiency of IL-1 antagonist) syndrome
- Other variants of psoriasis
- Atopic dermatitis
- Pyoderma gangrenosum
- PAPA syndrome
- Hidradenitis suppurativa
- Lamellar ichthyosis
- Sweet's syndrome
- Neutrophilic panniculitis
- Melanoma
- SAPHO syndrome
- Photoaging
- Cytophagic histiocytic panniculitis

Contraindications

- Active infections.
- Severe renal impairment
- Hypersensitivity to the drug

Pregnancy Prescribing Status: Category 'B'.
Safety in Lactation: Unknown.

Clinical Uses

Schnitzler's Syndrome (SS)

The therapeutic landscape has dramatically changed for patients with SS after the introduction of AK. Apart from resolving urticarial lesions in SS, AK helps in ameliorating other symptoms, as well as normalizing other inflammatory markers. There is resolution of anaemia, reactive leucocytosis and thrombocytosis following AK administration in SS. However, monoclonal IgM remains detectable [3–5].

The dose of AK in SS is 100 mg/day given subcutaneously (SC). However, some patients are able to maintain disease control with alternate day therapy. Most patients who skip doses rapidly experience resurgence of symptoms, but after reinstitution of therapy, therapeutic responses are again obtained [6].

Cryopyrin-Associated Periodic Syndrome

These include familial cold autoinflammatory syndrome, Muckle-Wells syndrome and neonatal onset multisystem inflammatory disease.

- Familial cold autoinflammatory syndrome (FCAS): AK is beneficial for both rheumatologic and cutaneous manifestations of FCAS. Dose of AK in FCAS is 100 mg SC administered on a daily basis [7–9].
- Muckle-Wells syndrome (MWS): AK has shown to be safe and effective for treating MWS. Dose of AK is similar to that in FCAS. Within 2 weeks of therapy initiation, noticeable improvement in disease symptoms is seen [10, 11].
- Familial Mediterranean Fever (FMF): In FMF, AK is used when therapy with colchicine has failed, impossibility of therapy with colchicine owing to its side effects, or if FMF is associated with vasculitis [12]. Dose of AK is 100 mg/day SC. At times, AK may also be combined with canakinumab (a human monoclonal antibody against IL-1β) [12].

Psoriasis

AK has been used for treating recalcitrant forms of psoriasis. It was approved by the FDA in the management of plaque psoriasis in 1998. Studies have also revealed its value for generalized pustular psoriasis and psoriatic arthropathy [13, 14]. The dose administered is 100 mg/day SC. Treatment can even extend up to 6 months at times to prevent relapse [14].

Atopic Dermatitis (AD)

It was demonstrated in an in vitro study that IL-1 production and physical contact of keratinocytes and T lymphocytes probably are critical for the development of AD. AK may help in suppressing IFNγ production by T cells in AD [15].

Pyoderma Gangrenosum (PG)

As there are only a few studies demonstrating AK as an effective therapeutic modality in PG, more controlled studies in this regard are warranted [16].

PAPA Syndrome (Pyogenic Arthritis, Pyoderma Gangrenosum and Acne Syndrome)

There has been a report by Brenner et al. [17] wherein quick and lasting response of PG was demonstrated in a patient of PAPA syndrome following treatment with AK.

Lamellar Ichthyosis (LI)

In LI, there is an increased expression of IL-1α and lack of loricrin cross-linking. It is suggested that AK enables a dose-dependent reduction in hyperkeratosis, without a decrease in nonpolar lipids in the horny cell layer of the epidermis. Therefore, taking this into consideration, AK can potentially reduce scaling without the need to constantly apply emollients [18].

Sweet's Syndrome

AK in sweet's syndrome acts on the IL-1/inflammasome pathway, an important pathway involved in disease pathogenesis. Though AK is not the first-line drug for sweet's syndrome, it may be of value in those cases refractory to conventional treatments [19].

Neutrophilic Panniculitis (NP)

A case report by Lepsker et al. [20] has demonstrated benefit from AK for NP. Here, the patient was administered 100 mg of AK SC for 15 days.

Melanoma

The role of AK in melanoma is perplexing. AK has shown, in various studies, to reduce ICAM-1 expression on tumour cells and may also modify myeloid suppressor cell populations [21, 22].

SAPHO Syndrome

Eleftheriou et al. [23] treated four children having refractory disease with AK. By 6 weeks, symptoms reduced. However, the response was not sustained and relapsed with cessation of therapy.

Photoaging

AK acts by reducing the production of matrix metalloproteinase (MMP)-1 and MMP-3 and in this way may prevent photoaging [24, 25]. However, this could be more of a theoretical significance, given the other safer therapeutic modalities currently being used for photoaging.

Cytophagic Histiocytic Panniculitis (CHP)

CHP is a rare panniculitis associated with fever, hepatosplenomegaly, lymphadenopathy, pancytopenia, hepatic abnormalities, triglyceridemia and coagulopathy without an elevated erythrocyte sedimentation rate. Recently, AK has been found to be useful for this indication [26].

Adverse Effects

- Infections
- Neutropenia
- Thrombocytopenia
- Increase in mast cell numbers [27]
- Interstitial granulomatous drug reaction
- Inflammatory lesions at the injection site

Drug Interactions

Avoid TNFα antagonists and live attenuated vaccines while administering AK.

Availability

AK is available as prefilled syringes containing 100 mg/0.67 mL solution for subcutaneous injection.

Conclusion

AK is a new addition to the treatment armamentarium of dermatologists. However, its use is limited because of its cost and associated adverse effects, especially in patients with comorbid factors.

References

1. Sujatha MB. Anakinra—an overview. Kerala J Orthop. 2012;25:51–4.
2. Mertens M, Singh JA. Anakinra for rheumatoid arthritis: a systematic review. J Rheumatol. 2009;36:1118–25.
3. Gilson M, Abed S, Larroche C, et al. Treatment of Schnitzler's syndrome with anakinra. Clin Exp Rheumatol. 2007;25:931.
4. Schuster C, Kranke B, Aberer E, et al. Schnitzler's syndrome: response to anakinra in two cases and review of literature. Int J Dermatol. 2009;48:1190–4.

5. Frischmeyer-Guerrerio PA, Rachamalla R, et al. Remission of Schnitzler's syndrome after treatment with anakinra. Ann Allergy Asthma Immunol. 2008;100:617–9.
6. Lipsker D. The Schitzler's syndrome. Orphanet J Rare Dis. 2010;5:38.
7. Ross JB, Finlayson LA, Klotz PJ, et al. Use of anakinra (kineret) in the treatment of familial cold autoinflammatory syndrome with a 16 month follow up. J Cutan Med Surg. 2008;12:8–16.
8. Leslie KS, Lachmann HJ, Bruning E, et al. phenotype, genotype and sustained response to anakinra in 22 patients with autoinflammatory disease associated with CIAS-1/NACP 3 mutations. Arch Dermatol. 2006;142:1591–7.
9. O'Connell SM, O'Regan GM, Bolger T, et al. Response to IL-1 receptor antagonist in a child with familial cold autoinflammatory syndrome. Pediatr Dermatol. 2007;24:85–9.
10. Madan V, Kingston H, Jamieson LA, et al. Muckle Wells syndrome/neonatal onset multisystem inflammatory disease overlap associated with myelodysplasia and cerebrovascular accident. Clin Exp Dermatol. 2010;35:752–5.
11. Kuemmerle-Deschner JB, Tyrrell PN, Koetter I, et al. Efficacy and safety of anakinra therapy in pediatric and adult patients with the autoinflammatory Muckle Wells syndrome. Arthritis Rheum. 2011;63:840–9.
12. Meinzer U, Quartier P, Alexandra JF, et al. Interleukin-1 targeting drugs in familial mediterranean fever. A case series and a review of literature. Semin Arthritis Rheum. 2011;41:265–71.
13. Viguier M, Guigue P, Pages C, et al. Successful treatment of generalized pustular psoriasis with the interleukin-1 receptor antagonist anakinra: lack of correlation with IL1RN mutations. Ann Intern Med. 2010;153:66–7.
14. Jung N, Hellmann M, Hoheisel R, et al. An open label pilot study of the efficacy and safety of anakinra in patients with psoriatic arthritis refractory to or intolerant to methotrexate. Clin Rheumatol. 2010;29:1169–73.
15. Renne J, Schafer V, Werfel T, et al. Interleukin-1 from epithelial cells fosters T cell dependant skin inflammation. Br J Dermatol. 2010;162:1198–205.
16. Wollina U, Haroske G. Pyoderma gangrenosum. Curr Opin Rheumatol. 2011;23:50–6.
17. Brenner M, Ruzicka T, Plewig G, et al. Targeted treatment of pyoderma gangrenosum in PAPA (pyogenic arthritis, pyoderma gangrenosum and acne) syndrome with the recombinant human interleukin-1 receptor antagonist anakinra. Br J Dermatol. 2009;161:1199–201.
18. O'Shaughnessy RF, Choudhary I, Harper JI. Interleukin-1 alpha blockade prevents hyperkeratosis in an in vitro model of lamellar ichthyosis. Hum Mol Genet. 2010;19:2594–605.
19. Kluger N, Gil-Bistes D, Guillot B, et al. Efficacy of anti-interleukin 1 receptor antagonist anakinra (kineret) in a case of refractory Sweet's syndrome. Dermatology. 2011;222:123–7.
20. Lipsker D, Perrigouard C, Foubert A, et al. Anakinra for difficult to treat neutrophilic panniculitis: IL-1 blockade as a promising treatment option for neutrophil mediated inflammatory skin disease. Dermatology. 2010;220:264–7.
21. McKenzie RC, Oran A, Dinarello CA, et al. Interleukin-1 receptor antagonist inhibits subcutaneous B16 melanoma growth in vitro. Anticancer Res. 1996;16:437–41.
22. Triozzi PL, Aldrich W. Effects of interleukin-1 receptor antagonist and chemotherapy on host tumor interactions in established melanoma. Anticancer Res. 2010;30:345–54.
23. Eleftheriou D, Gerschman T, Sebire N, et al. Biologic therapy in refractory chronic non-bacterial osteomyelitis of childhood. Rheumatology (Oxford). 2010;49:1505–12.
24. Wang X, Bi Z, Chu W, et al. Il-1 receptor antagonist attenuates MAP kinase/AP-1 activation and MMP-1 expression in UV-irradiated human fibroblasts induced by culture medium from UV-B irradiated human skin keratinocytes. Int J Mol Med. 2005;16:1117–24.
25. Karrer S, Bosserhoff AK, Weiderer P, et al. Keratinocyte derived cytokines after photodynamic therapy and their paracrine induction of matrix metalloproteinases in fibroblast. Br J Dermatol. 2004;151:776–83.
26. Aronson IK, Worobec SM. Cytophagic histiocytic panniculitis and hemophagocytic lymphohistiocytosis: an overview. Dermatol Ther. 2010;23:389–402.
27. Pazyar N, Feily A, Yaghobi R. An overview of interleukin-1 receptor antagonist, anakinra in the treatment of cutaneous diseases. Curr Clin Pharmacol. 2012;7:271–5.

Index

A. K. Bubna, *Therapeutics in Dermatology - Essentials for Clinical Practice*, https://doi.org/10.1007/978-981-95-3791-4

D

E

F

9789819537907